Pharmacotherapy and Pharmaceutics

Pharmacotherapy and Pharmaceutics

Edited by **Sean Boyd**

SYRAWOOD
PUBLISHING HOUSE
New York

Published by Syrawood Publishing House,
750 Third Avenue, 9th Floor,
New York, NY 10017, USA
www.syrawoodpublishinghouse.com

Pharmacotherapy and Pharmaceutics
Edited by Sean Boyd

International Standard Book Number: 978-1-68286-352-7 (Hardback)

Printed in China.

Contents

Preface

Over the recent decade, advancements and applications have progressed exponentially. This has led to the increased interest in this field and projects are being conducted to enhance knowledge. The main objective of this book is to present some of the critical challenges and provide insights into possible solutions. This book will answer the varied questions that arise in the field and also provide an increased scope for furthering studies.

Pharmacotherapy and pharmaceutics are branches of pharmaceutical science which purely deal with pharmaceutical drugs. Drug development is essential for research and discovering new drugs for better medical treatment. This book compiles case studies from all parts of the world in these fields. It focuses on the conception, design, manufacture, classification, etc. of existing as well as new drugs. This book will serve as a reference material for students and professionals alike.

I hope that this book, with its visionary approach, will be a valuable addition and will promote interest among readers. Each of the authors has provided their extraordinary competence in their specific fields by providing different perspectives as they come from diverse nations and regions. I thank them for their contributions.

Editor

Biochemical tolerance during low dose propylene glycol exposure in neonates: A formulation-controlled evaluation

Aida Kulo[1,2], Anne Smits[3], Gunnar Naulaers[3], Jan de Hoon[1] and Karel Allegaert[3,4*]

Abstract

Background and purpose of the study: Propylene glycol (PG) is a frequently co-administered solvent in formulations administered to neonates, but reports on its (in)tolerance are limited. We aimed to report on renal, metabolic and hepatic tolerance before, during and following intravenous (iv) PG-paracetamol exposure and compared these data with similar datasets reported in literature on neonates exposed to PG without paracetamol or paracetamol without PG.

Methods: Renal (diuresis, creatinemia, sodium), metabolic (Base Excess, Anion Gap, lactate, bicarbonate) and hepatic (liver enzymes, bilirubinemia) indicators before, during and following iv paracetamol-PG exposure in neonates as included in the PARANEO (*para*cetamol in *neo*nates) study (intra-individual trends, ANOVA) were collected and analysed. Comparison with observations collected in cases exposed to either iv phenobarbital-PG or iv paracetamol-mannitol (inter-individual comparison, Mann Whitney-*U* test) were made.

Results: PG exposure (median 34.1 mg/kg/24 h) did not affect postnatal renal, metabolic and hepatic adaptations in 60 cases exposed to paracetamol-PG. These indicators were similar when compared to 29 cases exposed to phenobarbital-PG or 172 cases exposed to paracetamol-mannitol.

Major conclusion: Based on observations in 89 neonates, low dose PG exposure was tolerated well. Studies on PG pharmacokinetics and its covariates are needed to estimate the upper level of PG tolerance in neonates.

Keywords: Propylene glycol, Solvent, Excipient, Formulation, Safety, Tolerance

Introduction

Propylene glycol (1,2 propanediol, PG) is a clear, colourless, odourless, water-soluble alcohol. Physically, it is similar to ethylene glycol but PG is claimed to be less toxic [1,2]. However, PG exposure can cause lactic acidosis, may result in an increase in Anion Gap or Osmolar Gap, hyponatremia or hepatic dysfunction. Other side effects such as hemolysis, mental status changes or renal toxicity (e.g. renal tubular acidosis, acute tubular necrosis resulting in increased serum creatinine and oliguria) were reported as manifestations of PG toxicity [1-3]. Most of these reports relate to continuous intravenous (iv) administration of benzodiazepines (e.g. lorazepam) containing PG as solvent in adult intensive care setting, resulting in PG exposure above 200 g/day or 2 g/kg/day [4].

Based on the current evidence, PG toxicity relates to its accumulation, and therefore is driven by the extent of exposure and the individual elimination capacity [5]. Median PG clearance following exposure to 3–15 g PG/m^2 in adults was 15.9 L/h, the estimated elimination half life 2–5 hours. About 45% was eliminated by renal route, 55% underwent hepatic metabolisation through lactate and pyruvate [3]. Consequently, impaired hepatic or renal clearance increases the likelihood of PG accumulation and subsequent toxicity. By virtue of their nature, infants combine limited renal elimination with limited hepatic metabolism.

Data on PG exposure in neonates have been reported by Shehab *et al.*, Chicella *et al.*, MacDonald *et al.* and by the Food and Drug Administration (FDA) [6-10]. Shehab *et al.* described PG exposure (median 426 mg/kg/day) in 82 neonates to raise awareness on PG exposure in neonates [6].

* Correspondence: karel.allegaert@uz.kuleuven.ac.be
[3]Neonatal Intensive Care Unit, University Hospitals Leuven, Leuven, Belgium
[4]Neonatal Intensive Care Unit, University Hospitals Leuven, Herestraat 49, Leuven, 3000 Belgium
Full list of author information is available at the end of the article

Chicella *et al.* published on PG accumulation associated with continuous infusion of lorazepam in 11 infants (age range 1–15 months) [7]. The authors hereby described PG accumulation during continuous infusion without clinical and laboratory abnormalities (Osmolar Gap, lactate). In contrast, toxicity related to PG has been reported in preterm neonates following exposure of up to 3000 mg/day for at least 5 days. This toxicity was clinical (seizures) and biochemical (hyperosmolarity, lactic acidosis, raised serum creatinine, bilirubin) [8,9]. Similarly, there is a recent FDA drug safety communication on serious health problems in preterm neonates exposed to an oral solution of lopinavir/ritonavir (Kaletra®, Abbott Laboratories Illinois, United States), containing ethanol (42.4% v/v) and PG (15.3% w/v) [10].

In the current paper, we focus on aspects of PG tolerance/toxicity by reporting on a further extended prospectively collected dataset [11] on renal, metabolic and hepatic tolerance following iv paracetamol-PG exposure in 60 neonates included in the PARANEO (*para*cetamol in *neo*nates) study [12]. We compared these observations during paracetamol-PG exposure with similar observations in neonates exposed to formulations containing PG without paracetamol [11] or paracetamol without PG [13,14].

Methods

PARANEO study, paracetamol-PG study

The study was conducted in Leuven NICU following approval by the local ethical board of the University Hospitals Leuven (B-32220084836) and study registration (EUdraCT 2009-011243-39, www.clinicaltrials.gov). Neonates were included after informed written parental consent. The decision to prescribe a source of intravenous PG, either paracetamol-PG or another PG containing formulation, was made by the attending physician and based on the clinical needs.

The Leuven Neonatal Intensive Care Unit has 35 intensive care beds and another 8 high care beds. The clinical part of the study was between September 2009 and December 2010. Observations were collected during repeated iv paracetamol-PG (Paracetamol Synthetica®, Treviso, Italy, 0.8 mg PG/mg paracetamol) administration in 60 neonates. Indications for iv paracetamol administration were medical (traumatic delivery, necrotizing enterocolitis, prostaglandin E_2 administration, fever) or postoperative (e.g. cardiac, thoracic, abdominal). The dosing regimen comprised a loading dose (20 mg/kg paracetamol), followed by a maintenance dose of 5 mg/kg, 7.5 mg/kg or 10 mg/kg every 6 hours for extreme preterm (i.e. born before 32 weeks gestational age), preterm (<37 weeks gestational age) and term (≥ 37 weeks gestational age) neonates and was maintained for 48 h [12]. Based on the formulation used (0.8 mg PG/mg paracetamol), this resulted in PG co-administration of 16 mg/kg, 4, 6 and 8 mg/kg.

Biochemical indicators of PG related toxicity were based on biochemical indicators earlier reported in literature and relate to renal [creatinaemia, plasma sodium, diuresis (ml/kg/h)], metabolic [Base Excess (BE), Anion Gap (AG), lactate, bicarbonate] or hepatic [aspartate transaminase (AST), alanine transaminase (ALT), direct bilirubinemia] disturbances [11]. To facilitate sampling, and to make observations throughout time comparable, only patients with an arterial line were included. All observations available in a time interval of 48 h before the first administration up to 48 h after the last PG exposure were collected.

Sampling and analysis of samples was performed based on the prescription of the attending physician since routinely collected biochemical data were used to evaluate PG (in) tolerance [11].

Other cohorts to compare with

Renal and metabolic observations collected in this group of 60 neonates exposed to paracetamol-PG were compared with similar observations prospectively collected in 29 neonates exposed to other sources of PG [11]. Luminal© Injektionslösung, (Desitin Arzneimittel, Hamburg, Germany) 700 mg PG/200 mg Phenobarbital, Lanoxin© (GlaxoSmithKline, Genval, Belgium), 828 mg PG/0.5 mg digoxin and Diphantoine iv© (Kela Pharma, Sint Niklaas, Belgium), 2 000 mg PG/250 mg phenytoin were identified as sources of intravenous PG in the Leuven NICU [11] (B-32220084836).

Similarly, observations on hepatic and renal tolerance during and following paracetamol-PG were compared with earlier reported observations on hepatic and renal tolerance following paracetamol-mannitol (Perfusalgan®, Bristol Myers Squibb, Braine L'Alleud, Belgium) exposure in 149 and 23 cases respectively [13,14]. All paracetamol exposed cases were treated with a similar amount of paracetamol (20–40 mg/kg/24 h after an initial loading dose of 20 mg/kg).

Statistics and analysis

Clinical characteristics and indicators of renal, metabolic or hepatic disturbances before, during and after paracetamol-PG exposure were described by median, standard deviation and range. Intra-individual trends of biochemical indicators were analysed using ANOVA (trend analysis, following logarithmic conversion if data were not normally distributed) and paired analysis (before, during and following). Observations (before, during, following exposure) collected in paracetamol-PG cases were compared (unpaired Mann Whitney-*U* test) with observations collected in cases exposed to other PG sources [11] or to paracetamol-mannitol [13,14]. (MedCalc®, Mariakerke, Belgium) was used. A $p\text{-value} < 0.05$ was considered significant.

Results

The clinical characteristics in 60 neonates included in the PARANEO study are provided in Table 1 and reflect the heterogeneous population of extreme preterm neonates (< 32 weeks gestational age) to term neonates with congenital malformations exposed to PG. In Table 2, observations as collected in PARANEO cases (colomn 1) were compared to observations reported in cases exposed to paracetamol-mannitol (column 2). Column 3 provides the same type of observations but compared to observations in 29 neonates exposed to other PG sources in the same neonatal unit and in the same time interval. Median PG exposure for both cohorts (n = 60 + 29) was 145.6 (17.5-591.5) mg, 62 (14.8-284) mg/kg or 34.1 (14–252) mg/kg/24 h respectively. There were no significant differences in PG exposure or clinical characteristics between both PG exposed cohorts.

Renal indicators of potential paracetamol-PG toxicity (Table 2, renal indicators) were diuresis (291 observations), creatinemia (295 observations) and sodium (322 observations). Using ANOVA, there is a progressive increase in diuresis (3.7 before to 4.7 and 4.8 ml/kg/h during and following paracetamol-PG exposure respectively, $p < 0.05$). When we focus on diuresis (n = 105) during PG exposure 48 h time interval, there is not a significant change in diuresis.

There are no significant differences between cases exposed to paracetamol-PG compared to other sources of PG (n = 139, median values 3.7, 5.2 and 4.8 ml/kg/day) and are similar to the 4.8 ml/kg/h reported in neonates exposed to paracetamol-mannitol. Similarly, there is a progressive, significant decrease in serum creatinine when observations collected before, PG exposure were compared with observations collected during or following exposure, irrespective of the PG source (column 3, $p < 0.05$). There is no significant trend in serum creatinine during exposure. Finally, serum creatinine during paracetamol-PG exposure is similar to paracetamol-mannitol cases (colomn 2).

Metabolic indicators of paracetamol-PG toxicity were Base Excess (987 observations), Anion Gap (292 observations), lactate (1041 observations) and bicarbonate (1361 observations). Using ANOVA, there is a progressive decrease - reflecting normal postnatal adaptations - in Base Excess, Anion Gap, lactate and bicarbonate (Table 2, all at least $p < 0.05$). Based on 606, 129, 611 and 767 observations to compare with cases exposed to other PG sources, there were no significant differences between both cohorts (Table 2, colomn 1 and 3).

Finally, *hepatic indicators* of potential paracetamol-PG toxicity were AST (136 observations), ALT (130 observations) and direct bilirubinemia (191 observations). Using ANOVA, no significant changes throughout consecutive time intervals were observed. When compared to a published dataset on hepatic tolerance before, during and following paracetamol-mannitol exposure, no significant differences were observed (Table 2, colomn 1 and 2).

Table 1 Clinical characteristics of 60 neonates included in the PARANEO study

clinical characteristics	*median*	*standard deviation, range*
Gestational age (wks)	37	4.1, 25 - 42
Postnatal age (days)	3	6.7, 1 - 28
early neonatal life (<7d)	44/60	
Birth weight (kg)	2.71	0.91, 0.6 - 4.3
VLBW (<1500 g)	10/60	
Current weight (kg)	2.7	0.92, 0.606 - 4.3
PG exposure, (total mg)	166	96, 21.6 - 466
PG exposure (mg/kg/24 h)	33.35	38, 14.8 - 252

(Data reported by median, standard deviation and range).
(PG = propylene glycol; VLBW = very low birth weight, < 1500 g at birth, at inclusion 9/60).

Discussion

Embedded in a prospective study on iv paracetamol disposition in 60 neonates, we documented that a median PG exposure of 34.1 (range 14–252) mg/kg/24 h for 2 days did not affect normal postnatal renal, metabolic and hepatic adaptations. These observations were similar to cohorts exposed to other sources of either iv PG or iv paracetamol.

Whittaker *et al.* refocused on the exposure to additives in medications used in describing the presence of several solvents - including PG - in drugs administered to neonates in the absence of any data on the safety level of exposure [14]. Similar to the established use of off-label drugs, we have to be aware that we are in a setting of established (co)administration of solvents in neonates [6,7,15]. PG toxicity relates to accumulation, and is therefore driven by exposure and elimination capacity [1-4]. Although conclusions on tolerance can only be based on biomarkers initially reported in adults and only focus on short term outcome, the current observations suggest that there is a lower limit of safe short term exposure to PG in neonates (< 35 mg/kg/24 h) similar to the spectrum concept of adult safe exposure level, claimed to be about 1000 mg/kg/24 h [5].

Information on PG pharmacokinetics in neonates is needed to estimate the level of PG tolerance in neonates. At present, the data on PG pharmacokinetics in neonates are very limited. The group of MacDonald estimated a PG serum elimination half life in preterm neonates (all < 1.5 kg) to be 10.8 to 30.5 h [8,9]. To compare observations in preterm neonates with more mature neonates, we recalculated PG pharmacokinetics in a dataset of 22 PG plasma (median PG concentration 31.9, range 15–46 mg/l)

Table 2 Indicators of propylene glycol (PG) (in) tolerance are summarized in 60 cases exposed to paracetamol-PG (PARANEO study), to paracetamol-mannitol or to other sources of PG (n = 29)

	paracetamol-PG			paracetamol-mannitol			other sources of PG		
	ref [12]			ref [13,14]			ref [11]		
	before	during	following	before	during	following	before	during	following
Renal indicators									
Diuresis (ml/kg/h)	3.7, SD 1.2	4.7,SD 1.3	4.8, SD 1.5	n.a.	4.8, SD 1.5	n.a.	3.7, SD 1.5	5.2, SD 1.6	4.8, SD 1.2
	(1.2-7.0)	(1.9-8.9)	(2.1-9.9)				(1.1-7.5)	(2.5-11)	(1.8-9.5)
Creatinemia(mg/dl)	0.62, SD 0.19	0.56, SD 0.18	0.49, SD 0.16	n.a.	0.57, SD 0.19	n.a.	0.62, SD 0.26	0.52, SD 0.28	0.66, SD 0.62
	(0.25-1.05)	(0.21-1.05)	(0.24-1.02)				(0.19-1.36)	(0.22-1.32)	(0.25-2.9)
Sodium (mEq/l)	139, SD 4.9	139, SD 3.8	139, SD 4.1	n.a.	n.a.	n.a.	138.5, SD 4.9	141, SD 6.6	140, SD 5.3
	(127–154)	(129–148)	(123–148)				(128–151)	(125.8-154.8)	(127–151.3)
Metabolic indicators									
Base Excess									
	−3.7, SD 4.0	−3.0, SD 3.5	−1.4, SD 4.3	n.a.	n.a.	n.a.	−3.6, SD 3.9	−2.8, SD 3.4	−4.0, SD 4.6
Anion Gap	(−14.5-10.1)	(−14.4-8.6)	(−16.7-7)				(−21.6-3.2)	(−13.5-7)	(−16.9-7.8)
	13.6, SD 3.1	12.8, SD 2.4	12.4, SD 2.3	n.a.	n.a.	n.a.	14.1, SD 4.3	11.1, SD 3.2	11.6, SD 2.6
Lactate (mg/l)	(7.2-21.7)	(7.2-20.9)	(7.9-18.9)				(8.4-27.3)	(6.3-22.5)	(7–21.3)
	1.1, SD 0.8	1, SD 0.9	0.9, SD 0.65	n.a.	n.a.	n.a.	2, SD 2.8	1.6, SD 0.8	1.0, SD 0.4
Bicarbonate (mEq/l)	(0.4-5.2)	(0.4-8.5)	(0.4-6.4)				(0.6-16)	(0.4-6.2)	(0.4-2.9)
	21.8, SD 3.8	22, SD 3.5	22.7, SD 3.8				21.7, SD 3.6	22.9, SD 3.5	21.7, SD 4.2
	(11.2-35.9)	(11.8-34.4)	(8.3-33.5)	n.a.	n.a.	n.a.	(7–29.6)	(15.1-31.5)	(12.1-35)
Hepatic indicators									
AST (IU/l)	33, SD 57	35, SD 35	30, SD 35	34, SD 68	30, SD 41	26, SD 38	n.a.	n.a.	n.a.
	(7–256)	(13–229)	(14–196)	(12–1 068)	(10–376)	(8–198)			
ALT (IU/l)	9, SD 58	11, SD 53	12, SD 88	13, SD 32	13, SD 32	13, SD 28	n.a.	n.a.	n.a.
	(4–411)	(4–318)	(5–489)		(4–216)	(4–117)			
Direct bilirubinemia (mg/dl)	0.43, SD 0.4	0.39, SD 0.4	0.47, SD 0.5	(4–216)	n.a.	n.a.	n.a.	n.a.	n.a.
	(0.01-2.39)	(0.01-2.2)	(0.01-2.7)	n.a.					

Observations collected before (−48 h until start), during, and after (until +48 h after the last administration are reported. Data are provided by median, standard deviation (SD) and range (n.a = not available).

samples collected in a cohort of 6 (near)term neonates (median weight 3.08 kg, median postmenstrual age 38 weeks) [16]. Assuming a one compartment model, with zero order input and first order output, the calculated PG elimination half life is 8.88 h, PG clearance is 0.0683 l/h. The differences in elimination half life at least suggest that age or weight will be one of these covariates [17,18].

In conclusion, based on renal, metabolic and hepatic indicators of PG toxicity collected in 89 neonates, a median exposure of 34.1 mg/kg/24 h, is tolerated well. Studies on PG pharmacokinetics and its covariates are needed to estimate the upper level of PG tolerance in neonates.

Competing interest
There are no other conflicts of interest related to this publication.

Acknowledgements
Aida Kulo was supported by a Join EU-SEE scholarship, Karel Allegaert by the Fund for Scientific Research, Flanders (Fundamental Clinical Investigatorship 1800209 N). This work has been facilitated thanks to the dr Monique Govaerts award 2006–2008 for clinical toxicology, Royal Academia of Medicine, Belgium.

Author details
[1]Center for Clinical Pharmacology, University Hospitals Leuven, Leuven, Belgium. [2]Institute of Pharmacology, Clinical Pharmacology and Toxicology, Faculty of Medicine, University of Sarajevo, Sarajevo, Bosnia Herzegovina. [3]Neonatal Intensive Care Unit, University Hospitals Leuven, Leuven, Belgium. [4]Neonatal Intensive Care Unit, University Hospitals Leuven, Herestraat 49, Leuven, 3000 Belgium.

Authors' contribution
All authors contributed to the concept and design, analysis and interpretation of data, drafting and revising and final approval. KA was responsible for the study registration, AK and AS for the data acquisition.

References
1. Wilson KC, Reardon C, Theodore AC, Farber HW: **Propylene glycol toxicity: a severe iatrogenic illness in ICU patients receiving iv benzodiazepines: a case series and prospective, observational pilot study.** *Chest* 2005, **128:**1674–1681.
2. Zar T, Graeber C, Perazella MA: **Recognition, treatment, and prevention of propylene glycol toxicity.** *Semin Dial* 2007, **20:**217–219.
3. Speth PA, Vree TB, Neilen NF, de Mulder PH, Newell DR, Gore ME, de Pauw BE: **Propylene glycol pharmacokinetics and effects after intravenous infusion in humans.** *Ther Drug Monit* 1987, **9:**255–258.
4. Nelsen JL, Haas CE, Habtemariam B, Kaufman DC, Partridge A, Welle S, Forrest A: **A prospective evaluation of propylene glycol clearance and accumulation during continuous-infusion lorazepam in critically ill patients.** *J Intensive Care Med* 2008, **23:**184–194.
5. Yahwak JA, Riker RR, Fraser GL, Subak-Sharpe S: **Determination of a lorazepam dose threshold for using the osmol gap to monitor for propylene glycol toxicity.** *Pharmacotherapy* 2008, **28:**984–991.
6. Shehab N, Lewis CL, Streetman DD, Donn SM: **Exposure to the pharmaceutical excipients benzyl alcohol and propylene glycol among critically ill neonates.** *Pediatr Crit Care Med* 2009, **10:**256–259.
7. Chicella M, Jansen P, Parthiban A, Marlowe KF, Bencsath FA, Krueger KP, Boerth R: **Propylene glycol accumulation associated with continuous infusion of lorazepam in pediatric intensive care patients.** *Crit Care Med* 2002, **30:**2752–2756.
8. MacDonald MG, Getson PR, Glasgow AM, Miller MK, Boeckx RL, Johnson EL: **Propylene glycol: increased incidence of seizures in low birth weight infants.** *Pediatrics* 1987, **79:**622–625.
9. Glasgow AM, Boeckx RL, Miller MK, MacDonald MG, August GP, Goodman SI: **Hyperosmolality in small infants due to propylene glycol.** *Pediatrics* 1983, **72:**353–355.
10. FDA notifications: **Kaletra revisions to packaging approved.** *AIDS Alert* 2010, **25:**34.
11. Allegaert K, Vanhaesebrouck S, Kulo A, Cosaert K, Verbesselt R, Debeer A, de Hoon J: **Prospective assessment of short-term propylene glycol tolerance in neonates.** *Arch Dis Child* 2010, **95:**1054–1058.
12. Allegaert K, Palmer GM, Anderson BJ: **The pharmacokinetics of intravenous paracetamol in neonates: size matters most.** *Arch Dis Child* 2011, **96:**575–580.
13. Allegaert K, Rayyan M, de Rijdt T, van Beek F, Naulaers G: **Hepatic tolerance of repeated intravenous paracetamol administration in neonates.** *Paediatr Anaesth* 2008, **18:**388–392.
14. Allegaert K, de Hoon J, Verbesselt R, Vanhole C, Devlieger H, Tibboel D: **Intra- and interindividual variability of glucuronidation of paracetamol during repeated administration of propacetamol in neonates.** *Acta Paediatr* 2005, **94:**1273–1279.
15. Whittaker A, Currie AE, Turner MA, Field DJ, Mulla H, Pandya HC: **Toxic additives in medication for preterm infants.** *Arch Dis Child Fetal Neonatal Ed* 2009, **94:**F236–F240.
16. Kulo A, Allegaert K, de Hoon J, Verbesselt R: **Determination of propylene glycol in low volume plasma and urine samples of neonates by LC with photodiode array detection.** *Chromatographia* 2011, **73:**463–470.
17. Allegaert K, Verbesselt R, van den Anker JN, Rayyan M, Debeer A, Naulaers G, de Hoon J: **Developmental pharmacology: neonates are not just small adults.** *Acta Clin Belg* 2008, **63:**16–24.
18. de Cock RF, Piana C, Krekels EH, Danhof M, Allegaert K, Knibbe CA: **The role of population PK-PD modelling in paediatric clinical research.** *Eur J Clin Pharmacol* 2011, **67**(Suppl 1):5–16.

2

Evaluation of parenteral nutritional support in the surgical and medical wards of a referral teaching hospital

Samaneh Bairami[2], Sepideh Elyasi[1], Hossein Khalili[1*] and Saeed Reza Jamali-Moghadam[3]

Abstract

Background and purpose: Malnutrition is a common problem in patients who are hospitalized in surgical and medical wards. Surgical patients, geriatric populations and individuals with severe illness are more vulnerable to malnutrition during their hospitalization course.

The purpose of this study was evaluation of parenteral nutrition services in a referral teaching hospital, Tehran, Iran.

Method: Medical records of 72 patients who received parenteral nutrition during one year period in different surgical and medical wards of Imam Khomeini hospital were reviewed retrospectively by clinical pharmacists. Criteria for initiation of parenteral nutrition, selection of appropriate formulation and monitoring parameters were assessed based on the American Society of Parenteral and Enteral Nutrition recommendations.

Results: Based on the patients' anthropometric parameters and serum albumin levels, 4.2%, 75% and 20.8% of the patients were well-nourished, moderately malnourished and severely malnourished respectively at the hospital admission and before nutritional support. Adequate calorie, protein, carbohydrate and lipid supports were achieved in 21.1%, 32.4%, 23.7% and 10.5% of the patients respectively. About 91% of the patients experienced at least one complication of the nutritional support.

Conclusion: In this evaluation, several errors in assessment, establishing goals, and monitoring of parenteral nutrition regimens have been detected. Approximately all of the patients did not receive to the trace elements supports goals.

Keywords: Parenteral nutrition, Errors, Medical and surgical wards

Background

Malnutrition is a common problem in hospitalized patients [1,2]. Surgical patients with malnutrition have around three times more postoperative complications and four times greater risk of death than well nourished patients with similar operations [3]. Metabolic support via parenteral nutrition (PN) has become an important intervention in a variety of medical and surgical conditions [4,5]. Although PN has improved patient outcomes, recent meta-analysis have raised questions about its safety and high rate of PN-associated complications [6]. Metabolic disturbances such as hyperglycemia, electrolyte abnormalities such as hypophosphatemia or hypokalemia, infection of PN catheters, liver dysfunction (presented as steatosis, steatohepatitis, cholestasis and cholelithiasis) and embolic events can occur following PN [5,7-10]. Re-feeding syndrome is a common and potentially dangerous metabolic complication of PN that can cause fatal cardiac arrhythmia, systolic heart failure, respiratory insufficiency, and hematologic derangements [11].

PN formulations are extremely complex admixtures and errors in PN can occur in selection of appropriate formulation, dose, administration method, labeling and compounding devices [12-15]. For prevention of these errors, appropriate evaluation of patient's metabolic needs, ordering, preparation, administration and monitoring of PN is essential. Nutritional support team is

* Correspondence: khalilih@tums.ac.ir
[1]Department of Clinical Pharmacy, Faculty of Pharmacy, Tehran University of Medical Sciences, Tehran, Iran
Full list of author information is available at the end of the article

responsible for evaluation and calculation of patient's metabolic needs, selecting appropriate route of nutritional support, ordering patient's specific admixture, and patient's monitoring for efficiency and complication of nutritional support [16-18]. The purpose of this study was evaluation of PN services in the surgical and medical wards of a referral teaching hospital, Tehran, Iran.

Methods

Medical records of 72 patients who received PN in the surgical and medical wards of Imam Khomeini Hospital were reviewed retrospectively by clinical pharmacists during one year period. The Institutional Review Board (IRB) and the Medical Ethics Committee of the hospital approved the study.

Patients' nutritional assessment prior to initiation of PN, daily PN formula, and monitoring parameters were extracted from the patients' medical charts. Criteria for initiation of PN, selection of appropriate formulation and monitoring parameters were assessed based on the American Society of Parenteral and Enteral Nutrition (ASPEN) recommendations [4]. These recommendations have been summarized in Table 1 [3]. Nutritional support was considered appropriate if the patient had received 90% of the recommended goals.

Statistical Package for the Social Sciences (SPSS) version 11.5 (SPSS Inc., USA) was used for descriptive statistical analysis. Categorical variables were expressed as percentage. Continuous data were reported as mean ± standard deviation (SD). Pair sample t-test was used for comparison of patients' laboratory parameters before and after initiation of PN. Pearson chi-square was used for evaluation of correlations.

Results

Seventy- two patients (43 males and 29 females) received PN during one year period in the surgical and medical wards of Imam Khomeini hospital. The patients were under nutritional support only from PN (total parenteral nutrition; TPN) route. Average age of the patients was 57.3±16.6 years old. Gastrointestinal surgeries (52.8%), tumor resection surgeries (27.1%) were the most common reasons of the patients' hospital admission followed by cardiac (8.6%) and renal (7.1%) disorders. Most of the patients were admitted in the surgical wards (73.6%). The most common baseline diseases of the patients have been shown in Table 2. Forty-eight (66.7%) and 24 (33.3%) of the patients received their PN supports through a central venous catheter and peripheral venous catheter respectively. Average length of the patients' hospitalization and duration of PN were 21.3±11.0 and 11.7±7.8 days respectively.

Based on the anthropometric parameters (weight, high, age, sex and body mass index) and patients' serum albumin levels, 4.2%, 75% and 20.8% of the patients were well-nourished, moderately malnourished and severely malnourished respectively at hospital admission and before PN initiation.

Average basal total energy expenditure, carbohydrate, protein and lipid requirements and intakes of the patients have been shown in Table 3. Sufficient energy, protein, carbohydrate and lipid support were met in 21.1%, 32.4%, 23.7% and 10.5% of the patients respectively. Patients' mortality rates were not significantly different between the patients with sufficient or insufficient metabolic support (p =0.7).

The mean volume of fluids that had administered for the patients was 3571.2±986.1 ml which was sufficient for 77.8% of the patients. Normal saline 0.9% (37%), dextrose water 10% (34%) and half saline (29%) were the most used fluids. Average intakes and adequacy of electrolytes support in the patients were reviewed in Table 4. There were no significant differences between the patients' serum calcium (p =0.7), magnesium (p =0.6) and phosphorus (p =0.7) concentrations before and after PN (Table 5). Although the mean of patients' serum albumin levels was elevated after PN but it was insignificant (p =0.2). The patients received 43.9±37.1 ml of the human albumin (20%) for mean duration of 12.9±8.3 days. The most common albumin indications in our patients were hypovolemia (16.6%), edema (7.2%) and cirrhosis (5.8%). In 76.7% of the patients who received albumin during PN period, did not had the FDA approved indications. Mortality rate in the patients who received albumin with approved indications was significantly less than those without indication (p =0.003).

All of the patients who vitamins were selected as a component of their PN regimen, received more than the recommended amounts of vitamin A, D, E and B_{12}. Only 13.15% and 15.8% of them received vitamin K and B-complex in appropriate doses respectively. They also received vitamin C significantly more than their requirements (p =0.003).

We have also evaluated adequacy of PN monitoring in the patients. The results have been shown in Table 6. About 91% of the patients experienced at least one complication of the nutritional supports (Table 7). The mean blood sugar of the patients before PN was 109.3±29.4 mg/dl. Hyperglycemia occurred in 23.2% of the patients as a complication of PN. Incidence of hyponatremia, hypomagnesemia and hypokalemia were 16.6%, 10.5% and 24.5% respectively in our patients. Just 1.4% and 5.8% of the patients experienced elevation of serum hepatic transaminases (≥ 3 times upper limit normal) and bilirubin concentrations respectively. There were no significant differences between the patients' serum urea and creatinine levels before and after PN. From the included patients, twelve (16.6%) of them died. We have not

Table 1 Recommended criteria for parenteral nutrition*

1. Assessment

A. Nutritional history

Medical & surgical history

Psychosocial history

Socioeconomic status

Diet history (include weight changes and food preferences and intolerances)

Medications

Functional capacity

B. Physical examination (include anthropometrics)

C. Biochemical assessment & other monitoring parameters

Body weight

Serum electrolytes (sodium, potassium, calcium, magnesium, phosphorus, chloride, bicarbonate, blood urine nitrogen (BUN), creatinine

Glucose

Albumin and prealbumin

Triglycerides

Complete blood count (CBC)

Liver function tests (AST, ALT, alkaline phosphatase, bilirubin)

International normalized ratio (INR), prothrombin time

2. Establish nutritional goals

A. Therapeutic plan

1. *Energy:* total calories 20–30 kcal/kg/day

(hospitalized patient 20–25kcal/kg/day

moderate stress/ malnourished 25–30 kcal/kg/day

severe stress, critically ill 30–35 kcal/kg/day)

2. *Protein:* maintenance 0.8-1 g/kg/day

catabolic patients 1.2-2 g/g/day

chronic renal failure (renal replacement therapy) 1.2-1.5 g/kg/day

acute renal failure + catabolic 1.5-1.8 g/kg/day

3. *Fat:* 15–30% of non-protein calories intake (≤ 2.5 g/kg/day)

4. *Carbohydrate*: 70–85% of non-protein calories intake (≤7 g/kg/day)

B. Fluid: 30–40 ml/kg

C. Additives

1. *Electrolyte and minerals:*

Sodium 1–2 mEq/kg/day

Potassium 1–2 mEq/kg/day

Calcium 10–15 mEq/day

Magnesium 8–20 mEq/day

Phosphorus 20–40 mmol/day

Acetate and chloride: as needed to maintain acid–base balance

2. *Trace elements:*

Chromium 10–15 mcg/day

Copper 0.3-0.5 mg/day

Table 1 Recommended criteria for parenteral nutrition* *(Continued)*

Manganese 60–100 mcg/day

Selenium 20–60 mcg/day

Zinc 2.5-5 mg/day

Iron: not routinely added

3. *Vitamins:*

Vitamin A 3300 IU/day

Vitamin D 200 IU/day

Vitamin E 10 IU/day

Vitamin K 150 mcg/day

Vitamin C (ascorbic acid) 200 mg/day

Vitamin B_{12} (cyanocobalamin) 5 mcg/day

Vitamin B_1 (thiamin) 6 mg/day

Vitamin B_2 (riboflavin) 3.6 mg/day

Vitamin B_3 (niacin) 40 mg/day

Vitamin pantothenic acid 15 mg/day

Vitamin B_6 (pyridoxine) 6 mg/day

Biotin 60 mcg/day

Folic acid 600 mcg/day

3. Monitoring

A. Daily

Body weight

Vital signs

Fluid intake

Nutritional intake

Output

Serum electrolytes (sodium, potassium, chloride, bicarbonate) BUN, creatinine

Glucose

B. Two or three times a week

CBC

Calcium, magnesium, phosphorus

C. Weekly

Albumin & prealbumin

liver Function tests

INR, prothrombin time

Nitrogen balance

*These criteria are based on the American Society of Parenteral and Enteral Nutrition recent recommendations. In this guideline baseline nutritional assessment of patients based on the anthropometric parameters, nutritional history, physical examinations, laboratory and biochemical parameters and pre-existing diseases were recommended. Nutritional requirements including calorie, carbohydrate, protein, lipid, vitamins and trace elements were considered with respect to severity of patients' illnesses and clinical status. Monitoring parameters during nutritional support course have been shown in the end of the table.

Table 2 Baseline diseases of the patients*

Disease	Frequency (%)
Cancer	60.5
Diabetes Mellitus	26.3
Cardiovascular Diseases	18.4
Renal diseases	5.3

*In this table baseline diseases of the patient have been shown. Most patients who required nutrition support, suffered from cancer (especially gastrointestinal one).

found significant correlation between adequate nutritional support (calorie, protein, lipid, electrolyte and vitamins) and the patients' mortality rate.

Discussion

The most common problem related to pharmaceutical preparation of PN formulations is day-to-day changes of patients' nutritional requirements following changing in their clinical and physiological conditions [16,19-21]. Improving the quality of patients' metabolic supports can be achieved with adequate nutritional assessment using a standard protocol. This is especially important in the settings such as a referral teaching hospital with high prevalence of nutritional support complexities [22].

The ASPEN standards for nutritional support, recommend that all patients who are candidate for PN should undergo nutritional assessment at baseline before initiation of metabolic support. Baseline nutritional assessments include gathering of patients' demographic data such as age, gender, weight, height, nutritional history, physical examinations including anthropometric information, and biochemical parameters (Table 1). These measurements can be used to differentiate between acute and chronic malnutrition and calculation of patients' nutritional requirements [4]. These assessment were done somewhat for most of the patients during hospitalization course and had been recorded in their medical charts.

Based on the patients' baseline nutritional assessment, a metabolic support's plan for fluids, calories, protein, fat, and carbohydrate should be designed for each patient [14]. We have used ASPEN criteria for evaluation of PN in the study. Approximately 21.1% of the patients received calorie goals, but we have not found any significant correlation between the patients' calorie intake and mortality. However sample size of the study was too small for evaluation of correlations between the parameters. Eighty percent of the patients received sufficient fluid (volume) and it seems that low calorie intake was not due to inadequate intake of volume.

Electrolytes, vitamins, minerals and other trace elements are necessary component of PN and metabolic complications can arise following inappropriate replacement of these nutrients [14,21]. From these elements, calcium was frequently replaced inappropriately for the patients. Sufficient calcium replacement is necessary as there is a significant urine calcium loss in patients who receiving PN [13,18].

Errors in replacement of vitamins were more frequent in the study and most of the patients did not receive nutritional goals with respect to these elements. Vitamin D

Table 3 Average basal energy expenditure and other macro-nutrients requirements of the patients*

Parameter	Patients' requirement	Patients' intake	P- value
Basal energy (kcal/day)	1844.2±345.1	1045.1±457.8	<0.001
Protein (g/day)	92.5±20.1	61.1±26.9	<0.001
Carbohydrate (g/day)	308.1±108.4	173.6±17.3	<0.001
Lipid (g/day)	513.1±748.7	496.1±76.5	0.9

*Basal energy, protein, carbohydrate, and lipid requirements of the patients were calculated based on the American Society of Parenteral and Enteral Nutrition recommendations and patients' clinical status and severity of the baseline illnesses. Amount of the patients' intake were calculated based on the administered solutions that had been recorded in the patients' medical charts.

Table 4 Average intakes and adequacy of electrolytes support in the patients*

Electrolyte	Average intake (meq)	% of the patients who received sufficient electrolyte support	% of the patients who received insufficient electrolyte support
Sodium	50	2.6	97.37
Magnesium	27.12	55.3	44.7
Potassium	69.14	92.1	7.9
Calcium	6.52	47.4	52.6

*Average electrolytes intake of the patients were collected from the patients' medical records and the administered solutions. Adequacy of the electrolytes supports were determined based on the American Society of Parenteral and Enteral Nutrition recommendations and patients' clinical status and severity of baseline illnesses.

Table 5 Comparison of the patients' serum electrolytes, total protein, albumin, creatinine and urea levels before and after parenteral nutrition*

Parameter	Before parenteral nutrition	After parenteral nutrition	P value
Calcium (mg/dl)	8.3±0.9	8.3±1.1	0.7
Magnesium (mg/dl)	2.3±0.5	2.2±0.4	0.6
Phosphorus (mg/dl)	2.9±0.9	2.9±1.1	0.7
Albumin (g/dl)	3.3±0.7	3.4±0.7	0.2
Protein (g/dl)	6.3±1.1	6.4±1.2	0.5
Urea (mg/dl)	53.2±47.3	50.3±47.2	0.3
Creatinine (mg/dl)	1.4±1.1	1.4±1.2	0.9

*The patients' laboratory and biochemical parameters before and after parenteral nutrition support were collected from the medical records and were compared with paired sample t-test analysis.

Table 6 Accuracy of parenteral nutrition monitoring in the patients*

Parameter	Correct monitoring (%)	Errors in monitoring (%)
Daily monitoring parameters (such as temperature, patient's intake and output)	13.2	86.8
CBC monitoring (semiweekly monitoring parameter)	81.6	18.4
Calcium, magnesium & phosphorus (semiweekly monitoring parameter)	21.1	78.9
Albumin (weekly monitoring parameter)	23.7	76.3
Liver function tests (weekly monitoring parameter)	39.5	60.5

*Accuracy of parenteral nutrition monitoring were determined based on the American Society of Parenteral and Enteral Nutrition recommendations and patients' clinical status and severity of baseline illnesses.

is recommended for patients receiving PN as well as other human subjects. Metabolic complications such as hypocalcemia, hypercalciuria and negative calcium balance have been reported following long-term PN [23,24]. Most of the patients received vitamin D more than their requirement, probably due to availability of one parenteral vitamin D preparation (300,000 IU) in our hospitals which contain more than even one week requirement of a patient.

Vitamin K (as phylloquinone or menaquinones) is an essential cofactor for coagulation cascade. Moreover, there are some evidences that show roles of vitamin K in the bone and vascular health. However the only generally accepted indication in the PN regimens is prevention of bleeding. The natural phylloquinone content of commercial PN products varies extensively depending on their fat sources. High levels of this element were reported in the PN formulations with soybean oil (150–300 μg per 100 g) fat origin [25]. In year 2000, the US Food and Drug Administration (FDA) organization revised their guidelines and recommend that adult parenteral multivitamin preparations should supply 150 μg phylloquinone per day [26]. In our study most of the patients did not receive vitamin K in their PN regimen.

Baseline laboratory and biochemical parameters should be assessed prior to initiation of PN. These parameters were assessed appropriately in 60% of the patients. Except sodium and potassium, other electrolytes such as calcium and magnesium were not evaluated at baseline for 89% of the patients. Vital signs (temperature, blood pressure, respiratory rate, pulse rate), weight, and fluid input and output, serum electrolytes (sodium, potassium, chloride, bicarbonate), BUN, serum creatinine and blood glucose are recommended to be monitored daily. In more than 80% of the patients these parameters were monitored semiweekly. It may be related to limited laboratory facilities, nursing staff workload, and patient's preferences [16,27].

Table 7 Common parenteral nutrition complications in the patients*

Complication	Frequency (%)
Hyperglycemia (%)	23.3
Hyponatremia	16.6
Hypomagnesemia	10.5
Hypokalemia	24.5
Hypophosphatemia (%)	5.3
Rise of liver function tests (%)	7.2
Catheter infection (%)	2.7

* Parenteral nutrition complications were detected based on the patients' physical examinations, clinical evaluations, and monitoring of laboratory and biochemical parameters.

Complete blood count monitoring was performed semiweekly in most of the patients, but serum electrolytes levels were not monitored appropriately in more than 70% of the patients. Serum albumin levels and hepatic enzymes that are recommended to be monitored as weekly intervals were assessed more frequently in 35% of the patients. In another study conducted by Macfarlane et al. the same results were obtained [16]. These differences may somewhat related to the recommendations. For example monitoring of these parameters as daily for 2 to 3 days, then every other day for 4 days, and then every week was recommended by another guideline [28]. ASPEN guidelines recommend the weekly monitoring of these values as it is simple, less expensive and requires less-frequent blood sampling. This criterion should be changed if patient's clinical condition needs close monitoring [4,16].

In this evaluation, we have found several deficiencies in assessment, establishing goals, and monitoring of the PN regimens in the medical and surgical wards. Complete nutritional assessments were performed only for 11% of the patients and many of them did not receive nutritional goals. About 25% of the patients received sufficient calorie and protein. Due to cost and availability issues of the parenteral trace elements products, approximately all of the patients did not receive their requirements.

This study has some limitations that must be considered. First, the data cannot be generalized to other teaching hospitals because of their different settings. Second, the study was retrospective and other factors such as exact nutrition status of the patients and effects of the patients' demographic data such as socio-economic status were not evaluated. Small sample size is another limitation of the study. Also we have not followed the patients for consequence of adequate or inadequate of the nutritional support.

Conclusion

Errors in nutritional support processes, especially in era of PN are common in the medical and surgical wards. Development of an internal PN protocol for each hospital under observation and monitoring of a nutritional support team consisted of a physician, dietitian, pharmacist and nurse can prevent these errors. Education of hospital staff about appropriate patient's nutritional assessment at hospital admission, ordering, and administration of PN solutions are also helpful.

Competing interests

The authors have not any conflict of interest about this work and have not any financial support.

Authors' contributions

The manuscript is results of a hospital pharmacy project. SB is main investigator of the study and was responsible for data gathering and review of the patients' charts. SE as a clinical pharmacy resident was responsible for data analysis and preparation of the manuscript draft. HK is supervisor of the study and responsible for editing and revising of the manuscript. Clinical evaluation of the patients during course of the study was done by SRJM. All authors read and approved the final manuscript.

Acknowledgement

We must appreciate staffs of the Central Pharmacy of Imam Khomeini Hospital especially Roza Rafiee and Mamak Nikroe for their kindly supports.

Author details

[1]Department of Clinical Pharmacy, Faculty of Pharmacy, Tehran University of Medical Sciences, Tehran, Iran. [2]Central Hospital Pharmacy of Imam Khomeini Hospital, Tehran, Iran. [3]Department of Infectious Diseases, Imam Khomeini Hospital, Tehran, Iran.

References

1. Pablo AR, Izaga MA, Alday LA: **Assessment of nutritional status on hospital admission: nutritional scores.** *Eur J Clin Nutr* 2003, **57**:824–831.
2. Mojtahedzadeh M, Khalili H, Oveisi MR, Tavakolli F, Abdollahi M: **Quality of nutrition in critically ill patients.** *Biomed Res* 2003, **14**:161–165.
3. National Collaborating Centre for Acute Care: *Nutrition support in adults oral nutrition support, enteral tube feeding and parenteral nutrition.* London: National Collaborating Centre for Acute Care; 2006. Available from www.rcseng.ac.uk.
4. Mirtallo J, Canada T, Johnson D, Kumpf V, Petersen C, Sacks G, Seres D, Guenter P: **Safe Practices for Parenteral Nutrition.** *J Parenter Enteral Nutr* 2004, **28**:39–70.
5. Parrish CR: **Liver dysfunction associated with parenteral nutrition: what are the options?** *Pract Gastroenterology* 2006, **45**:49–68.
6. Buchman AL: **Complications of long-term home total parenteral nutrition; Their Identification, Prevention and Treatment.** *Dig Dis Sci* 2001, **46**:1–18.
7. Abrishami R, Ahmadi A, Abdollahi M, Moosivand A, Khalili H, Najafi A, Gholami K, Hamishehkar H, Peivandi Yazdi A, Mojtahedzadeh M: **Comparison the inflammatory effects of early supplemental parenteral nutrition plus enteral nutrition versus enteral nutrition alone in critically ill patients.** *DARU J Pharm Sci* 2010, **18**:103–106.
8. Rosmarin DK, Wardlaw GM, Mirtallo J: **Hyperglycemia associated with high, continuous infusion rates of total parenteral nutrition dextrose.** *Nutr Clin Pract* 1996, **11**:151–156.
9. Hartl WH, Jauch KW, Parhofer K, Rittler P: **Complications and Monitoring. Guidelines on Parenteral Nutrition.** *German Med Sci* 2009, **7**:1–12.
10. Lee H, Koh SO, Park MS: **Higher dextrose delivery via TPN related to the development of hyperglycemia in non-diabetic critically ill patients.** *Nutr Res Pract* 2011, **5**:450–454.
11. Marinella MA: **Re-feeding syndrome: an important aspect of supportive oncology.** *J Support Oncol* 2009, **7**:11–16.
12. Food and Drug Administration: **Safety Alert: Hazards of precipitation associated with parenteral nutrition.** *Am J Hosp Pharm* 1994, **51**:1427–1428.
13. Ribeiro DO, Lobo BW, Volpato NM, Veiga VF, Cabral LM, Sousa VP: **Influence of the calcium concentration in the presence of organic phosphorus on the physicochemical compatibility and stability of all-in-one admixtures for neonatal use.** *Nutr J* 2009, **8**:1–13.
14. Sacks GS, Rough S, Kudsk KA: **Frequency and severity of harm of medication errors related to the parenteral nutrition process in a large university teaching hospital.** *Pharmacotherapy* 2009, **29**:966–974.
15. Ali A, Walentik C, Mantych GJ, Sadiq HF, Keenan WJ, Noguchi A: **Iatrogenic acute hypermagnesemia after total parenteral nutrition infusion mimicking septic shock syndrome: two case reports.** *Pediatrics* 2003, **112**:70–72.
16. Macfarlane K, Bullock L, Fitzgerald JF: **A usage evaluation of total parenteral nutrition in pediatric patients.** *J Parenter Enteral Nut* 1991, **15**:85–88.
17. Martinez Olmos MA, Martinez Vazquez MJ, Montero Hernandez M, Siquier Homar P, Valdueza Beneitez J, Morales Gorria MJ, Arbones Fernandez-Vega MJ, Pena Gonzalez E, Inaraja Bobo MT: **Assessment of activity of care of a nutritional support multidisciplinary team in the follow-up of total parenteral nutrition.** *Nutr Hosp* 2006, **21**:57–63.
18. Gervasio JM, Ash JN: **Adult parenteral nutrition.** In *Applied Therapeutics.* Edited by Young LY, Koda-Kimble MA. Vancouver: Applied Therapeutics, Inc; 2008. 37 (1–22).
19. Gallagher B, Allred CR, Voss AC: **Malnutrition and clinical outcomes; The case of medical nutrition therapy.** *J Am Diet Assoc* 1996, **96**:361–366.
20. Kim DY, Lee SM, Lee KE, Lee HR, Kim JH, Lee KW, Lee JS, Lee SN: **An evaluation of nutrition support for terminal cancer patients at teaching hospitals in Korea.** *Cancer Res Treat* 2006, **38**:214–217.
21. Font-Noguera I, Cercós-Lletí AC, Llopis-Salvia P: **Quality improvement in parenteral nutrition care.** *Clin Nutr* 2001, **20**:83–91.
22. Gales BJ, Riley DG: **Improved total parenteral nutrition therapy management by a nutritional support team.** *Hosp Pharm* 1994, **29**:469–470.
23. Oka R, Nakagawa Y, Shoji T, Matsuda Y, Hamamoto Y, Takeshita M: **Usefulness of a nutrition assessment system for parenteral/enteral nutrition therapy.** *Yakugaku Zasshi* 2006, **126**:1351–1356.
24. Deluca HF: **Vitamin D, and the parenteral nutrition patient.** *Gastroenterology* 2009, **137**:79–91.
25. Singh H, Duerksen DR: **Vitamin K and nutrition support.** *Nutr Clin Pract* 2003, **18**:359–365.
26. Shearer MJ: **Vitamin K, in parenteral nutrition.** *Gastroenterology* 2009, **137**:105–118.
27. Heyland DK, Macdonald S, Keefe L, Drover JW: **Total parenteral nutrition in the critically ill patient.** *J Am Med Assoc* 1998, **280**:2013–2019.
28. Cochran EG, Phelps SJ, Helms RA: **Parenteral nutrition in pediatric patients.** *Clin Pharm* 1988, **7**:351–366.

Overexpression of aldo-keto-reductase in azole-resistant clinical isolates of *Candida glabrata* determined by cDNA-AFLP

Shirin Farahyar[1], Farideh Zaini[1*†], Parivash Kordbacheh[1], Sassan Rezaie[1], Mahin Safara[1], Reza Raoofian[3] and Mansour Heidari[2†]

Abstract

Background: *Candida glabrata* causes significant medical problems in immunocompromised patients. Many strains of this yeast are intrinsically resistant to azole antifungal agents, and treatment is problematic, leading to high morbidity and mortality rates in immunosuppressed individuals. The primary goal of this study was to investigate the genes involved in the drug resistance of clinical isolates of *C. glabrata*.

Methods: The clinical isolates of *C. glabrata* were collected in an epidemiological survey of candidal infection in immunocompromised patients and consisted of four fluconazole and itraconazole resistant isolates, two fluconazole and itraconazole sensitive isolates, and *C. glabrata* CBS 138 as reference strain. Antifungal susceptibility patterns of the organisms were determined beforehand by the Clinical and Laboratory Standards Institute (CLSI). The potential gene(s) implicated in antifungal resistance were investigated using complementary DNA- Amplified Fragment Length Polymorphism (cDNA-AFLP). Semi-quantitative RT-PCR was carried out to evaluate the expression of gene(s) in resistant isolates as compared to sensitive and reference strains.

Results and conclusions: The aldo-keto-reductase superfamily (*AKR* gene) was upregulated in the resistant clinical isolates as assessed by cDNA-AFLP. Semi-quantitative RT-PCR revealed AKR mRNA expression approximately twice that seen in the sensitive isolates. Overexpression of the *AKR* gene was associated with increased fluconazole and itraconazole resistance in *C. glabrata*. The data suggest that upregulation of the *AKR* gene might give a new insight into the mechanism of azole resistance.

Keywords: Azole, Aldo-keto-reductase, cDNA-AFLP, *Candida glabrata*, Semi-quantitative RT-PCR

Background

The incidence of fungal infections has increased over the past two decades. Opportunistic fungal infections occur in immunocompromised hosts [1], particularly among patients infected with human immunodeficiency virus (HIV), individuals receiving immunosuppressive therapy for organ or stem cell transplantation, and cancer patients [2]. *Candida glabrata* has emerged as a common fungal pathogen in many countries and is often reported as the second most prevalent species after *C. albicans* [3]. *Candida glabrata* appears to be innately resistant to fluconazole [4,5] and is less sensitive to it than *C. albicans*, *C. parapsilosis*, or *C. tropicalis.* Studies have shown that mechanisms of azole resistance in *C. glabrata* are often associated with the upregulation of the genes *CgCDR1* (*C. glabrata Candida* drug resistance), *CgCDR2* (formerly *PDH1*) [6,7], and *CgSNQ2* (*C. glabrata* sensitivity to 4-nitroquinoline N-oxide) which encode proteins belonging to ATP binding cassette (ABC) transporters [8]. *CgSNQ2* was controlled by *CgPDR1* (*C. glabrata* pleiotropic drug resistance 1) [9]. A further azole resistance mechanism in *C. glabrata* has been shown to be the mutation or overexpression of the *ERG11* gene (*CgERG11*) that encodes cytochrome P-450 lanostrol 14-α demethylase, the azole target enzyme, and increases *CYP51* (the *ERG11* orthologue) activity, enhancing azole resistance [10].

* Correspondence: Fzaini@tums.ac.ir
†Equal contributors
[1]Department of Medical Mycology and Parasitology, School of Public Health, Tehran University of Medical Sciences, Tehran, Iran
Full list of author information is available at the end of the article

ERG11 is a well-characterized gene implicated in the fluconazole resistance of *Candida krusei* and *Candida albicans* [6,11,12]. The molecular mechanisms in the resistant strains of *C. glabrata* are not completely understood. In this study, antifungal resistance mechanisms were investigated using cDNA-AFLP, a genome-wide expression analysis method that does not require prior sequence knowledge of the genes [13]. This technology is an ideal alternative to microarrays [14].

Materials and methods

Yeast isolates

Four fluconazole and itraconazole resistant isolates, two fluconazole and itraconazole sensitive isolates, and one reference strain of *C. glabrata* were used. The isolates of *C. glabrata* were obtained from clinical samples collected in an epidemiological survey of candidal infections in immunocompromised patients conducted at the Department of Medical Mycology and Parasitology, Tehran. The clinical isolates were recovered from oropharynx of patients. The reference *C. glabrata* strain, CBS 138, was provided by Professor Koichi Makimura, Teikyo University Institute of Medical Mycology-Tokyo, Japan (Table 1). The clinical isolates were identified using standard mycological methods, including assimilation patterns.

Culture conditions and drug susceptibility testing

The isolates and reference strain were cultured on a yeast extract peptone-glucose (YEPD) agar plate containing 5 g/l yeast extract (Baltimore Biological Laboratory, USA), 10 g/l peptone (Merck, Germany), 20 g/l glucose (Merck, Germany), 0.5 g/l chloramphenicol; and 20 g/l agar (Biolife, Italy) incubated at 37°C for 72 h. A single colony of each isolates and reference strain was selected and subcultured in YEPD broth for 24 h at 37°C. Resistant isolate No. 51 was cultured in YEPD broth with fluconazole (128 μg/ml) for 48 h at 37°C. Susceptibility to fluconazole and itraconazole drugs was determined by microdilution according to the criteria for Clinical and Laboratory Standards Institute (CLSI) M27–A2 (formerly NCCLS) [15,16].

Table 1 Number of isolates, site of isolation and azole susceptibility of *Candida glabrata* clinical isolates used in this study

Isolate no.	Site of isolation	MIC(μg/ml)	
		Fluconazole	Itraconazole
91	Oropharynx	0.25	0.5
45	Oropharynx	0.5	0.25
51	Oropharynx	64	2
153	Oropharynx	64	4
137	Oropharynx	64	2
219	Oropharynx	64	2

RNA extraction

Total RNA was extracted from the exponential phase using the RNeasy Protect Mini Kit (Qiagen, Germany). For mechanical disruption, the yeast cells were sonicated with acid-washed glass beads (0.45–0.52 mm diameter). The released RNA was treated through an RNase-free DNase step (Qiagen, Germany) and quantity and quality of RNA was measured with the Nanodrop 1000 spectrophotometer (Thermo Scientific, USA).

cDNA-AFLP

Complementary DNA Amplified Fragment Length Polymorphism (cDNA-AFLP) was conducted with minor modifications. For complementary DNA (cDNA) synthesis, 6 μg of total RNA from each isolate was heated at 65°C for 10 min, followed by cooling on ice. A master mixture contained 7.5 μl of 5X reverse transcriptase (RT) buffer comprising Tris–HCl (pH 8.3 at 25°C) (Fermentas, Canada); 1 μl Oligo dT (20 pmol/μl); all four dNTPs (10 mM) 1.5 μl; Ribolock (20 U) 1.5 μl (Fermentas, Canada); and DEPC treated water. Two hundred units of Moloney Murine Leukemia Virus (M-MuLV) reverse transcriptase enzyme (Fermentas) were added. The RT temperature was 42°C for 60 min and 70°C for 10 min. cDNA was checked with the reference gene *URA3* (orotidine-5'-phosphate decarboxylase) with the following PCR conditions: 5 min at 94°C; 30 cycles of 30 s at 94°C, 30 s at 55°C, 45 s at 72 °C, and 7 min at 72°C. Primers were designed with the NCBI primer–BLAST (Basic Local Alignment Search Tool) program http://www.ncbi.nih.gov/primer-BLAST (Table 2). DNA polymerase I (Fermentas, Canada) was used for second strand cDNA synthesis at 16°C for 3 h and was precipitated with ethanol. The quality of dscDNA was evaluated with the Nanodrop 1000 spectrophotometer (Thermo Scientific). Two micrograms dscDNA were digested with the MboI restriction enzyme (Fermentas) for 4 h at 37°C, and the enzyme was inactivated at 80°C for 20 min. Eight μg of ADMbo1 and 4 μg of adMbo1 cDNA-AFLP adaptors (Table 3) were ligated to MboI digested dscDNA fragments by T4 DNA Ligase (Takara Bio Inc. Japan) conducted at 1 min at 50°C, decreasing to 10°C over the course of 1 h (1°C per 90 s). T4 DNA ligase was added, and the mixture was incubated at 16°C for 16 h. The pre-amplification was performed with the PreAmp adaptor as primer with the following PCR conditions: 5 min of denaturation at 94°C; 30 cycles of 94°C for 30 s, 55°C for 30 s, 72°C for 30 s; and a final extension at 72°C for 5 min. The sensitive adaptors used in sensitive amplification were designed with one selective base at the 3′end (Table 3). Ten PCRs were performed utilizing all sensitive adaptor combinations, and the PCR products were separated by 8% non-denaturated poly acrylamide gel electrophoresis (PAGE) and stained with silver nitrate.

Table 2 Primers used in this study

Gene	Primer	Sequence	Gene location (5'-3')	Product size (bp)
URA3	URA3 F	GGGCTCTTTAGCTCATGGTG	432-451	173
	URA3 R	CAAGTGCATCGCCTTTATCA	604-585	
AKR	AKR F	GGTCTCGGGCCTCGGCTACA	321-340	289
	AKR R	TGGGGCATACGCCTCGACCA	609-590	

The differentiated transcription-derived fragments (TDFs) were observed.

Isolation, cloning, and sequencing of cDNA-AFLP fragments

Selected bands were isolated from the PAGE and re-amplified using appropriate sensitive adaptors. The TDFs were cloned using a TA-cloning kit (Invitrogen, USA) and the recombinant plasmids were screened using M13 forward (−20) (5′-GTAAAACGACGGCCAG-3′) and M13 reverse (5′-CAGGAAACAGCTATGAC-3′) primers with the following PCR protocol: 30 cycles of 94°C for 1 min, 55°C for 1 min; 72 C for 1 min; and 72°C for 7 min. PCR products were analyzed by agarose gel electrophoresis . The recombinant plasmids containing unknown DNA were sequenced by M13 forward (−20) and M13 reverse primers. Some TDFs were verified with direct sequencing (Macrogene, Korea). Sequence data were analyzed in non-redundant nucleic and protein databases BLAST (http://www.ncbi.nim.nih.gov/BLAST/).

Semi-quantitative RT-PCR

Semi-quantitative RT-PCR was carried out to evaluate the mRNA overexpression level of TDFs, which were identified by cDNA-AFLP [17] using specifically designed primers (Table 2). An equal amount (6 μg) of total RNA from each of the clinical isolates and the CBS 138 reference strain was used for first strand cDNA synthesis, and the expression pattern in cDNA-AFLP was determined with the primers on RNA of clinical isolates. The *URA3* gene was used as internal control and negative controls were prepared with sterile water as template. The gel image was captured digitally with a Sony XC-ST50CE camera (Sony, Japan).

Table 3 Adaptors used in cDNA-AFLP method

Adaptors	Sequence (5'-3')
ADMbo1	AGCACTCTCCAGCCTCTCACCGCA
adMbo1	GATCTGCGGTGA
Pre Amp	AGCACTCTCCAGCCTCTCACCGCAGATC
S1Mbo1	AGCACTCTCCAGCCTCTCACCGCAGATCC
S2Mbo1	AGCACTCTCCAGCCTCTCACCGCAGATCG
S3Mbo1	AGCACTCTCCAGCCTCTCACCGCAGATCA
S4Mbo1	AGCACTCTCCAGCCTCTCACCGCAGATCT

The band intensity was analyzed and quantified with gel analysis software UVI (Roche, Germany).

Results

Antifungal susceptibility

Susceptibility to fluconazole and itraconazole was determined by the broth microdilution method described in the CLSI (document M27-A2). The minimum inhibitory concentration (MIC) of fluconazole and itraconazole obtained against clinical isolates of *C. glabrata* showed four strains resistant to fluconazole (MIC 64 μg/ml) and itraconazole (MIC 2–4 μg/ml), while two strains were susceptible to fluconazole (MIC 0.25–0.50 μg/ml) and itraconazole (MIC 0.25–0.50 μg/ml) (Table 1).

cDNA-AFLP

The cDNA-AFLP products of clinical isolates and reference strain

Fragments of cDNA-AFLP were observed on 8% non-denaturing PAGE using silver staining. Over 100 TDFs were produced using 10 primer combinations. Twenty fragments were identified as differentially regulated. High expression TDFs were observed in the resistant isolates, with lower levels of cDNA-AFLP fragments detected in the sensitive isolates. Ten TDFs ranging from 120 bp to 600 bp were isolated from the cDNA-AFLP profile and identified by cloning and DNA sequencing (Table 4). A differentially expressed TDF was produced at approximately 550 bp when using S3Mbo1 and S4Mbo1 as sensitive primers (Figure 1). Sequencing showed that the TDF was consistent with the gene associated with aldo-keto-reductase (*AKR* gene: Gene ID: 2886902; Gene Symbol: CAGL0C04543g; XM_445372.1). Other clones contained two unknown function sequences observed at about 320 bp and 360 bp using S2Mbo1/S2Mbo1 and S2Mbo1/S3Mbo1 as sensitive primers, respectively (Figure 2).

Table 4 Sequences identified by cDNA-AFLP

Accession no.	Size (bp)	Identity
XM_445372.1	550	aldo-keto-reductase
XM_446417.1	320	unknown function
XM_444814.1	360	unknown function

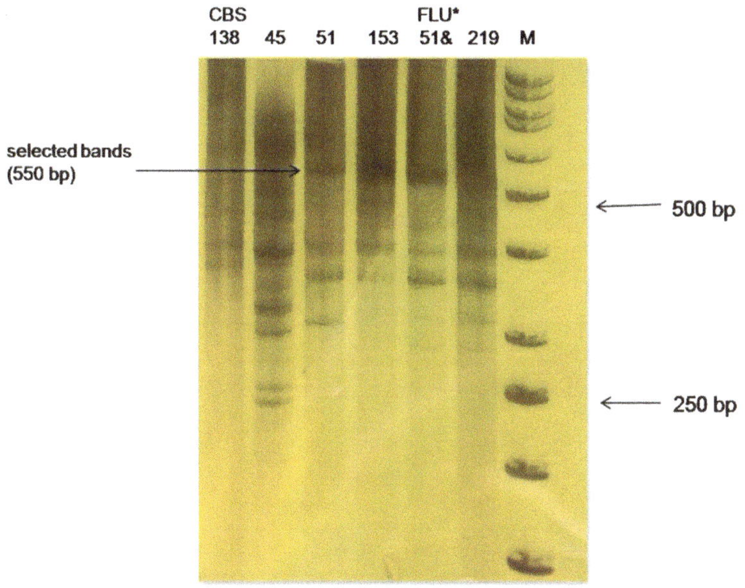

Figure 1 Expression pattern of TDFs of cDNA-AFLP PAGE. Sensitive amplification of cDNA-AFLP on a PAGE from S3Mbo1/S4Mbo1 as primers. The lanes numbered correspond to the clinical isolates presented in Table 1. The arrows point to a differentially expressed TDFs. M: Marker 50 bp; * FLU: Fluconazole.

Semi-quantitative RT-PCR

To confirm AKR as a potential gene for azole resistance, a semi-quantitative RT-PCR technique was performed on the cDNAs from resistant and sensitive clinical isolates as well as on the CBS 138 reference strain. Figure 3 represents the upregulation of AKR mRNA expression levels in these samples. Semi-quantitative RT-PCR showed that AKR mRNA expression was about twice that seen in the sensitive isolates (Figure 4). AKR transcript level in the resistant isolate treated with fluconazole was the same as the one observed in the resistant clinical isolates (data not shown).

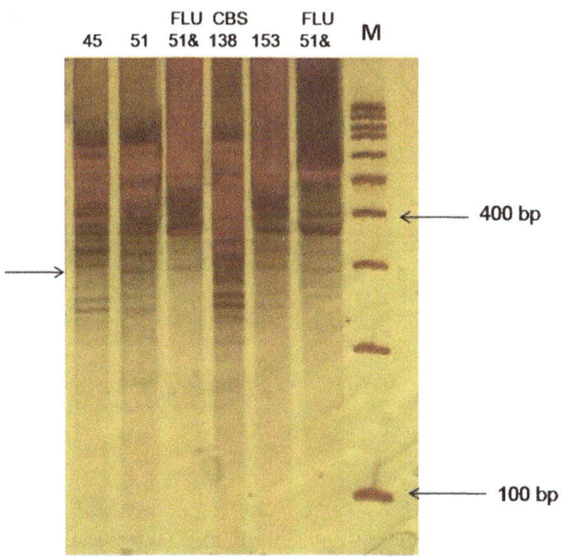

Figure 2 Expression pattern of TDFs of cDNA-AFLP PAGE using silver staining. Sensitive amplification of cDNA-AFLP on a PAGE from primer combinations S2Mbo1/S2Mbo1 and S2Mbo1/S3Mbo1. The lanes numbered correspond to the clinical isolates presented in Table 1. The arrows point to differentially expressed TDFs. DNA ladder; M: (100 bp) molecular weight marker. *FLU: Fluconazole.

Discussion

Candida glabrata, second only to *C. albicans* as an infectious pathogen in candidiasis, contributes to an average of 11% of candidal infections, varying from 7% to 20% depending on geographic location [18]. In the survey providing data for the present study of immunocompromised patients, *C. glabrata* accounted for about 15% of candidal infections. Twenty-five percent of the isolates were resistant to fluconazole (Zaini *et al.*, unpublished data). Although several genes may be implicated in azole resistance, the molecular pathways involved are not completely understood.

We report, for the first time using cDNA-AFLP, AKR transcripts upregulated in resistant clinical isolates. The *AKR* gene is not the first suggested to be involved in azole resistance. Upregulation of *CgCDR1* and *CgCDR2* genes associated with increased expression of the ABC transporter has been well documented [19,20]. The *PDR1* gene is important in acquired azole resistance [21], and so-called gain-of-function mutations of the *CgPDR1* gene have been shown to play an essential role in azole resistance by *C. glabrata* [22-25]. These mutations indicate that many genes are differentially regulated in azole resistant isolates as compared to the wild type. Multiple genes (from 27–235)

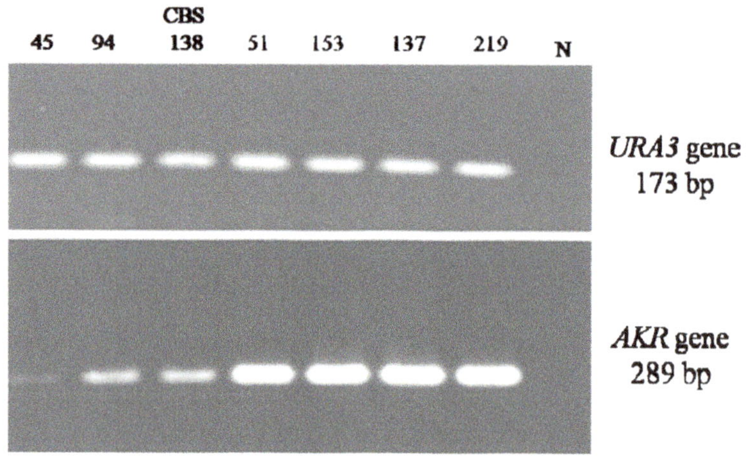

Figure 3 Semi quantitative RT-PCR analysis of *AKR* gene mRNA expression. The lanes numbered correspond to the clinical isolates presented in Table 1. N, negative control (water). *URA3* gene (173 bp) was used as internal control.

show increased expression, and aldo-keto-reductase (CAGL0C04543g: XM_445372.1) is upregulated (1.5 to 2-fold) [25]. The results of the present study also demonstrated that *AKR* mRNA expression in azole resistance reaches levels of about twice that found in sensitive strains. The molecular mechanisms of azole resistance in *C. albicans* are connected with overexpression of ATP-binding cassette (ABC) transporters or major facilitator superfamily, and upregulation of these genes can also be brought about by exposure to benomyl and fluphenazine. In the presence of benomyl, some genes belonging to the aldo-keto reductase family, such as *IFD* genes, *IPF5987*, and *GRP2*, can be activated with the oxido-reductase function [26].

The aldo-keto-reductase superfamily (AKR) comprises several proteins with similar kinetic and structural properties and has been found in a wide range of phyla, including both prokaryotes and eukaryotes [27]. AKRs catalyze the reduction of aldehydes and ketones to their corresponding alcohol products by reducing nicotinamide adenine dinucleotide phosphate (NADPH) cofactor [28]. Several drugs and pharmaceuticals are reactive carbonyls and aldehydes or are converted to carbonyls during *in vivo* metabolism. An important role of AKRs is in preventing carbonyl toxicity [27]. The physiological roles of this superfamily have been studied in the yeast *Saccharomyces cerevisiae*, a simple eukaryote containing various *AKR* genes that encode proteins similar in structure and function to mammalian AKRs, including those of humans. The physiological activity of yeast AKRs is largely unclear. Prior studies have identified six open reading frames (YHR104W, YOR120W, YDR368W, YBR149W, YJR096W, YDL124W) in the *S. cerevisiae* genome that encode proteins with activity overlapping human aldose reductase [29]. YHR104W and YDR368W are stress response proteins [30]. The product of YOR120W is a galactose-inducible crystalline-like yeast protein, and YBR149W encodes a dehydrogenase that plays a role in the direction of arabinose oxidation rather than reduction [31]. Numerous studies have demonstrated that aldo-keto-reductases are active in stress conditions. Another important role of the yeast *AKR* genes is to protect against heat shock stress [32]. In

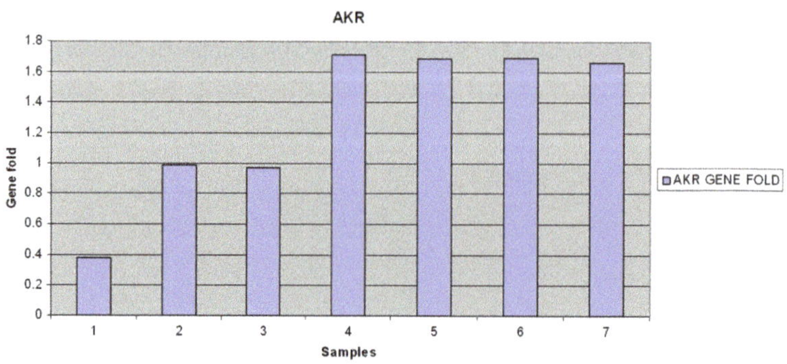

Figure 4 *AKR* gene showed increased expression level after normalization with internal control (*URA3*). Samples 1 and 2 show clinical isolates of *C. glabrata* sensitive to fluconazole and itraconazole; 3 shows CBS 138, and samples 4,5,6,7 are resistant clinical isolates.

addition, AKRs potentially play roles in oxidative defense and transcriptional regulation [33]. AKR function has also been reported in drug metabolism and detoxification of pharmaceuticals, drugs, and xenobiotics in humans [27], and it seems that the physiological roles of the *AKR* gene in yeast are similar to those in humans. Our results suggest upregulation of *AKR* gene is involved in the molecular mechanism of drug resistance in *C. glabrata*.

Conclusion

Aldo-keto-reductases are important in intermediary metabolism, detoxification, and stress conditions. The *AKR* gene was highly expressed in azole resistant *C. glabrata*, and may be associated with the biological networks of drug resistance factors of *C. glabrata*. To the best of our knowledge, this study is the first to report the implication of AKR in azole resistance among *C. glabrata* clinical isolates, using the cDNA-AFLP technique. Further investigations are needed to clarify the role of this gene.

Abbreviations

ABC: ATP binding cassette; AKR: Aldo-keto-reductase; cDNA-AFLP: Complementary DNA-amplified fragment length polymorphism; *CgCDR1*: *Candida glabrata Candida* drug resistance 1; *CgCDR2*: *Candida glabrata Candida* drug resistance 2; *CgPDR1*: *Candida glabrata* pleiotropic drug resistance; *CgSNQ2*: *Candida glabrata* sensitivity to 4-nitroquinoline N-oxide; MFS: Major facilitator superfamily; TDFs: Transcript-derived fragments.

Competing interests

The authors declare they have no competing interests.

Authors' contributions

FZ, MH, and SF contributed to concept and study design, analysis of data, and supervision of sections of the study. SF carried out experimentation and was responsible for the molecular studies, sequence alignment, and analysis of the data. RR assisted with molecular genetics. MS helped in susceptibility testing of antifungal drugs. PK and SR provided scientific advice. SF prepared the manuscript which FZ and MH critically revised. All authors read and approved the final manuscript.

Acknowledgments

The authors thank Dr. Hossein Mirhendi, Professor in Department of Medical Mycology & Parasitology, School of Public Health, Tehran University of Medical Sciences, and Professor Koichi Makimura of Teikyo University Institute of Medical Mycology for kindly providing the reference strain (CBS 138). This research was supported by Tehran University of Medical Sciences and Health Services grants 11438. This study represents a part of the PhD dissertation by Shirin Farahyar.

Author details

[1]Department of Medical Mycology and Parasitology, School of Public Health, Tehran University of Medical Sciences, Tehran, Iran. [2]Department of Medical Genetics, School of Medicine, Tehran University of Medical Sciences, Tehran, Iran. [3]Department of Medical Genetics, School of Medicine, Mashhad University of Medical Sciences, Mashhad, Iran.

References

1. Pfaller M, Diekema D: **Epidemiology of invasive candidiasis: a persistent public health problem.** *Clin Microbiol Rev* 2007, **20**:133–163.
2. Richardson M, Lass-Flörl C: **Changing epidemiology of systemic fungal infections.** *Clin Microbiol Infect* 2008, **14**:5–24.
3. Ruhnke M: **Epidemiology of *Candida albicans* infections and role of non-*Candida-albicans* yeasts.** *Curr Drug Targets* 2006, **7**:495–504.
4. Fidel PL Jr, Vazquez JA, Sobel JD: ***Candida glabrata*: review of epidemiology, pathogenesis, and clinical disease with comparison to *C. albicans*.** *Clin Microbiol Rev* 1999, **12**:80–96.
5. Perea S, Patterson TF: **Antifungal resistance in pathogenic fungi.** *Clin Infect Dis* 2002, **35**:1073–1080.
6. Akins RA: **An update on antifungal targets and mechanisms of resistance in *Candida albicans*.** *Med Mycol* 2005, **43**:285–318.
7. Sanguinetti M, Posteraro B, Fiori B, Ranno S, Torelli R, Fadda G: **Mechanisms of azole resistance in clinical isolates of *Candida glabrata* collected during a hospital survey of antifungal resistance.** *Antimicrob Agents Chemother* 2005, **49**:668–679.
8. Sanglard D, Ischer F, Bille J: **Role of ATP-binding-cassette transporter genes in high-frequency acquisition of resistance to azole antifungals in *Candida glabrata*.** *Antimicrob Agents Chemother* 2001, **45**:1174–1183.
9. Torelli R, Posteraro B, Ferrari S, La Sorda M, Fadda G, Sanglard D, Sanguinetti M: **The ATP binding cassette transporter–encoding gene *CgSNQ2* is contributing to the *CgPDR1* dependent azole resistance of *Candida glabrata*.** *Mol Microbiol* 2008, **68**:186–201.
10. Marichal P, Vanden Bossche H, Odds FC, Nobels G, Warnock DW, Timmerman V, Van Broeckhoven C, Fay S, Mose-Larsen P: **Molecular biological characterization of an azole-resistant *Candida glabrata* isolate.** *Antimicrob Agents Chemother* 1997, **41**:2229–2237.
11. Lamping E, Ranchod A, Nakamura K, Tyndall JDA, Niimi K, Holmes AR, Niimi M, Cannon RD: **Abc1p is a multidrug efflux transporter that tips the balance in favor of innate azole resistance in *Candida krusei*.** *Antimicrob Agents Chemother* 2009, **53**:354–369.
12. Tavakoli M, Zaini F, Kordbacheh M, Safara M, Raoofian R, Heidari M: **Upregulation of the ERG11 gene in *Candida krusei* by azoles.** *DARU J Pharm Sci* 2010, **18**:276–280.
13. Jayaraman A, Puranik S, Rai NK, Vidapu S, Sahu PP, Lata C, Prasad M: **cDNA-AFLP analysis reveals differential gene expression in response to salt stress in *foxtail millet* (*Setaria italica L.*).** *Mol Biotechnol* 2008, **40**:241–251.
14. Reijans M, Lascaris R, Groeneger AO, Wittenberg A, Wesselink E, van Oeveren J, Wit E, Boorsma A, Voetdijk B, van der Spek H: **Quantitative comparison of cDNA-AFLP, microarrays, and GeneChip expression data in *Saccharomyces cerevisiae*.** *Genomics* 2003, **82**:606–618.
15. National Committe for Clinical Laboratory Standards: *Reference method for broth dilution antifungal susceptibility testing of yeasts*, NCCLS document M27-A2 National Committee for Clinical Laboratory Standards 2002. Wayne, Pa: NCCLS; 2002.
16. Falahati M, Shabani M, Rodaki MMA, Jahaniani F, Bagheri KP, Ebrahimi SA: **Interaction between ketoconazole, amphotericin B and terbinafin and three diazenumdiolates in concomitant uses against some fugal species.** *DARU J Pharml Sci* 2006, **14**:87–92.
17. Saffari M, Dinehkabodi OS, Ghaffari SH, Modarressi MH, Mansouri F, Heidari M: **Identification of novel p53 target genes by cDNA AFLP in glioblastoma cells.** *Cancer Lett* 2009, **273**:316–322.
18. Pfaller MA, Diekema DJ, Gibbs DL, Newell VA, Barton R, Bijie H, Bille J, Chang SC, da Luz Martins M, Duse A: **Geographic variation in the frequency of isolation and fluconazole and voriconazole susceptibilities of Candida glabrata: an assessment from the ARTEMIS DISK Global Antifungal Surveillance Program.** *Diagn Microbiol Infect Dis* 2010, **67**:162–171.
19. Bennett JE, Izumikawa K, Marr KA: **Mechanism of increased fluconazole resistance in *Candida glabrata* during prophylaxis.** *Antimicrob Agents Chemother* 2004, **48**:1773–1777.
20. Prasad R, Gaur N, Gaur M, Komath S: **Efflux pumps in drug resistance of *Candida*.** *Infect Disord Drug Targets* 2006, **6**:69–83.
21. Vermitsky JP, Earhart KD, Smith WL, Homayouni R, Edlind TD, Rogers PD: **Pdr1 regulates multidrug resistance in *Candida glabrata*: gene disruption and genome-wide expression studies.** *Mol Microbiol* 2006, **61**:704–722.
22. Berlla N, Borecka S, Dzugasova V, Bojnansky J, Subik J: **Mutations in the *CgPDR1* and *CgERG11* genes in azole-resistant *Candida glabrata* clinical isolates from Slovakia.** *Int J Antimicrob Agents* 2009, **33**:574–578.
23. Berila N, Subik J: **Molecular analysis of *Candida glabrata* clinical isolates.** *Mycopathologia* 2010, **170**:99–105.
24. Ferrari S, Ischer F, Calabrese D, Posteraro B, Sanguinetti M, Fadda G, Rohde B, Bauser C, Bader O, Sanglard D: **Gain of function mutations in *CgPDR1* of *Candida glabrata* not only mediate antifungal resistance but also enhance virulence.** *PLoS Pathog* 2009, **5**:e1000268.

25. Ferrari S, Sanguinetti M, Torelli R, Posteraro B, Sanglard D: **Contribution of *CgPDR1*-regulated genes in enhanced virulence of azole-resistant *Candida glabrata*.** *PLoS One* 2011, **6**:e17589.
26. Karababa M, Coste AT, Rognon B, Bille J, Sanglard D: **Comparison of gene expression profiles of *Candida albicans* azole-resistant clinical isolates and laboratory strains exposed to drugs inducing multidrug transporters.** *Antimicrob Agents Chemother* 2004, **48**:3064–3079.
27. Barski OA, Tipparaju SM, Bhatnagar A: **The aldo-keto reductase superfamily and its role in drug metabolism and detoxification.** *Drug Metab Rev* 2008, **40**:553–624.
28. Mindnich RD, Penning TM: **Aldo-keto reductase (AKR) superfamily: genomics and annotation.** *Hum Genomics* 2009, **3**:362–370.
29. Petrash JM, Murthy B, Young M, Morris K, Rikimaru L, Griest TA, Harter T: **Functional genomic studies of aldo-keto reductases.** *Chem Biol Interact* 2001, **130**:673–683.
30. Garay-Arroyo A, Covarrubias AA: **Three genes whose expression is induced by stress in *Saccharomyces cerevisiae*.** *Yeast* 1999, **15**:879–892.
31. Kim ST, Huh WK, Lee BH, Kang SO: **D-arabinose dehydrogenase and its gene from *Saccharomyces cerevisiae*.** *Biochim Biophys Acta* 1998, **1429**:29–39.
32. Chang Q, Griest TA, Harter TM, Mark Petrash J: **Functional studies of aldo-keto reductases in *Saccharomyces cerevisiae*.** *Biochim Biophys Acta* 2007, **1773**:321–329.
33. Chang Q, Petrash JM: **Disruption of aldo-keto reductase genes leads to elevated markers of oxidative stress and inositol auxotrophy in *Saccharomyces cerevisiae*.** *Biochim Biophys Acta* 2008, **1783**:237–245.

4

Reporting of adverse drug reactions: an exploratory study among nurses in a teaching hospital, Ajman, United Arab Emirates

Lisha Jenny John[1*], Mohamed Arifulla[2], Jenny John Cheriathu[3] and Jayadevan Sreedharan[4]

Abstract

Background and the purpose of the study: Adverse drug reactions (ADRs) are important public health problem associated with morbidity, mortality and financial burden on the society. Nurses play important role in medication safety surveillance through the spontaneous voluntary reporting of ADRs. Nurses' knowledge, attitude and practice towards ADR reporting and factors affecting reporting was assessed in the study.

Methods: All nurses working in a tertiary care hospital, Ajman, UAE participated in this cross-sectional survey. A self administered questionnaire of four domains (knowledge, attitude, practice, factors affecting reporting) was distributed among nurses after obtaining informed consent. The knowledge and attitude components were assigned score of one for correct response. Data was analyzed using SPSS (version 19). Mann–Whitney *U* test was used to compare knowledge and attitude scores between subgroups; Spearman's correlation for any relationship between knowledge and attitude.

Results: Of the total participants, females constituted 92.3%; average duration of clinical experience 6.5 ± 3.3 years; mean age 28.9 ± 4.1 years. Median score for knowledge components of ADR reporting was 11(total score: 17) and for attitude components was 4(total score: 8). No difference noted in knowledge and attitude scores between gender, age group, educational qualification. A positive correlation between knowledge and attitude components was observed (r = 0.38). ADRs are important cause for morbidity and mortality was reported by (54.9%). 49.5% were aware of Pharmacovigilance centers'. Uncertainty of ADRs (49.5%); concern that the report may be wrong (46.2%) and inadequate knowledge of ADR reporting procedure were the major barriers to reporting. Training in ADR reporting as the key measure to improve reporting was suggested by (86.8%).

Major conclusion: The results of the study strongly point out the need for interventional program among nurses focusing on the importance of ADR reporting and reporting procedure to encourage their active, voluntary participation in drug safety surveillance.

Introduction

Adverse drug reactions (ADRs) are one of the major drug related problems associated with pharmacotherapy. ADRs are important public health problem imposing a considerable economic burden on the society and health-care systems. It is one of the important causes of hospitalization varying between 5-13% [1-4]. Spontaneous and voluntary reporting system is an integral component of drug safety surveillance program and also the most effective methods of acquiring ADR information especially the new and serious ADRs. The spontaneous reporting system of the pharmacovigilance program has contributed significantly to improve the ADR reporting rates worldwide [5,6]. Nevertheless, under-reporting is the major shortcoming of spontaneous reporting system [7,8]. Under-reporting delays early detection of ADRs and can increase associated morbidity, mortality in the patient. Health care professionals play an important role in the detection, assessment and spontaneous reporting of ADRs. Several studies have established the role of health care providers in spontaneous reporting of ADRs [9-11].

* Correspondence: drlishaj@yahoo.com
[1]Lecturer, Department of Pharmacology, Gulf Medical University, Ajman, United Arab Emirates
Full list of author information is available at the end of the article

Among the health care providers, nurses are in a unique position to monitor and report ADRs. Knowledge and attitude of nurses towards reporting of ADRs play a significant role in the spontaneous reporting system. Several factors influence reporting behaviour among health care providers such as; financial incentives for reporting; fear of litigation; belief that serious ADRs are well documented; uncertainty of an ADR, a single ADR report may not contribute and lack of interest or lack of time [12]. Identifying the factors influencing reporting is essential to suggest measures to enhance reporting. Several studies carried out to assess the knowledge, attitude, and practice among nurses have documented that the knowledge of ADR reporting procedure are inadequate among nurses [11,13-17]. There have been no empirical studies from United Arab Emirates evaluating the knowledge, attitude, and practice of ADR reporting among nurses. Hence the present study aimed to assess the knowledge, attitude, and practice of nurses to ADR reporting and factors that influence reporting in a multispecialty teaching hospital.

Methods

Study design and setting

Nurses working at Gulf Medical College Hospital and Research Center (GMCHRC), Ajman, UAE participated in this cross-sectional survey. GMCHRC is the first private multi-specialty teaching hospital in the Emirate of Ajman.

Study population

During the study period (March 2011- May 2011) there were a total of 110 nurses working in the hospital and they were approached to participate in the study. The nurses who were not willing to participate in the study and those on leave during the study period were excluded.

Study tool

The knowledge, attitude, and practice of ADR reporting among the nurses were assessed by using a self administered questionnaire which included both open-ended and closed-ended questions. It included the following domains:

1. Demographic information of participants.
2. Seventeen questions about the knowledge of nurses regarding adverse drug reaction, pharmacovigilance, importance of ADR reporting, location of ADR monitoring center, and ADR reporting system.
3. Eight questions related to the attitude of nurses towards pharmacovigilance.
4. Practice of reporting of ADRs. The questions on practice in the questionnaire included whether they have reported any ADR, number of times they have reported ADR to Pharmacovigilance center.
5. Factors encouraging and discouraging reporting of ADRs.
   Knowledge questions mainly centered on general concept of pharmacovigilance and adverse drug reaction reporting system. Attitude questions focused on the nurses' viewpoint regarding different aspects of ADR reporting. The nurses response ranged from strongly agree, strongly disagree and not sure for the attitude questions. A score of one was assigned to the correct response to questions. Thus the maximum possible score for knowledge component was 17 and eight for attitude questions.

Data collection

The approval from the Institutional Ethics Committee was sought before the initiation of the study. The questionnaires were distributed to nurses in all the hospital wards and outpatient departments after obtaining their informed consent. The anonymously filled in questionnaires were collected back on the same day.

Data management and statistical analysis

The collected data were entered into the Microsoft Excel spread sheet, and analyzed using SPSS statistical software (version 19). Mann–Whitney *U* test was used for comparing the median scores for knowledge and attitude components among different subgroups of respondents such as gender, age group variation and educational qualification. Spearman's correlation was used to determine any relationship between knowledge and attitude. All tests were carried out at significance level of less than or equal to 0.05.

Results

Demographic characteristics

A total of 91 nurses (response rate of 82.7%) were included in the study. The vast majority of respondents 84 (92.3%) were females, with males representing 7.7% of the total; this reflects the gender imbalance within health care services especially in the nursing field. Considering years of experience in the field of nursing, the experience ranged from one year to eighteen years with average clinical experience of 6.5 ± 3.3 years. Respondents' ages ranged from 20 to 45 years, with a mean of 28.9 ± 4.1 years. Table 1 shows the demographic distribution of the participants.

Knowledge and attitude scores

The total possible score for knowledge component was 17. The median score for knowledge on ADR reporting was 11 and the scores ranged from five to 16. In about 27 nurses (29.7%), the scores varied from 11 to 13 (65-76% of the total knowledge score); and 26 (28.5%) nurse's the scores varied from 14 to 16 (82-94% of the total knowledge score). The correct definition of

Table 1 Demographic characteristics of the participants

Item	Sub group	Number	Percentage
Age group			
	< 30 years	55	60.4
	> = 30 years	36	39.6
Years of experience			
	</=5 years	39	42.9
	>5 years	52	57.1
Qualification			
	BSc Degree	21	23.1
	Diploma	70	76.9
Gender			
	Male	7	7.7
	Female	84	92.3
Nationality			
	Pakistani	2	2.2
	Indian	84	92.3
	Egyptian	1	1.1
	Filipino	4	4.4

pharmacovigilance and ADR was identified by 76(83.5%) of the nurses. Of the total, only 50(54.9%) nurses knew that ADRs are important cause for morbidity and mortality and 24(26.4%) responded that they were not aware of this fact.

The total possible score for attitude components was eight; the median score for attitude components was four and the minimum score was zero and maximum eight. A total of 37(40.7%) nurses stated ADR reporting is a professional obligation.

The comparison of median scores for the knowledge and attitude with demographic variables is shown in Table 2. Nurses less than 30 years of age had a slightly higher knowledge scores than those above 30 years of age which was not statistically significant. Similarly the nurses with BSc degree had slightly higher median knowledge score than the Diploma holders. The median attitude score was similar in both age groups as well as level of education. The knowledge and attitude scores of nurses with previous experience in reporting ADRs and those not reported, were similar in the two groups; implying that their previous experience of reporting did not improve their knowledge or attitude towards reporting (Table 2).

The Spearman correlation was applied for knowledge and attitude components and the co-efficient obtained was 0.38 which suggests a positive correlation; as the knowledge of ADR reporting increases among the nurses, their attitude towards reporting also improves accordingly.

Practice component

A total of 85(82.4%) nurses had observed ADRs in their nursing practice. Even though ADR reporting is not mandatory, eight (8.8%) nurses had reported ADRs to the Pharmacovigilance centers. All the nurses had reported the ADRs to the concerned doctor as soon as they noticed. 45(49.5%) respondents were aware of the existence of Pharmacovigilance centers.

Factors encouraging ADR reporting

The factors that promote reporting of ADRs stated by the participants were; patient safety 80(87.9%), the seriousness of the ADR 69(75%) and new ADRs 69(75%).

Table 2 Demographic characteristics and the knowledge, attitude scores

Item	Subgroup	Knowledge component	p value	Attitude component	p value
Age					
	< 30 years	12		4	
	>/=30 years	10.5	0.23	4	0.95
Nursing experience					
	<=5 years	12		4	
	>5 years	11	0.07	4	0.63
Qualification					
	B.Sc degree	12		4	
	Diploma degree	11	0.16	4	0.47
Gender					
	Male	12		3	
	Female	11	0.51	4	0.18
Previous experience in ADR reporting					
	Yes	10		3.5	
	No	12	0.23	4	0.58

Barriers to ADR reporting

The factors that hinder reporting among the nurses were; uncertainty of the ADRs 45(49.5%); concern that the report may be wrong 42(46.2%) and inadequate knowledge of the ADR reporting procedure 41(45%). The other factors that discourage nurses from reporting ADRs are listed in Table 3.

The most common strategic approaches suggested by the respondents to enhance the reporting frequency were; training to report ADRs and easy accessibility to ADR reporting forms. The other measures suggested by the participants have been depicted in the Figure 1.

Only five of the nurses had received training in the reporting process, but majority of the nurses were willing to be trained 79 (86.8%).

Discussion

Health care providers play an integral role in the Pharmacovigilance program especially the nurses due to their close interaction with the patients. Nurses are often the primary source of possible ADR alerts to the clinicians.

Majority of the respondents in the study were females (92.3%). This finding was similar to previous studies [16,17]. Generally it is observed that the females opt for nursing career than the males which explains this finding on gender disparity. Majority of the nurses in our study were Diploma holders in Nursing, unlike Hanafi et al. where in, majority were Graduates (BSc degree) [16]. The average age of nurses in our study ranged between 20-45 years, which was similar to the earlier studies among the nurses [16,17].

In the present study, about half of the respondents were aware that ADRs are an important cause for morbidity and mortality. In contrast, Fadare et al. noted that 93.8% of their study participants were aware of this fact regarding ADRs [18].

The knowledge scores for more than 50 percent of the nurses were above 65% of the total score. The attitude scores of ADR reporting for about 28% of the participants were above 50%. One of the important finding in the present study was the positive correlation between knowledge and attitudes towards ADR reporting. Thus if the knowledge on ADR reporting is improved then the nurses' attitude also improves which would be reflected on the ADR reporting schemes in a positive manner. In distinction, Hanafi et al. reported poor knowledge level among the nurses and positive attitude to towards Pharmacovigilance [16]. Palaian et al. noted low scores for both knowledge and attitude components of ADR reporting among the nurses [15].

The correct definition of the terms 'pharmacovigilance' and 'adverse drug reaction' was identified by 76(83.5%) of the nurses, similar to an earlier study from Iran [16]. In contradiction, Rajesh R et al. and Hanafi et al. studies reported that 21.3% and 32% of the nurses (pre intervention) identified the correct definition of pharmacovigilance respectively [14,17] and only 1.6% of nurses in a study from China [13].

Hajebi G et al. reported that nurses with prior familiarity to ADR center had greater knowledge and positive attitude to towards ADR reporting [17]. However in the present study comparing the scores of nurses who have had previously reported ADR and those not reported, the knowledge and attitude scores were similar suggesting that the previous experience of reporting did not improve their knowledge or attitude towards reporting. The probable reason for this finding could be the lack of continuum in the reporting process; ADR reporting is a continuous process among the health care providers in the hospital.

Considerable number of the nurses (80%) had observed ADRs during their nursing practice, and all of them had reported to the concerned doctors and 8.8% of the nurses had reported ADRs to Pharmacovigilance center in spite of ADR reporting not being mandatory similar to other reports [13,17,19,20]. This shows the nurses concern towards their patients' safety. In contradiction, Fadare et al. noted that about 74% of the nurses had observed ADRs [18]. Soleymani et al., demonstrated the significant role of spontaneous reporting system in the health care system [21]. Soleymani et al. reported that the overall reporting frequency of tramadol induced ADRs reduced drastically over a period of 5 years (2006-2010) which was attributed to the initiatives taken by the National Pharmacovigilance center. High reporting frequency of tramadol induced severe ADRs and poisoning cases (dose dependent) to the Iranian Pharmacovigilance Center by spontaneous reporting lead to the implementation of new guidelines to limit the distribution of tramadol to hospital use only and also changed the potency of available injectable form from100mg to 50 mg [21]. These examples can be presented to understand importance of spontaneous reporting in patient safety.

According to the results, 50% of the participants were aware of the existence of ADR monitoring centers. This finding was comparable to Khalili et al. from Iran [20]. This observation further emphasizes

Table 3 Barriers to reporting of ADRs by the nurses

Barriers to reporting	Number	Percentage
Uncertainty of the ADRs	45	49.5
Report may be wrong	42	46.2
Unaware of the reporting procedure	41	45.1
Lack of time to fill-in a report	30	33.0
Need not report a recognized ADR	29	31.9
Reporting may generate extra work	24	26.4

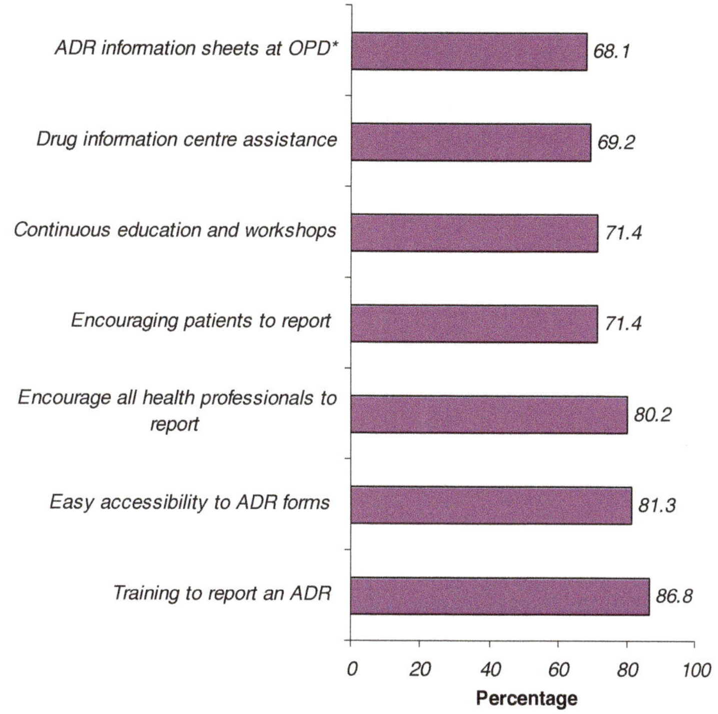

Figure 1 Strategic approaches suggested by the respondents to enhance ADR reporting. * OPD: Out Patient Department; ADR: Adverse drug reaction.

the need for awareness of the ADR reporting system among the nurses.

About 40% of the nurses in the present study felt ADR reporting is a professional obligation. Similar observation was noted by a previous report from Iran (16). Patient safety is the prime responsibility of the nurses and by the active and voluntary participation in the Pharmacovigilance program they contribute towards their patient's safety and medical ethics.

The major barriers to under-reporting, from the present study were uncertainty of the ADRs, the concern of the report may be wrong and inadequate knowledge of the reporting procedure. These observations were consistent with the earlier reports [13,18,20]. These observations reflect the common anxieties among the reporters. An ADR report need not be confirmatory of the relationship between the drug and ADR. When an ADR is suspected, even those not known to the drug it should be reported. In order to address the problem of under-reporting, ADR reporting procedure can be made available as small booklets, posters, electronic flashes at various locations in the hospital to serve as constant reminders. Regular sensitization programs such as continued nursing education and workshops should be carried out among nurses to stress the importance of pharmacovigilance. These training programs clear all misconceptions associated with the ADR reporting.

The strategic approaches suggested by the respondents to enhance reporting included training in ADR reporting and easy accessibility to ADR reporting forms which is in line with Li et al. Training and educational interventions would increase the knowledge and as knowledge is directly related to the attitude, this would in turn motivate nurses to reports the ADRs they encounter. Previous reports have reported significant improvement of knowledge, attitude and perception of healthcare workers about ADR after intervention [20,22,23] Educational program can include presentations, workshops, small group discussions, providing information about pharmacovigilance for healthcare workers by mail, newsletters, reminders, advertisement and continuous education of nurses, and involvement of clinical pharmacists in the medical wards [20]. Pharmacovigilance can be included in the nursing curriculum to introduce them to this concept early in their career. Nursing supervisors and administrators can monitor and actively initiate these program and workshops to improve reporting in the hospitals. Regular feed back of the reports and presentations of the reported ADRs can be a motivational force to continue reporting process among the health care professionals.

The limitations of the study include; the results are of a single-centre and small sample size which may be. The study can be further extended to other hospitals in the country to generalize the findings. Another limitation is those inherent to questionnaire-based studies such as subjective response and recall bias.

In conclusion, the results of the study strongly point out the need for interventional program among nurses focusing on the importance of ADR reporting and reporting procedure to encourage their active, voluntary participation in drug safety surveillance.

Competing interests

The authors declare that they have no competing interests.

Authors' contributions

LJ designed the study, deduced the data, drafted the manuscript, and revised it. JC acquired the data. LJ, JA, MA planned the study, conducted the data analysis, interpreted the data, and revised the manuscript. JS participated in statistical analysis, interpreted the data, and revised the manuscript. MA, JC, JS critically revised the manuscript. All the authors approved the final document.

Acknowledgements

We sincerely thank Dr. Jayakumary Muttappallymyalil for editing the manuscript, Research Division of Gulf Medical University for data entry and Reprography Department for printing of the survey forms.

Author details

[1]Lecturer, Department of Pharmacology, Gulf Medical University, Ajman, United Arab Emirates. [2]Professor and Head, Department of Pharmacology, Gulf Medical University, Ajman, United Arab Emirates. [3]Lecturer and Specialist, Department of Pediatrics, Gulf Medical College Hospital and Research Center, Ajman, United Arab Emirates. [4]Professor and Assistant Director, Research Division, Gulf Medical University, Ajman, United Arab Emirates.

References

1. Kongkaew C, Noyce PR, Ashcroft DM: **Hospital admissions associated with adverse drug reactions: a systematic review of prospective observational studies.** *Ann Pharmacother* 2008, **42:**1017–1025.
2. Mjörndal T, Danell Boman M, Hägg S, Bäckström M, Wiholm BE, Wahlin A, *et al*: **Adverse drug reactions as a cause for admission to a department of internal medicine.** *Pharmacoepidemiol Drug Saf* 2002, **11:**65–72.
3. Janaje Munasinghe TM, Singer DRJ: **Costs and preventing of adverse drug reactions.** *Eur J Intern Med* 2001, **12:**403–405.
4. Wu WK, Pantaleo N: **Evaluation of outpatient adverse drug reactions leading to hospitalization.** *Am J Health Syst Pharm* 2003, **60:**253–259.
5. Waller PC: **Making the most of spontaneous adverse drug reaction reporting.** *Basic Clin Pharmacol Toxicol* 2006, **98:**320–323.
6. Vallano A, Cereza G, Pedròs C, Agustí A, Danés I, Aguilera C, *et al*: **Obstacles and solutions for spontaneous reporting of adverse drug reactions in the hospital.** *Br J Clin Pharmacol* 2005, **60:**653–658.
7. Lexchin J: **Is there a role for spontaneous reporting of adverse drug reactions?** *CMAJ* 2006, **174:**191–192.
8. Lopez-Gonzalez E, Herdeiro MT, Figueiras A: **Determinants of under-reporting of adverse drug reactions: a systematic review.** *Drug Saf* 2009, **32:**19–31.
9. Morrison-Griffiths S, Pirmohamed M: **Specialist nurse reporting of adverse drug reactions.** *Prof Nurse* 2000, **15:**300–304.
10. Ulfvarson J, Mejyr S, Begman U: **Nurses are increasingly involved in pharmacovigilance in Sweden.** *Pharmacoepidemiol Drug Saf* 2007, **16:**532–537.
11. Backstrom M, Mjorndal T, Dahlqvist R: **Spontaneous reporting of adverse drug reactions by nurses.** *Pharmacoepidemiol Drug Saf* 2000, **11:**647–650.
12. Inman WH: **Attitudes to adverse drug-reaction reporting.** *Br J Clin Pharmacol* 1996, **41:**433–435.
13. Li Q, Zhang SM, Chen HT, Fang SP, Yu X, Liu D, *et al*: **Awareness and attitudes of healthcare professionals in Wuhan, China to the reporting of adverse drug reactions.** *Chin Med J* 2004, **117:**856–861.
14. Rajesh R, Vidyasagar S, Varma DM: **An Educational Intervention to assess Knowledge Attitude Practice of pharmacovigilance among Health care professionals in an Indian tertiary care teaching hospital.** *International Journal of PharmTech Research* 2011, **3**(2):678–692.
15. Palaian S, Ibrahim MI, Mishra P: **Health professionals' knowledge, attitude and practices towards pharmacovigilance in Nepal.** *Pharmacy Practice (Internet)* 2011, **9**(4):228–235.
16. Hajebi G, Mortazavi SA, Salamzadeh J, Zian A: **A Survey of Knowledge, Attitude and Practice of Nurses towards Pharamacovigilance in Taleqani Hospital.** *Iranian Journal of Pharmaceutical Research* 2010, **9**(2):199–206.
17. Hanafi S, Torkamandi H, Hayatshahi A, Kheirollah G, Javadi M: **Knowledge, attitudes and practice of nurses regarding adverse drug reaction reporting.** *IJNMR* 2012, **17**(1):1–7.
18. Fadare JO, Enwere OO, Afolabi AO, Chedi BAZ, Musa A: **Knowledge, Attitude and Practice of Adverse Drug Reaction Reporting among Healthcare Workers in a Tertiary Center in Northern Nigeria.** *Trop J Pharm Res* 2011, **10**(3):235–242.
19. Salehifar E, Ala SH, Gholami KH: **Knowledge, attitude and performance of pharmacists and nurses in Mazandaran province, Iran regarding adverse drug reaction and its reporting, 2005.** *Mazandaran University of Medical Sciences Journal* 2007, **16**(56):115–125.
20. Khalili H, Mohebbi N, Hendoiee N, Keshtkar AA, Dashti-Khavidaki S, Khalili H, Mohebbi N, Hendoiee N, Keshtkar AA, Dashti-Khavidaki S: **Improvement of knowledge, attitude and perception of healthcare workers about ADR, a pre- and post-clinical pharmacists' interventional study.** *BMJ Open* 2012, **13**(2). doi:10.1130.bmjopen-2011-000367. e000367.
21. Soleymani F, Shalviri G, Abdollahi M: **Pattern of use and Adverse Drug Reactions of Tramadol; A Review of 336, 610, 664 Insured Prescriptions During 5 Years.** *Int J Pharmacol* 2011, **7:**757–760.
22. Tabali M, Jeschke E, Bockelbrink A, Witt CM, Willich SN, Ostermann T, *et al*: **Educational intervention to improve physician reporting of adverse drug reactions (ADRs) in a primary care setting in complementary and alternative medicine.** *BMC Publ Health* 2009, **31**(9):274.
23. Pedrós C, Vallano A, Cereza G, Mendoza-Aran G, Agustí A, Aguilera C, *et al*: **An intervention to improve spontaneous adverse drug reaction reporting by hospital physicians: a time series analysis in Spain.** *Drug Saf* 2009, **32**(1):77–83. doi:10.2165/00002018-200932010-00007.

5

In-vitro/In-vivo comparison of leuprolide acetate release from an in-situ forming plga system

Roya Mashayekhi[1,2], Hamid Mobedi[2*], Jamal Najafi[3] and Marjan Enayati[4]

Abstract

A poly (lactide-co-glycolide) (PLGA) implant was used to control the release profile of leuprolide acetate (LA) drug. The system is an in-situ polymeric precipitation system. And the formulation consisted of PLGA polymer, LA drug and N-methyl-2-pyrrolidon solvent with no additives. First, the formulation was injected into PBS solution for in-vitro studies and then it was administered to the animal models (female rats) for in-vivo release studies. The release profiles of leuprolide acetate were measured by UV spectrophotometry for a period of 28 days. The initial burst release of LA was 14% in in-vitro whereas it was 7% in in-vivo. In-vitro and in-vivo release profiles of LA had similar trends after 72 hours. However, the rate of LA release was slower in-vivo. This might be attributed to the limited diffusion process of solvent and the drug molecules. This could be due to presence of an additional pressure caused by the surrounding tissue and also the presence of small amount of water between cells in the subcutaneous site. Cross-section and surface of the implants were studied via scanning electron microscopy. Morphology of both in-vitro and in-vivo implants confirmed the release behaviours. No toxicity effects were reported in the histopathological assay. Furthermore, the pharmacological analysis showed more inactive ovaries due to release of LA.

Keywords: Drug delivery system, In-vitro, In-vivo, Biodegradable polymer, Rat, Poly (lactide-co-glycolide) (PLGA)

Introduction

An injectable in-situ polymeric system forms a solid or semisolid drug reservoir upon the parenteral injection of a drug solution [1]. This is due to the permeation of water molecules into the implant, solvent removal process and coagulation of the polymer after injection [2,3]. These systems have many advantages such as; ease of administration, having less complicated fabrication, increasing effective pharmacological duration, preserving the effectiveness of short lifetime drugs and reducing the need for repeated daily injection. However, they suffer from one major disadvantage, which is their high burst release defined as the amount of drug released during the first 24 hours [4,5]. An undesirable high burst release may exhaust the loaded drug from the implants too rapidly and cause severe toxicity problems. It can also lead to an overall shorter drug release duration, and subsequently less therapeutic efficiency and cost-effectiveness.

Leuprolide acetate has been utilised for the treatment of the various diseases such as: advanced prostate cancer, breast cancer, uterine fibroids, endometriosis, and Alzheimer [6]. LA is a synthetic analog of endogenous Gn-RH agonist and a non-apeptide drug. It increases the circulating levels of the luteinizing hormone (LH) and follicle-stimulating hormone (FSH) leading to a transient increase of gonadal steroids. In females, continuous administration of LA reduces the level of LH and FSH. But in males, the level of the testosterone increases right after the initial drug administration and then falls below the castrate threshold for the next 2–4 weeks. LA can be administered via parenteral and pulmonary routes [7,8]. And it can be incorporated in different types of drug carriers such as nano/micro particles, capsules and in-situ forming implants. For instance, LA was successfully loaded in PLGA/PLA microspheres as an osmotical driven implantable system [9,10].

PLGA is a FDA approved biodegradable alpha polyester. It has been used in several therapeutic applications and can be utilised in various forms of controlled release devices. For instances, it has been used as a suture mesh for a guidance around nerve defects, as a scaffold

* Correspondence: h.mobedi@ippi.ac.ir
[2]Iran Polymer and Petrochemical Institute, P.O. Box:14185/458, Tehran, Iran
Full list of author information is available at the end of the article

for cell proliferation [11] and as drug delivery carriers with various forms. Moreover, N-methyl-2-pyrrolidone (NMP) is a water-soluble, water-miscible, biocompatible, and inert organic solvent with low toxicity potential in animal and human studies [12].

The main objective of this study is to investigate the release profile of leuprolide acetate from a PLGA injectable implant using in-vitro and in-vivo studies. PLGA implants were prepared and were injected into phosphate buffer saline (PBS) solution for the in-vitro studies. Subsequently, the same formulations were administered subcutaneously to the rat animal model for in-vivo studies. Drug release profiles were characterised using UV spectroscopy method. Structure and morphology of the PLGA implants were investigated in-vitro and in-vivo via scanning electron microscopy. The toxicity effects of the implants on the living tissues were investigated by a histopathological assay on sexual and non-sexual organs. Furthermore, the pharmacological analysis was conducted to study the influence of the LA release on the ovaries and the uterine of the animal models within 28 days.

Materials and methods

Materials

Poly (lactide-co-glycolide) (50:50), Resomer® RG 504, (Mw=48,000 Da) as a biodegradable copolymer, was obtained from Boehringer Inc. (Ingelheim, Germany) for sterilization. Leuprolide acetate (Mw 1209 Da) was supplied by Bachem Inc. (Bubendorf, Switzerland). Analytical grade N-methyl-2-pyrrolidon was purchased from Merck (Riedel-deHaen Company, German).

Methods

Sample preparation

The RG 504 PLGA polymer and NMP as a solvent were used. First, the polymer was mixed with NMP in the specific ratio of PLGA (28 wt %) to NMP (69 wt %) by a glass mixer. Subsequently, the mixture was placed on a continuous shaker in order to obtain clear solutions after 1 hour. The PLGA solutions were gamma irradiated (dose of 25kGy). Then 3 wt % leuprolide acetate was dissolved in the polymer solution [13]. The sample preparation was performed at ambient temperature (23°C ± 3°C).

In-vitro studies

0.5 g of the formulations were injected into 15 ml PBS (0.2 M, pH 7.4) through a 20 gauge needle and were stored at 37°C in an incubator. 15 ml PBS released media was taken and replaced at the determined time points (0, 1, 2, 3, 7, 14, 18, 21, 25, 28 days). The concentration of the leuprolide acetate was calculated by UV spectrophotometer.

In-vivo studies

Female Sprauge-Dawley rats (8 weeks old, 150±5 g) were used. The formulation was injected subcutaneously on the back using 16 gauge needle. The animal models were divided into 3 groups (Group A, B and C). Group A (n=21) were administered with 100 (μg/kg/day) of LA [14], and Group B (n=21), received the formulation without drug 10 (μg/kg/day) of formulation. Group C (n=3) was the control group and they were sacrificed in the first day. This point is important that the research on animals was acted in pathology department in "Iran Veterinary Organization" with ethical approval (ISO 17025) from TUV (Germany).

Determination of leuprolide acetate (LA)

UV spectrophotometer (CECIL 1000 SERIES, England) was used for in-vitro and in-vivo release studies. In in-vitro release studies, the amounts of drug released in PBS were measured at discrete time intervals. For in-vivo release studies, the remainder PLGA implants were first dissolved in 10 ml NMP. Then, the amounts of the leuprolide acetate in the implants were calculated. Samples without LA were also monitored so that any contributions to the measured absorbance from the polymer could be evaluated.

The UV-spectroscopy method was carried out at wavelength of 279 nm. The developed method was validated with respect to linearity, accuracy (recovery), precision and specificity in accordance with ICH (International Conference on Harmonisation) requirements for assay method determination [15].

Specificity was investigated by determining the blank dissolution media and the dissolution media containing LA and any other potential excipients by UV, then spiking the drug substance and examining any interference between peaks. To determine the linearity and range of the assay method, standard solutions of LA having known concentrations were used; these standards have been analysed with the UV method as described. For each concentration, 3 runs have been performed. Accuracy was evaluated by analysing synthetic mixtures spiked with known quantities of drugs. Linearity was studied in the range of 1–25 μg/ml of the analyte content. The calibration curve obtained had a R2 value of 0.998, an intercept of 0.004 and a slope of 0.007; the intervals at 95% confidence level, calculated for the intercept included the zero value. Accuracy was determined at three levels of content in placebo. Recovery ranged from 98 to 103.5 with a mean value of 101.3 a RSD % of 0.85 and finally in the specificity term we have not seen any interference between API and other excipients. Thus the method showed an acceptable degree of linearity, accuracy and precision according to the validation requirements and can be considered valid.

Scanning electron microscopy (SEM)

The surface morphologies and the cross-sections of the PLGA implants were studies by SEM (Cambridge S360, England) at predetermined times (24 h, 3, 7, and 14 days). Samples were frozen and mounted on metal stubs with double-sided carbon tape and coated with gold (30 mA for 5 min) by a sputter coater (E 5200 AUTO, BioRAD Polaron Devision, England). The morphologies of the in-vivo samples after the day 14 were not studied because of significant degradation of the implants.

Pharmacological and histopathological analysis

The animal models were scarified at the defined time points. Their non-sexual organs (lung, liver, kidney) and sexual organs (four layers of uterine and ovaries) were fixed with 10% neutralised formalin. The paraffin method was utilised for preparation of paraffin blocks and sections were cut and mounted on microscope slides. The sections were stained by hematocyline and eosin for histological investigation and these were studied using a light microscope.

Statistical analysis

The in-vivo and in-vitro release data were analysed statistically, with ANOVA using Minitab 14.

Results and discussions

In-vitro studies

Release profile of the PLGA implant is shown in Figure 1. It was observed that 14% of the drug was released initially in the first 24 hours. This initial fast release phase may be attributed to the porous surface structure and interconnected channels [16] which were observed in the SEM micrographs (Figure 2). These types of structures have been observed in previous studies utilising injectable in-situ forming PLGA implants [17].

The release profile was followed by a slow release phase with the rate of 1% over the next 3 days (Figure 3). These results are confirmed in the SEM micrographs (Figure 2). The degradation of the implant was not noticeable in this stage. The surface was smooth and had much less interconnected channels. However, the diameters of these channels were larger than before. The rate of the drug release was increased significantly after 72 hours. This fast release trend was maintained till day 7 and more than 50% of the loaded drug was released within this period of time (Figure 1). The surface structure of the implant showed more pores. Also, the cross-section of the implant had large tear–like structure (Figure 2) that may cause the fast release of the therapeutic agent [18]. The rate of the drug release was reduced afterward and in this final stage only 23.4 wt. % of the LA was released (Figure 3). The surface and cross-section morphologies of the prepared implants showed relatively larger interconnected channels with more pores on the surface of the implants. The PLGA implants were degraded in 28 days. And the number and size of the porosities were increased as a function of time (Figure 2).

PLGA degrades by means of hydrolysis including surface hydrolysis, bulk hydrolysis, and bulk catalysed hydrolysis. The inwards diffusion of the aqueous phase causes degradation of the polymer chains which in turn facilitates the diffusion of the entrapped drug. The biodegradation products of PLGA (lactic and glycolic acid) are common body metabolites, which are non-toxic, non-immunogenic, non-carcinogenic, and non-teratogenic.

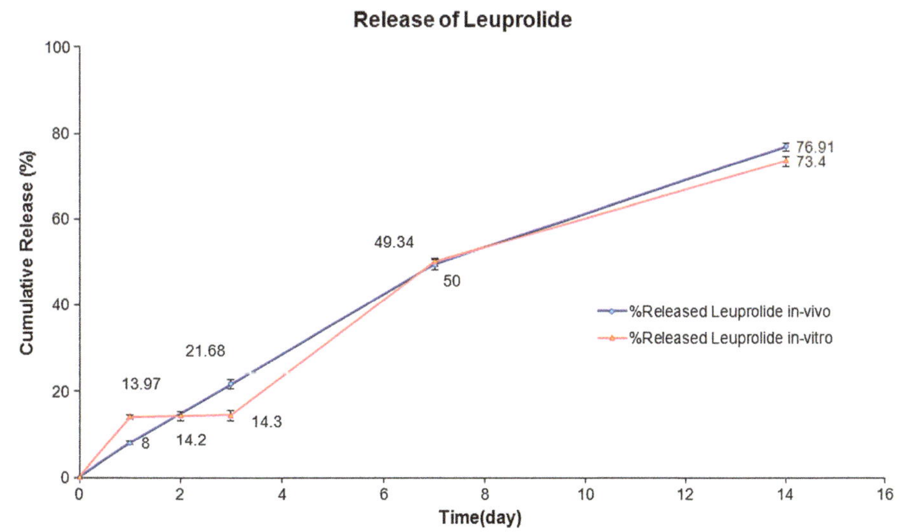

Figure 1 A comparison of the in-vitro and in-vivo cumulative release of LA from PLGA (50:50) systems (Mean±S.D., n=3).

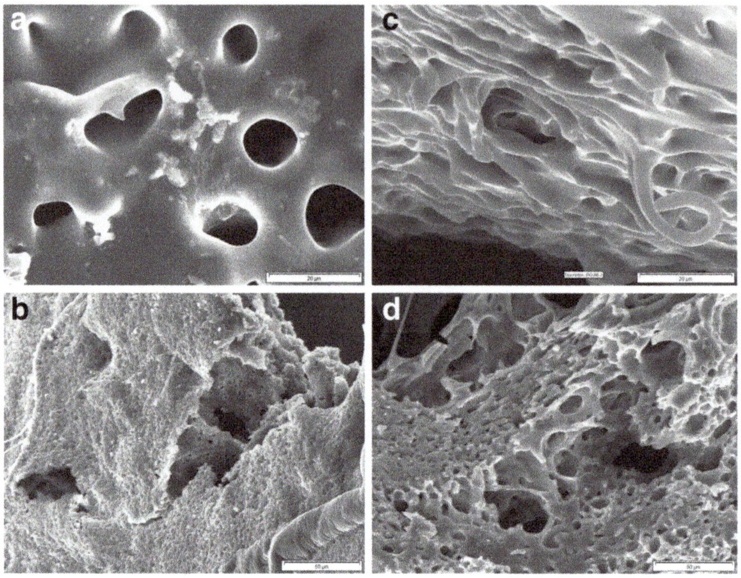

Figure 2 SEM images of surfaces and cross sections of the in-situ formed implants of PLGA/NMP/LA in the in-vitro environment: surface morphology after (a) 24 hours, (c) 7 days (1500x), and cross-section structure after: (b) 24 hours, (d) 3 days (500x).

However, the products of polymer degradation can be trapped in the internal structure, which can change the localised pH within the polymer matrix. This phenomenon accelerates the polymer degradation due to autocatalysis [19].

Furthermore, PLGA erosion was determined by monitoring the pH changes and lactic acid formation as a reaction of the degradation. There was a lag-phase in formation of lactic acid in the first 4 days. The pH of the release medium was 7 and the drug release rate was not noticeable at this stage. The pH of the environment decreased afterward due to the degradation of the PLGA implant and the presence of lactic acid in the release medium [20].

In this study, the mechanism of the LA release had 4 stages: (i) diffusion of drug through the polymer; (ii) surface erosion of the polymer and continuous release of the physically entrapped drug; (iii) cleavage of the covalent bonds between the polymer bulks followed by the drug diffusion; and (iv) slow diffusion of LA through the polymer and degradation of the polymer until drug depletion.

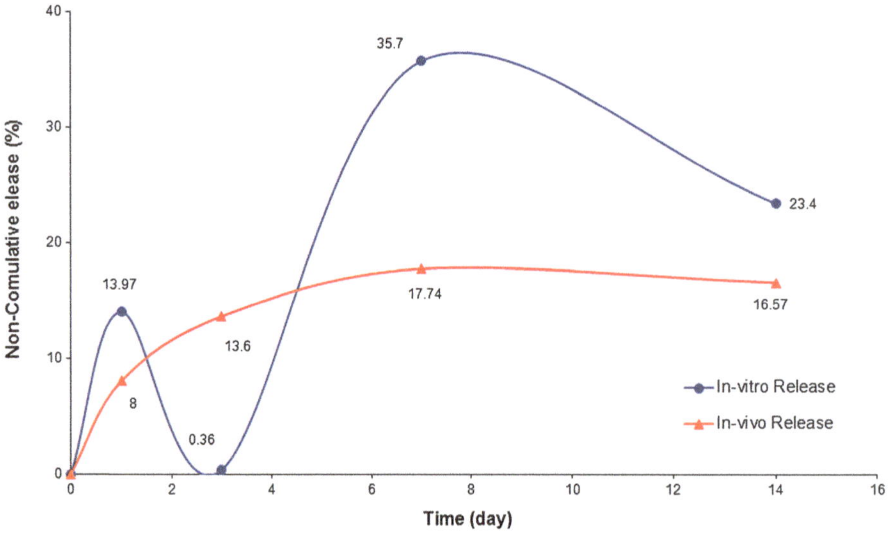

Figure 3 Non-cumulative in-vitro and in-vivo release profiles of the LA from PLGA implants (Mean± S.D., n=3).

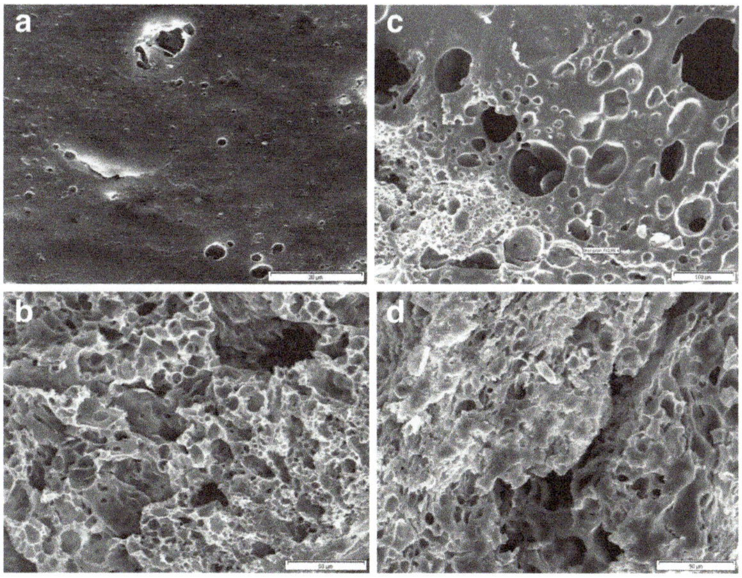

Figure 4 Surface and cross-section of the drug loaded PLGA implants in the in-vivo environment: surface morphology after (a) 24 hours, (c) 7 days (1500x), and cross-section structure after (b) 24 hours and (d) 3 day (500x).

In-vivo studies

The in-vivo release profile of the formulation is shown in Figure 1. It was observed that only 8% of the drug was released within the first 24 hours. This initial release was 6% less than the initial release in the in-vitro study. The surface and cross-section morphologies of the implant were also studied (Figure 4). The implant had a smooth surface whereas, many small interconnected channels were observed in the cross-section in the first 24 hours. Overall, the surfaces and the cross-sections of the implants were similar in both in-vitro and in-vivo studies. After the initial release phase, 21.6% and 49% of the drug were released in the next 3 and 7 days, respectively. SEM micrographs confirmed the in-vivo release results (Figure 4). The rate of degradation was increased significantly and more pores were observed on the surface structures of the implants. The diameters of the interconnected channels were increased throughout the bulk of the implant which results to the formation of tear-like structures. In the last stage of the release profile (from day 7 to day 14), the release rate for the sample increased significantly as degradative hydrolysis of the polymer implant took place and the central region, which would be expected to contain a higher concentration of drug, was exposed.

The morphology and structure of a blank PLGA implant (with no drug) was also studied. The SEM micrographs were similar to the SEM micrographs of the implant loaded with LA in terms of the degree of their porosities and their internal structures. These similarities were observed throughout the 28 days of the studies, except from day 3. The surface of the implant had much less pores during this period in the blank implant.

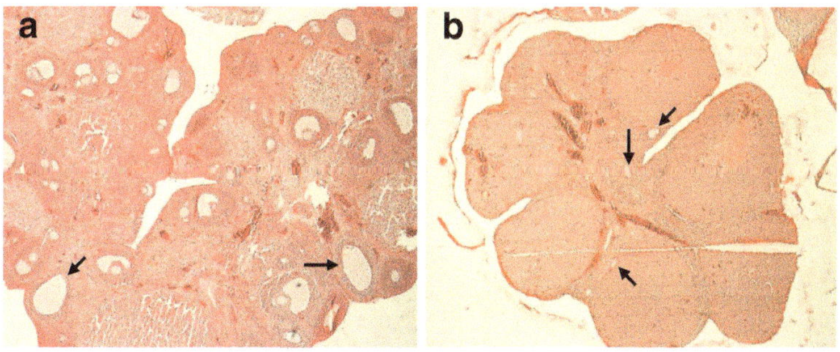

Figure 5 Histology images of (a) inactive ovary (control group), and (b) active ovary (injected LA formulation group) (Mean ± S.D., n=3).

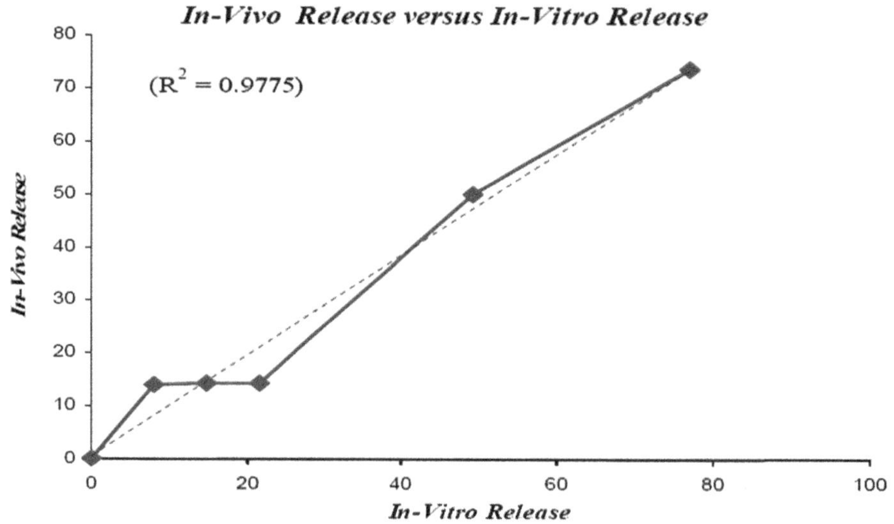

Figure 6 In-vivo release of LA vs. in-vitro release.

Histopathology study

All implants used in human body should be biocompatible and non-toxic. In this study, it was observed that all tissue samples had normal structures with no necrotic tissues. And the implant does not possess any toxicity effects on the living tissues and organs including the tissues at the injection site and sexual/non-sexual organs.

Pharmacology study

Pharmacological studies showed that all the animal models, injected with the PLGA formulations with LA drug, had inactive ovaries in the first 28 days. Whereas, the ovaries of the animals injected with the formulation without the drug were completely active. These results showed that LA suppressed gonadotropin receptors effectively and stopped the ovaries functioning in the first 24 hours (Figure 5). Big white spheres in Figure 5a show activity of ovaries bacause absent of LA and in Figure 5b small white spheres showed inactivity of ovaries with the release of LA.

Comparison of in-vitro and in-vivo results

The main objective of this study was to evaluate the release profiles of the injectable PLGA implants in both in-vitro and in-vivo environments. The release results were compared and analysed statistically via Minitab 14 software. The amount of released leuprolide in-vitro and in-vivo are shown in Table 1. The drug release rates were 6% slower in the first 24 and 72 hours in the in-vivo environments. This could be due to the presence of an additional pressure caused by the surrounding tissue and also presence of small amounts of water between cells in the subcutaneous site. Afterwards, the differences between the release rates in the two environments were reduced and similar trends in release profiles were observed after day 7. The in-vivo release rate vs. in-vitro release rate graph was constructed (Figure 6). R2 of the graph was 0.9775 suggesting that the kinetics of the release profile was linear.

Conclusion

The release profiles of LA from injectable in-situ forming PLGA implants were studied in in-vitro and in-vivo environments. The release profiles had four phases in the in-vitro study. It started with a burst release phase where 14% of the loaded drug was released in the first 24 hours. The rate of the drug release in the initial phase was lower in the in-vivo environment and the amount of release drug was only 8% in the first 24 hours. However, the release profiles had similar trends after day 3 in both in-vitro and in-vivo environments. Histopathology studies confirmed that the implants were biocompatible and no toxicity effects were observed on the various living tissues and organs. Pharmacology studies revealed that the LA loaded implants were effective in suppressing the gonadotropin receptors and halting the ovaries function.

Table 1 The amount of leuprolide acetate released in in-vitro and in-vivo environments

	In vitro					*In vivo*				
	Day 1	Day 2	Day 3	Day 8	Day 14	Day 1	Day 2	Day 3	Day 8	Day 14
Test 1	13	13.1	13.2	49.9	75.2	8.1	13.1	20.1	48	76.7
Test 2	14.7	15.1	15.3	47	68.1	9.1	13.9	22.1	51	74.8
Test 3	14.2	14.6	14.7	51.2	76.9	6.8	15.6	22.9	51.2	79.2
Mean	14.0	14.3	14.4	49.4	73.4	8.0	14.2	21.7	50.1	76.9

Competing interests

We declare that we have no competing interests.

Authors' contributions

RM, HM, and ME in studies and experimental laboratories, also JN carried out histopathological. All authors read and approved the final manuscript.

Author details

[1]Faculty of Biomedical Engineering Department, Islamic Azad University, Science and Research Branch, Tehran, Iran. [2]Iran Polymer and Petrochemical Institute, P.O. Box:14185/458, Tehran, Iran. [3]Center of Veterinary, Tehran, Iran. [4]Pharmaziezentrum, Althanstrasse 14, Universität Wien, Raum 2D177, Wien, Austria.

References

1. Hammer KS, Boisclair J, Schuetz H, Petersen H, Goepferich A: **Biocompatibility of an Injectable in-situ Forming Depot for Peptide Delivery.** *Pharm Sci* 2010, **99:**4390–4399.
2. Fogueri LR, Singh S: **Smart Polymers for Controlled Delivery of Proteins and Peptides.** *A Review of Patents* 2009, **3**(7):40–48.
3. Kranz H, Brazeau GA, Napaporn J, Martin RL, Millard W, Bodmeier R: **Myotoxicity studies of injectable biodegradable in-situ forming drug delivery system.** *Int J Pharm* 2001, **212:**11.
4. Bodmeier S, López Esguerra V, Körber M, Dong WY: **Stability of poly (D,L-lactide-co-glycolide) and leuprolide acetate in in-situ forming drug delivery systems.** *JCR* 2006, **115**(2):158–167.
5. Dunn RL, Garrett JS, Ravivarapu H, Chandrashekar BL: **Polymeric delivery formulations of Leuprolide with improved efficacy.** *US Patent* 2004, **6:**773,714.
6. Okada H, Doken Y, Ogawa Y: **Persistent Suppression of the Pituitary-Gonadal System in Female Rats by Three-Month Depot Injectable Microspheres of Leuprorelin Acetate.** *J Pharm Sci* 1996, **85**(10):1045.
7. Hatano T: **Incidence of bone fracture in patients receiving luteinizing hormone-releasing hormone agonists for prostate cancer.** *BJU Int* 2000, **86:**449–452.
8. Eligard SO: **leuprolide acetate in a novel sustained-release delivery system.** *Urology* 2003, **61**(2Suppl 1):25–31.
9. Bari H: **Inter A, prolonged release parenteral drug delivery system.** *Inter J Pharm Sci Rev Res* 2010, **3**(1):1–11.
10. Zare M, Mobedi H, Barzin J, Mivehchi H, Jamshidi A, Mashayekhi R: **Effect of Additives on Release Profile of Leuprolide Acetate in an In-situ Forming Controlled-Release System: In-vitro Study.** *J Appl Poly Sci* 2008, **107:**3781–3787.
11. Krogman NR, Singh A, Nair LS, Laurencin CT: **Allcock HR.** *Biomacromolecules* 2007, **8:**13106–13125.
12. Dunn RL, Garrett JS, Ravivarapu H, Chandrashekar B: **Polymeric delivery formulations of leuprolide with improved efficacy.** *US Patent* 2003, **656:**5874.
13. Strickley RG: **Solubilizing excipients in oral and injectable formulations.** *Pharm Res* 2001, **21:**201–230.
14. Okada H, Inoue Y, Heya T, Ueno H, Ogawa Y, Toguchi H: **Pharmacokinetics of once-month injectable microspheres of leuprolide acetate.** *Pharm Res* 1991, **8**(6):787–791.
15. Guideline, I.C.H.H.T: **Validation of analytical procedures: Methodology.** *ICH* 1996.
16. Luan X, Bodmeier R: **Influence of the poly (lactide-co-glycolide) type on the Leuprolide release from in-situ forming microparticle systems.** *JCR* 2006, **110:**266–272.
17. Bakhshi R, Vasheghani-Farahani E, Mobedi H, Jamshidi A, Khakpour M: **The effect of additives on naltrexone hydrochloride release and solvent removal rate from an injectable in-situ forming PLGA implant.** *Poly Adv Tech* 2006, **17:**354–359.
18. Luan X, Bodmeier R: **Modification of the tri-phasic release pattern of Leuprolide Acetate-loaded poly (lactide-co-glycolide) microparticles.** *Euro J Pharm Biopharm* 2006, **63:**205–214.
19. Khang G, Kyuang JE, Rhee JM: **Controlled release of nerve growth factor from sandwiched poly (D, L-lactide-co-glycolide) films for the application in neural tissue engineering.** *Macromol Res* 2003, **11**(5):334–340.
20. Astaneh R, Moghimi HR, Erfan M, Mobedi H: **Formulation of an injectable implant for peptide delivery and mechanistic study of the effect of polymer molecular weight on its release behavior.** *DARU* 2006, **14**(2):65–70.

Coumarin compounds of *Biebersteinia multifida* roots show potential anxiolytic effects in mice

Hamid Reza Monsef-Esfahani[1], Mohsen Amini[2], Navid Goodarzi[3,4], Fatemeh Saiedmohammadi[1,5], Reza Hajiaghaee[6], Mohammad Ali Faramarzi[7], Zahra Tofighi[1] and Mohammad Hossein Ghahremani[4,5*]

Abstract

Background: Traditional preparations of the root of *Biebersteinia multifida* DC (Geraniaceae), a native medicinal plant of Irano-Turanian floristic region, have been used for the treatment of phobias as anxiolytic herbal preparation.

Methods: We utilized the phobic behavior of mice in an elevated plus-maze as a model to evaluate the anxiolytic effect of the plant extract and bio-guided fractionation was applied to isolate the active compounds. Total root extract, alkaline and ether fraction were administered to mice at different doses 30 and 90 min prior to the maze test. Saline and diazepam were administered as negative and positive controls, respectively. The time spent in open and closed arms, an index of anxiety behavior and entry time, was measured as an index of animal activity.

Results: The total root extract exhibited anxiolytic effect which was comparable to diazepam but with longer duration. This sustained effect of the crude extract was sustained for 90 min and was even more after injection of 45 mg/kg while the effect of diazepam had been reduced by 90 min. The anxiolytic effect factor was only present in the alkaline fraction and displayed its effect at lower doses than diazepam while pure vasicinone as the previously known alkaloid did not shown anxiolytic effect. The effect of the alkaline fraction was in a dose dependent manner starting at 0.2 mg/kg with a maximum at 1.0 mg/kg. Bio-guided fractionation using a variety of chromatographic methods led to isolation and purification of three coumarin derivatives from the bioactive fraction, including umbelliferone, scopoletin, and ferulic acid.

Conclusion: For the first time, bio-guided fractionation of the root extract of *B. multifida* indicates significant sustained anxiolytic effects which led to isolation of three coumarin derivatives with well-known potent MAO inhibitory and anti-anxiety effects. These data contribute to evidence-based traditional use of *B. multifida* root for anxiety disorders.

Keywords: Biebersteinia multifida, Coumarin, Anxiolytic, Scopoletin, Umbelliferone

Background

Biebersteinia multifida DC (Geraniaceae), a native plant of Irano-Turanian floristic regions [1], is known traditionally as Chelleh-Dagh or Adamak in Iran. All four species of Biebersteinia distributed geographically from central Asia to Greek in temperate mountain zones. Among these pharmacologically active species, only *B. multifida* and *B. orphanidis* have tuberous roots. In folk medicine, the tuberous roots of *B. multifida* have been used topically for the relief of inflammation and pain of musculoskeletal disorders [2,3] and orally in the treatment of nocturia in children and of phobia and anxiety in humans and domestic animals [4] with no systematic approach to characterize the observed ethnopharmacological effects. Thus far, isolation of an alkaloid, vasicinone, and number of polysaccharides and peptide substances has been reported [5]. Flavonoids including 7-glucosides of apigenin, luteolin, and tricetin, as well as the 7-rutinoside of apigenin and luteolin have been isolated from its leaves which in part are responsible for antioxidant and antihemolytic activities [6-8]. Recently, essential oil composition of *B. multifida*

* Correspondence: mhghahremani@tums.ac.ir
[4]Nanotechnology Research Centre, Faculty of Pharmacy, Tehran University of Medical Sciences, Tehran, Iran
[5]Department of Pharmacology and Toxicology, Faculty of Pharmacy, Tehran University of Medical Sciences, Tehran, Iran
Full list of author information is available at the end of the article

was studied which exhibited that the main components were (E)-nerolidol, phytol, 6,10,14-trimethyl-2- pentadecanone and hexadecanoic acid [9].

Ethnopharmacological studies have revealed that the root extract of this plant has anti-inflammatory and analgesic activities that confirm the traditional use of *B. multifida* for the treatment of joint disturbances as well as in restoring bone fractures [10]. However, no report has yet been made on the anti-anxiety effects of the plant.

The elevated plus-maze has been developed as an ethological model of provoked anxiety and its use for the study of animal anxiety-like behavior has been pharmacologically validated and widely used for rats and mice [11-13]. In the present study, we have utilized the phobia behavior of mice in the elevated plus-maze as a model to evaluate the anxiolytic effect of the plant. For this purpose, the anxiolytic effects of the total root extract of *B. multifida* and its fractions were evaluated in mice and the chemical composition of the active fraction was identified.

Materials and methods

Chemicals

All chemicals were obtained from Merck (Darmstadt, Germany). Solvents used in chromatography methods were HPLC-grade. Diazepam (purity: not less than 98.0%) was obtained from Chemidarou Pharmaceutical Company (Tehran, Iran). Vasicinone (purity ≥97%) was a generous gift from Dr. Vahid Ziaee in Department of Medicinal Chemistry, Tehran University of Medical Sciences.

Plant materials

The plant materials were collected from the region of Ruine, located in North Khorasan Province of Iran following the national rule on biodiversity by local agent of Iran Department of Environment. A voucher specimen has been deposited at the Herbarium of the Faculty of Pharmacy, Tehran University of Medical Sciences (Voucher No. 6691 TEH) by Prof. GR Amin. The root of the plant was used in this study.

Chromatographic apparatus

A high performance liquid chromatography (HPLC) instrument equipped with K-1001 pump (Knauer, Germany), a D-14163 manual injector valve (Rheodyne), and a K-2600 UV detector for peak detection was used in the analytical studies. Another HPLC instrument (Knauer, Germany) including preparative K-1800 pumps (Double), two switching valves and a K-2501 UV detector were used for preparative purification. Solvents were filtered through a Millipore system and separation was performed on Knauer Eurosphere 100 C18 columns (150 mm × 4.0 mm, I.D. 5 μm) and (120 mm × 16 mm, I.D. 5 μm) for analytical and preparative HPLC, respectively.

Spectroscopy instruments

The ^{1}H-NMR and ^{13}C-NMR spectra of the isolated compounds were measured in DMSO-d_6 or $CDCl_3$ at 500 and 125 MHz, respectively, using a Bruker AC 500 spectrophotometer (Germany). Mass spectra were prepared on Finnigan-Mat TSQ-70 spectrometer (CA, USA). Fourier-transform infrared (FTIR) spectra were obtained with a Nicolet Magna-FTIR 550 spectrometer (WI, USA).

Extraction procedures

The roots were collected from the field, cleaned, dried for two weeks in the shade, then powdered and stored in airtight containers. The total extract was prepared from the powdered root refluxed with methanol for 72 hours using a Soxhlet apparatus, followed by filtration. The filtrate was concentrated using low-pressure distillation at 45°C and evaporated to dryness. We obtained 690±1 g of total extract solids from 4900 g powdered root (14.08%). To prepare the fractions, an aliquot of 300 g of the extract solids were re-suspended in 1400 mL of water/acetic acid (95:5) solution and further extracted with light petroleum ether (4 × 1000 mL) to separate the lipophilic compounds (ether fraction, 4.3% of total extract). The remaining aqueous part was treated with ammonia 25% and sequentially partitioned in chloroform and ethyl acetate (4 × 1000 mL for each of them). The solvent was removed under reduced pressure and the total alkaline residue (1.6%) was used for the experiments (alkaline fraction). All extracts were analyzed by thin layer chromatography (TLC). Plant total extract was prepared in 1% carboxymethylcellulose (CMC) in saline prior to animal testing. The alkaline and ether fractions were dissolved in saline containing 2% DMSO.

Pharmacological studies

Male Swiss white mice, 20–25 g, were obtained from the Animal Care Facility (Faculty of Pharmacy, Tehran, Iran). The animals were housed six per cage in a temperature-controlled (22 ± 1°C) colony room. They were maintained in a 12h light/dark schedule with *ad libitum* food and water except during experimental procedures. All trials were carried out in the light phase. Subjects were experimentally naïve and each mouse was used only once. Animals were allowed 7 days to acclimatize to the laboratory environment including handling before testing began. All procedures were carried out in accordance with institutional guidelines for animal care and use. The protocol (No. 357) had been approved by the Committee of Ethics of the Faculty of Sciences of Tehran University.

Plant extracts and fractions were injected intraperitoneally (*i.p.*) in a single dose. Control groups received vehicle in saline (saline group) or diazepam 1 mg/kg, as a known anti-anxiety drug. The elevated plus maze consisted two open arms (6 × 30 × 2 cm) and two closed arms (6 × 30 × 10 cm), having an open roof, elevated 40 cm with a central platform of 8 × 8 cm. The test was performed 30 and 90 min after injection. Each mouse was placed in the central platform facing toward a closed arm and the cumulative time spent in open or closed arms was recorded for 5 min. The percent time spent was used as the measure of plus-maze performance. The ratio of percent time spent in open to closed arm (Ratio = % time spent in open arms/% time spent in closed arms) was indexed as the anxiolytic effect of various groups. Based on this calculation, when the animal had equal preference for open and closed arms at ratio = 1, this was an indicator of loss of anxiety. A ratio < 1 indicated that the animal avoided the open arm, indicating anxiety behavior. The entry time into each arm and the total entry time for each mouse were used as an index of activity for each animal. There were 4 mice in each group and the experiment was repeated 3 times, independently (n = 12).

Isolation, purification, and structure elucidation

The alkaline fraction (2 g) was subjected to column chromatography (100 g silica gel) for clean-up and initial fractionation. Elution with 1200 mL of $CHCl_3$/EtOAC (80:20) gave a fraction that contained major compounds of the chloroform extraction. This fraction was further purified by HPLC to yield compounds 1 and 2 as described below. Compound 3 eluted from the column with an Rf value greater than 1 and 2. This compound was further purified by preparative TLC by $CHCl_3$/EtOAC (65:35) as the mobile phase.

For further purification, the $CHCl_3$/EtOAC (80:20) fraction from column chromatography was subjected to preparative HPLC. Initially, a small amount of the fraction was injected into the analytical HPLC and the composition of the mobile phase was optimized by varying the percent of acetonitrile in phosphate buffer for separation of compounds 1 and 2. The best purification was obtained using the following conditions: acetonitrile/0.1 M phosphate buffer/glacial acetic acid (6:94:1 v/v/v), pH 4.15; flow rate: 1.2 mL/min; detector wavelength 300 nm. After optimizations using analytical HPLC, scale-up was performed for preparative separation. A flow rate of 14 mL/min was applied for preparative separation; other conditions were identical with the analytical method. The $CHCl_3$/EtOAC (80:20) fraction was subjected to preparative HPLC and pure compounds 1 (32 mg) and 2 (12 mg) were separated collected in the mobile phase. The purity of these two compounds was re-checked by analytical HPLC and structure elucidation of the purified compounds was carried out by spectroscopic methods (MS, FTIR, ^1H and ^{13}C-NMR).

Statistical analysis

The data obtained from independent pharmacological experiments were pooled and reported as mean ± SEM. The data were analyzed by one-way ANOVA followed by Tukey post hoc multiple comparison. $P < 0.05$ was considered significant.

Results

The anxiolytic effect of total extract in mice

In animals receiving the total extract of the roots and tested 30 min after injection, the time spent in open arm was prolonged compared to the animals that received saline (Figure 1). The effect was first seen at a dose of 25 mg extract/kg body weight and increased in a dose dependent

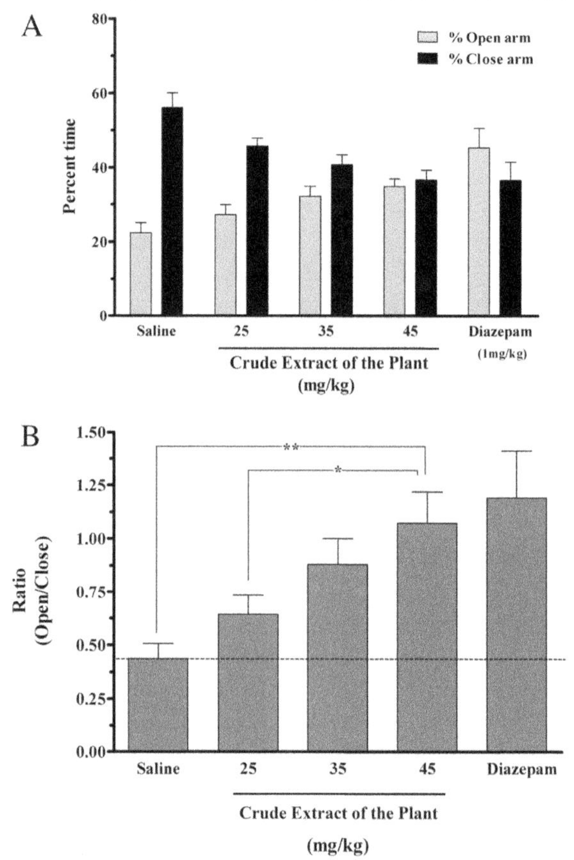

Figure 1 Evaluation of the effects of a crude extract from *Biebersteinia multifida* roots on mouse behavior on an elevated plus-maze. A) The percent time spent in each arm and **B)** The anxiolytic ratio as ratio of percent time spent in open arms to the close arms (Ratio = % time in open arms/% time in closed arms). The animals were injected 30 min prior to the test with saline (vehicle), diazepam (1 mg/kg) or different doses of crude extract. Data are presented as mean ± SE for each group (n = 12 in each group). The dotted line indicates the Ratio (open/close) of the vehicle (saline). *p value < 0.05, **p value < 0.01.

Table 1 The effect of total extract of *Biebersteinia multifida* on the behavior of mice on an elevated plus-maze

	Total entry		Percent entry into open arms	
Treatment	30 min	90 min	30 min	90 min
Saline	14.5 ± 1.5[a]	14.5 ± 0.9	41.2 ± 3.8	39.2 ± 4.3
Diazepam (1 mg/kg)	24.2 ± 2.7	18.3 ± 2.2	57.2 ± 3.55	44.2 ± 2.4
Extract (25 mg/kg)	15.7 ± 1.3	16.1 ± 1.3	41.2 ± 2.4	46.4 ± 2.2
Extract (35 mg/kg)	12.4 ± 1.3	14.3 ± 0.8	43.1 ± 1.7	44.2 ± 3.5
Extract (45 mg/kg)	16.4 ± 1.0	12.8 ± 1.4	50.5 ± 2.2	52.1 ± 2.8
Extract (50 mg/kg)	15.5 ± 3.6	10.0 ± 2.2	48.8 ± 1.9	44.0 ± 12.3
Extract (75 mg/kg)	8.2 ± 1.2	ND[b]	53.0 ± 6.2	ND

[a]The data are presented as mean ± SE (n = 12).
[b]*ND* not determined.
The table indicates the total entry and percent entry into open arms as an indicator of the activity of the animal. The entry to each arm was measured at 30 and 90 min after administration of the total extract.

manner to its maximum level at 45 mg/kg, where the animals spent equal time in the open and closed arms. The effect of 45 mg/kg of the total extract was comparable to that of diazepam at 1 mg/kg, where the mice showed a slightly more, but not significant, preference for the open arm (Figure 1A). At lower dose (10 mg/kg), the animals behaved similar to those given the saline treatment. At higher doses (50 and 75 mg/kg), the animals continued to show equal preference for the open and closed arms. The extract had very little effect on the activity of the animals at the doses used. As indicated in Table 1, the total entries into the closed and open arms are equal in all groups. In animals receiving 50 and 75 mg/kg of the extract, the entries were lower and they were mostly in sleep (Table 1). To compare the anxiolytic effect in various groups, we calculated the ratio of percent time spent in open arm to closed arm (see *Materials and Methods*) for each group (Figure 1B). The ratio = 1 indicates an equal preference for the open and the closed arms, representing loss of anxiety; and the ratio lower than 1 implies less preference for the open arm and an increase in anxiety behavior. This ratio in animals receiving 25 mg/kg of the total extract was higher (0.64±0.09) than in the saline group (0.44±0.07), indicating a trend toward preference for the open area although the difference was not statistically significant (Figure 1B). The anxiolytic ratio increased with increases in the dose of total extract and reached 1.07±0.15 in the mice that received 45 mg/kg of the total extract ($p < 0.01$ compared to saline), suggesting a lack of anxiety. This ratio was comparable to that obtained with diazepam (1.19±0.22, $p < 0.01$ compared to saline, Figure 1B). In order to evaluate the duration of anxiolytic effect, we also tested the effect of total extract 90 min after injection. As seen in Figure 2, the anxiolytic effect of the plant extract was sustained for 90 min. This anxiolytic ratio was even higher at 90 min after injection of 45 mg/kg of the total extract ($p < 0.05$ compared to 30 min, Figure 2). On the other hand, the effect of diazepam had been reduced considerably by 90 min. This observation suggests a longer duration of action for the extract compared to that of diazepam (Figure 2).

The anxiolytic effect of alkaline and ether fractions

To further isolate the active compounds in *B. multifida*, the total root extract was fractionated as mentioned in *Materials and Methods.* Alkaloids of this plant may be responsible for its pharmacological activities [10]; thus we examined the anxiolytic activity of the alkaline and ether (lipophilic compounds) fractions of the root extract. Figure 3 shows the effects of various doses of the alkaline fraction on animal performance on elevated plus-maze 30 min after injection. An increase in tendency toward presence in the open arm was seen as the dose of the alkaline fraction was increased (Figure 3). The anxiolytic ratio calculated for these experiments

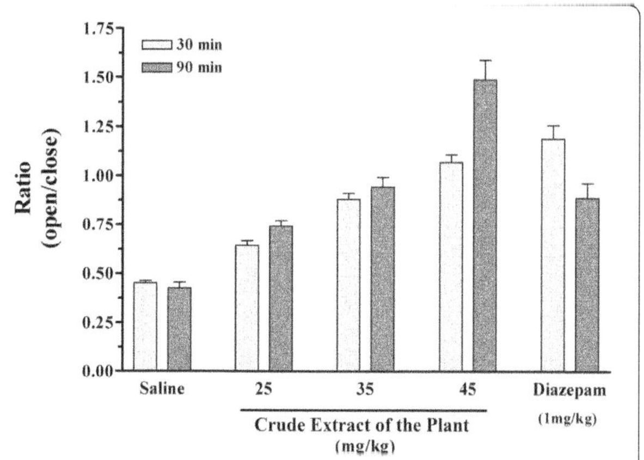

Figure 2 The time dependency of the anxiolytic effect of total extract. Effects were analyzed by performing the test at 30 min and 90 min after injection. The animals were injected 30 min prior to the plus maze test with saline (vehicle), diazepam (1 mg/kg) and different doses of crude extract of the plant. The ratio of percent time spent in open arms to close arms was calculated and plotted as mean ± SE for each group (n = 12 in each group).

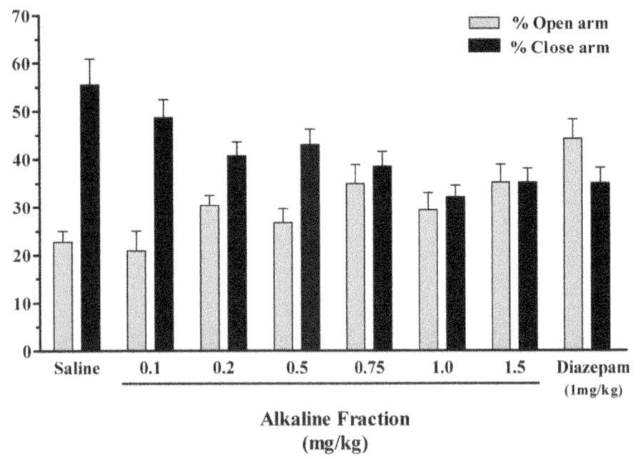

Figure 3 The effect of an alkaline fraction of a *Biebersteinia multifida* root extract on the behavior of mice on an elevated plus-maze by the percent time spent in each arm. The animals were injected 30 min prior to the test with saline (vehicle), diazepam (1 mg/kg) or different doses of alkaline fraction. Data are presented as mean ± SE for each group (n = 12 in each group).

indicated that this effect was dose dependent; it began at a dose of 0.2 mg/kg and the maximum effect was obtained at 1.0 mg/kg of the alkaline fraction. The activity of the animals indicated as total entries into the arms show no significant differences among the various groups (Table 2). We also studied the effect of the alkaline fraction 90 min after injection. As Figure 4 shows, unlike the diazepam treated group, the anxiolytic effect of alkaline fraction continued to be seen 90 min after injection, suggesting a sustained effect for this fraction.

We also tested the ether fraction of plant extract, which contained lipophilic compounds. At doses of 3 and 6 mg/kg of the ether fraction, the animals showed no significant anxiolytic effects compared to saline treated group (Figure 5A). The 3 and 6 mg of ether fraction were equivalent to 69.7 and 139.5 mg of total extract, respectively. The effect of the ether fraction was similar to saline and did not show any anxiolytic effect at either 30 or 90 min after injection (Figure 5B).

Collectively, the alkaline fraction produced an anxiolytic effect in a dose dependent manner starting at 0.2 mg/kg and reaching a maximum effect at 1.0 mg/kg. This effect was comparable to that seen for diazepam (1.0 mg/kg). Doses of 0.2 and 1.0 mg/kg of alkaloid fraction were equivalent to 12.5 and 62.5 mg/kg of the total root extract.

Isolation, purification, and structure elucidation of chemicals present in the alkaline fraction

The alkaline fraction that showed the anxiolytic effect was subjected to different chromatography methods, as mentioned in *Materials and Methods*, which led to isolation and purification of three compounds.

Structure elucidation of compounds 1, 2, and 3 was carried out by spectroscopic methods (MS, FTIR, ^{1}H and ^{13}C-NMR) and by comparison of acquired data with those reported in the literature [14-17]. Compounds 1, 2, and 3 were identified as umbelliferone, scopoletin, and ferulic acid, respectively (Figure 6, Additional file 1: Table S1 and Additional file 2: Figure S1, Additional file 3: Figure S2, Additional file 4: Figure S3, Additional file 5: Figure S4, Additional file 6: Figure S5, Additional file 7: Figure S6) as the major components of alkaloid fraction.

Discussion

The anti-inflammatory and analgesic activities of *B. multifida* have been reported before [10]. We have employed a bio-guided fractionation to study the anxiolytic effect of the extracts. This approach has been successfully applied as a valuable strategy for the finding of new lead compounds in phytochemical studies [18].

The use of the elevated plus-maze to study animal anxiety-like behavior has been comprehensively studied and pharmacologically validated for rats [11] and mice

Table 2 The effect of alkaline fraction of *Biebersteinia multifida* on the behavior of mice on an elevated plus-maze

	Total entry		Percent entry to open arms	
Treatment	**30 min**	**90 min**	**30 min**	**90 min**
Saline	14.2 ± 1.7[a]	8.8 ± 1.5	41.5 ± 3.3	39.9 ± 3.6
Diazepam (1 mg/kg)	32.2 ± 4.1	25.8 ± 6.2	60.5 ± 2.4	54.0 ± 6.4
Alkaline fraction (0.1 mg/kg)	19.2 ± 1.2	15.4 ± 1.7	42.3 ± 4.1	41.7 ± 6.9
Alkaline fraction (0.2 mg/kg)	14.8 ± 0.7	13.8 ± 1.4	48.8 ± 2.3	36.2 ± 2.5
Alkaline fraction (0.5 mg/kg)	13.8 ± 1.64	9.5 ± 1.3	41.0 ± 4.4	37.7 ± 4.9
Alkaline fraction (0.75 mg/kg)	16.5 ± 1.5	12.1 ± 1.1	51.2 ± 3.9	51.6 ± 3.6
Alkaline fraction (1.0 mg/kg)	23.0 ± 1.7	13.0 ± 4.3	48.4 ± 2.0	59.9 ± 3.1
Alkaline fraction (1.5 mg/kg)	18.2 ± 2.7	ND[b]	51.5 ± 2.7	ND

[a]The data are presented as Mean ± SE (n = 12).
[b]*ND* not determined.
The table indicates the total entry and percent entry into open arms as an indicator of the activity of the animal. The entry to each arm was measured at 30 and 90 min after administration of the alkaline fraction.

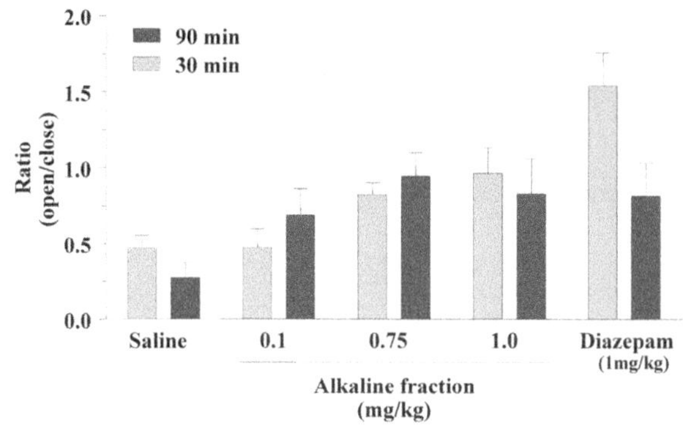

Figure 4 The time dependency of the anxiolytic effect of an alkaline fraction from *Biebersteinia multifida* roots on mice. The elevated plus-maze test was performed 30 min and 90 min after injection. The animals were injected 30 min prior to the test with saline (vehicle), diazepam (1 mg/kg) or different doses of alkaline fraction. The ratio of percent time spent in open arms to close arms was calculated and plotted as mean ± SE for each group (n = 12 in each group).

[13]. In various studies, the open arm entry to total entry or open time ratio were used as an indicator of anxiety behavior in mice and rats [11,13]. Since locomotion is an important factor in the elevated plus-maze, the total entry time has been used as an indicator of activity [11,13]. In this study, the time spent in each arm, the open and closed time ratio, was used to evaluate the anxiety behavior, while the total entry time considered as an index of animal activity.

A bio-guided phytochemical analysis of *B. multifida* has not previously been reported. Although other reports have thus far identified a number of flavonoids, a few polysaccharides and one alkaloid (vasicinone) from root extract, in which vasicinone considered as the responsible molecule for observed pharmacological activities [5-7,9], there were no direct relation between the isolated compounds to traditional use of *B. multifida*. Thus, to identify the active anxiolytic components, the total extract is fractioned into alkaline and ether fractions and subjected to anxiety alleviation studies. The anxiolytic compounds act readily in alkaline fraction form while the ether fraction showed little anxiolytic effect. This bio-guided fractionation indicates that the active compounds are present in the alkaline fraction. Furthermore, the results suggest that the alkaloid extract has a sustained anxiolytic effect compared to that observed with diazepam. Diazepam is a known anxiolytic used as control in various pharmacological studies. In this study, our results indicate a strong anti anxiety effect in animals receiving diazepam (Figures 1 and 2). Interestingly, the anxiolytic effect of diazepam has been reduced considerably by 90 min (Figure 2). Thus compared to diazepam, the plant extract has a longer duration of action.

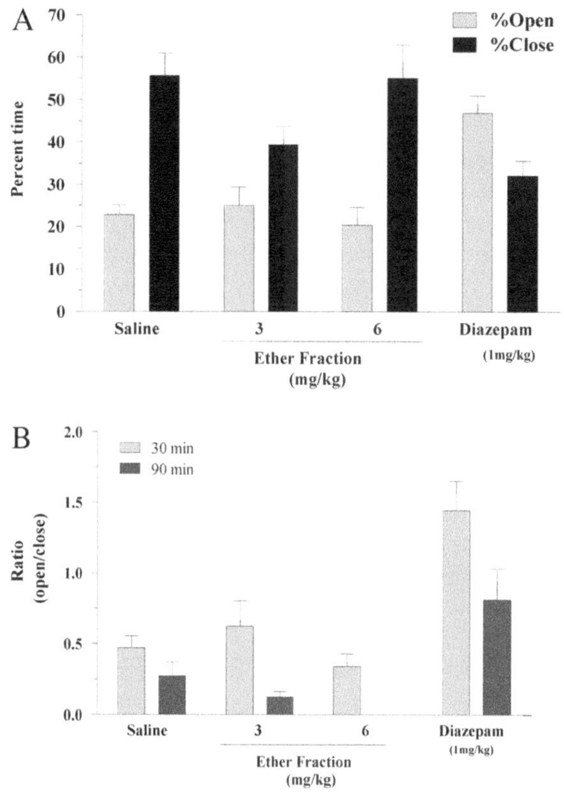

Figure 5 The effect of an ether fraction of a *Biebersteinia multifida* root extract on the behavior of mice on an elevated plus-maze. The animals were injected with ether fraction and the percent time spent in each arms of the plus maze test was plotted for each group. The ratio of time spent in open arms to close arms was calculated as an indicator of anxiety and fear of open and elevated area, and plotted for each group (Ratio = % time in open arms/% time in closed arms). The graph presents the results of three independent experiments (n =8 in each group).

Before any further chromatographic studies, the effects of pure vasicinone -as the suspected active compound in the alkaloid fraction- on mouse performance is tested by the same experimental procedure as described above. The analysis of vasicinone, at doses as high as 10 mg/kg, had no significant effect on open time ratio (data not shown). Thus, the alkaline fraction is further characterized for the major components present which lead to isolation and structure elucidation of three compounds of coumarin derivatives including umbelliferone, scopoletin, and ferulic acid. However the presence of ferulic acid after alkaline

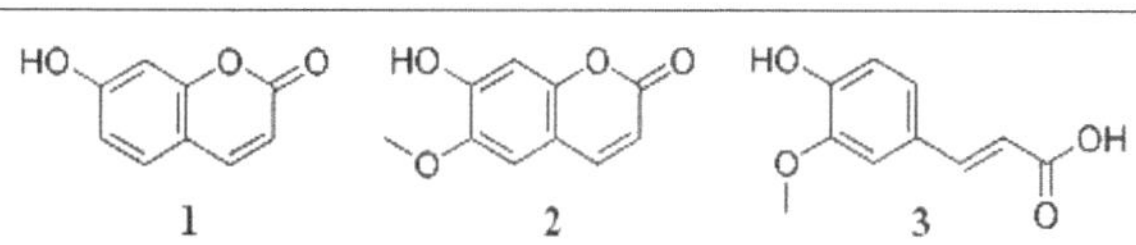

Figure 6 Chemical structures of compounds isolated from a *Biebersteinia multifida* root extract, including umbelliferone (1), scopoletin (2) and ferulic acid (3).

extraction could be a consequence of ring opening of scopoletin after extraction.

According to previous reports, coumarin derivatives, including scopoletin and umbelliferone, are potent inhibitors of monoamine oxidases (MAOs) [19,20]. Scopoletin shows MAO inhibition activity in a dose-dependent fashion, with IC_{50} values of 19.4 μg/mL [19]. In addition, daphnoretin a bicoumarin of scopoletin and umbelliferone exhibits significant anxiolytic activity in EPM model [21-23]. It has been also suggested that coumarin derivatives interact with the benzodiazepine binding site of the GABA-A receptor [24]. This may explain the effects observed in the present study and may confirm at least a partial role of these coumarins anxiolytic effects of *B. multifida*.

In addition to the anxiolytic effect, scopoletin is also a known potent anti-inflammatory agent [25,26], which can explain, in part, the anti-inflammatory and anti-nociceptive effects of *B. multifida* extracts. The ability of low molecular weight substances to cross the blood–brain barrier could explain the reported central anti-nociceptive effect [10]. However, this needs further specific pure substance studies in validated pharmacological models.

In conclusion, for the first time, bio-guided fractionation of the root extract of *B. multifida* indicates significant sustained anxiolytic effects which led to isolation of three coumarin derivatives of those scopoletin and umbelliferone with known MAO inhibitory and anti-anxiety effects. These data contribute to evidence-based traditional medicines using root of *B. multifida* for anxiety disorders.

Additional files

Additional file 1: Table S1. NMR chemical shift assignments of umbelliferone (1), scopoletin (2) and ferulic acid (3).

Additional file 2: Figure S1. Mass spectrum of Umbelliferone.

Additional file 3: Figure S2. FTIR spectrum of Umbelliferone.

Additional file 4: Figure S3. Mass spectrum of Scopoletin.

Additional file 5: Figure S4. FTIR spectrum of Scopoletin.

Additional file 6: Figure S5. Mass spectrum of Ferulic acid.

Additional file 7: Figure S6. FTIR spectrum of Ferulic acid.

Competing interests

The authors declare that they have no conflicts of interest.

Authors' contributions

HRM participated in the design of the study and carried out the phytochemical studies. MA carried out the structure elucidation. NG carried out the extraction, isolation and HPLC analysis and wrote the manuscript. FS carried out the animal studies and drafted the manuscript. RH participated in extraction and chromatography studies. MAF participated in the phytochemical analysis. ZT participated in experimental coordination and helped to draft the manuscript. MHG designed the study, performed the statistical analysis and finalized the manuscript. All authors read and approved the final manuscript.

Acknowledgments

This study was financially supported by a grant from Research Council of Tehran University of Medical Sciences and a grant from Center of Excellence for Toxicology, Ministry of Health and Medical Education of Iran. We gratefully acknowledge Professor Gholam Reza Amin, head of the Herbarium of Faculty of Pharmacy, Tehran University of Medical Sciences, and Dr. Vahid Ziaee for providing synthetic Vasicinone generously.

Author details

[1]Department of Pharmacognosy, Faculty of Pharmacy, Tehran University of Medical Sciences, Tehran, Iran. [2]Department of Medicinal Chemistry, Faculty of Pharmacy, Tehran University of Medical Sciences, Tehran, Iran. [3]Department of Pharmaceutics, Faculty of Pharmacy, Tehran University of Medical Sciences, Tehran, Iran. [4]Nanotechnology Research Centre, Faculty of Pharmacy, Tehran University of Medical Sciences, Tehran, Iran. [5]Department of Pharmacology and Toxicology, Faculty of Pharmacy, Tehran University of Medical Sciences, Tehran, Iran. [6]Pharmacognosy & Pharmaceutics Department of Medicinal Plants Research Center, Institute of Medicinal Plants, ACECR, Karaj, Iran. [7]Department of Pharmaceutical Biotechnology, Faculty of Pharmacy & Biotechnology Research Center, Tehran University of Medical Sciences, Tehran, Iran.

References

1. Muellner AN, Vassiliades DD, Renner SS: **Placing Biebersteiniaceae, a herbaceous clade of Sapindales, in a temporal and geographic context.** *Plant Syst Evol* 2007, **266:**233–252.
2. Amin G: *Popular Medicinal Plants of Iran.* 1st edition. Tehran: Research Deputy, Ministry of Health, Treatment and Medical Education; 1991.
3. Amirghofran Z: **Medicinal plants as immunosuppressive agents in traditional Iranian medicine.** *Iran J Immunol* 2010, **7:**65–73.
4. Aboutorabi H: ***Ethnobotanic and phytochemical study of plants in Rouin region.*** *PharmD Thesis.* Tehran: Tehran University of Medical Sciences; 2001.
5. Arifkhodzhaev AO, Rakhimov DA: **Polysaccharides of saponin-bearing plants. V. Structural investigation of glucans A, B, and C and their oligosaccharides from Biebersteinia multifida plants.** *Chem Nat Compd* 1994, **30:**655–660.
6. Greenham J, Vassiliades DD, Harborne JB, Williams CA, Eagles J, Grayer RJ, Veitch NC: **A distinctive flavonoid chemistry for the anomalous genus Biebersteinia.** *Phytochemistry* 2001, **56:**87–91.
7. Omurkamzinova VB, Maurel ND, Bikbulatova TN: **Flavonoids of Biebersteinia multifida.** *Chem Nat Compd* 1991, **27:**636–637.
8. Nabavi SF, Ebrahimzadeh MA, Nabavi SM, Eslami B, Dehpour A: **Antihemolytic and antioxidant activities of Biebersteinia multifida.** *Eur Rev Med Pharmacol Sci* 2010, **14:**823–830.
9. Javidnia K, Miri R, Soltani M, Khosravi AR: **Essential oil composition of biebersteinia multifida DC. (Biebersteiniaceae) from Iran.** *J Essent Oil Res* 2010, **22:**611–612.
10. Farsam H, Amanlou M, Dehpour AR, Jahaniani F: **Anti-inflammatory and analgesic activity of Biebersteinia multifida DC. root extract.** *J Ethnopharmacol* 2000, **71:**443–447.
11. Pellow S, Chopin P, File SE, Briley M: **Validation of open: closed arm entries in an elevated plus-maze as a measure of anxiety in the rat.** *J Neurosci Methods* 1985, **14:**149–167.
12. Rabbani M, Sajjadi SE, Jalali A: **Hydroalcohol extract and fractions of Stachys lavandulifolia vahl: effects on spontaneous motor activity and elevated plus-maze behaviour.** *Phytother Res* 2005, **19:**854–858.
13. Lister RG: **The use of a plus-maze to measure anxiety in the mouse.** *Psychopharmacology* 1987, **92:**180–185.
14. Yan J, Tong S, Sheng L, Lou J: **Preparative isolation and purification of two coumarins from Edgeworthia chrysantha Lindl by high speed countercurrent chromatography.** *J Liq Chromatogr Related Technol* 2006, **29:**1307–1315.
15. Aplin RT, Page CB: **The constituents of native umbelliferae. Part I. Coumarins from dill (Anetheum graveolens L.).** *J Chem Soc C* 1967, **2593:**2596.
16. Torres R, Urbina F, Morales C, Modak B, Delle Monache F: **Antioxidant properties of lignans and ferulic acid from the resinous exudate of Larrea nitida.** *J Chil Chem Soc* 2003, **48:**61–63.

17. Dobhal MP, Hasan AM, Sharma MC, Joshi BC: **Ferulic acid esters from Plumeria bicolor.** *Phytochemistry* 1999, **51**:319–321.
18. Pieters L, Vlietinck AJ: **Bioguided isolation of pharmacologically active plant components, still a valuable strategy for the finding of new lead compounds?** *J Ethnopharmacol* 2005, **100**:57–60.
19. Yun BS, Lee IK, Ryoo IJ, Yoo ID: **Coumarins with monoamine oxidase inhibitory activity and antioxidative coumarino-lignans from Hibiscus syriacus.** *J Nat Prod* 2001, **64**:1238–1240.
20. Seon HJ, Xiang HH, Seong SH, Ji SH, Ji HH, Lee D, Myung KL, Jai SR, Bang YH: **Monoamine oxidase inhibitory coumarins from the aerial parts of Dictamnus albus.** *Arch Pharm Res* 2006, **29**:1119–1124.
21. Herrera-Ruiz M, Gonzalez-Carranza A, Zamilpa A, Jimenez-Ferrer E, Huerta-Reyes M, Navarro-Garcia VM: **The standardized extract of Loeselia mexicana possesses anxiolytic activity through the gamma-amino butyric acid mechanism.** *J Ethnopharmacol* 2011, **138**:261–267.
22. Navarro-García VM, Herrera-Ruiz M, Rojas G, Zepeda LG: **Coumarin derivatives from Loeselia mexicana. Determination of the anxiolytic effect of daphnoretin on elevated plus-maze.** *J Mex Chem Soc* 2007, **51**:193–197.
23. Kumar D, Bhat ZA, Kumar V, Shah MY: **Coumarins from Angelica archangelica Linn. and their effects on anxiety-like behavior.** *Prog Neuropsychopharmacol Biol Psychiatry* 2013, **40**:180–186.
24. Singhuber J, Baburin I, Ecker GF, Kopp B, Hering S: **Insights into structure–activity relationship of GABAA receptor modulating coumarins and furanocoumarins.** *Eur J Pharmacol* 2011, **668**:57–64.
25. Moon PD, Lee BH, Jeong HJ, An HJ, Park SJ, Kim HR, Ko SG, Um JY, Hong SH, Kim HM: **Use of scopoletin to inhibit the production of inflammatory cytokines through inhibition of the IκB/NF-κB signal cascade in the human mast cell line HMC-1.** *Eur J Pharmacol* 2007, **555**:218–225.
26. Meotti FC, Ardenghi JV, Pretto JB, Souza MM, D'Ávila Moura J, Cunha A Jr, Soldi C, Pizzolatti MG, Santos ARS: **Antinociceptive properties of coumarins, steroid and dihydrostyryl-2- pyrones from Polygala sabulosa (Polygalaceae) in mice.** *J Pharm Pharmacol* 2006, **58**:107–112.

Comparing the effects of fluoxetine and imipramine on total cholesterol, triglyceride, and weight in patients with major depression

Esmaeil Shahsavand Ananloo[1], Padideh Ghaeli[2*], Mohammad-Zaman Kamkar[3] and Majid Sadeghi[4]

Abstract

Background: There are some reports on the effects of antidepressants on metabolic syndrome. However, our search in the previously published literature showed a lack of information on the comparison of the effects of different classes of antidepressants on lipid profile. Therefore, this study was aimed to compare the effects of fluoxetine and imipramine on serum total cholesterol (TC) and triglyceride (TG) as well as body weight (BW) in patients with major depressive disorder.

Methods: Fifty one patients, 18 to 70 years of age, with major depressive disorder complied with the criteria of this preliminary, open-label clinical trial. Subjects received either imipramine (75–200 mg/day) or fluoxetine (20–40 mg/day) for 8 weeks. Total cholesterol and TG levels, as well as BW were compared at baseline with those at weeks 4 and 8. Data was analyzed by SPSS software version 16.0.

Results: In the fluoxetine group, TC levels decreased from 165.71 mg/dL to 156.71 mg/dL at week 4 ($P = 0.07$), and to 143.94 mg/dL at week 8 ($P = 0.16$); TG levels decreased from 129.35 mg/dL to 115.88 mg/dL at week 4 ($P < 0.001$), and to 110.41 mg/dL at week 8 ($P = 0.56$). In the imipramine group, TC levels increased from 169.10 mg/dL to 178.69 mg/dL at week 4 ($P = 0.07$), and to 208.69 mg/dL at week 8 ($P < 0.001$) while TG levels increased from 111.73 mg/dL to 128.83 mg/dL at week 4 ($P = 0.005$), and to 160.90 mg/dL at week 8 ($P < 0.001$). BW was significantly increased in the imipramine group at weeks 4 and 8. In the fluoxetine group, BW was non-significantly decreased from 75.69 ± 7.97 Kg (baseline) to 75.67 ± 8.01 Kg at week 4 ($P = 0.88$), and to 75.22 ± 8.67 Kg at week 8 ($P = 0.20$), while in the imipramine group, BW had significant increases from 72.53 ± 8.55 Kg (baseline) to 73.95 ± 8.61 mg/dL at week 4 ($P < 0.001$), and to 75.13 ± 8.34 mg/dL at week 8 ($P < 0.001$).

Repeated measures ANOVA showed significant effects on both TC and TG levels as well as on BW in all patients receiving imipramine. However, in patients on fluoxetine, repeated measures ANOVA showed significant effects of this medication only on TC levels in males.

Conclusions: Monitoring TC and TG and BW is recommended before starting imipramine in depressed patients with increased risk for cardiovascular disease. Fluoxetine may be the preferred agent in those with high or borderline high lipid levels.

Keywords: Tricyclic antidepressants, Serotonin reuptake inhibitors, Cholesterol, Triglyceride, Body weight

* Correspondence: mmppg@yahoo.com
[2]Roozbeh Hospital, Tehran University of Medical Sciences (TUMS), Tehran, IRAN
Full list of author information is available at the end of the article

Background

The lifetime prevalence of depressive disorders has been reported to be high. National Comorbidity Survey (NCS), conducted in 1990–1992, noted that the lifetime prevalence of major depressive disorder in the United States was 14.9% for lifetime and 8.6% for 12-month [1]. However, after the introduction of the DSM-IV criteria, the National Comorbidity Survey Replication (NCS-R) reported the prevalence of MDD as 16.2% for lifetime and 6.6% for 12-month by using World Health Organization's Composite International Diagnostic Interview (CIDI) [2,3].

Fluoxetine, a specific serotonin reuptake inhibitor (SSRI) and imipramine, a tricyclic antidepressant (TCA) have been successfully used in the treatment of major depression for many years. These drugs differ in their pharmacology, adverse effects, and drug-drug interactions. Fluoxetine is well absorbed after oral administration and has a large volume of distribution. It is extensively metabolized in the liver, and is highly protein bound. Fluoxetine has an elimination half-life (t ½) of 24 to 96 hours; its metabolite t ½, norfluoxetine, ranges between 168 and 360 hours. Therefore, this drug should be used with caution in patients with decreased liver function and metabolic activity [4,5]. On the other hand, imipramine is highly metabolized in the liver with a t ½ of 6 to 28 hours; its major active metabolite is desipramine. This drug blocks histamine-1 and alpha-1 receptors and therefore may cause sedation, increase appetite, and orthostatic hypotension. It may also cause constipation, blurred vision, and urinary retention due to its anticholinergic effects [5].

Cipriani et al. analyzed data from 102 randomized clinical trials (RCTs) that compared SSRIs and TCAs, and noted no overall difference in efficacy between these two classes of antidepressants. However, SSRIs were shown to be better tolerated than TCAs according to the results of this analysis [6].

Since weight changes are among the criteria of depression and may result in related consequences such as alteration in lipid profile, this preliminary study was aimed to observe and compare the effects of fluoxetine and imipramine (representatives of the two classes of SSRIs and TCAs) on serum total cholesterol (TC) and triglyceride (TG), as well as body weight (BW) in depressed patients.

On the other hand, a number of factors such as medications, appetite, exercise, and medical illnesses may be of importance regarding weight changes associated with depression [7].

After searching Medline, and PsychLit from 1970 to 2012, we found that there are a few studies on the effects of fluoxetine or imipramine on serum TC, TG, and BW in animals and even fewer reports in depressed patients. For instance, one study in 1976 reported that prolonged intragastric administration of imipramine in rabbits resulted in a significant increase in serum cholesterol after 4, 8 and 12 weeks [8]. Additionally, association between TCAs and weight gain as well as association between SSRIs with abdominal obesity and hypercholesterolemia have been noted in the literature [9–12].

Activation of sterol regulatory element-binding protein (SREBP) may be important in understanding metabolic side effects of psychiatric drugs. Raeder et al. exposed cultured human glioma cells to some psychotropics. Some antidepressants including Imipramine and fluoxetine resulted in activation of SREBP system. Subsequently, it was noted that downstream genes that were involved in the biosynthesis of cholesterol and fatty acid were upregulated by studied antidepressants but to a different extent [13].

Based on the knowledge of the authors of the present study, no previous published study looked at the comparison of any SSRIs with TCAs regarding their effects on TG and TC levels and their relationships with BW in patients with major depressive disorder. Therefore, this preliminary study was designed to compare the effects of short-term use of fluoxetine and imipramine on TC and TG levels as well as BW in patients who suffered from major depressive disorder.

Methods

Fifty eight patients, 18 to 70 years of age, with major depressive disorder (based on DSM-IV criteria) accepted to enter this preliminary, open-label, clinical trial. Subjects received either imipramine or fluoxetine for 8 weeks in private psychiatric offices in Tehran, Iran. Patients did not receive any antidepressant or any other medication (s) that was reported to affect lipid levels or BW (e.g., TCAs, antipsychotics, etc.) for 2 weeks before the initiation and during the study. Patients with TC levels above 250 mg/dL (according to the reference of the laboratory values), and TG levels above 200 mg/dL (according to the reference of the laboratory values), diabetes mellitus, a history of any major cardiovascular diseases, and pregnant women were excluded from this study. Additionally, none of the patients should have received electroconvulsive therapy within 6 months before the initiation of the antidepressants. Participants were asked to report any changes in their diet or appetite during the study. Patients were assigned to receive oral fluoxetine (20 to 40 mg/d) or imipramine (75 to 200 mg/d) for 8 weeks. Benzodiazepines were allowed when needed for anxiety, agitation, or sleep problems. Total cholesterol and TG levels as well as BW were measured at the initiation time as well as 4 and 8 weeks after starting antidepressants.

Fifty one out of the 58 patients, who signed informed consent forms, fulfilled the criteria of and participated in the study. The study was approved by the Ethics Committee of the Faculty of Pharmacy at Tehran University of Medical Sciences (TUMS) and was conducted in accordance with the Declaration of Helsinki 1975 as revised in 2000.

SPSS software version 16.0 was used to analyze the data. Independent-sample t-test was performed to compare the means of TC, TG, and BW measures between the 2 groups at baseline, weeks 4 and 8. Additionally, paired sample t-test was performed to compare the means of TC and TG levels, and also BW at weeks 0, 4, and 8 for each group.

Linear regression was used for each group to find whether or not the sex or age has any significant effects on TC or TG levels as well as BW. Repeated measures ANOVA was used to compare the results of TC and TG levels as well as BW between weeks 0, 4, and 8 in each groups. Results are presented as mean ± standard deviation (SD); standard error mean (SEM). Differences were considered significant when $P < 0.05$.

Results

Fifty one patients complied with the study criteria and completed the study. Nineteen patients including 11 males and 8 females (mean age ± SD; SEM = 42.58 ± 15.19; 3.48 years) received fluoxetine while 32 patients including 13 males and 19 females (mean age ± SD; SEM = 41.97 ± 14.79; 2.61 years) received imipramine. The difference in age between the two groups was not significant ($F = 0.017$, $P = 0.888$). Baseline clinical characteristics of patients are shown in Table 1. As shown in this table, the differences between fluoxetine and imipramine groups at baseline for TC and TG levels as well as for BW were not statistically significant.

We did not find any reportable changes in patients' appetite and food intake during the study; this finding was based on patients' responses to a set of formatted questions about hydrocarbate, lipid and protein intake as well as appetite at every visit.

The results of repeated measure ANOVA and paired t-test for TC or TG level as well as for BW are shown in Table 2.

As shown in Table 2, repeated measures ANOVA showed significant effects on both TC and TG levels as well as on BW in all patients receiving imipramine and also in males or females on the same antidepressant. However, in patients on fluoxetine, repeated measures ANOVA showed significant effects of this medication only on TC levels in males.

TC levels analysis

Mean TC levels were significantly different between fluoxetine and imipramine groups at both week 4 ($F = 3.11$, $P = 0.04$; two-tailed) and week 8 ($F = 0.07$, $P < 0.001$; two-tailed).

All samples

Paired sample t-test showed that in the fluoxetine group, TC level had a trend toward the significant decrease from 165.71 ± 35.80 mg/dL (baseline) to 156.71 ± 35.53 mg/dL at week 4 ($P = 0.07$), and a non-significant decrease to 143.94 ± 44.71 mg/dL at week 8 ($P = 0.16$). On the other hand, in the imipramine group, TC level had a trend toward the significant increase from 169.10 ± 36.20 mg/dL (baseline) to 178.69 ± 42.78 mg/dL at week 4 ($P = 0.07$), and a significant increase to 208.69 ± 43.33 mg/dL at week 8 ($P < 0.001$).

Male sample

Paired sample t-test showed that in the fluoxetine group, TC level had a non-significant decrease from 154.60 ± 29.39 mg/dL (baseline) to 147.80 ± 27.93 mg/dL at week 4 ($P = 0.39$), and a significant decrease to 128.70 ± 34.96 mg/dL at week 8 ($P = 0.006$). On the other hand, in the imipramine group, TC level had a non-significant increase from 159.92 ± 33.18 mg/dL (baseline) to 171.46 ± 39.49 mg/dL at week 4 ($P = 0.21$), and a significant increase to 194.38 ± 40.42 mg/dL at week 8 ($P < 0.001$).

Female samples

Paired sample t-test showed that in the fluoxetine group, TC level had a significant decrease from 181.57 ± 40.29 mg/dL (baseline) to 169.43 ± 43.30 mg/dL at week 4 ($P = 0.036$), and a non-significant decrease to 165.71 ± 50.58 mg/dL at week 8 ($P = 0.86$). On the other hand, in the imipramine group, TC level had a non-significant increase from 176.56 ± 37.85 mg/dL (baseline) to 184.56 ± 45.68 mg/dL at week 4 ($P = 0.22$), and a significant increase to 220.31 ± 43.31 mg/dL at week 8 ($P = 0.003$).

Table 1 Baseline clinical characteristics of patients

	Imipramine	Fluoxetine	Statistics
Age (years); Mean ± SD	41.97 ± 14.79	42.58 ± 15.19	F = 0.017, P = 0.888
Age Range (years)	18 - 70	18 - 68	
TC (mg/dL)	169.10 ± 36.20	165.71 ± 35.80	F = 0.088, P = 0.715
TG (mg/dL)	111.73 ± 36.52	129.35 ± 26.61	F = 0.088, P = 0.715
BW (Kg)	72.53 ± 8.55	75.69 ± 7.97	F = 0.059, P = 0.114

TC = Total Cholesterol; TG = Triglyceride; BW = Body Weight.

Table 2 Effects of Imipramine and Fluoxetine on serum TC and TG levels, and BW

Groups	Paired t-test; Within groups changes between weeks 0 and 4 (p value)	Paired t-test; Within groups changes between weeks 4 and 8 (p value)	Repeated measures ANOVA; F (p value)
TC level (mg/dL)			
Imipramine			
√ All subjects	9.59 (0.07**)	30.00 (**<0.001***)	24.68 (**<0.001***)
o Male	11.54 (0.21)	22.92 (**<0.001***)	11.07 (**<0.001***)
o Female	8.00 (0.22)	35.75 (**0.003***)	13.88 (**<0.001***)
Fluoxetine			
√ All subjects	9.00 (0.07**)	12.77 (0.16)	2.93 (0.07**)
o Male	6.80 (0.39)	19.10 (**0.006***)	6.67 (**0.027***)
o Female	12.14 (**0.04***)	3.72 (0.86)	0.22 (0.810)
TG level (mg/dL)			
Imipramine			
√ All subjects	17.10 (**0.005***)	32.07 (**<0.001***)	18.88 (**<0.001***)
o Male	11.75 (**0.013***)	26.75 (**<0.001***)	24.06 (**<0.001***)
o Female	20.66 (**0.036***)	35.62 (**0.007***)	9.53 (**0.001***)
Fluoxetine			
√ All subjects	13.47 (**<0.001***)	5.47 (0.56)	2.59 (0.09)
o Male	14.27 (**0.016***)	9.36 (0.30)	3.24 (0.06**)
o Female	12.00 (**<0.001***)	1.67 (0.94)	0.26 (0.78)
BW (Kg)			
Imipramine			
√ All subjects	1.42 (**<0.001***)	1.18 (**<0.001***)	29.70 (**<0.001***)
o Male	1.07 (**0.009***)	1.00 (**0.007***)	11.56 (**<0.001***)
o Female	1.66 (**<0.001***)	1.31 (**0.008***)	18.54 (**0.001***)
Fluoxetine			
√ All subjects	0.02 (0.88)	0.45 (0.20)	1.51 (0.24)
o Male	0.18 (0.44)	0.05 (0.85)	0.41 (0.54)
o Female	0.36 (0.25)	1.21 (0.14)	4.06 (0.05**)

* Statistically significant effect ** Trend towards significant effect.

It should be mentioned that the changes in TC levels were not dependent on age when analyzing the data for all subjects.

TG levels analysis

Mean TG levels were not significantly different between fluoxetine and imipramine groups at week 4 ($F = 1.88$, $P = 0.20$; two-tailed) but were significant at week 8 ($F = 1.33$, $P = 0.002$; two-tailed).

All samples

Paired sample t-test showed that in the fluoxetine group, TG level had a significant decrease from 129.35 ± 26.61 mg/dL (baseline) to 115.88 ± 26.87 mg/dL at week 4 ($P < 0.001$), and a non-significant decrease to 110.41 ± 48.30 mg/dL at week 8 ($P = 0.56$). On the other hand, in the imipramine group, TG level had significant increases from 111.73 ± 36.52 mg/dL (baseline) to 128.83 ± 35.27 mg/dL at week 4 ($P = 0.005$), and to 160.90 ± 56.04 mg/dL at week 8 ($P < 0.001$).

Male samples

Paired sample t-test showed that in the fluoxetine group, TG level had a significant decrease from 130.45 ± 32.92 mg/dL (baseline) to 116.18 ± 33.20 mg/dL at week 4 ($P = 0.016$), and a non-significant decrease to 106.82 ± 50.84 mg/dL at week 8 ($P = 0.30$). On the other hand, in the imipramine group, TG level had significant increases from 115.42 ± 37.55 mg/dL (baseline) to 127.17 ± 40.54 mg/dL at week 4 ($P = 0.013$), and to 153.92 ± 42.94 mg/dL at week 8 ($P < 0.001$).

Female samples

Paired sample t-test showed that in the fluoxetine group, TG level had a significant decrease from 127.33 ± 9.52 mg/dL (baseline) to 115.33 ± 10.25 mg/dL at week 4

(P = 0.001), and a non-significant decrease to 117.00 ± 46.98 mg/dL at week 8 (P = 0.94). On the other hand, in the imipramine group, TG level had significant increases from 109.28 ± 36.69 mg/dL (baseline) to 129.94 ± 32.50 mg/dL at week 4 (P = 0.036), and to 165.56 ± 64.08 mg/dL at week 8 (P = 0.007). The changes in TG levels were not dependent on age when analyzing the data for all samples.

Body weight analysis

Mean BW were not significantly different between fluoxetine and imipramine groups at week 4 (F = 0.05, P = 0.41; two-tailed) and week 8 (F = 0.02, P = 0.87; two-tailed).

All samples

Paired sample t-test showed that in the fluoxetine group, BW was non-significantly decreased from 75.69 ± 7.97 Kg (baseline) to 75.67 ± 8.01 Kg at week 4 (P = 0.88), and to 75.22 ± 8.67 Kg at week 8 (P = 0.20). On the other hand, in the imipramine group, BW had significant increases from 72.53 ± 8.55 Kg (baseline) to 73.95 ± 8.61 mg/dL at week 4 (P < 0.001), and to 75.13 ± 8.34 mg/dL at week 8 (P < 0.001).

Male samples

Paired sample t-test showed that in the fluoxetine group, BW had non-significant increases from 78.68 ± 7.71 Kg (baseline) to 78.86 ± 7.53 Kg at week 4 (P = 0.44), and to 78.91 ± 7.62 Kg at week 8 (P = 0.85). On the other hand, in the imipramine group, BW had significant increases from 76.85 ± 8.08 Kg (baseline) to 77.92 ± 7.88 Kg at week 4 (P = 0.009), and to 78.92 ± 7.61 Kg at week 8 (P = 0.007).

Female samples

Paired sample t-test showed that in the fluoxetine group, BW had non-significant decreases from 71.00 ± 6.24 Kg (baseline) to 70.64 ± 6.24 Kg at week 4 (P = 0.25), and to 69.43 ± 7.21 Kg at week 8 (P = 0.14). On the other hand, in the imipramine group, BW had significant increases from 69.58 ± 7.73 Kg (baseline) to 71.24 ± 8.20 mg/dL at week 4 (P < 0.001), and to 72.53 ± 7.97 mg/dL at week 8 (P = 0.008).

It should be mentioned that the changes in BW measures were not dependent on age when analyzing the data for all patients. Using regression analysis did not detect any association between BW (independent variable) and either TC or TG levels (dependent variables) in weeks 0, 4, and 8; no significant association was found between these parameters.

Discussion

Even though there are some literature on the effects of antidepressants on lipid factors and BW, our study was designed to compare the effects of fluoxetine with imipramine on these factors simultaneously.

In a letters to the editor, Roessner and colleagues reported a case in which TC level was increased in a woman with severe recurrent depression who was taking doxepin [14]. In another study in 1994 by Pollack et al., consumption of nortriptyline after 7 months showed significant elevation in TG and very-low-density lipoproteins (VLDL) levels in 26 elderly patients suffering depression [15].

A case of a hypercholesterolemic female, with postpartum depression, who started receiving fluoxetine two weeks after her labour, was previously reported. The woman's TC and TG levels was measured prior to as well as 4 and 8 weeks after the initiation of the fluoxetine. Serum TC level was decreased from 242 mg/dL at the baseline to 224 mg/dl after 4 weeks and to 202 mg/dl after 8 weeks [16]. Similarly, triglyceride level was decreased from 516 mg/dL at week 0 to 448 mg/dL at week 4 and further to 404 mg/dL at week 8 [16]. Even though this patient was started on fluoxetine after labour, it should be noted that a part of the change in TC and TG levels may have been due to the nature of pregnancy and the related physiological changes during and after this time.

In a study by Raeder et al. on patients on SSRIs who were based on a cross-sectional survey in Hordaland county in Norway (The Hordaland Health Study '97-'99), it was noted that use of most SSRIs may be associated with some metabolic changes. This study reported that sertraline, fluoxetine, or fluvoxamine, in 131 patients, was associated with both abdominal obesity and hypercholesterolemia. However, in 187 patients on paroxetine, the use of the drug showed association with obesity but not with hypercholesterolemia. Additionally, it was noted that there was no association between the use of citalopram in 142 patients with any metabolic factor or lipid profile [12].

On the other hand, association between TCAs (e.g. imipramine) and weight gain has been reported in the literature. Fernstrom et al. examined weight gain in patients taking imipramine 200–250 mg per day for 16 weeks and noted statistically significant increases in weight and body mass index of the patients [17].

Frank et al. reported weight changes in patients with recurrent major depression who were receiving about 215 mg of imipramine per day for over 5 months [18]. This study noted non-significant, minimal changes in body weight during the first 9 weeks of the treatment. On the other hand, different results regarding weight gain have been reported with different agents in SSRI family. Several studies have reported weight loss with short-term use of fluoxetine [19,20]. The literature was reviewed regarding the relative risk for antidepressant-induced weight gain by Fava [21]. This study suggested that TCAs may cause more weight gain than SSRIs. It also noted that long-term use of paroxetine increases weight more than the use of other SSRIs.

Interestingly, a study by Sep-Kowalikowa and colleagues, in 1992, on 329 depressed and neurotic patients noted increases in weight of patients receiving amitriptyline or doxepin but reduction in this factor in those receiving imipramine [22].

Fava et al. evaluated weight changes in patients on 26 to 32 weeks treatment with, paroxetine, sertraline, or fluoxetine. This long-term study noted that paroxetine resulted in significant weight increase, however, sertraline increased and fluoxetine decreased BW in non-significant manners [23].

To our knowledge, no previous study compared the alterations in TC and TG levels as well as BW in patients on imipramine with those on fluoxetine at the same time. The present study compared the effects of short-term use of fluoxetine and imipramine on the above factors in patients with major depressive disorder.

Our study noted a trend toward a significant decrease in TC serum levels of patients on fluoxetine after 4 weeks and a non-significant decrease at the eighth week. Imipramine showed a trend toward a significant increase in TC levels after 4 weeks and a significant increase in this parameter at the eighth week. In addition, our study noted a significant decrease in TG serum levels of patients on fluoxetine after 4 weeks and a non-significant decrease at the eighth week. On the other hand, Imipramine showed significant increases in TG levels at weeks 4 and 8. The changes in TC and TG levels in both groups were in the normal range and did not seem to be clinically significant. However, these changes can become clinically important in patients with high or low normal TC and TG levels or in those with risk factors for developing hypercholesterolemia. There are a few studies that have evaluated the effects of SSRIs or TCAs on lipid profile. TCAs have been noted to have unfavourable effects on TG and low-density lipoprotein cholesterol, probably, because of the weight gain associated with TCAs [24]. Raeder et al. reported that SSRIs as a group were associated with hypercholesrterolemia [12]. However, our study showed the opposite effects for fluoxetine.

It should also be noted that the duration of this study may not have been long enough to show the chronic effects of the studied antidepressants on lipid profile.

There were some other limitations in our study that could have affected the results. Originally, we planned to perform a randomized, double-blind trial. Due to the fact that imipramine was available in tablet form and fluoxetine in capsule form, we were not able to get these medications in the same form at the time. However, since our study primarily was looking into the effects of the drugs on serum TC and TG levels that are not considered as subjective values, we did not think an open-label study would significantly interfere with the results. Another reason was that when we initiated the study, many psychiatrists in Iran preferred TCAs over SSRIs for the treatment of major depression. For this reason, the number of patients on imipramine was much more than those on fluoxetine.

Conclusions

Clinicians should consider medical conditions of patients and the changes in weight, TC and TG levels of patients, especially those with cardiovascular risk, and any drug-drug interaction before initiating fluoxetine or imipramine. Fluoxetine may be suggested to be used in depressed patients with high normal TC or in individuals with a high risk to develop hypercholesterolemia. Further studies are needed to evaluate the effects of long-term use of imipramine and fluoxetine on lipid profile and BW in depressed patients.

Competing interest
The authors declare that they have no competing interests.

Authors' contributions
ESA was responsible for recruiting patients, visiting and evaluating them; he was also involved in designing the study, analyzing the data and writing the manuscript. PG (the corresponding author) was involved in all aspects of the study from designing the trial and coordination of the study through the statistical analysis and drafting the manuscript. This study was a continuation of MZK's thesis toward graduation from the residency program in psychiatry (proposal registration #245-78/04/16 at Tehran University of Medical Sciences, Faculty of Medicine); he continued visiting and evaluating patients and was involved in original drafting of the manuscript. MS was consulted for different aspects of the study; he also introduced depressed patients and evaluated them during the study. All authors read and approved the final manuscript.

Acknowledgements
The authors would like to thank Mr. Abbas Kamalipour, RN at the Department of Pharmacy, Mrs. Fattaneh Abdi, RN at the Department of Nursing at Roozbeh Hospital, Mrs. Farzaneh Zarei, MS coordinator at the pychiatrists' offices, and Hassan Torkamandi, PharmD at Shariati Hospital for their valuable help.

Author details
[1]Department of Genomic Psychiatry (DGP), Roozbeh Hospital, Tehran University of Medical Sciences (TUMS), Tehran, IRAN. [2]Roozbeh Hospital, Tehran University of Medical Sciences (TUMS), Tehran, IRAN. [3]Fifth of Azar Hospital, Golestan University of Medical Sciences, Gorgan, IRAN. [4]Psychiatry and Psychology Research Center, Roozbeh Hospital, Tehran University of Medical Sciences (TUMS), Tehran, IRAN.

References
1. Kessler RC, Nelson CB, McGonagle KA, Liu J, Swartz M, Blazer DG: **Comorbidity of DSM-III-R major depressive disorder in the general population.** *Br J Psychiatry* 1996, **168**(Suppl 30):17–30.
2. Kessler RC, Walters EE: **The National Comorbidity Survey: Psychiatric Epidemiology.** In. 2nd edition Edited by Tsaung MT, Tohen M. New York, NY: John Wiley & Sons; 2002:343–362.

3. Kessler RC, Berglund P, Demler O, Jin R, Koretz D, Merikangas KR, *et al*: **The epidemiology of major depressive disorder: results from the National Comorbidity Survey Replication (NCS-R).** *JAMA* 2003, **289**:3095–3105.
4. Altamura AC, Moro AR, Percudani M: **Clinical pharmacokinetics of fluoxetine.** *Clin Pharmacokinet* 1994, **26**:201–214.
5. Devane LC: **Cyclic antidepressants: Clinical Pharmacokinetics Pocket Handbook.** In Edited by Murphy EJ. Bethesda, MD: American Society of Health-System Pharmacy (ASHP); 1993.
6. Cipriani A, Brambilla P, Furukawa T, Geddes J, Gregis M, Hotopf M, *et al*: **Fluoxetine versus other types of pharmacotherapy for depression.** *Cochrane Database Syst Rev* 2005, **4**:CD004185.
7. Michelson D, Amsterdam JD, Quitkin FM, Reimherr FW, Rosenbaum JF, Zajecka J, Sundell KL, Kim Y, Beasley CM: **Changes in weight during a 1 year trial of fluoxetine.** *Am J Psychiatry* 1999, **156**(8):1170–1176.
8. Bala S, Garg KN: **Effect of prolonged trifluoperazine, imipramine and haloperidol administration on serum cholesterol. An experimental study in rabbits.** *Pharmacology* 1976, **14**:385–389.
9. Paykel ES, Mueller PS, De la Vergne PM: **Amitriptyline, weight gain and carbohydrate craving: a side effect.** *Br J Psychiatry* 1973, **123**:501–507.
10. Berken GH, Weinstein DO, Stern WC: **Weight gain: a side-effect of tricyclic antidepressants.** *J Affect Disord* 1984, **7**:133–138.
11. Garland EJ, Remick RA, Zis AP: **Weight gain with antidepressants and Raeder lithium.** *J Clin Psychopharmacol* 1988, **8**:323–330.
12. Raeder MB, Bjelland I, Emil Vollset S, Steen VM: **Obesity, dyslipidemia, and diabetes with selective serotonin reuptake inhibitors: the Hordaland health Study.** *J Clin Psychiatry* 2006, **67**:1974–1982.
13. Raeder MB, Ferno J, Glambek M, Stansberg C, Steen VM: **Antidepressant drugs activate SREBP and up-regulate cholesterol and fatty acid biosynthesis in human glial cells.** *Neurosci Lett* 2006, **395**:185–190.
14. Roessner V, Demling J, Bleich S: **Doxepin increases serum cholesterol levels.** *Can J Psychiatry* 2004, **49**(1):74–75.
15. Pollock BG, Perel JM, Paradis CF, Fasiczka AL, Reynolds CF 3rd: **Metabolic and physiologic consequences of nortriptyline treatment in the elderly.** *Psychopharmacol Bull* 1994, **30**:145–150.
16. Ghaeli P, Shahsavand E, Sadeghi M, Khalili H: **Fluoxetine decreased serum total cholesterol and triglyceride levels in a hypercholesterolemic patient with postpartum depression.** *Iranian Journal of Psychiatry* 2006, **1**:84–85.
17. Fernstrom MH, Krowinski RL, Kupfer DJ: **Chronic imipramine treatment and weight gain.** *Psychiatry Res* 1986, **17**:269–273.
18. Frank E, Kupfer DJ, Bulik CM, Levenson JA: **Imipramine and weight gain during the treatment of recurrent depression.** *J Affect Disord* 1990, **20**:165–172.
19. McGuirk J, Silverstone T: **The effect of the 5-HT re-uptake inhibitor fluoxetine on food intake and body weight in healthy male subjects.** *Int J Obesity Relat Metab Disord* 1990, **14**(4):361–372.
20. Harto NE, Spera KF, Branconnier RJ: **Fluoxetine-induced reduction of body mass in patients with major depressive disorder.** *Psychopharmacol Bull* 1988, **24**:220–223.
21. Fava M: **Weight gain and antidepressants.** *J Clin Psychiatry* 2000, **61**(Suppl 11):37–41.
22. Sep-Kowalikowa B, Prokopowicz A, Pankiewicz P: **Weight gain during antidepressant therapy.** *Psychiatr Pol* 1992, **26**(1–2):37–43.
23. Fava M, Judge R, Hoog SL, Nilsson ME, Koke SC: **Fluoxetine versus sertraline and paroxetine in major depressive disorder: changes in weight with long-term treatment.** *J Clin Psychiatry* 2000, **61**:863–867.
24. McIntyre RS, Soczynska JK, Konarski JZ, Kennedy SH: **The effect of antidepressants on lipid homeostasis: a cardiac safety concern?** *Expert Opin Drug Saf* 2006, **5**:523–537.

Urease inhibitory activities of β-boswellic acid derivatives

Sanaz Golbabaei[1], Roya Bazl[1], Sahand Golestanian[1], Farzaneh Nabati[1], Zinat Bahrampour Omrany[1], Behnam Yousefi[2], Reza Hajiaghaee[3], Shamsali Rezazadeh[3] and Massoud Amanlou[1*]

Abstract

Background and the purpose of the study: *Boswellia carterii have* been used in traditional medicine for many years for management different gastrointestinal disorders. In this study, we wish to report urease inhibitory activity of four isolated compound of boswellic acid derivative.

Methods: 4 pentacyclic triterpenoid acids were isolated from *Boswellia carterii* and identified by NMR and Mass spectroscopic analysis (compounds **1**, 3-O-acetyl-9,11-dehydro-β-boswellic acid; **2**, 3-O-acetyl-11-hydroxy-β-boswellic acid; **3**. 3-O- acetyl-11-keto-β-boswellic acid and **4**, 11-keto-β-boswellic acid. Their inhibitory activity on Jack bean urease were evaluated. Docking and pharmacophore analysis using AutoDock 4.2 and Ligandscout 3.03 programs were also performed to explain possible mechanism of interaction between isolated compounds and urease enzyme.

Results: It was found that compound **1** has the strongest inhibitory activity against Jack bean urease ($IC_{50} = 6.27 \pm 0.03$ μM), compared with thiourea as a standard inhibitor ($IC_{50} = 21.1 \pm 0.3$ μM).

Conclusion: The inhibition potency is probably due to the formation of appropriate hydrogen bonds and hydrophobic interactions between the investigated compounds and urease enzyme active site and confirms its traditional usage.

Keywords: *Boswellia carterii*, Urease inhibitor, Boswellic acid, Docking, Autodock

Introduction

Inhibition of enzymes by natural products which are proven to be the source of therapeutic agents, have increasingly attracted the interests of scientists as a valuable strategy in drug discovery. *Boswellia carterii* is widely distributed in the Indian subcontinent and Africa. The gum exudates of *Boswellia spp.* comprise of several pentacyclic triterpenoid acids, which are known as boswellic acids (BA's) and reported to have different biological activities. Their ability to induce apoptosis choose them as potent compounds in treatment of colon, prostate and breast cancers [1-7] and a broad range of neurodegenerative conditions such as Alzheimer's and Parkinson's disease [8-11]. Also their inhibitory effect through topoisomerase I and II has been reported [12].

* Correspondence: amanlou@tums.ac.ir
[1]Department of Medicinal Chemistry, Faculty of Pharmacy and Medicinal Plants Research Center, Tehran University of Medical Sciences, Tehran, Iran
Full list of author information is available at the end of the article

In addition, a number of extracted organic acids of this plant show other biological activities such as inhibition of peptic ulcer formation, probably by increasing the gastric mucosal resistance which its exact molecular mechanism is still not clear. In the recent report, it was shown that methanolic extract of *B. carterii* has urease inhibition activity [13,14].

Enzyme inhibition has already led to the discovery of the wide variety of useful drugs in the treatment of several diseases. It is found that *Helicobacter pylori* infection is the main cause of gastritis, peptic ulcer disease and gastric cancers [15,16].

Urease of *H. pylori* producing abundant amounts of ammonia (10–15% of total proteins by weight), make the growth and survival of bacteria possible, by increasing the pH of environment [17]. Therefore, it plays the major role in gastric diseases. Accordingly, urease inhibition has recently attracted much attention in pharmaceutical applications and discovery of potent anti-ulcer drugs. *H. pylori* has become resistant to many antibiotics, thus introducing new agents, like natural urease inhibitors, is of special importance. In addition, urease activity not only participates in the formation of kidney stones [18], but also involves in the development of urolithiasis, pyelonephritis, hepatic encephalopathy [19].

Throughout our work to search for natural urease inhibitor's compounds from medicinal plants, we now report the isolation of four derivatives of boswellic acids to test their inhibitory activities through Jack bean urease. We employed Jack bean urease instead of bacteria's one because it was previously found out that the mechanism and kinetics of inhibition for bacteria urease and Jack bean urease are comparable [20].

Molecular docking and simulation studies improve the reliability, accuracy of biological test, and show possible interactions between molecules and their target receptors. So the extracted compounds were subjected to molecular docking for better recognition of their interaction with urease.

Material and methods

Materials

Jack bean urease (EC 3.5.1.5 from Fluka Co, Switzerland), thiourea and all other chemicals used were of analytical grade (Merck Co, Germany). All solutions were prepared in MilliQ (Millipore, USA) water.

Preparation of extract

An earlier report claimed that acetyl-keto-β-boswellic acid could not be separated from a mixture of acetyl-β-boswellic acid and acetyl keto-β-boswellic acid by any of the chemical methods, such as ketal formation [21] or semi-carbazide formation. In another method, methanol was found to be the most appropriate solvent for extraction, and used for simultaneous quantitative estimation of major BA's from *Boswellia spp.*

In this research, solvent-solvent extraction, thin-layer (TLC) and column chromatography were performed to isolate the main active constituent of *B. carterii.* A total of 10 g of oleo-gum resin was grounded. Of this, extraction performed in 100 ml methanol three times. After filtration, the extract was concentrated and solvent was removed. KOH 2% was added to separate the acidic fraction and extraction was performed by ethyl acetate five times. In the next step, the aqueous phase was acidified with HCl 2%, and previous step was repeated. Then the organic phase washed with distilled water to obtain fractions containing BA's compounds. Liquid chromatography was used to obtain related derivatives in organic fraction. The organic layers were dried, filtered and concentrated under vacuum on a rotary evaporator. Liquid chromatography of 5 g of sample which dissolve in chloroform is performed on 100 g of silica gel 60 (0.063 - 0.2 mm). Solvent partitioning of the crude extracts was used to divide the extract into eight fractions with different polarities. The fractions were combined based on similarity of the chemical composition determined by TLC analysis.

Crude fractions 1-5 were concentrated under vacuum on the rotary evaporator. Fractions 6-7 were combined based on similarity of their TLC profile and subjected to further column chromatography and eluted with a methanol/chloroform gradient solvent mixture (3; 5; 7; 10 ml of methanol) to give fractions K, L, M and O. pure compound was identified using spectroscopic analysis which their structures are shown in Figure 1. The ^{1}H and ^{13}C-NMR spectra were recorded on a Bruker Avance 300-MHz NMR spectrophotometer, with internal standard tetramethylsilane (TMS). The structures were further confirmed by mass-spectral analysis and comparing with reported data for all the compounds.

Biological evaluation

For urease inhibition assays after addition of phosphate buffer pH = 6.8, sonication was performed for 3 min, followed by centrifugation and evaluating absorbance of upper solution in $\lambda = 278$ nm which is attributed to the urease. By using following equation $A = \lambda bc$, where c is the concentration of solution (mol/L), b the Length of the UV cell, we can calculate the concentration of initially urease solution in this way. After appropriate

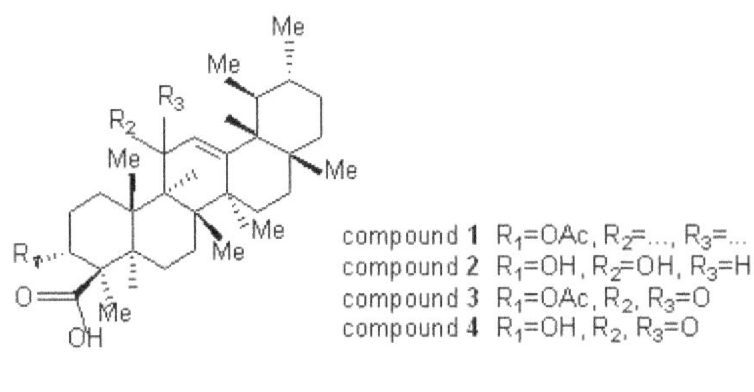

Figure 1 Structure of isolated boswellic acid derivatives.

Table 1 Percent of inhibition, IC_{50} and ΔG° of four isolated boswellic acids derivatives

Compounds	Percent of inhibition (50 μg/ml)	IC_{50} ± S.E.M (μM)	ΔG° (Kcal/mol)
1	60.5	6.27 ± 0.037	−7.49
2	56.2	9.21 ± 0.069	−7.20
3	37.4	16.34 ± 0.063	−7.11
4	39.1	85.23 ± 0.065	−5.84
Thiourea	88.0	21.10 ± 0.3	−6.42

dilution, the concentration of enzyme solution adjusted 2 mg/ml.

The assay mixture, containing 50 μl (2 mg/ml) of Jack-bean urease and 100 μl of different concentration of test compounds, which were dissolved in ethanol 20% previously, was added to 850 μl of 25mM urea and pre-incubated for 0.5 h in water bath at 37°C. The urease reaction was stopped after 30 min incubation by following procedure.

Urease activity was determined by measuring ammonia production using the indophenol method as described by Weatherburn [18]. After pre-incubation, 500 μl of phenol reagent (1% w/v phenol and 0.005% w/v sodium nitroprusside) and 500 μl of alkali reagent (1% w/v NaOH and 0.075% active chloride NaOCl) were added to 100 μl of incubation mixture and kept at 37°C for 30 min.

The absorbance was measured at 625 nm. All experiments were performed in triplicate in a final volume of 1 ml, and thiourea was used as a standard urease inhibitors. Percentage inhibitions were calculated using the formula (100 − (OD sample / OD control) × 100).

The concentration that provokes an inhibition halfway between the minimum and maximum response of each compound (relative IC_{50}) was determined by monitoring the inhibition effect of various concentrations of compounds in the assay. The IC_{50} values were then calculated using GraphPad Prism 5 software.

Molecular docking

The newly compounds were subjected for molecular docking. To validate observed activities and designing new inhibitors based on choosing the appropriate pharmacophore molecular docking was performed using AutoDock 4.2 along with AutoDockTools 1.4.5 using Lamarckian genetic algorithm on PDB structure (3LA4) http://www.pdb.org with resolution of 2°A [22].

In the present study, non-standard protein residues (KCX and CME) and the metal ions were included in the binding site specification. The docking calculations adopted in this work yield favorable orientations of ligands in a receptor. The graphical user interface ADT was employed to set up the enzymes: all hydrogen calculated and nonpolar hydrogens were merged to carbons. For determination of pharmacophore, Ligandscout 3.03 program was used [23].

Four potent inhibitors have sketched by Marvin sketch applet (Marvin package, Chemaxon company). Then adding polar hydrogens and rotatable bonds were done with Openbabel and AutodockTools, respectively [24,25]. Docking with a maximum number of 25 × 10^6 energy evaluations were performed. After clustering analysis, conformation with the most favorable binding energy was selected.

Result and discussion

Plants are the important source of new drug developments. Current study presents an investigation on urease

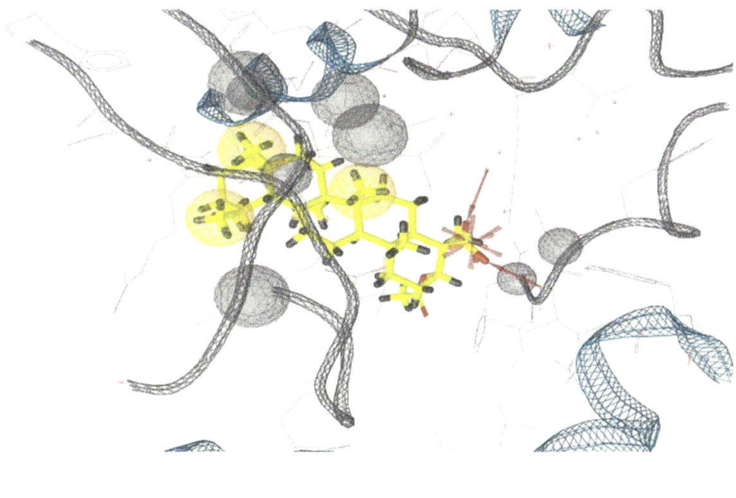

Figure 2 Molecular docking of compound 1, a 3D aspect.

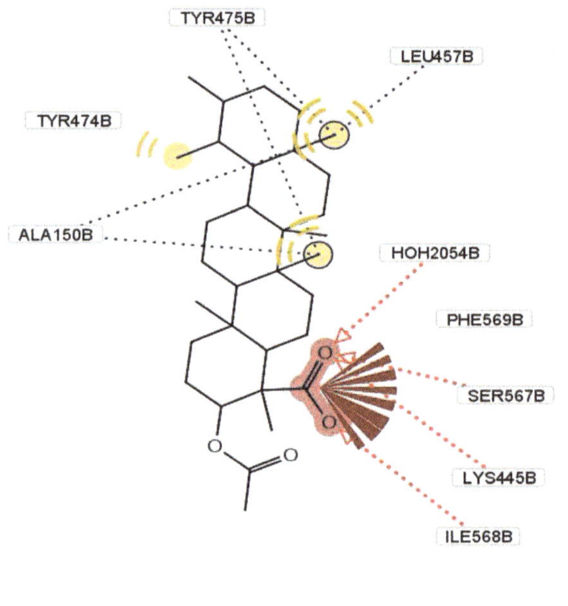

Figure 3 Molecular docking of compound 1 and its interaction with different residue of urease enzyme active site involved in interaction. Formation of hydrogen bonds between carbonyl of Phe 569, Ser 567, Ile 568 and Lys 445 from B-domain of enzyme and oxygen of the carboxyl moiety in compound **1**. Hydrophobic interactions with Ala 150, Leu 457, Try 474 and Try 475 of urease.

inhibition of four isolated compounds from *B. carterii* which has been numbered as medicinal plant and had been used in stomach and colon disorders [26,27], on the other hand, detection of urease inhibitors, have been regarded as targets for new anti-ulcer drugs.

The aim of the present study is to confirm the possible anti-ulcer activity of the olibanum through inhibition of urease enzyme to support for its use as gastrointestinal agents in traditional medicine. Isolated compounds (Figure 1) were screened for urease inhibition activity against jack bean urease, and their relative IC_{50} values were depicted in Table 1.

Out of four BA's tested for their urease inhibitory activity, compound **4** was the only weakly active ($IC_{50} = 85.23 \pm 0.06$ μM) and compound **1** ($IC_{50} = 6.27 \pm 0.03$ μM) was found to be the most potent compound, compared to the standard inhibitor (thiourea, $IC_{50} = 21.1 \pm 0.3$ μM). In this series, compounds **2** and **3** ($IC_{50} = 9.21 \pm 0.06$, 16.34 ± 0.06 μM, respectively) are exhibited remarkable inhibition toward urease.

It could be seen that the dehydro-substituted compound has stronger activity against urease than the hydroxy or keto-substituted ones. To investigate the binding effects between extracted BA's and the Jack bean urease the molecular docking study was performed. The 3D binding model of compound **1** is depicted in Figure 2.

In the binding model, carbonyl of Phe 569, Ser 567, Ile 568 and Lys 445 from B-domain of enzyme forms hydrogen bonds with oxygen of the carboxyl moiety in compound **1**. Moreover, the compound may form hydrophobic interactions with Ala 150, Leu 457, Try 474 and Try 475 of urease (Figure 3). This potential inhibitory property possessed by this compound, may be attributed to the above hydrogen bonds and hydrophobic interactions.

The docking calculations also reveal that the complex has the lower free energy of binding (-7.49 kcal/mol) compared with other extracted compounds, which may also explain the excellent inhibitory activity of it. As a

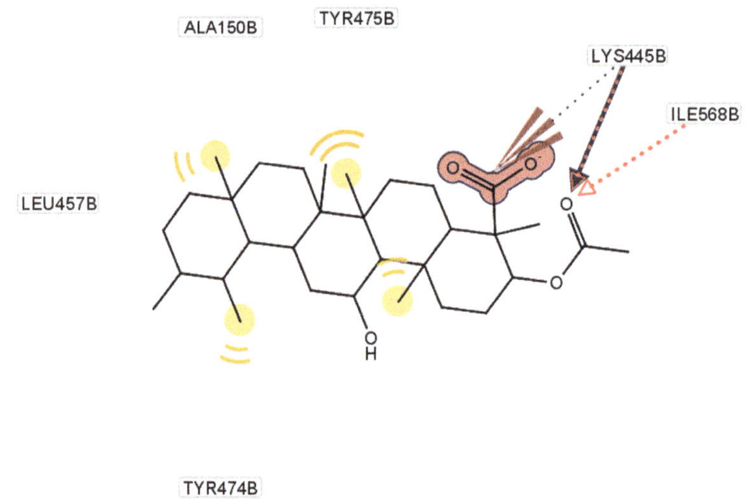

Figure 4 Molecular docking of compound 2 and its interaction with different residue of urease enzyme active site involved in interaction.

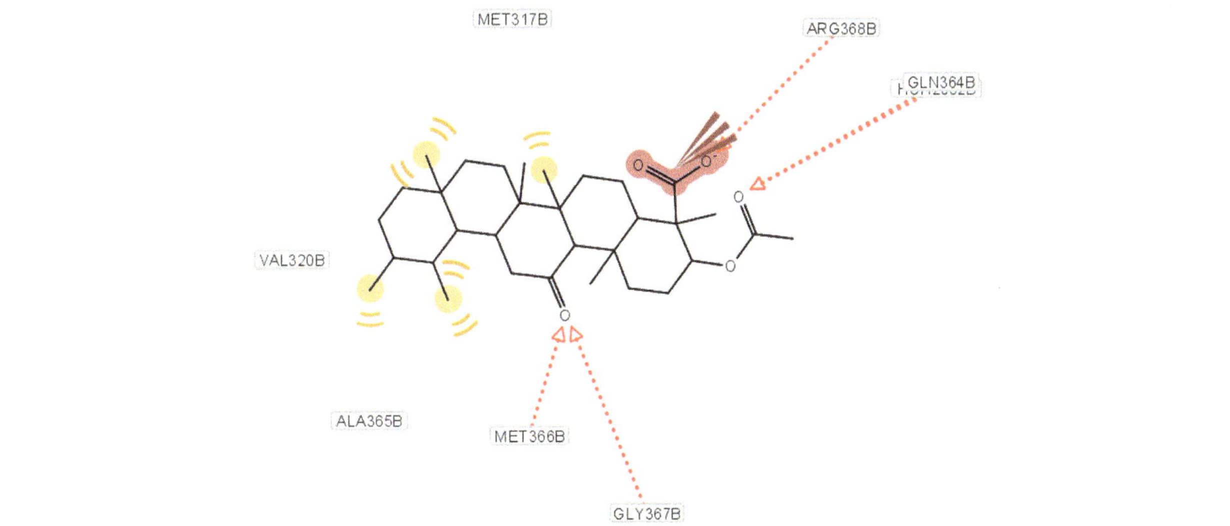

Figure 5 **Molecular docking of compound 3 and its interaction with different residue of urease enzyme active site involved in interaction.**

comparison, a molecular docking study on the other compounds was also carried out, as it shown in Figures 4, 5, 6.

As it has shown, the enhanced percentage of urease inhibitory activity of compounds **1**, **2** and **4** with 60.5, 56.2 and 39.1%, respectively, compared to the structurally related compound **3** (37.4%) may either be due to the presence of methyl group and hydrophobic interaction of them with adjacent amino acids. This interaction becomes lower in the case of compound **3** because of steric factors. This phenomenon is depicted clearly in Figure 5.

As it has shown in Figure 5, for compound **3**, due to hydrogen bonding between oxygen of carboxyl group and Arg 368 and Gln 364, conformational locking happened, which possibly make the approach of the compound difficult towards the enzyme's binding site and results in a sharp decline in inhibitory potential as compared to compound **4** (Figure 6). In another word, substitution at ortho position of C ring with different groups such as hydroxyl and ketone result to diminish of the inhibition potency. This effect explains the lower hydrophobic interaction between methyl group and amino acids present at interacting site.

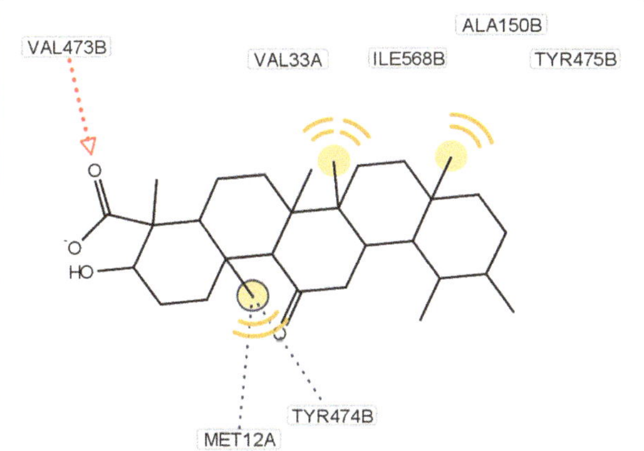

Figure 6 **Molecular docking of compound 4 and its interaction with different residue of urease enzyme active site involved in interaction.**

Besides, presence of three kinds of hydrogen bonds formed by the carboxyl group of compound **1**, two kinds of hydrogen bonds in compound **2** and one kind in compound **4** with respective amino acids in the hydrophobic pocket can explain their percent of inhibition activity order against urease (Table 1). For compound **3**, despite the existence of four hydrogen bond's percent of inhibition decrease dramatically. This observation can be explained by existing steric hindrance, which prevents the compound to interact with the hydrophobic site appropriately.

Conclusion

In this research isolated compounds from *B. carterii* has been tested against urease, which may confirm its potential traditional use for stomach problems. Based on the above study, we can preliminarily conclude that the substituted C ring of BA's may result to decreased inhibition concentration compared with the reference inhibitor thiourea. In addition, hydrophobic interactions between methyl group of compounds and near residues play an important role in the inhibition. This observation can be applied to the development of new antiulcer agents.

Competing interest

There are no other conflicts of interest related to this publication.

Authors' contributions

All authors contributed to the concept and design, making and analysis of data, drafting, revising and final approval. MA is responsible for the study registration, financial and administrative support. SG, FN & ZBO are responsible for biological assays. RB, SaG & BY were involved for docking studies. RH & ShR were responsible for preparation of extract and isolation of compounds 1-4. SG, RB& MA were participated in data assembly and analysis, interpretation and manuscript writing. All authors read and approved the final manuscript.

Acknowledgement

This project was supported by grants from the Research Council of Tehran University of Medical Sciences and Iran National Science Foundation.

Author details

[1]Department of Medicinal Chemistry, Faculty of Pharmacy and Medicinal Plants Research Center, Tehran University of Medical Sciences, Tehran, Iran. [2]School of Advanced Medical Technologies, Tehran University of Medical Sciences, Tehran, Iran. [3]Pharmacognosy & Pharmaceutics Department of Medicinal Plants Research Center, Institute of Medicinal Plants, ACECR, Karaj, Iran.

References

1. Han RJ: **Highlight on the studies of anticancer drugs derived from plants in China.** *Stem Cells* 1994, **12**:53-63.
2. Bhushan S, Kumar A, Malik F, Andotra SS, Sethi VK, Kaur IP, Taneja SC, Qazi GN, Singh JJ: **A triterpenediol from *boswellia serrata* induces apoptosis through both the intrinsic and extrinsic apoptotic pathways in human leukemia HL-60 cells.** *Apoptosis* 2007, **12**:1911–1926.
3. Janssen G, Bode U, Breu H, Dohrn B, Engelbrecht V, Gobel UJ: **Boswellic acids in the palliative therapy of children with progressive or relapsed brain tumors.** *Klin Padiatr* 2000, **212**:189–195.
4. Winking M, Sarikaya S, Rahmanian A, Jodicke A, Boker DK: **Boswellic acids inhibit glioma growth: a new treatment option?** *J Neurooncol* 2000, **46**:97–103.
5. Glaser T, Winter S, Groscurth P, Safayhi H, Sailer E-R, Ammon HPT, Schabet M, Weller MJ: **Boswellic acids and malignant glioma: induction of apoptosis but no modulation of drug sensitivity.** *Br J Cancer* 1999, **80**:756–765.
6. Liu JJ, Nilsson A, Oredsson S, Badmaev V, Zhao WZ, Duan R-D: **Boswellic acids trigger apoptosis via a pathway dependent on caspase-8 activation but independent on Fas/Fas ligand interaction in colon cancer HT-29 cells.** *J Carcinogenesis* 2002, **23**:2087–2093.
7. Hoernlein RF, Orlikowsky T, Zehrer C, Niethammer D, Sailer ER, Simmet T, Dannecker GE, Ammon HP: **Acetyl-11-keto-beta-boswellic acid induces apoptosis in HL-60 and CCRF-CEM cells and inhibits topoisomerase I.** *J Phamacol Exp Ther* 1999, **288**:613–619.
8. Shen Y, Hu Y, Chen B, Yao SJ: **Screening of enzyme inhibitors from traditional Chinese medicine.** *Comb chem high throughput screening* 2010, **13**:885–899.
9. Frank MB, Yang Q, Osban J, Azzarello JT, Saban MR, Saban R, Ashley RA, Welter JC, Fung K, Lin H-KJ: **Frankincense oil derived from *boswellia carteri* induces tumor cell specific cytotoxicity.** *BMC Complementary Altern Med* 2009, **9**:6–17.
10. Akihisa T, Tabata K, Banno N, Tokuda H, Nishihara R, Nakamura Y, Kimura Y, Yasukawa K, Suzuki TJ: **Cancer chemopreventive effects and cytotoxic activities of the triterpene acids from the resin of *boswellia carteri*.** *Biol Pharm Bull* 2006, **29**:1976–1979.
11. Vivek R, Yadav L, Prasad S, Sung B, Juri G, Gelovani J, Guha S, Krishnan S: **Boswellic acid inhibits growth and metastasis of human colorectal cancer in orthotopic mouse model by downregulating inflammatory, proliferative, invasive and angiogenic biomarkers.** *Int J Cancer* 2012, **130**:2176–2184.
12. Syrovets T, Buchele B, Gedig E, Slupsky JR, Simmet TJ: **Acetyl-boswellic acids are novel catalytic inhibitors of human topoisomerases I and II alpha.** *Mol Pharmacol* 2000, **58**:71–81.
13. Singh S, Khajuria A, Taneja SC, Khajuria RK, Singh J, Johri RK, Qazi GNJ: **The gastric ulcer protective effect of boswellic acids, a leukotriene inhibitor from boswellia serrata, in rats.** *Phytomedicine* 2008, **15**:408–415.
14. Biglar M, Soltani K, Bazl R, Amanlou M: **A preliminary investigation of the jack-bean urease inhibition by randomly selected traditional used herbal medicine.** *IJPR* 2012, **11**:831–837.
15. Devesa SS, Blot WJ, Fraumeni JF: **Changing patterns in the incidence of esophageal and gastric carcinoma in the United States.** *J Cancer* 1998, **83**:2049–2053.
16. Howson CP, Hiyama T, Wynder EL: **The decline of gastric cancer: epidemiology of an unplanned triumph.** *J Epidemiol Rev* 1986, **8**:1–27.
17. Ha N-C, Oh S-T, Sung JY, Cha KA, Lee MH, Oh BH: **Supramolecular assembly and acid resistance of *helicobacter pylori* urease.** *J Nat Struct Biol* 2001, **8**:505–509.
18. Mobley HLT, Hausinger RP: **Microbial ureases: significance, regulation, and molecular characterization.** *J Microbial Rev* 1989, **53**:85–108.
19. Lodhi MA, Hussain J, Abbasi MA, Jassbi AR, Choudhary MI, Ahmad VJ: **A new bacillus pasteurii urease inhibitor from *euphorbia decipiens*.** *J Enzyme Inhib Med Chem* 2006, **21**:531–535.
20. Ciurli S, Benini S, Rypniewski WR, Wilson KS, Miletti S, Mangani S: **The complex of Bacillus pasteurii urease with acetohydroxamate anion from X-ray data at 1.55 Å resolution.** *J Coord Chem Rev* 1999, **190**:331–355.
21. Magerlein BJ, Levin RHJ: **Chemical studies with 11-oxygenated steroids. V. 3α,20β-Dihydroxypregnan-11-one 11-ethylene ketal.** *J Am Chem Soc* 1955, **77**:1904.
22. Azizian H, Nabati F, Sharifi A, Siavoshi F, Mahdavi M, Amanlou M: **Large-scale virtual screening for the identification of new helicobacter pylori urease inhibitor scaffolds.** *J Mol Model* 2011, **18**:2917–2927.
23. Wolber G, Langer T: **LigandScout: 3-D pharmacophores derived from protein-bound ligands and their use as virtual screening filters.** *J Chem Inf Model* 2005, **45**:160–169.
24. Wolber G, Dornhofer AA, Langer T: **Efficient overlay of small organic molecules using 3D pharmacophores.** *J Comput Aided Mol Des* 2007, **20**:773–788.
25. Morris GM, Goodsell DS, Halliday RS, Huey R, Hart WE, Belew RK, Olson AJ: **Distributed automated docking of flexible ligands to proteins: parallel applications of autodock 2.4.** *J Comput Chem* 1996, **19**:1639–1662.
26. Gerhardt H, Seifert F, Buvari P, Vogelsang H, Repges RZ: **Therapy of active crohn disease with *boswellia serrata* extract H 15.** *Gastroenterol* 2001, **39**:11–17.
27. Gupta I, Parihar A, Malhotra P, Singh GB, Lüdtke R, Safayhi H, Ammon HP: ***Boswellia serrata* gum resin in patients with ulcerative colitis.** *J Eur Med Res* 1997, **2**:37–43.

Antiproliferative activity of methanolic extracts from two green algae, *Enteromorpha intestinalis* and *Rizoclonium riparium* on HeLa cells

Subhabrata Paul and Rita Kundu*

Abstract

Background: Natural compounds can be alternative sources for finding new lead anti-cancer molecules. Marine algae have been a traditional source for bioactive compounds. *Enteromorpha intestinalis* and *Rhizoclonium riparium* are two well distributed saline/brackish water algae from Sundarbans. There's no previous report of these two for their anti-proliferative activities.

Methods: Cytotoxicity of the algal methanolic extracts (AMEs) on HeLa cells were assayed by 3-(4, 5-dimethylthiazol-2-yl)-2, 5- diphenyltetrazolium bromide (MTT) reduction assay. Morphological examinations were done by Haematoxylin, Hoechst 33258 and Acridine orange staining. DNA fragmentation was checked. Gene expressions of Cysteine aspartate protease (Caspase) 3, Tumor protein (TP) 53, Bcl-2 associated protein X (Bax) were studied by Reverse transcription- polymerase chain reaction (RT-PCR) keeping Glyceraldehyde 3-phosphate dehydrogenase (GAPDH) as internal control. Protein expressions were studied for Caspase 3, phospho-p53, Bax, Microtubule associated proteins-1/ light chain B (MAP1/LC3B) by western blot.

Results: The AMEs were found to be cytotoxic with Inhibitory concentration 50 (IC50) values 309.048 ± 3.083 μg/ml and 506.081 ± 3.714 μg/ml for *E. intestinalis* and *R. riparium* extracts respectively. Treated cells became round with blebbings with condensed nuclei. Acidic lysosomal vacuoles formation occurred in treated cells. Expression of apoptotic genes in both mRNA and protein level was lowered. Expression of LC3B-II suggested occurrence of autophagy in treated cells.

Conclusions: These two algae can be potent candidates for isolating new lead anticancer molecules. So they need further characterization at both molecular and structural levels.

Keywords: *Enteromorpha intestinalis*, *Rhizoclonium riparium*, HeLa, MTT, Acridine orange, LC3B

Background

Cancer is considered to be the second leading cause of death [1]. An estimated 12.7 million new cases are registered each year with 7.6 million deaths and 24.6 million persons living with cancer worldwide [2]. According to a recent report of World Health Organization (WHO), cervical cancer ranks as the most frequent cancer among women between 15–44 years age group in India and all over the world. Currently a population of more than 366 million women of India (age group of 15 or more), are at a risk of developing cervical cancer. Every year 529828 women are diagnosed with the disease and 275128 die from this cancer throughout the world. The scenario is not very different in India also. Here, each year, the estimated number of new cases is 134420 and number of mortality is 72825. Considering the growth rate of population, the projected new cases of cervical cancer by 2025 will be 720060 and projected number of death will be 395095 in the global context, whereas , in India, the projected new cases will be 115171 which is very alarming [3,4].

Chemotherapy is still the standard treatment method along with surgery and radiation therapy. Most of the available treatments cause severe side effects such as bleeding, cognitive impairment, sensory abnormalities, infertility, damage to hoemopoetic tissue, hair-loss due to their non-

* Correspondence: kundu_rita@yahoo.co.in
Department of Botany, University of Calcutta, 35, Ballygunge Circular Road, Kolkata 700019, India

selective cytotoxicity. Emerging cancer drug resistance is another serious problem regarding chemotherapy [5]. Search for a new anticancer drug with lesser side effects and selective cytotoxicity has been one of the main thrust of cancer research worldwide. In this context, natural products, derived from plants, marine organisms and microorganisms, have drawn attentions of many scientists. According to WHO; 80% of world's population, especially in developing countries rely on plant derived medicines [6]. In the few decades natural products from higher plants were explored in great extent for possible anticancer activities, while other groups (algae, fungi) were not given proper attention. But, there is a tremendous scope to obtain novel bioactive compounds from the algae. Algae are a promising group to furnish various bioactive compounds as they are a group of diverse (unicellular to multicellular, prokaryotic to eukaryotic) members with diverse (freshwater to brakish/marine) habitats. They have been traditionally used as food and medicine in India, China, Japan, Korea, Ireland and Wales. Brown seaweeds (macroalgae) like *Laminaria, Undaria* are utilized as sources of iodine [7]. Alginate produced by brown algae (seaweeds) is used in food and pharmaceutical industries due to its ability to chelate metal ions. Carrageenans (water soluble sulfated galactans with an alternating backbone of α(1–4)-3,6 anhydro- D-galactose and ß(1–3) D galactose used as emulsifier/ stabilizers in milk based food products (ice-cream, pudding, desert gels, jams) are also obtained from macro algae (*Kappaphycus alvarezii*) [8]. Though, marine algae are rich source of pharmacologically active metabolites [9-13], having antimicrobial, antineoplastic, antiviral, anti-inflammatory and immunostimulant [14-16] activities, they were not exploited so far for their antiproliferating properties till today. Only few reports are available regarding the anticancer activities of algae. *Spirulina, Anabaena* and *Aphanizomenon*, members of Cyanophyceae (blue green algae) were reported to induce apoptosis in HL-60 and MCF7 cell lines [17-19]. But reports regarding the anticancer properties of Chlorophyta (green algae) are sparse. Extracts of *Udotea flabellum* was reported to have antiproliferative activity on HeLa, SiHa and KB cell lines [20].

In the present study, we have evaluated the cytotoxic potential of methanolic extracts of two green algae *Enteromorpha intestinalis* and *Rhizoclonium riparium*, using MTT assay on cervical cancer cell line (HeLa) followed by DNA fragmentation assay. Role of Caspase 3, p53 and Bax were studied in transcriptional and translational level to investigate their role in inducing cell death. Role of LC3B was studied at the translational level.

Methods

Chemicals and reagents

Methanol (Merck) was used to extract the algal materials. Dulbecco's Modified Eagle Medium (DMEM), Fetal Bovine Serum (FBS) and antibiotic-antimycotic solution [Penicillin, Streptomycin & Amphotericin], Sodium bicarbonate ($NaHCO_3$) (Himedia) were used in cell culture. 3-(4, 5-dimethylthiazol-2-yl)-2, 4-diphenyltetrazolium bromide (MTT) (Sigma) and Dimethyl sulfoxide (DMSO) (Merck) were used in cell viability assays. Haematoxylin (Gurr), Hoechst 33258 (Sigma), Paraformaldehyde (PFA)(HiMedia) were used in cellular and nuclear morphology study. Acridine orange (Sigma) was used in acidic vacuole staining. Non idet P-40 (NP40) (Sigma) was used in DNA isolation. Tris(hydroxymethyl)aminomethane (Tris), Ethylenediaminetetraacetic acid (EDTA), Acetic acid (Merck); Agarose, Ethidium bromide (EtBr) (Sigma) were used in Agarose gel electrophoresis. TRI reagent, Chloroform and Isopropanol (Sigma) were used for total RNA isolation. Sodium hypochlorite (NaClO) (Merck) used in RNA gel electrophoresis. First strand cDNA synthesis kit [MuLv RT kit] (Fermentas); Taq Polymerase, dNTPs (Chromus Biotech) were used in semi quantitative RT-PCR reactions. 100× protease inhibitor cocktail (G-Biosciences) was used at the time of protein isolation. Sodium hydroxide (NaOH), Sodium carbonate (Na_2CO_3), Sodium potassium tartrate ($C_4H_4KNaO_6 \cdot 4H_2O$), Copper sulfate ($CuSO_4 \cdot 5H_2O$) (Merck); Bovine serum albumin (BSA), Folin phenol reagent (Sigma) were used in protein quantification. Acrylamide, Bis-acrylamide, Ammonium persulfate (APS), Sodium dodecyl sulfate (SDS) (Merck) and Tetramethylethylenediamine (TEMED) (Sigma) were used in polyacrylamide gel electrophoresis (PAGE). Caspase3 (Imgenex); LC3B, ß-tubulin (Sigma); IgG-AP (Santa Cruz Biotechnology); Bax, phospho-p53 (Cell Signalling Technology); nitro-blue tetrazolium/5-bromo-4-chloro-3'-indolyphosphate (NBT/BCIP) (Sigma) and nitrocellulose paper (NC) (Schleicher & Schuell) were used in western blot analysis.

Algal material

Two green algae, *Rhizoclonium riparium* (Roth) Harvey and *Enteromorpha intestinalis* (Linnaeus) [21] were collected during January 2012, from different blocks (Sandeshkhali and Jharkhali) of Sundarbans mangrove ecosystem (Indian part). Collected samples were properly identified and voucher specimens were deposited in the Calcutta University Herbarium (CUH). Accession numbers issued by CUH against *R. riparium* was CUH/AL/MW-48 and for *E. intestinalis* was CUH/AL/MW-50.

Preparation of algal extracts

10 gm of algal samples were excised to small pieces and extracted with methanol (3 times) for 72 hours at room temperature. The extract was concentrated and dried with freeze dryer (Eyela). The dried mass was weighed and again dissolved in appropriate volume of methanol to make the concentration of the AMEs as 20 μg/μl. The

extract was further filtered through a 0.22 μm sterile filter (Pall) and stored at −20°C for future use.

Cell line

For the *in vitro* assay HeLa cell line was used. HeLa cells are Human Papilloma virus (HPV) 18 positive human cervical cancer cell line, expressing high risk E6 and E7 oncoproteins [22] and low level of p53. 293 T cells are normal human embryonic kidney (HEK) cell line expressing large T antigen of Simian virus 40 (SV-40), often used as transfection host.

Cell culture

HeLa and 293 T cells were maintained in monolayer cultures in DMEM supplemented with 0.15% $NaHCO_3$, 5% FBS, 2 mM L-glutamine, 0.45% L-glucose, 100units/ml penicillin, 100 μg/ml streptomycin and 250 ng/ml Amphotericin B at 37°C in a humidified incubator having 5% Carbon dioxide (CO_2).

MTT assay

Cytotoxicity of the AMEs was evaluated by standard MTT assay [23]. 2×10^4 HeLa and 293 T cells /well were seeded in 96 well flat bottom culture plates along with negative control sets (without cells). After overnight incubation cells were treated with different concentrations (in a range of 0–500 μg/ml) of the AMEs in triplicate along with a vehicle control set (2.5% of the growth medium). After 24 hours, the medium with treatments were removed and replaced with fresh medium along with 100 μg of MTT in each well and incubated for another 4 hours. Then the medium was removed and the formazan crystals were dissolved in 100 μl DMSO and absorbance was taken at 490 nm [24] in an Elisa reader (BioRad). The extent of cytotoxicity was determined using the following formula:

$$\%inhibition = [1-(Absorbance_{treated}/Absorbance_{non-treated})] \times 100$$

IC50 values were calculated subsequently. All the experiments were done with this IC50 doses.

Morphological studies

AMEs treated HeLa cells were stained with Haematoxylin and Hoechst 33258 to study cellular and nuclear morphology. Treated and control cells were stained with supravital stain Acridine orange to study the formation of acidic vacuoles. $5x10^4$ HeLa cells/ coverslip were seeded and after overnight incubation, treated with IC50 values of the AMEs for 24 hours along with a non-treated set. Then fixed in 4% PFA and subsequently Haematoxylin and Hoechst staining were done.

For cellular morphology study, the fixed cells were stained with 1% acidic Mayer's Haematoxylin for 5 minutes at room temperature. For nuclear morphology, 2 μg/ml of Hoechst 33258 was used to stain the nuclei for 15 minutes in dark at room temperature. For Acridine orange staining, after 24 hours of AME treatment, cells were additionally incubated in fresh media containing Acridine orange (1 μg/ml) for 15 minutes without fixation.

After the staining procedures were over, extra stain was drained out, washed briefly in phosphate buffered saline (PBS) and mounted in PBS containing 10% glycerol, 2% N-propyl gallate. Cells were visualized under both bright field and fluorescence {excitation 356 nm, emission 465 nm for Hoechst and excitation 488 nm, emission 530(green) 650 (red) for Acridine orange} in an epi-fluorescence microscope (Olympus).

DNA fragmentation

10^7 HeLa cells were seeded in T25 flask. After overnight incubation, medium was replaced and fresh medium was added along with IC50 doses of AMEs. After 24 hours of treatment, cells were harvested and lysed with lysis buffer containing 20 mM EDTA, 50 mM Tris, 1%SDS and 1% NP-40 for 2 hours in ice. Then the total genomic DNA was purified and treated with RNase treatment (20 μg/ml) at 37°C for 1 hour. DNA was then precipitated, washed with 75% ethanol, briefly air-dried, dissolved in Tris-EDTA buffer (pH8) and electrophoresed in 1.5% agarose gel containing EtBr (0.5 μg/ml), Tris acetate EDTA (TAE) buffer at 4 V/cm, and subsequently visualized under ultra violet (UV) trans-illuminator and photographed in gel documentation system (UVP Multidoc-It).

Gene and protein expression studies

10^7 HeLa cells were seeded in T25 flask. After overnight incubation, medium was replaced and fresh medium was added along with IC50 doses of AMEs. After 24 hours of treatment, cells were harvested and RT-PCRs and Western blots were done.

Semi quantitative RT-PCR

Total RNA was isolated from the cells using TRI reagent following manufacturer's protocol. RNA integrity was checked in 1.5% agarose gel containing 0.3% NaClO [25], EtBr (0.5 μg/ml), TAE buffer at 4 V/cm with subsequent visualization under UV.

First strand cDNA synthesis was carried out taking 2 μg RNA using 1st strand cDNA synthesis kit [MuLv RT kit] following manufacturer's protocol. Taking 2 μl of cDNA as template, PCRs were conducted for Caspase-3, Bax and TP53 gene while GAPDH serves as an internal control. The PCR products were subsequently subjected to agarose gel electrophoresis (AGE), visualized under ultra violet (UV) trans-illuminator and photographed in gel documentation system (UVP Multidoc-It). Densitometric analysis of the bands was done using UVP Doc-ItLS image analysis software.

The primers used were designed by Primer-3 software using FASTA sequences from NCBI-Nucleotide. The forward and reverse primer sequences along with their respective PCR profiles are listed in Table 1.

Western blot

Total protein was isolated by lysing HeLa cells using 1xSDS gel loading buffer (50 mM Tris-Cl pH 6.8, 2% SDS, 10% 2-Mercaptoethanol, 0.01% Bromophenol blue, 10% Glycerol) along with 1× protease inhibitor (with EDTA) followed by incubation in boiling water bath for 10 min. Then the lysates were centrifuged at 14000 g for 15 minutes at 4°C. Supernatants stored at −20°C for further uses.

Extracted protein samples were quantified following micro-Lowry method with slight modifications. To 2 µl of lysates 200 µl of 10% TCA was added and incubated 30 minutes at −20°C and the centrifuged at 15000 g for 15 minutes at 4°C. The precipitated protein pellets then re-dissolved in 100 µl of 1(N) NaOH and subsequently incubated in 1 ml Lowry reagent (2% Na_2CO_3:2% $C_4H_4KNaO_6.4H_2O$: 1% $CuSO_4.5H_2O$ = 100:1:1) for 10 minutes at room temperature. Then 100 µl of Folin phenol reagent (diluted 1:1 with milli Q grade water) added to the samples and further incubated in dark at room temperature for 30 minutes. O.D of the samples was taken at 750 nm in a double beam spectrophotometer (Hitachi) and concentration of the samples was determined using a standard curve prepared with BSA.

100 µg of each protein samples were separated in 12% polyacrylamide gels. Semi dry transfer of the protein samples were done using 0.45 µm nitrocellulose paper, incubated in blocking buffer (5% BSA) for 2 hours at room temperature. Then the membrane was incubated at 4°C with appropriate dilutions of primary antibodies (1:2000 for anti ß-tubulin, 1:1000 for anti Bax, 1:500 for anti phospho-p53 and anti LC3B, 1:250 for anti Caspase 3) for overnight. After subsequent incubation of 2 hours with AP conjugated IgG (1:5000) at room temperature, NBT-BCIP solution was added and incubated until bands appeared. Pictures of the membranes were taken in gel documentation system (UVP Multidoc-It). Densitometry analysis of the bands was done using UVP Doc-ItLS image analysis software.

Statistical analysis

All the experiments were carried out thrice in triplicates. All numerical data were expressed as mean of triplicates ± standard error (SE). Statistical analysis and generation of histograms were performed using Graphpad Prism 5.02 software. All datasets obtained from the experiments were subjected to grouped analysis by two-way analysis of variance (ANOVA) followed by Bonferroni post tests keeping $p < 0.05$ in all cases.

Results

MTT assay

To study the antiproliferative potential of the methanolic extract of these two algae on Hela cells and 293 T cells, MTT assays were done. Reduction of the substrate (MTT) by cellular dehydrogenase to form water insoluble formazan is the basis of the cytotoxicity test. Reduction in colour intensity in the treated sets than the non treated ones clearly indicated cytoxicity of the AME's on HeLa cells. From the experiment it was observed that cell death was concentration dependent, number of nonviable cells increased with increased concentration of AMEs.

Table 1 Primer sequences and PCR profiles for the genes Caspase 3, Bax, TP53 and GAPDH

A	Primer sequence (5′ → 3′)	
Gene	Forward	Reverse
Caspase 3	ATTGTGGAATTGATGCGTGA	GGCAGGCCTGAATAATGAAA
TP53	ATGGCCATCTACAAGCAG	ACAGTCAAGAGCCAACCTCAG
Bax	GTGGCAGCTGACATGTTTTC	GGAGGAAGTCCAATGTCCAG
GAPDH	CAAGGTCATCCATGACAACTTTG	GTCCACCACCCTGTTGCTGTAG

B	PCR profile						
PCR steps / Gene	Initial denaturation	Denaturation	Annealing	Extension	No. of cycles	Final extension	Product length (bp)
Caspase 3	94°C – 4 m	94°C – 60s	52°C – 45 s	72°C – 60s	35	72°C – 7 m	205
TP53		94°C – 30s	58°C – 30s	72°C – 45 s			210
Bax		94°C – 60s	57°C – 30s	72°C – 45 s			151
GAPDH		94°C – 30s	58°C – 30s	72°C – 45 s			496

(A) Primer sequences, designed by Primer3 software tabulated.
(B) PCR profiles after optimization for single band for a target.

We have observed that the IC50 doses of the AMEs in HeLa cells were 309.048 ± 3.083 μg/ml and 506.081 ± 3.714 μg/ml for *E. intestinalis* and *R. riparium* extracts respectively. For 293 T cells, the IC50 doses were 651.183 ± 1.198 μg/ml and 905.727 ± 4.034 μg/ml. The vehicle control set showed 4.345 ± 0.594 percent inhibition. From the study it was observed that methanolic extract of *E. intestinalis* was more cytotoxic than *R. riparium* (Figure 1a & b).

Cell and nuclear morphology

Both the AMEs treated HeLa cells showed distinct differences in their cellular and nuclear morphology in

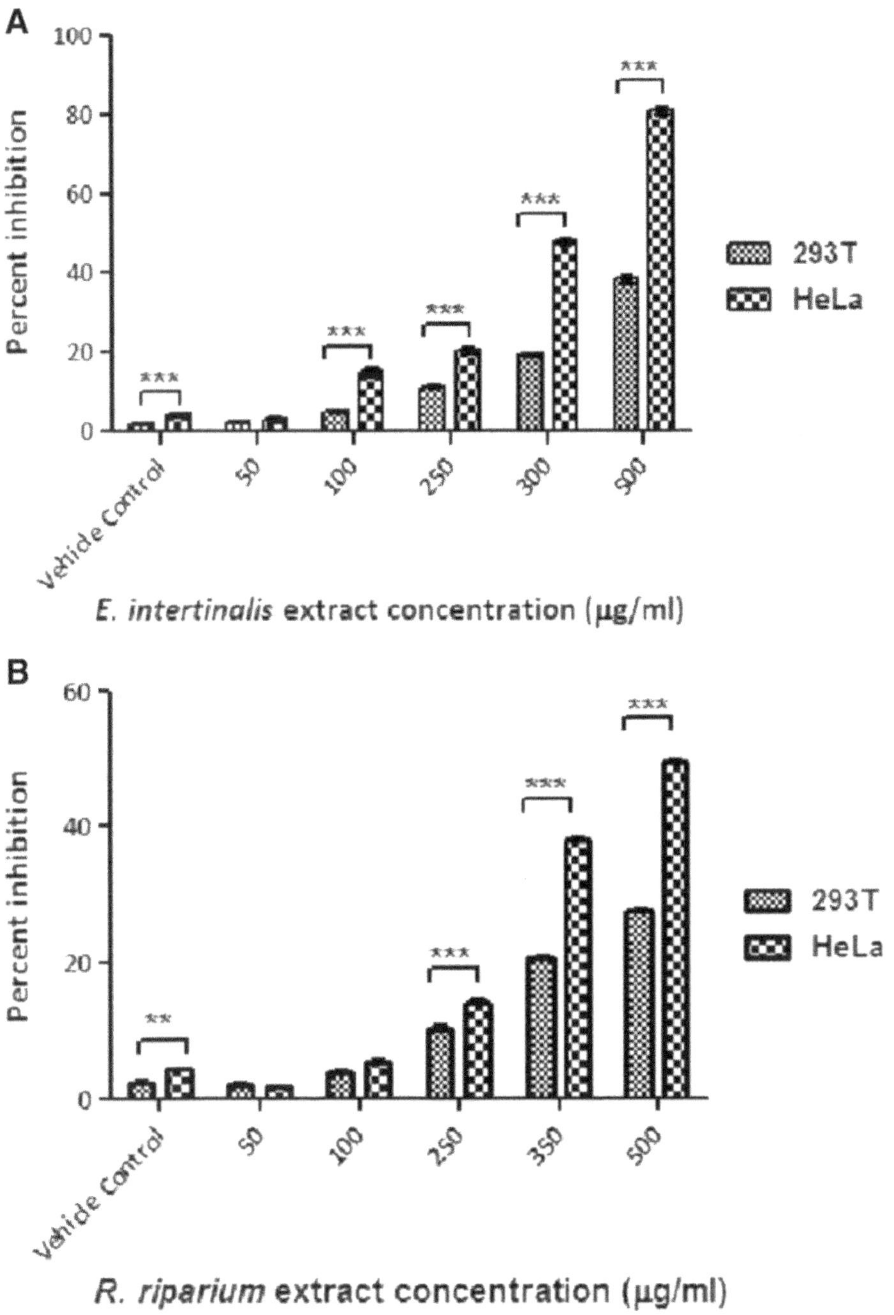

Figure 1 Histograms showing the antiproliferative effects of the AMEs on HeLa and 293 T cell lines. The cells were treated with increasing concentration of AMEs for 24 hours. Cytotoxicity of the AMEs was evaluated by MTT assay. Results showed percent inhibition of cell growth against increasing concentration of the extracts. **(A)** *E. intestinalis* extract treated, **(B)** *R. riparium* extract treated.Columns with bars represent mean ± SE of triplicates. Percent inhibitions of the AMES at each concentration point were compared between the two cells lines. According to the significance levels found, they were further categorized using various symbols as follows, ******: $p < 0.01$; *******: $p < 0.001$.

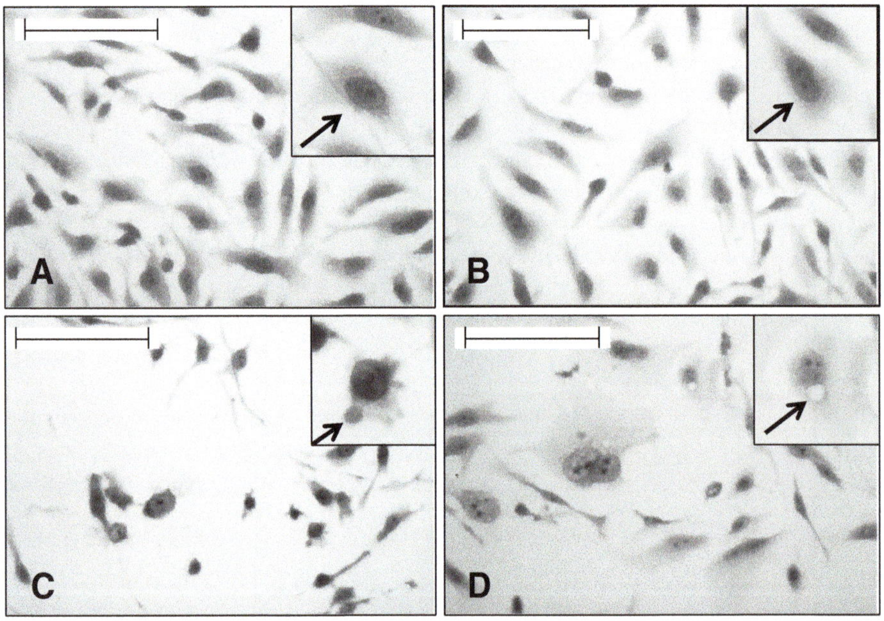

Figure 2 HeLa cells grown on sterile cover slips were treated with IC50 doses of the AMEs for 24 hours. Then they were stained with Haematoxylin to study the cellular morphology. Scale indicates 50 μm. Inset shows magnified view. **A)** Non-treated cells, the arrow shows normal cellular morphology **B)** Vehicle control cells, the arrow shows normal cellular morphology **C)** Cells treated with *E. intestinalis* extract, the arrow shows cytoplasmic blebbings **(D)** Cells treated with *R. riparium* extract, the arrow shows cytoplasmic vacuolation.

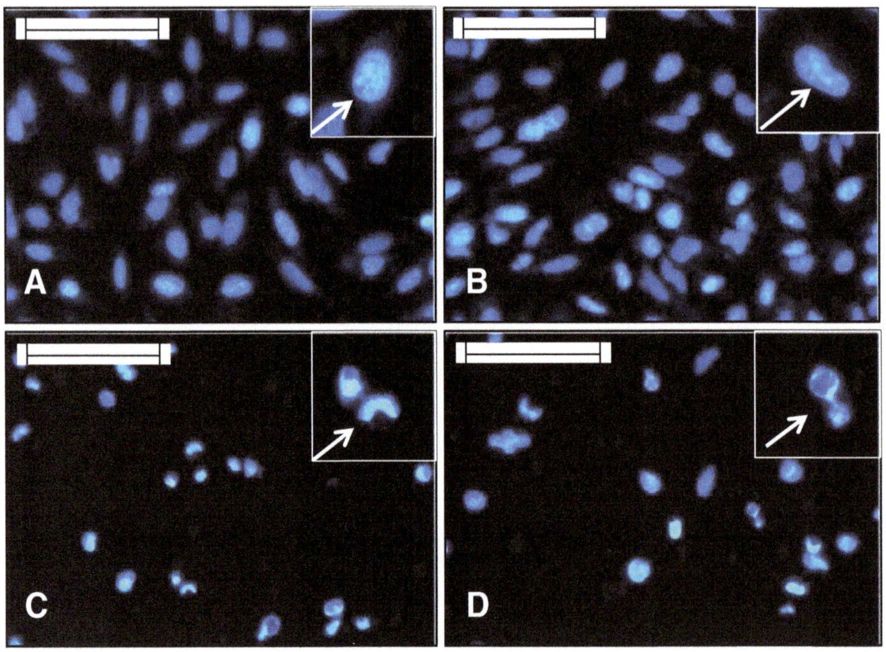

Figure 3 HeLa cells grown on sterile cover slips were treated with IC50 doses of the AMEs for 24 hours. Then they were stained with Hoechst 33258 to study the nuclear morphology. Scale indicates 50 μm. Inset shows magnified view. **(A)** Non-treated cells, the arrow shows normal looking nucleus; **(B)** Vehicle control cells, the arrow shows normal elliptical nucleus; **(C)** *E. intestinalis* extract treated sets, the arrow shows nuclei with deformity; **(D)** *R. riparium* treated cells, the arrow shows highly condensed nuclei.

comparison to the untreated cells. In the treated sets, cells became round, lost their characteristic stretched appearance, showed clear cytoplasmic blebbings and vacuolation. Cells stained with Hoechst, observed under fluorescence microscope showed nuclear morphology. Nuclei of the control sets were elliptical in shape, but the treated nuclei were somewhat different. In the treated cells nuclear condensation was pronounced with deformed appearances. Vehicle sets in both cases showed characteristic morphological features as the non-treated ones (Figures 2 and 3).

Acidic vacuole localization

Acridine orange in uncharged form, stain both cytoplasm and nucleic acids which fluoresce bright green. Whereas in protonated form it accumulates in the lysosomal acidic vacuoles, form aggregates and fluoresce bright red [26]. When studied under a fluorescence microscope, it was observed that in the non-treated and vehicle control sets minimal red fluorescence was found, whereas, increased red fluorescence were observed in the treated cells. In *R. riparium* extract treated cells almost the whole cytoplasm became red (Figure 4) indicating the merging of all the acidic vacuoles.

DNA fragmentation assay

DNA fragmentation is a classical hallmark of apoptosis. But in the treated cells no sign of DNA laddering was observed (Figure 5). Intact genomic DNA was found in all the cells which implied that apoptosis might not be the mechanism for inducing cell death in the treated ones.

Semi-Q RT-PCR

To investigate the role of Caspase 3, Bax and p53 in AMEs induced cell death in HeLa cells, expression profile of these genes were studied by semi q RT-PCR. For the gene expression studies, RT-PCR gave us a qualitative estimation of up regulation/down regulation of some apoptotic genes (Figure 6). Caspase 3 expression was found to be downregulated in both *E. intestinalis* treated (75.45%) and *R. riparium* treated (85.54%) cells. Bax expression was down regulated in both the treated samples, which was more pronounced in *E. intestinalis* (58.13%) extract treated cells than *R. riparium* (46.34%) treated cells. TP53 expression also decreased in both the samples, slightly higher in *E. intestinalis* (58.22%) extract treated cells than *R. riparium* (53.22%) treated cells. The down regulated expression profiles of caspase 3 and Bax

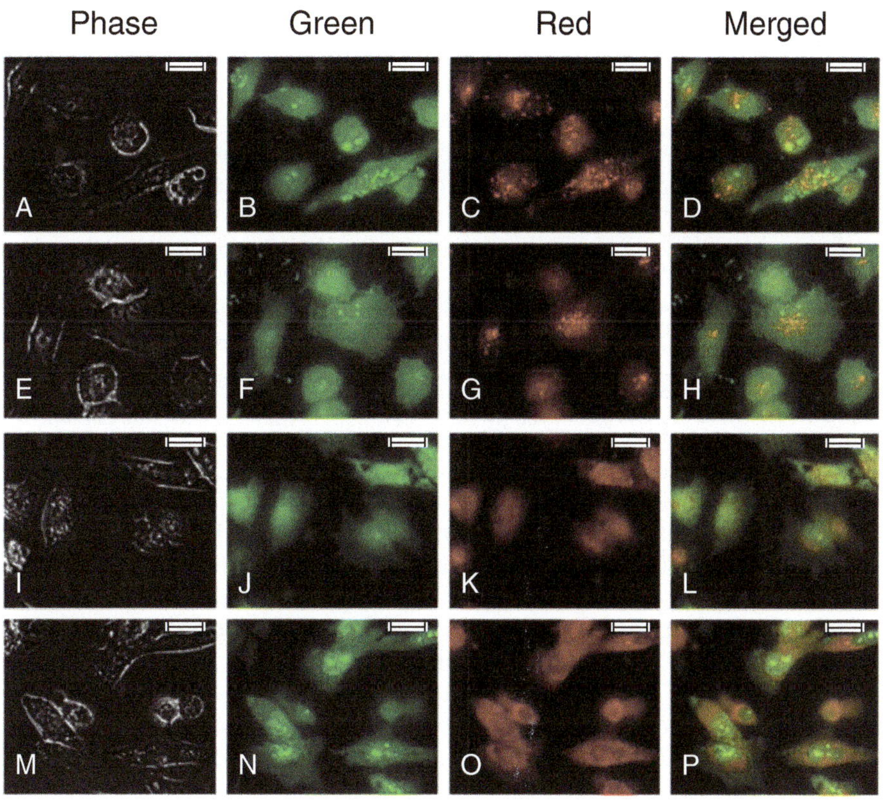

Figure 4 HeLa cells grown on sterile cover slips were treated with IC50 doses of AMEs for 24 hours. Then they were stained with Acridine orange (1 μg/ml) to study the formation of acidic vacuoles. Scale indicates 50 μm. **A-D)** Non-treated, **E-H)** Vehicle control, **I-L)** *E. intestinalis* extract treated, **M-P)** *R. riparium* treated HeLa cells.

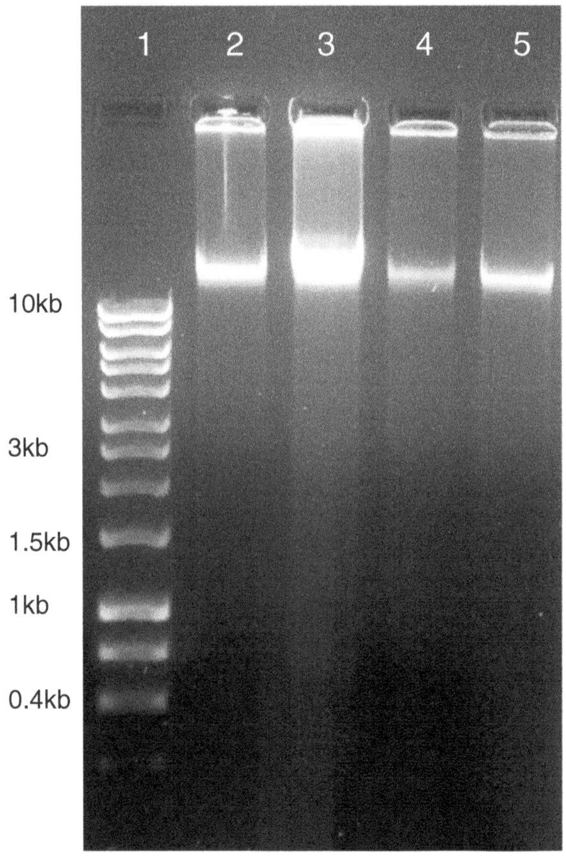

Figure 5 HeLa cells grown in T25 flask were treated with IC50 doses of AMEs for 24 hours along with a control set. Genomic DNA was isolated from all the sets and electrophorased in 1.5% agarose gel. Lane **1)** Molecular marker (0.4-10 kb, Lane **2)** Non-treated, Lane **3)** Vehicle control, Lane **4)** *E. intestinalis* extract treated, Lane **5)** *R. riparium* extract treated.

in the treated cells indicate that cell death was not mediated by Bax and caspase3.

Immunoblotting

Expression level of some apoptotic and autophagic proteins were monitored at the translational level (Figure 7). In all the samples cleaved caspase3 expression was absent while Pro-Caspase 3 expression was less down regulated in *E. intestinalis* (17.35%) than *R. riparium* (26.85%) treated cells. Bax expression on the other hand was found to be more down regulated in *E. intestinalis* (27.83%) than *R. riparium* (18.86%) treated cells. Expression of phospho-p53 was absent in all the samples. Expression of LC3B-I and LC3B-II was found in both the treated samples while absent in non-treated and vehicle control sets. LC3B-I and LC3B-II expressions were higher (8.07% and 19.79% respectively) in *R. riparium* extract treated cells than the *E. intestinalis* treated cells.

Discussion

In this study, we have evaluated the methanolic extracts of two green algae, *E. intestinalis* and *R. riparium* for their antiproliferative activity in human cervical cancer cell line HeLa. These two green algae are found widely in the water bodies of Sundarbans mangrove ecosystem and commonly used as fish feed. There were no previous reports about their antiproliferative property on cervical cancer cell lines. An alkali extracted polysachharide (DAEB) from *E. intestinalisis* was found to be capable of preventing formation of Sarcoma 180 tumor and had some antitumor activity which was mediated by immunoenhancement of immune system instead of direct cytotoxicity [27].

To determine the IC50 doses of these two AMEs, MTT assays were done. Along with HeLa cells, a non-cancerous cell line, 293 T (human embryonic kidney cell line) were treated with the AMEs. From the results, it was observed that IC50 doses of the AMEs were significantly much higher for the 293 T cell line that the HeLa cell line. Which indicates that the AMEs were less cytotoxic to the non-cancerous cell line. Grouped analysis using Two-way ANOVA followed by Bonferroni posttests revealed that with respect to the control 293 T cells cytotoxicity of the AMEs in HeLa cells were significant above 50 μg/ml for *E. intestinalis* extract and above 100 μg/ml for *R.riparium* extract. This implies that *E.intestinalis* extract is more potent than *R.riparium* extract.

Cellular and nuclear morphology observed in the treated cells showed clear indication of cytotoxicity. But the responses were different for the two extracts. In *E. intestinalis* extract treated cells, cytoplasmic blebbings were observed along with deformed nuclei, while cytoplasmic vacuolation with condensed nuclei was observed in *R. riparium* treated cells. Chromatin condensations into compact figures, which are often globular or crescent shaped, are defined as stage II chromatin condensation, and occurs in apoptosis. Cytoplasmic blebbings are generally associated with apoptosis where cells undergoing apoptosis breaks down into apotosomes/apoptotic bodies, which were further absorbed by macrophages (*in vivo*), whereas cytoplasmic vacuolation is associated with autophagic cell death, a type II programmed cell death. During autophagy, portions of the cytoplasm and subcellular organelles are sequestered by endoplasmic reticulum, resulting in vesicular bodies which acted as autophagosomes. They are further fused with the lysosomes to form autophagosomal vesicles where the contents are enzymatically degraded [28]. For detecting the acidic compartments, lysosomotropic agent acridine orange was used for staining. Cells treated with *R. riparium* extract showed higher amount of acidic vacuole formation. On the other hand cells treated with *E. intestinalis* extract showed lesser number of acidic vacuole formation. In *R. riparium* treated cells,

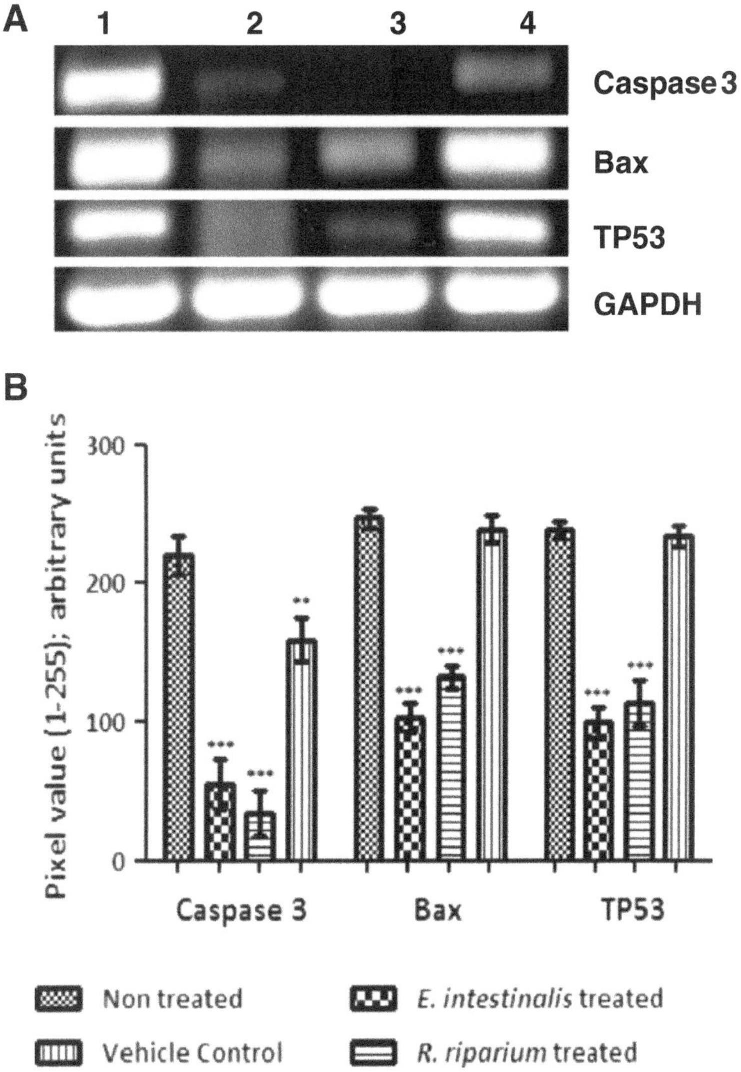

Figure 6 Gene expression profiles of Caspase 3, Bax, TP53, GAPDH in HeLa cells treated with AMEs (IC50 doses) by semi quantitative RT-PCR. (A) Representative pictures of three independent experiments. Lane 1) Non-treated, Lane 2) *E. intestinalis* extract treated, Lane 3) *R. riparium* treated, 4) Vehicle control. **(B)** Relative levels of gene expressions after normalization for GAPDH were determined by densitometry analysis of the bands, represented by histogram. Columns with bars represent mean ± SE of triplicate pixel values for the bands. Intensity for each band in the treated sets was compared with that of in non treated sets. According to the significance levels found, they were further categorized using various symbols as follows, **: $p < 0.01$; ***: $p < 0.001$.

all most the whole cell became red, due to merging of all the acidic vacuoles. The observation was further validated by immunoblot results.

DNA fragmentation is a classical hallmark of apoptosis. In response to apoptotic signals (DNA damage/ stress) proapoptotic Bcl2 family protein Bax becomes activated resulting in mitochondrial membrane permeabilization. As a result cytochrome C and APAF-1 (apoptotic protease activating factor 1) are released from the inter-membrane space and activate caspase 9 through cleavage. Caspase 9 generates a signaling cascade of caspase cleavage that results in DNA fragmentation into 180 basepairs and multiples of it. The effecter caspase is caspase 3. p53 has a major role in cell survival . In healthy cells the nuclear amount of p53 is very low. Due to binding of adapter protein MDM2, p53 is subsequently exported to cytosol and degraded. Whereas in the cells with damaged DNA, p53 becomes phosphorylated. As MDM2 cannot recognize phosphorylated p53, the nuclear p53 is stabilized and induce pro-apoptotic proteins (Bax, Puma and Noxa etc.). We have found some signs of apoptotic features (nuclear and cellular) in the AMEs treated cells, so we have undertaken the DNA fragmentation assay and the same time assessed the expressions of caspase 3, Bax and p53 at the transcriptional level. From our observation we found that DNA fragmentation was

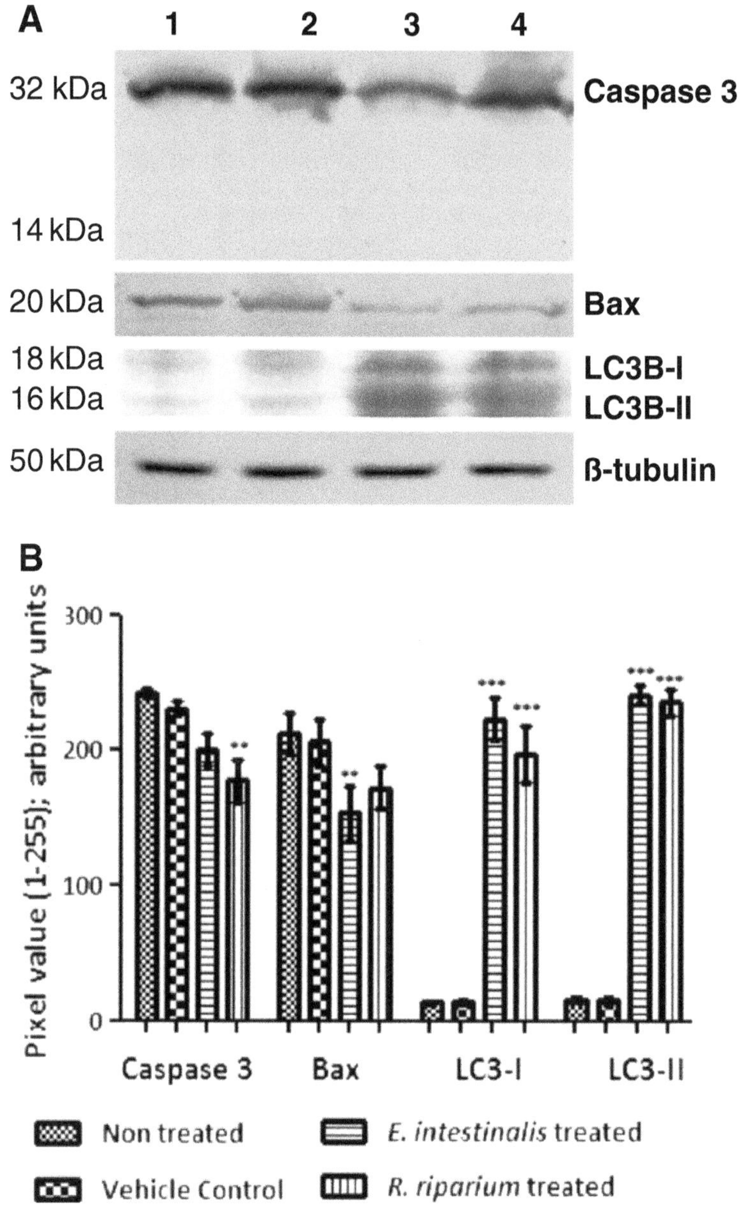

Figure 7 Protein expression profiles of Caspase 3, Bax, LC3B-I & II and ß-tubulin in HeLa cells treated with AMEs (IC50 doses) by Western blot. (A) Representative pictures of three independent experiments. Lane 1) Non-treated, Lane 2) Vehicle control 3) *E. intestinalis* extract treated, Lane 4) *R. riparium* treated. **(B)** Relative levels of gene expressions after normalization for ß-tubulin were determined by densitometry analysis of the bands, represented by histogram. Columns with bars represent mean ± SE of triplicate pixel values for the bands. Intensity for each band in the treated sets was compared with that of in non treated sets. According to the significance levels found, they were further categorized using various symbols as follows, **: $p < 0.01$; ***: $p < 0.001$.

absent indicating a cell death process not mediated by caspase 3 or Bax.

RT-PCR observation also validates the findings. Here Bax and caspase 3 expressions were found to be less in comparison to the controlled cells and expression of p53 was down regulated in all the samples. In translational levels, the expression of cleaved pro-caspase 3 and Bax were found to be down regulated in both the samples whereas no expressions of cleaved caspase 3 and phospho-p53 (data not shown) were observed. Absence of DNA fragmentation, down regulation of Bax, p53 and absence of cleaved caspase 3 strongly indicated a cell death pathway other than apoptosis or type I cell death.

As the AMEs treated samples showed some signs positive (vacuolation in cytosol) for autophagy or type-II cell death, role of LC3 was studied by western blot. LC3 (MAP1) is a mammalian homolog of the yeast ATG8 protein, a ubiquitin like protein that becomes lipidated and tightly associated with autophagosomal membranes. LC3 proteins are specifically cleaved at their carboxy terminal to form LC3-I, which has an exposed carboxy terminal glycine that is conjugated to phosphatidylethanolamine to form LC3-II. This LC3-II protein bounds tightly with the autophagosomal membranes and serves as an autophagic marker protein [29]. Our results clearly showed the presence of LC3-I in both the treated samples, while the presence of LC3-II was distinct in *R. riparium* treated samples. All these observations strongly suggest that these two algal extracts are capable of inducing cell death by autophagy. Previously autophagy was considered as a pro-survival mechanism of the cell. But recent studies suggest that autophagy result in cell deaths and sometimes activates apoptosis.

Conclusions

From the results it was quite evident that, both the AMEs had potent cytotoxicity on HeLa cells. With the lesser IC50 value, *E. intestinalis* extract was found to be more antiproliferative (usage of Methanol as vehicle exert negligible amount of cytotoxicity to the cells). The cellular morphological examinations revealed presence of vacuoles which may be due to formation of auto lysosomal vacuoles. In case of nuclear morphology study, though nuclear condensation was observed, absence of fragmented nuclei along with absence of DNA laddering indicated that any other mechanism than apoptosis is responsible for the cell death. Whereas increase in acidic vacuoles and expression of LC3B-II had suggested autophagic cell death in the treated samples.

Both the *E. intestinalis* and *R. riparium* methanolic extracts were found to be cytotoxic to HeLa cells, most probably by the involvement of autophagy. So they were potent candidates for further characterization of their chemical constituents and the molecular pathway by which they worked.

Abbreviations

AGE: Agarose gel electrophoresis; AME: Algal methanolic extract; APS: Ammonium persulfate; Bax: Bcl-2 associated protein X; BSA: Bovine serum albumin; $C_4H_4KNaO_6.4H_2O$: Sodium potassium tartrate; Caspase 3: Cysteine aspartate protease 3; CUH: Calcutta university herbarium; $CuSO_4.5H_2O$: Copper sulfate; DMEM: Dulbecco's modified eagle medium; DMSO: Dimethyl sulfoxide; EDTA: Ethylenediaminetetraacetic acid; EtBr: Ethidium bromide; FBS: Fetal bovine serum; GAPDH: Glyceraldehyde 3-phosphate dehydrogenase; HPV: Human papilloma virus; IC50: Inhibitory concentration 50; MAP1/LC3B: Microtubule associated proteins-1/ light chain B; MTT: 3-(4, 5-dimethylthiazol-2-yl)-2, 5- diphenyltetrazolium bromide; Na_2CO_3: Sodium bicarbonate; NaClO: Sodium hypochlorite; NaHCO3: Sodium bicarbonate; NaOH: Sodium hydroxide; NBT/BCIP: Nitro-blue tetrazolium/5-bromo-4-chloro-3'-indolyphosphate; NC: Nitrocellulose; NP-40: Non idet P40; PAGE: Polyacrylamide gel electrophoresis; PBS: Phosphate buffered saline; PFA: Paraformaldehyde; RT-PCR: Reverse transcription- polymerase chain reaction; SE: Standard error; SDS: Sodium dodecyl sulfate; TAE: Tris acetate EDTA buffer; TCA: Trichloro acetic acid; TEMED: Tetramethylethylenediamine; TP53: Tumor protein 53; Tris: Tris(hydroxymethyl)aminomethane; WHO: World health organization.

Competing interest

The authors declare that they have no competing interest.

Author's contributions

SP: Collected algae, prepared extracts and performed all the experiments; RK: conceived the experiment, and participated in its design and coordination and helped to draft the manuscript. All authors read and approved the final manuscript.

Acknowledgements

The research was supported by Centre of Advance Study (CAS) - Department of Botany, University of Calcutta. SP is thankful to University Grant Commission (UGC), Government of India for his fellowship. Authors are thankful to Department of Biotechnology & Department of Biochemistry, University of Calcutta for the instrumentation facilities. HeLa and 293 T cells were kind gifts from Dr. R. N. Baral, Chittaranjan National Cancer Institute, Kolkata. Authors would like to express their sincere gratitude to Dr.Ruma Pal, Associate Professor, Department of Botany, University of Calcutta for identifying the algal specimens. Authors are also thankful to Mr. Chinmoy Saha and Mr. Gour Gopal Satpati for their help in statistical analysis and algal voucher specimen preparation respectively.

References

1. Xu H, Yao L, Sung H, Wu L: **Chemical composition and antitumor activity of different polysaccharides from the roots Actinidia eriantha.** *Carbohydr Pol* 2009, **78**:316–322.
2. Jemal A, Bray F, Center MM, Ferlay J, Ward E, Forman D: **Global cancer statistics.** *Ca Cancer J Clin* 2011, **60**:69–90.
3. *WHO/ICO Information Centre on HPV and Cervical Cancer (HPV Information Centre). Human Papillomavirus and Related Cancers in India. Summary Report 2010.* www.hpvcentre.net/statistics/reports/IND.pdf.
4. *Globocan 2008.* globocan.iarc.fr/pages/fact_sheets_cancer.aspx.
5. Gottesman MM: **Mechanisms of cancer drug resistance.** *Annu Rev Med* 2002, **53**:615–627.
6. Gurib-Fakim A: **Medicinal plants: traditions of yesterday and drugs of tomorrow.** *Mol Aspects Med* 2006, **27**(1):1–93.
7. Boopathy NS, Kathiresan K: **Anticancer drugs from marine flora: an overview.** *J Oncol* 2010, **2010**:1–18.
8. Cardazo KHM, Guaratini T, Barros MP, Falcao VR, Tonon AP, Lopes NP, Campos S, Torres MA, Souza AO, Colepicolo P, Pinto E: **Metabolites from algae with economic impact.** *Comparative Biochemistry and Physiology Part C* 2007, **146**:60–78.
9. Cannell JPR: **Algae as a source of biologically active products.** *Pestic Sci* 1993, **39**:147–153.
10. Nekhoroshev MV: **The black sea algae are potential source of antitumor drugs.** *Al'-gologiya* 1996, **6**(1):86–90.
11. Mayer A, Lehmann V: **Marine pharmacology in 1999: antitumor and cytotoxic compounds.** *Anticancer Res* 2001, **21**:2489–2500.
12. Mayer AMS, Gustafson KR: **Marine pharmacology in: antitumor and cytotoxic compounds.** *Int J Cancer* 2000, **2003**(105):291–299.
13. Faulkner DJ: **Marine natural products.** *Nat Prod Rep* 2000, **17**:7–55.
14. Rinehart KL Jr, Shaw PD, Shield LS, Gloer JB, Harbour GC, Koker MES, Samain D, Schwartz RE, Tymiak AA, Weller DL, Carter GT, Munro MHG: **Marine natural products as sources of antiviral, antimicrobial, and antineoplastic agents.** *Pure and Appl Chem* 1981, **53**:795–871.
15. Tziveleka LA, Vagias C, Roussis V: **Natural products with anti-HIV activity from marine organisms.** *Curr Top Med Chem* 2003, **3**(13):1512–1535.
16. Konig GM, Wright AD: **Marine natural products research. Current directions and future potential.** *Planta Med* 1995, **62**:193–211.
17. Bechelli J, Coppage M, Rosell K, Liesveld J: **Cytotoxicity of algae extracts on normal and malignant cells.** *Leuk Res Treatment* 2011, **2011**:Article ID 373519, 7 pages.
18. Li B, Chu X, Gao M, Li W: **Apoptotic mechanism of MCF-7 breast cells in vivo and in vitro induced by photodynamic therapy with C-phycocyanin.** *Acta Biochim Biophys Sin* 2010, **42**:80–89.
19. Oftedal L, Selheim F, Wahlsten M, Sivonen K, Døskeland SO, Herfindal L: **Marine benthic cyanobacteria contain apoptosis-inducing activity**

synergizing with daunorubicin to kill leukemia cells, but not cardiomyocytes. *Mar Drugs* 2010, **8**:2659–2672.
20. Moo-puck R, Robledo D, Fredle-Pelegrin Y: **In vitro cytotoxic and antiproliferative activities of marine macroalgae from Yucatan, Maxico.** *Ciencias Marinas* 2009, **35**(4):345–358.
21. *Algaebase.* http://www.algaebase.org.
22. DeFilippis RA, Goodwin EC, Wu L, DiMaio D: **Endogenous human papillomavirus E6 and E7 proteins differentially regulate proliferation, senescence, and apoptosis in HeLa cervical carcinoma cells.** *J Virol* 2003, **77**:1551–1563.
23. Carmicheal J, DeGraff WG, Gazder AF: **Evaluation of a tetrazolium-based semiautomated colorimetric assay: assessment of chemosensitivity testing.** *Cancer Res* 1987, **47**:936–942.
24. Pang M, Gao Wu Z, Lv N, Wang Z, Tang X, Qu P: **Apoptosis induced by yessotoxins in Hela human cervical cancer cells in vitro.** *Molecular Medicine Reports* 2010, **3**:629–634.
25. Aranda PS, LaJoie DM, Jorcyk CL: **Bleach gel: a simple agarose gel for analyzing RNA quality.** *Electrophoresis* 2002, **33**:366–369.
26. Paglin S, Hollister T, Delohery T, Hackett N, McMahill M, Sphicas E, Domingo D, Yahalom J: **A novel response of cancer cells to radiation involves autophagy and formation of acidic vacicles.** *Cancer Res* 2001, **61**:439–444.
27. Jiao L, Li X, Li T, Jiang P, Wu M, Zhang L: **Characterization and anti-tumor activity of alkali-extracted polysaccharide from *Enteromorpha intestinalis*.** *Int Immunopharmacol* 2009, **9**:324–329.
28. Yang Y, Liang Z, Gu Z, Qin Z: **Molecular mechanism and regulation of autophagy.** *Acta Pharmacol Sin* 2005, **26**(12):1421–1434.
29. Hansen TE, Johansen T: **Following autophagy step by step.** *BMC Biol* 2011, **9**:39.

10

Trend analysis of the pharmaceutical market in Iran; 1997–2010; policy implications for developing countries

Abbas Kebriaeezadeh[1,2*], Nasser Nassiri Koopaei[1], Akbar Abdollahiasl[1*], Shekoufeh Nikfar[1] and Nafiseh Mohamadi[3]

Abstract

Background: So far, no detailed study of the Iranian pharmaceutical market has been conducted, and only a few studies have analyzed medicine consumption and expenditure in Iran. Pharmaceutical market trend analysis remains one of the most useful instruments to evaluate the pharmaceutical systems efficiency. An increase in imports of medicines, and a simultaneous decrease in domestic production prompted us to investigate the pharmaceutical expenditure structure. On the other hand, analyzing statistics provides a suitable method to assess the outcomes of national pharmaceutical policies and regulations.

Methods: This is a descriptive and cross-sectional study which investigates the Iranian pharmaceutical market over a 13-year period (1997–2010). This study used the Iranian pharmaceutical statistical datasheet published by the Iranian Ministry of Health. Systematic searches of the relevant Persian and English research literature were made. In addition, official government documents were analyzed as sources of both data and detailed statements of policy.

Results: Analysis of the Iranian pharmaceutical market in the 13-year period shows that medicine consumption sales value growth has been 28.38% annually. Determination of domestic production and import reveals that 9.3% and 42.3% annual growth, respectively, have been experienced.

Conclusions: The Iranian pharmaceutical market has undergone great growth in comparison with developing countries and the pharmerging group, and the market is expanding quickly while a major share goes to biotechnology drugs, which implies the need to commercialization activities in novel fields like pharmaceutical biotechnology. This market expansion has been in favor of imported medicine in sales terms, caused by the reinforcement of suspicious policies of policy makers that necessitates fundamental rearrangements.

Keywords: Pharmaceutical market trends, Therapeutic categories, Pharmaceutical biotechnology, Commercialization

Background

Total expenditure on health in Iran is increasing, while the public sector's share is decreasing. Private sector expenditure as out-of-pocket payment is remarkably high as it accounts for more than 50% of the whole expenditure [1]. The modern Iranian pharmaceutical system commenced 100 years ago with the opening of the first modern-style pharmacy by German, French, and Austrian pharmacists in Tehran. Pharmacy training was initiated by European instructors at Darolfonoon, which was remodeled with the inauguration of the Tehran Faculty of Pharmacy in 1934 which undertook a very important role in the Iranian pharmaceutical industry. Established in 1946, Abidi was the first Iranian pharmaceutical company, followed by Tolid Darou and Darou Pakhsh in 1958 and 1963, respectively [2]. After the Islamic revolution, two major motions caused fundamental changes: nationalization of the pharmaceutical industries, and generic scheme. Governmental industry privatization and transition to the semi-governmental sector was one of the major actions taken by the government in the 1988 to 1993 period. This study examines the present situation of the pharmaceutical system

* Correspondence: kebriaee@tums.ac.ir; abdollahiasl@gmail.com
[1]Department of Pharmacoeconomics and Pharmaceutical Administration, Faculty of Pharmacy, Tehran University of Medical Sciences, P.O. Box 14155–6451, Tehran 14174, Iran
[2]Department of Toxicology and Pharmacology, Faculty of Pharmacy, Tehran University of Medical Sciences, P.O. Box 14155–6451, Tehran 14174, Iran
Full list of author information is available at the end of the article

in Iran, including the domestic production companies, importing companies, distribution, regulations, human resources in the pharmaceutical system, and market trend analysis [3].

Present situation of the Iranian pharmaceutical industry

Pharmaceutical production consisted mainly of 89 companies in 2010. The market concentration ratio is low. In 2010, the Herfindahl–Hirschman Index (HHI) was 295.11 for the domestic production companies, indicating little market power. Raw and packaged materials are provided by the domestic and import suppliers. Regarding sales, ten top pharmaceutical companies in 2009–2010 are shown in Table 1. Tamin Pharmaceutical Investment Company (Social Security Organization), Sobhan Pharma Group, and Shafadarou corporation (Melli Bank Investment Corporation) are the most important public owners of the pharmaceutical industry. Based on these structures, pharmaceutical holdings (Groups) sales are shown in Table 2. Data reveals an increasing rate of privatization in pharmaceutical sector.

Import companies

There are 93 private companies engaged in importing medicine, and 30 designated emergency medicine centers besides national medicine and medical equipment corporations. There is Red Crescent (Ministry of Health), Darou pakhsh trade development (Tamin Investment Corporation), and KBC (Sobhan Pharmaceutical Group), which are all public. In 2010, the HHI was 781, which is higher in comparison with that of the domestic production companies. Ten top importer companies in 2009–2010 are shown in Table 3.

Table 1 Ten top domestic production pharmaceutical companies in Iran; 2009-2010

Rank	Company name	Market share	Cumulative market share
1	Darou Pakhsh Pharma	6.6%	6.6%
2	Exir Pharma	6.1%	12.7%
3	Jaber Ebne Hayyan	5.8%	18.5%
4	Farabi	5.3%	23.8%
5	Tehran Chemie	5.2%	29.0%
6	Alborz Darou	3.8%	32.8%
7	Sobhan Darou	3.7%	36.5%
8	Osvah	3.6%	40.1%
9	Dana	2.9%	42.9%
10	Aboureihan	2.8%	45.7%

Distribution

There were 35 nationwide drug distribution companies, among which the first four distribute approximately 70% of the entire market's drugs. All major holdings have their own nationwide drug distribution companies that are ranked in the top four. HHI was 1387, which was significantly higher than that of the domestic production.

Regulations

Passed in 1955, the medicine, drug, food, and drink affairs law act is the cornerstone for the current pharmaceutical procedures in Iran. Most of the bylaws and ordinances are designed and approved in the drug affairs department [2].

Licensing

Production, importation, and distribution of medicinal products are performed under strict control by the authorities, and involve registration and licensure by the food and drug organization (formerly, Undersecretary of Food and Drug).

Pricing

Medicine price is controlled by the food and drug organization through pricing commission regulations in a cost plus basis through comparison with selected companies according to published regulations.

Reimbursement

Medicine cost reimbursement is mainly undertaken by three major organizations: Social Security Organization (public), Medical Services Insurance Organization (governmental), and Medical Insurance Services Organization of Armed Forces (governmental), all of which reimburse the cheapest medicine registered. The emerging supplementary insurance companies are putting constraints on pharmaceutical expenditure. There is a positive list of medicines fully covered by the government that contains specialty drugs.

Human resources

Pharmacists are considered a major source for the pharmaceutical system. Most of the 13000 pharmacist society members are involved in pharmacies. About 6%

Table 2 Major holdings in domestic pharmaceutical production in Iran; 2009-2010

Rank	Pharmaceutical holdings	Market share	Cumulative market share
1	Tamin Investment Corporation	29%	29%
2	Sobhan Pharmaceutical Group	16%	45%
3	Shafadarou Corporation	10%	55%
4	Tehran Chimi Corporation (Private)	10%	65%

Table 3 Ten top importer companies in Iran; 2009-2010

Rank	Company name	Market share	Cumulative market share
1	Cobel	17.2%	17.2%
2	Akbarieh	12.3%	29.6%
3	Behestan Darou	11.6%	41.2%
4	Shafayab Gostar	8.4%	49.6%
5	Jahan Behbood	5.7%	55.3%
6	Ahran Tejarat	5.0%	60.3%
7	Gostaresh Bazargani Daroupakhsh	4.8%	65.1%
8	Actover	3.4%	68.4%
9	KBC	2.6%	71.0%
10	Kavosh Gostar Darou	2.2%	73.2%

of the pharmacists work in the industry. In the industry itself, less than 2% of the trained and scientific workforce is engaged in research and development.

Active pharmaceutical ingredients

A growing number of companies are engaged in the production of Active Pharmaceutical Ingredient (API). Each holding has its own API-producing branch, and there are more than 30 companies engaged in production of APIs. Formal policies of the Ministry of Health actively promote motions towards independence in the API industry. Companies active in the field of API production are mainly possessed by the private sector, contrary to the finished products and distribution companies [4].

Methods

This is a descriptive and cross-sectional study which investigates the Iranian pharmaceutical market over a 13-year period (1997–2010). This study used the Iranian pharmaceutical statistical datasheet published by the Iranian Ministry of Health. Drug consumption statistics are collected by the Food and Drug Organization (FDO) through the data received from the drug distribution companies. All distribution companies deliver their data on drug sales to the pharmacies as a unified format to the food and drug organization on a monthly basis. That data, after revision, is published as the Iranian pharmaceutical statistical datasheet yearly as sales volume (by unit) for any medicine delivered, and cost per medicine unit. Although that data does not represent real drug consumption and the subsidy paid by the government and only reveals the sales of drug to the pharmacies, it is the most unique and convenient method to monitor the pharmaceutical market. Systematic searches of the relevant Persian and English research literature were made, using electronic databases in addition to written reports. Official government documents were also analyzed as sources of data and detailed statements of policy. Different sources, such as statistics published by the Iranian Ministry of Health, pharmaceutical production companies syndicate, and the national medicine assemblies were also researched for statistics and data on medicine consumption in a domestic production and importation separation basis, production and importation statistics, pharmaceutical expenditure, medicine consumption per capita, and drug utilization by sales value in different therapeutic categories.

Results

The trend analysis shows that Iranian pharmaceutical medicine market has been drastically grown in the recent decade. In the period, the population of the country has grown from 61 to 74 million, namely a total and annual growth of 21.3% and 1.53%, respectively. Total medicine market sales value reached $2.467 billion in 2010 from $0.139 billion in 1997, representing a 1669% increase (Figure 1). The annual growth rate was 28.38%. Domestic pharmaceutical production sales value reached $1.639 billion in 2010 in comparison with $0.125 billion in 1997, a 1213% growth. The average annual sales value growth is 9.3%. The correlation coefficient (R^2) of 0.9293 shows a fairly consistent growth, though the 2011 estimate shows a decrease in market sales value. The imported medicine market sales value rose to $0.828 billion in 2010 from $0.015 in 1997, showing a dramatic total growth of 5499%, and an annual growth of 42.3%. In the period under investigation, sales value percentile proportion of imports to total drug consumption has reached 39% from 10.59% in the base year, showing a huge growth of 28.41%. The average sales value percentile proportion of imports to total medicine consumption has been 2.1% (R^2: 0.9612) (Figure 2). The sales value percentile proportion of domestic production to total medicine consumption has reduced from 89.41% to 61% in 2010, revealing a significant decrease of 28%.

Per capita drug consumption sales value

Over the 13-year period, the data indicates that the index has reached $34.43 from $2.28 in 1997, which shows an overwhelming growth of 1405%, and an annual average growth of 10.8% (R^2: 0.9235) (Figure 3). These figures show marked growth in comparison to population growth (20%).

Per capita value of domestic pharmaceutical medicine consumption

This index has reached $22.86 from $2.05 in 1997, with a total and an annual growth of 1018% and 10.8%, respectively (R^2: 0.9397).

Per capita value of the imported medicine consumption

This index has reached $11.57 from $0.24 in 1997, with a total growth of 4373% (R^2: 0.8907).

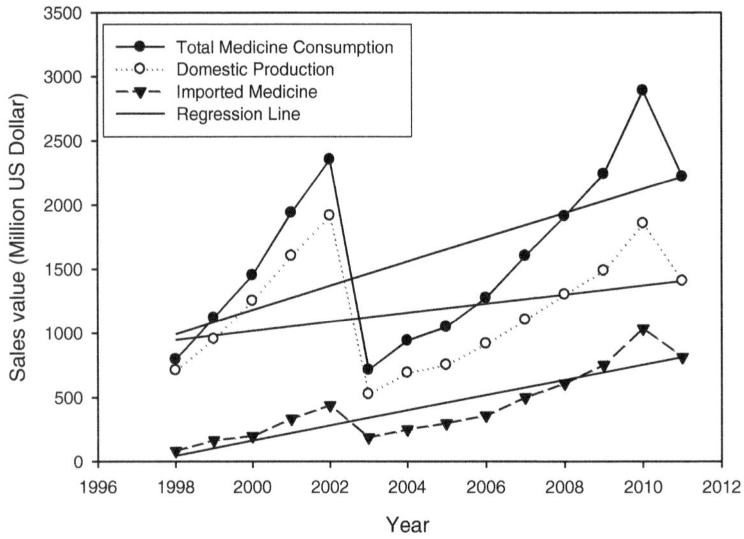

Figure 1 **Total, domestic production and imported medicine consumption by value; 1998–2011.**

Average sales value of the medicines by unit

The index reached an estimated $0.084 in 2011 from $0.009 in 1997, with a growth rate of 847% (R^2: 0.9407) (Figure 4). The average sales value of domestic and imported medicines by unit also shows a total growth rate of 631% (R^2: 0.9506) and 1930% (R^2: 0.8345), respectively.

Drug consumption by therapeutic categorization (by ATC codes)

As the graph depicts, the market shows a point drop in the year 2000 that was due to the nationwide currency exchange rate variation (Figure 5). The data shows that antiinfectives preparations for systemic use and then

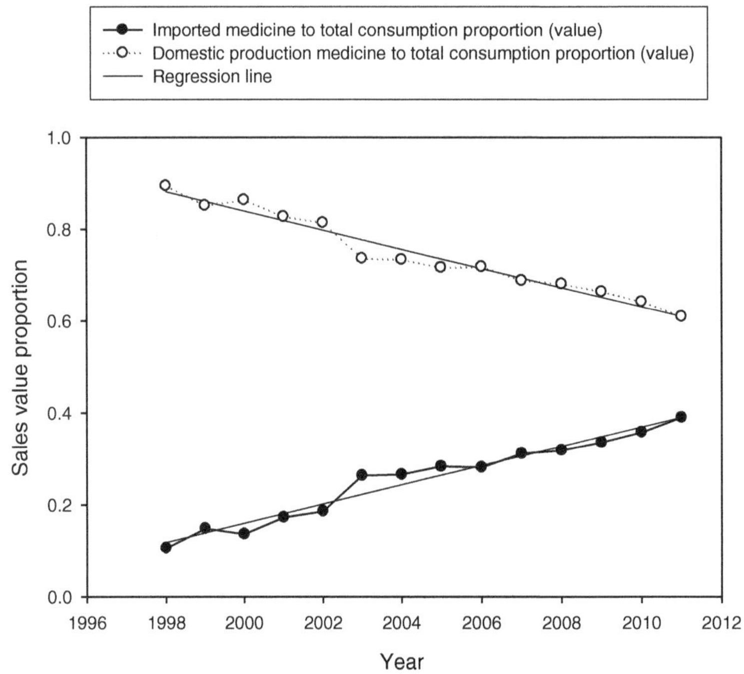

Figure 2 **Sales value percentile proportion of imports and domestic production to the total medicine consumption; 1998–2011.**

antineoplastics and immunomudulating agents seize the most shares in the market and have had the steepest slope among the categories. Alimentary tract and metabolism and nervous system products also show high growth rates. The two recently mentioned categories contain the most prevalent utilization among all in terms of volume (data not shown).

Discussion

This study presents the market environment of the pharmaceutical sector in Iran, and highlights its challenges and future prospects. In order to study a country's medicine market systematically, various indicators can be applied, e.g. market behavior about specific dosage forms or quantity or quality trends [3]. Most owners of the pharmaceutical industry were either dependent on the former regime or foreigners who left Iran after the revolution, so young domestic pharmacists began to manage the pharmaceutical system of the country. Iran-Iraq War (1980–1988) also prompted the need for strict monitoring of the market. The revolutionary government exerted fundamental changes in the food and drug organization in order to assess the need for pharmaceuticals in both general society and for the military forces. With the establishment of the planning office in the food and drug organization, some experts were ascribed to closely monitor the needs and prepare the production and the import scheme. In 1986, the government in office assumed private ownership and liberalization in the economic system, which resulted in magnificent growth in the market. In 1999, the government allowed domestic production companies usage of their free capacity to cross the borders of planning by the food and drug organization. In 2001, further liberalization in the pharmaceutical system and the lack of subsidized currency caused an increase in prices. This liberalization in the pharmaceutical system also augmented imports. Throughout the period, domestic production constituted a major share in the market [3]. The major reasons for the growing demand are as follows [4,5]:

- Iran's demographic structure and population growth;
- increased insurance coverage of the population;
- increased level of income and gross domestic product (GDP) per capita;
- incidence of new diseases and epidemiologic transition, e.g. types of cancer and multiple sclerosis;
- intentionally lowered medicine price; and
- medical sciences advances.

In the period under investigation, accessibility to health services and insurance coverage has grown remarkably, possibly as a result of GDP growth. The government has approached the medicine accessibility positively, and a number of medicines have been included in the medicine list. However, insurance coverage has not expanded simultaneously and proportionately. Health sector budget share in the GDP did not develop acceptably, causing a drastic increase in the public's out-of-pocket payment. Insurance coverage expansion was through three major organizations: the Social Security Organization, Medical Services Insurance Organization, and Medical Insurance Services Organization of Armed Forces. The universal insurance coverage act obliges the population to register for an insurance service which contributes to the goal. Iranian pharmaceutical industries mostly manufacture traditional medicines, and deficiency in the investments needed for monoclonal antibodies and other biotechnology-derived

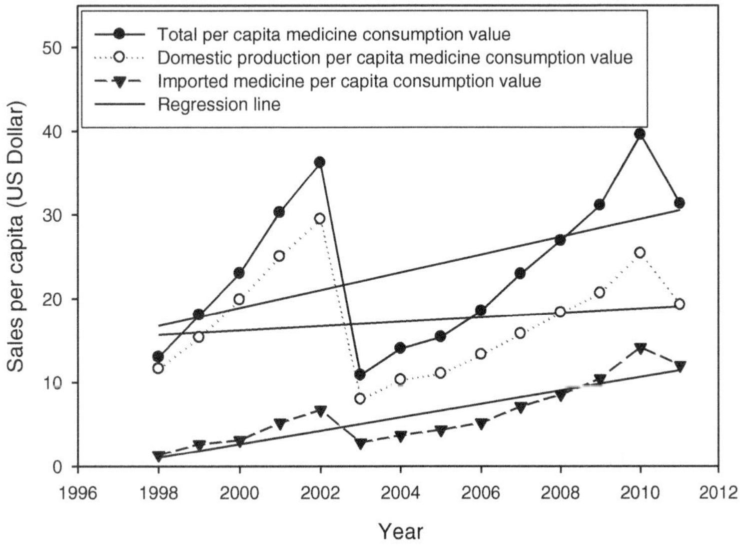

Figure 3 Total, domestic production and import value per capita medicine consumption; 1998–2011.

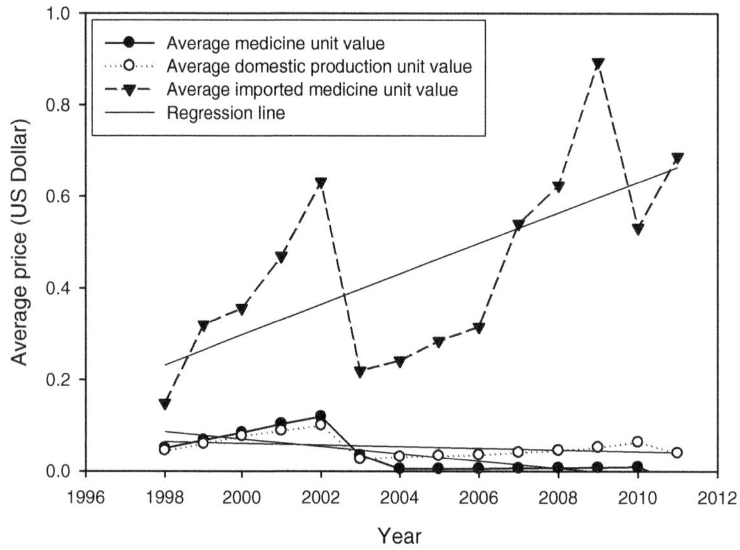

Figure 4 Average sales value of the total, domestic production and imported medicines by unit; 1998–2011.

products, as a consequence, helped the higher share of imported medicine. The Iranian pharmaceutical industry's private sector has not yet developed as much as required. More than 70% of the domestic industries are owned by the government and its related bodies or the public organizations. As evidenced by the two existing biotechnology companies, both of which are privately-owned, privatization can lead to greater sustainable development in domestic industries [6,7]. Currently, total pharmaceutical market value is about $3.2 billion, or as much as $4-4.5 billion according to some estimates on the real market size [8]. The present difference between real and estimated value is attributed to the price suppression policies of the authorities [9]. It should also be noted that national currency has experienced a drastic devaluation against USD. Iran experiences an average growth rate of 28.38%, which is significantly more than developing countries such as China and India which have around 11 to 15% growth [10,11]. The results show that the domestic production sales value has grown, but not in concordance with that of the imported medicine sales value. The results also imply that the current pharmaceutical policies are in favor of imports, as the slope of the import and domestic production lines illustrate. The rise in Iranian pharmaceutical expenditure is expected to continue at a significant, even higher rate than expected from developing countries, based on factors mentioned above and the deliberate deficiencies of pharmaceutical policy [12,13]. Medicines are regarded as both public and industry goods. Iranian patients are entitled to have access to high-quality, timely, and cost-effective medicine [14,15]. The Iranian

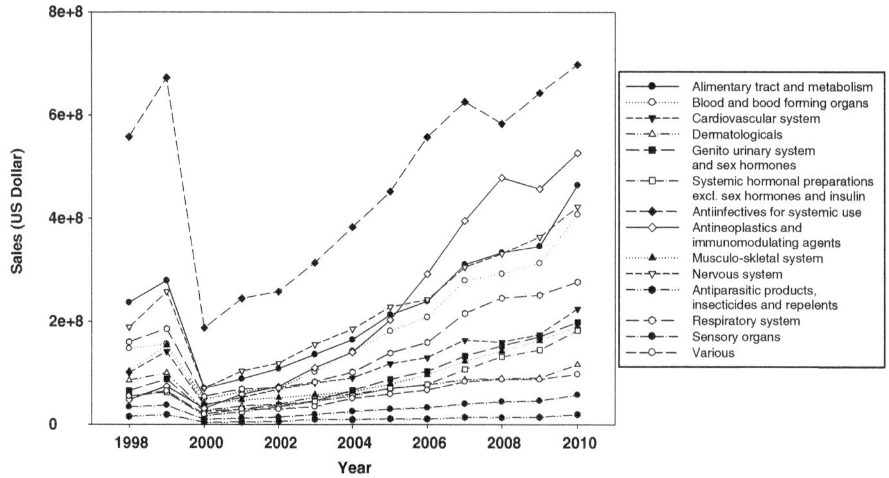

Figure 5 Medicine consumption by value in therapeutic categories; 1998–2010.

pharmaceutical market is predicted to maintain its growth for years to come. Currently, 20% of Iran's total health expenditure, on average, goes on medicine (reimbursed by the insurance organizations, based on their reports to the supreme insurance council for last year). Antibiotics, antineoplastics and immunomudulating agents (medicines mostly used for organ transplantation rejection prohibition), antidiabetics, and alimentary tract medications gain the most value in the market (Figure 5). Regarding sales volume, analgesics, antibiotics, and second generation antidiabetics are the best sellers. Investigating the mostly used products among the two top categories it is obvious that pharmaceutical biotechnology derived medicines such as proteins and monoclonal antibodies take major positions (results not presented). Considering the items mentioned, it is concluded that new and high tech medicines are seizing a large share of the market; which should incite policy makers to change for the better. If the market continues its growth, a great financial load will be imposed on the health system. Iran contains nearly 1% of the world's population, but only about 0.3% of the world market, so if the two are in an agreement, Iran should assume $7-8 billion in 2010, and $10-12 billion in 2020. Generic medicine use is an important component of the government's health plan that was obligatory through the generic scheme shortly after the revolution. The policy assisted the country pass the constraints of the 1980s, but vitally restricted research and development in the domestic industry, while exerting severe price containment policies [16]. Current issues of interest for the Iranian pharmaceutical market include a rise in imports and simultaneous fall in domestic production. Low rates of investment, capital asset substitution, scarce attention to modern technologies like pharmaceutical biotechnology, and a branded medicine market are possible reasons for this domestic medicine market shrinkage [17,18]. The investment activity of pharmaceutical companies is dependant mainly on product demand, profits, technological developments, and capital availability. It is vital to notice the steady decrease in investment rate for capital equipment replacement. This is associated with the market shift towards imported medicines and the lack of well-designed, long-term policies to support the domestic pharmaceutical industry that would potentiate reasonable conditions to encourage domestic production [19]. Meanwhile vast research projects have been conducted in the universities and research centers but few of them have been commercialized into medicines. Performing studies aligned with the needs of the biopharmaceutical industry could be seen as a choice. Policy makers and authorities could contribute the national production capabilities by establishing the basements to commercialize the researches, revising the policies, forming close relationships and cooperative committees with the biopharmaceutical industries and applying evidence based decision making procedures.

Conclusions

The absence of significant basic and applied biopharmaceutical research that can result in industrial breakthroughs and attain competitive advantage in Iran has induced a state of regression in the domestic industry that has accelerated a drain on the capital and energy of the industry. Such conditions, along with price suppression, increase imports [20,21]. It is advised that policy makers take all necessary measures towards establishing an appropriate pharmaceutical business environment that favors domestic production, as well as controlling rising expenditure in the pharmaceutical sector [22]. We can conclude that the average value of imported medicine per unit is growing, which suggests technological content is in continuous improvement in comparison with domestic ones [23-25]. Medicine consumption per capita shows that this index is high in Iran. Therefore, it is proposed that conducting applied research projects ordered by the biopharmaceutical industries along with preparing the requirements for commercialization of novel fields like pharmaceutical biotechnology which assigns a great share in the national pharmaceutical expenditure be in the top agenda.

Abbreviations

HHI: Herfindahl–Hirschman Index; API: Active Pharmaceutical Ingredient; FDO: Food and Drug organization; GDP: Gross Domestic Product; ATC: Anatomical Therapeutic Chemical Classification System.

Competing interests

The authors declare that they have no competing interests.

Authors' contributions

AK conceived the strategy of study and supervised the project, NNK conceived and implemented the strategy, performed the data analysis and statistical interpretation and drafted the paper, AA gave consultation on designing the study, complemented the data and statistical analysis, SN gave consultation on the study methodology and edited the draft, NM performed the data analysis. All authors read and approved the final manuscript.

Acknowledgements

The authors are thankful to the Food and Drug Organization (FDO) and Department of Planning and Statistics for providing the data for the project.

Author details

[1]Department of Pharmacoeconomics and Pharmaceutical Administration, Faculty of Pharmacy, Tehran University of Medical Sciences, P.O. Box 14155-6451, Tehran 14174, Iran. [2]Department of Toxicology and Pharmacology, Faculty of Pharmacy, Tehran University of Medical Sciences, P.O. Box 14155-6451, Tehran 14174, Iran. [3]Management Information System Division, Osvah Pharmaceutical Company, Tehran, Iran.

References

1. Ensor T, Weinzierl S: **Regulating health care in low- and middle-income countries: Broadening the policy response in resource constrained environments.** *Soc Sci Med* 2007, **65**:355–366.
2. Kebrieezadeh A, Eslamitabar S, Khatibi M: *Iranian pharmaceutical law and regulations.* 2nd edition. Tehran: Razico; 2009.
3. Reinhardt UE: **An information infrastructure for the pharmaceutical market.** *Health Aff* 2004, **23**(1):107–112.

4. Davari M, Walley T, Haycox A: **Pharmaceutical policy and market in Iran: past experiences and future challenges.** *J Pharm Health Serv Res* 2011, **2**:47–52.
5. Cheraghali AM: **Pharmacoeconomics: An Effective Tool for Prioritization in Iran Healthcare System.** *Iranian J Pharm Res* 2008, **7**(2):89–91.
6. Kebriee-zadeh A: **Overview of National Drug Policy of Iran.** *IJPR* 2003:1–2.
7. Faden L, Vialle-Valentin C, Ross-Degnan D, Wagner A: **Active pharmaceutical management strategies of health insurance systems to improve cost-effective use of medicines in low- and middle-income countries: A systematic review of current evidence.** *Health Policy* 2011, **100**:134–143.
8. Cheraghali AM: **Pharmaceutical Market.** *IJPR* 2006, **1**:1–7.
9. Rusu A, Kuokkanen K, Heier A: **Current trends in the pharmaceutical industry - A case study approach.** *Eur J Pharm Sci* 2011, **44**:437–440.
10. Drews J: **Strategic trends in the drug industry.** *Drug Discov Today* 2003, **8**(9):411–420.
11. Nikfar S, Kebriaeezadeh A, Majdzadeh R, Abdollahi M: **Monitoring of National Drug Policy (NDP) and its standardized indicators; conformity to decisions of the National Drug Selecting Committee in Iran.** *BMC Int Health Hum Rights* 2005, **5**:5.
12. Kontozamanis V, Mantzouneas E, Stoforos C: **An overview of the Greek pharmaceutical market.** *Eur J Health Econ* 2003, **4**:327–333.
13. Eisenberg DM, Davis RB, Ettner SL, Appel S, Wilkey S, Rompay MV, *et al*: **Trends in alternative medicine use in the United States, 1990–1997, results of a follow-up national survey.** *JAMA* 1998, **280**(18):1569–1575.
14. Tokgöz T: **The Turkish pharmaceutical market.** *JGM* 2010, **7**:270–274.
15. Tetteh EK: **Providing affordable essential medicines to African households: The missing policies and institutions for price containment.** *Soc Sci Med* 2008, **66**:569–581.
16. Cameron A, Ewen M, Ross-Degnan D, Ball D, Laing R: **Medicine prices, availability, and affordability in 36 developing and middle-income countries: a secondary analysis.** *Lancet* 2009, **373**:240–249.
17. Oortwijn W, Mathijssen J, Banta D: **The role of health technology assessment on pharmaceutical reimbursement in selected middle-income countries.** *Health Policy* 2010, **95**:174–184.
18. Kutaini D: **Pharmaceutical industry in Syria.** *J Med Life* 2010, **3**(3):348–350.
19. Ghislandi S, Krulichova I, Garattini L: **Pharmaceutical policy in Italy: towards a structural change?** *Health Policy* 2005, **72**:53–63.
20. Merkur S, Mossialos E: **A pricing policy towards the sourcing of cheaper drugs in Cyprus.** *Health Policy* 2007, **81**:368–375.
21. Aaserud M, Dahlgren AT, Kosters JP, Oxman AD, Ramsay C, Sturm H: **Pharmaceutical policies: effects of reference pricing, other pricing, and purchasing policies.** *Cochrane Database Syst Rev* 2006, **2**:.
22. Lockhart M, Babar ZUD, Garg S: **Evaluation of policies to support drug development in New Zealand.** *Health Policy* 2010, **96**:108–117.
23. Kisa A: **Analysis of the pharmaceuticals market and its technological development in Turkey.** *Int J Technol Assess Health Care* 2006, **22**(4):537–542.
24. Abdollahiasl A, Kebriaeezadeh A, Nikfar S, Farshchi A, Ghiasi G, Abdollahi M: **Patterns of antibiotic consumption in Iran during 2000–2009.** *Int J Antimicrob Agents* 2011, **37**:489–490.
25. Abdollahiasl A, Nikfar S, Kebriaeezadeh A, Dinarvand R, Abdollahi M: **A model for developing a decision support system to simulate national drug policy indicators.** *Arch Med Sci* 2011, **5**:744–746.

Induction of G1 cell cycle arrest and cyclin D1 down-regulation in response to pericarp extract of *Baneh* in human breast cancer T47D cells

Parisa Fathi Rezaei[1,2], Shamileh Fouladdel[1,3], Seyed Mahmood Ghaffari[4], Gholamreza Amin[5] and Ebrahim Azizi[1*]

Abstract

Background and the purpose of the study: Natural products from plants have an important role in the development and production of new drugs mainly for cancer therapy. More recently, we have shown that the pericarp methanolic extract of *Pistacia atlantica sub kurdica* (with local name of *Baneh*) as a rich source of active biological components with high antioxidant and radical scavenging activities, has ability to cease proliferation and induce apoptosis in T47D human breast cancer cells. The present study aimed to clarify whether *Baneh* extract able to alter cell cycle progression of T47D cells or not.

Methods: In order to study the possible effect of *Baneh* extract on cell cycle of T47D cells, we evaluated cell cycle distribution and its regulatory proteins by flow cytometry and western blot analysis respectively.

Results: *Baneh* extract induced G_0/G_1 cell cycle arrest in conjunction with a marked decrease in expression of cyclin D1 and cdk4 that was strongly dependent on time of exposure. In parallel, Dox-treated T47D cells in early time points were accumulated on S phase, but after 48 h cell cycle progression was inhibited on G_2/M. Dox promoted striking accumulation of cyclin B1 rapidly and enhanced cyclin A abundance.

Conclusion: Taken together, our results establish that the antitumor activity of the pericarp extract of *Baneh* partly is mediated via cell cycle arrest and downregulation of cyclin D1 and cdk4 expression. These findings warrant further evaluation regarding the mechanism(s) of action of this promising anticancer agent.

Keywords: Pistacia atlantica, Breast carcinoma, Cell cycle, Cyclins, Doxorubicin

Introduction

Breast cancer is one of the most common cancers in women worldwide and Iran in particular. Each year over 1.15 million women are diagnosed with breast cancer and nearly half of them die [1]. Thus, new therapeutic steps should be taken both to prevent the development of cancer and to lower mortality rates related to it.

The characteristic feature of tumor cells is uncontrolled cell growth as a result of alterations in a variety of molecules and regulatory pathways involved in cell cycle control [2]. Mitogenic signals induce cyclin D1 expression and binding to cdk4/ or cdk6 in G1 phase of the cell cycle. Then cyclin E/cdk2 activated in late G_1 phase. Cdk2 forms complex with cyclin A in S phase to induce proteins which involved in DNA replication. Cdk1/cyclin A is necessary for initiation of prophase and finally cdk1/cyclin B complex takes part in and completes mitosis [3].

Lately, a significant increase has been seen in the search for new effective cancer chemopreventive and chemotherapeutic agents, particularly for those that have a natural origin and relatively low toxicity [4]. Polyphenolic compounds, in addition to their antioxidant activity, could regulate the genes that are critical for the control of proliferation, cell cycle and apoptosis in cancer cells. Based on epidemiological and preclinical data, polyphenolic phytochemicals possess cancer chemopreventive properties [5]. The cancer preventive effects of polyphenols are due to the regulation of signaling pathways including; nuclear factor-kB (NF-kB), activator protein-1 (AP-1) or mitogen-activated protein kinases (MAPK) [6].

* Correspondence: aziziebr@tums.ac.ir
[1]Molecular Research Lab, Department of Pharmacology and Toxicology, Faculty of Pharmacy, Tehran University of Medical Sciences, Tehran, Iran
Full list of author information is available at the end of the article

Pistacia atlantica sub *kurdica*, known as *Baneh* by the natives, is an Iranian plant from *Anacardiaceae* family; grow in large populations in the western, central and eastern parts of Iran. Its nuts are used by the natives and its gum is used in the production of chewing gum [7]. *Pistacia* species has medicinal applications in different countries [8]. Only phytochemical analysis and apoptosis induction of *Baneh* pericarp extract on T47D and HT29 cells were reported by our group [9,10]. A wide range of investigations have exhibited anticancer potency of mastic gum of *P. lentiscus var. chia* in different cell culture systems including; prostate cancer, colon cancer, human colorectal xenografts, leukemia and Lewis lung carcinoma [9].

In view of the previously mentioned effects of *Baneh* extract on cell viability and apoptosis induction of T47D cells, we investigated whether the *Baneh* extract is involved in cell cycle progression of T47D cells.

Materials and methods

Materials

RPMI 1640 and FBS were obtained from Biosera (East Sussex, UK). Pen-strep and Trypsin-EDTA were purchased from Gibco (Paeiley, UK). Doxorubicin (EbeDoxo) was purchased from Ebewe (Unterach, Austria). Methanol was obtained from Merck (Darmstadt, Germany). The cell culture petridishes were obtained from Greiner Bio-one (Frickenhausen, Germany). DAPI (4,6-diamidino-2-phenylindole) and Nonidet P40 were purchased from Roche (Mannheim, Germany).

Plant materials and extraction

Fresh unripe fruits from *P. atlantica subsp kurdica* were gathered from Kurdestan province of Iran in June and recognized by Dr. Amin, Department of Pharmacy, Tehran University of Medical Sciences *(6673-THE)*. The pericarp methanolic extract of *Baneh* and its working concentrations were prepared as previously described by our group [9].

Cell culture

The human breast cancer cell line T47D (ATCC, HTB-133) was obtained from Pasteur institute (Tehran, Iran) and maintained in RPMI 1640 medium supplemented with 10% heat-inactivated fetal bovine serum, 100 μg/ml streptomycin and 100 U/ml penicillin under conditions of 5% CO_2 atmosphere at 37°C.

Cell cycle analysis

DAPI staining was used to determine the distribution of cells in different phases of the cell cycle by flow cytometry analysis [11]. Briefly, cells were treated with IC_{50} of *Baneh* extract (1 mg/ml) and Dox (250 nM) which was previously determined and reported by our group [9]. Treated and untreated cells were trypsinized, resuspended in DAPI staining solution and analyzed by Partec flow cytometer then data analysis was done using FloMax software.

Western blotting

Alteration in cell cycle regulatory proteins in presence of the *Baneh* extract and Dox was investigated by western blot as previously explained [12]. Briefly, the cells were lysed in lysis buffer. Then the total proteins were electrophoresed on a 12% SDS-PAGE, transferred to nitrocellulose membranes (Amersham pharmacia Biotech, Germany) and probed with following primary antibodies: mouse monoclonal cyclin D1 (BD Bioscience, USA); cyclin A, cyclin B1, cyclin E, cdk1, cdk2, cdk4, cdk6 (Santa Cruz Biotechnology, USA) and β-actin (Sigma, Germany); rabbit polyclonal cdk4 (Santa Cruz Biotechnology). We also used goat-anti-mouse IgG and goat-anti-rabbit IgG (Santa Cruz Biotechnology) conjugated to horseradish peroxidase as secondary antibodies. Immunoreactive polypeptides were detected by chemiluminescence using enhanced electrochemiluminescence (ECL) reagents (Amersham bioscience, Germany) and subsequent autoradiography.

Statistical analysis

All cell cycle analysis data were shown as mean±SE of three independent experiments. Data were statistically compared using one-way ANOVA with Tukey post hoc and $P<0.05$ were considered statistically significant.

Results

Effects on cell cycle distribution

Flow cytometry method showed that by increasing the time, *Baneh* treated cells were accumulated in G_0/G_1 phase compared to the control cells. Within 48 h ~ 80% of the cells were at the G_0/G_1 phase versus ~58% in the control cells. Dox exposed cells exhibited accumulation of the cells in S and by increasing the time, the cell cycle pattern was changed to G_2/M accumulation of the cells and after 48 h 91% of the cells were at the G_2/M phase against 19% in the control cells (Table 1).

Effects on cell cycle regulation

To further ascertain the molecular mechanisms involved in cell cycle block of T47D cells, western blot analysis was performed. As shown in Figure 1, the G_0/G_1 block of the cell cycle in *Baneh* treated cells was supported by the intensive down-regulation of cyclin D1 and cdk4, according to the exposure time. Cyclin E protein level was increased at early time points but strong down-regulation of cyclin E was happened after 48 h. Also cyclin A and cdk2 levels were decreased, but not in a time dependent manner, showing considerable decrease at 72 h. In addition, cyclin B1 level was decreased strongly at early time points and approximately disappeared after 48 h. Furthermore, in Dox-exposed cells, the G_2/M delay of cell cycle progression

Table 1 Alteration in the cell cycle distribution of T47D cells

	Groups	12 h	24 h	48 h	72 h
	CTRL	58.44 ± 0.056	58.74 ± 0.403	58.085 ± 0.96	51.96 ± 0.056
G_0/G_1	B	64.63 ± 0.5*	68.25 ± 1.9**	79.90 ± 0.91**	80.77 ± 31**
	DOX	36.91 ± 2.63**	14.97 ± 0.45**	4.59 ± 0.69**	3.95 ± 0.11**
	CTRL	23.35 ± 0.42	25.39 ± 1.86	22.92 ± 2.54	28.45 ± 2.27
S	B	24.99 ± 1	21.25 ± 0	12.85 ± 1.04*	12.17 ± 0.67**
	DOX	34.71 ± 1.45	49.69 ± 2.55*	4.98 ± 0.74**	4.51 ± 0.92**
	CTRL	18.21 ± 0.36	15.86 ± 2.26	18.99 ± 1.57	19.58 ± 2.34
G_2/M	B	10.41 ± 1.45	10.88 ± 0.73	7.24 ± 0.13*	7.05 ± 0.36*
	DOX	27.93 ± 3.46	35.35 ± 2.05*	90.9 ± 2.19**	91.51 ± 1.03**

CTRL: untreated cells.
B: *Baneh* extract-treated cells.
All data were shown as mean ± SE of three independent experiments. Data were statistically compared using one-way ANOVA with Tukey post hoc and $P<0.05$ were considered statistically significant.
*p<0.05 and **p<0.001 in comparison to control RPMI (CTRL).

was confirmed by the induction of cyclin B1 accumulation in comparison to the control cells. Cdk1 protein expression level showed strong increase within 24–48 h in comparison to the control cells. On the other hand, cyclin A and cdk2 levels in Dox exposed cells were higher than control cells. The expression of cdk4 and cdk6 were quietly similar to their expression in control cells. Dox induced upregulation of cyclin E at early time points but its expression was decreased after 48 h. Cyclin D1 expression in *Baneh* treated cells was higher than its expression in control cells within 12 and 24 h but was reduced after 48 h (Figure 1).

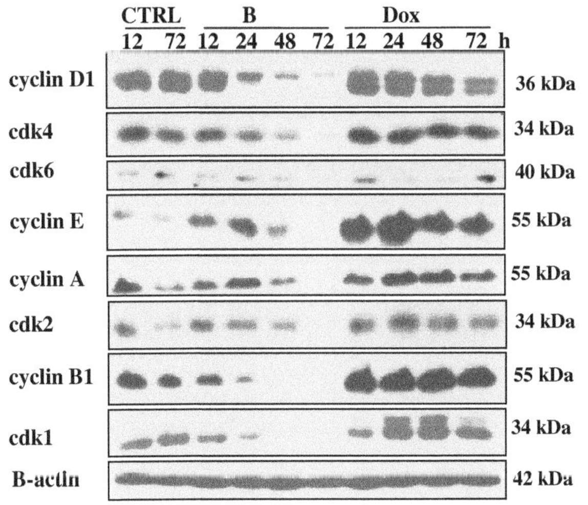

Figure 1 Expression of cell cycle-regulatory proteins. Cells were treated with RPMI (CTRL), *Baneh* 1 mg/ml (B) and Dox 250 nM for 12–72 h. Expression of cell cycle-regulatory proteins for indicated time points were analyzed by western blotting. B-actin is showed as loading control. A representative experiment of three independent experiments is shown.

Discussion

Chemotherapeutic approach which uses various natural (plant-derived) agents has become the focus of widespread attention for managing cancers in recent years; it is hoped that such studies will show a positive outcome to provide a scientific basis as to being efficient and useful in chemoprevention/chemotherapy of various cancers.

Reduction in metabolic activity of the cell is due to reduction in number of the cells for cell cycle block and/or cell death. Since the 30% induction of apoptosis in *Baneh*-treated T47D cells could not be enough to explain the reduction in cell viability observed with MTT assay, we decided to check the effect of *Baneh* extract on the cell cycle progression.

Uncontrolled cell cycle has a pivotal role in cancer incidence. Our results demonstrated that *Baneh* extract blocked the cell cycle in G_0/G_1 phase in a time dependent manner up to 48 h (Table 1) accompanied by down regulation of positive regulators of G_1/S transition including cyclin D1 and cdk4, depending on the time of exposure (Figure 1).

With respect to the phytochemical evaluation, the extract possesses considerable amounts of polyphenolic compounds including flavonoids and anthocyanins [10]. Dietary flavonoids inhibit the proliferation of various cancer cells and tumor growth in animal models [5]. Recent studies have shown that polyphenols directly or indirectly can inhibit different cells at different cell cycle phases [6]. Recently, S phase delay of *Baneh*-treated HT29 cells was reported by our group [10]. Pc-3 (prostate cancer cells) treated with gum mastic of *P. lentiscus* showed cyclin D1 downregulation and G1 block of the cell cycle [13]. Treatment of LNcap cells with Gum mastic led to downregulation of cyclin D1 [14]. HCT116-treated cells with chios mastic gum (CMG) were shown G_1cell cycle arrest [15]. It is established that a single polyphenol is capable of interacting with several protein kinases [16].

Polyphenolic compounds have phytoestrogenic activity [17]. T47D cells are known as ER+ (Estrogen Receptor) cells [18]. Estrogenic estradiols, act through the regulation of expression and function of the G_1 phase regulatory proteins and promote transition through G_1 phase. Cyclin D1, c-Myc, p21 and cyclin E-cdk2 are estrogen downstream targets [19]. Estradiol can increase cyclin D1 expression by stimulating cyclin D1 transcription via PI3-Kinase/Akt pathway [20]. The inhibitory effect of anti-estrogens on estrogen receptor activity leads to decreased cyclin D1 expression and dissociation of p21 and p27 from the cyclin D1-cdk4/6 complex then association with cyclinE-cdk2 complexes [21]. Because of the promoting effects of estrogen on expression of the cycling D1, it is conceivable that *Baneh* extract involves component(s) which act as anti-estrogenic agent in T47D cells. It has been established that anti-estrogen treatment of MCF7 breast cancer cells induced reduction of c-Myc expression, resulting in cyclin D1 downregulation and eventually cell cycle arrest [19]. In tamoxifen-treated T47D cells, G_0/G_1 delay of cell cycle was reported [22]. Cyclin D1 expression and p53 status, both at the gene and protein level, revealed a highly significant association. Cyclin D1 may be one of the downstream effectors of p53 [23]. Loss of G_1/S control and loss of p53 are two serious factors in tumor formation which directly affect cell-cycle checkpoints [24]. The status of p53 and ER affect the response of breast cancer cells to exogenous agents. T47D cells express mutated and nonfunctional form of p53 [25].

It is reported that NF-κB promotes G_1-to-S phase transition in mouse embryonic fibroblasts and in T47D carcinoma cells. Inhibition of NF-κB induces pRb phosphorylation and inhibits G_1-to-S phase transition. NF-κB can functionally interact with other transcription factors which regulate cyclin D1 promoter including; c-Fos/c-Jun, SP1, E2F1 [26]. According to the findings, inhibition of signal transduction proteins in the pathways linked to activation of NF-κB, in part is responsible for the cell cycle arrest and remarkable cyclin D1 reduction induced by *Baneh* extract in T47D cells.

Cyclin D1 is amplified and or overexpressed in a subset of human cancers including breast cancer [27]. Due to the astonishing downregulation effect of *Baneh* extract on cyclin D1 abundance it could be a good candidate for malignancies with deregulated expression of this protein.

Doxorubicin is one of the most common anticancer drugs and is used for the treatment of human cancers. The main anticancer effect of Dox is due to DNA damage and resulting growth arrest or cell death [28]. Dox treated cells shown G_2/M type of cell cycle arrest associated with cyclin B1enhancment (Table 1 and Figure 1). Increased expression of cyclin B1 and G2/M delay of cell cycle in Dox-treated HT29 cells was reported by our group [10]. Increased cyclin A expression, accumulation of cells at G_2/M and number of apoptotic cells in Dox-treated k562 cells were described [29]. Maximized level of cyclin B1 protein in T47D exposed cells with Dox (10 ng/ml) has been shown [18]. Previously, Ling et al., demonstrated that in p388 murine leukemia cells, Dox caused G_2/M cell cycle arrest, reduced p34 kinase activity, increased cyclin B1, alteration of cyclin B1/cdk1 complex function and/or DNA damage may trigger apoptosis [30]. Recently, induction of apoptosis in Dox-treated T47D cells was shown by our group [9]. This is the first report to show that *Baneh* extract can cease cell cycle progression of T47D cells.

Conclusion

Overall, our results clearly indicate that *Baneh* extract as a potent and novel natural anticancer agent able to cease cell cycle progression of T47D cells at G_0/G_1 phase associated with downregulation of cyclin D1 by increasing the exposure time. Therefore decreased cyclin D1 expression could be a potential mechanism of growth inhibition by *Baneh* extract. Based on these findings, *Baneh* extract might be a good candidate for cancer therapy but further studies are necessary for in depth investigations of mechanism(s) of action of *Baneh* extract.

Competing interests

The authors declare that they have no competing interests.

Authors' contribution

FRP: Conducting experiments and manuscript preparation, FSh: Conducting molecular experiments Ghaffari SM: Supervising experiments. AGh: Supervising herbal experiments AE: Project design, supervising experiments and manuscript preparation. All authors read and approve the final manuscript.

Acknowledgement

Authors would like to thank the office of Vice-Chancellor for research of Tehran University of Medical Sciences (TUMS) for financial support of this PhD research project.

Author details

[1]Molecular Research Lab, Department of Pharmacology and Toxicology, Faculty of Pharmacy, Tehran University of Medical Sciences, Tehran, Iran. [2]Department of Microbiology and Molecular cell biology, Faculty of Science, University of Maragheh, Maragheh, Iran. [3]Research Institute for Islamic and Complementary Medicine, Tehran University of Medical Sciences, Tehran, Iran. [4]Department of Biochemistry, IBB, University of Tehran, Tehran, Iran. [5]Department of Pharmacognosy, Faculty of Pharmacy, Tehran University of Medical Sciences, Tehran, Iran.

References

1. Montazeri A, Vahdaninia M, Harrirchi I, Harrirchi A, Khaleghi F: **Breast cancer in Iran: need for greater women awareness of warning signs and effective screening methods.** *Asia Pacific Family Medicine* 2007, **7**:1–6.

2. Graf F, Kohler L, Kniess T, Wuest F, Mosch B, Pietzsch J: **Cell cycle regulating kinase cdk4 as a potential target for tumor cell treatment and tumor imaging.** *J Oncol* 2009, **2009:**1–12.
3. Coqueret O: **Linking cyclins to transcriptional control.** *Gene* 2002, **299:**35–55.
4. Greenwald P: **Clinical trials in cancer prevention: current results and perspectives for the future.** *J Nutr* 2004, **134:**3507–3512.
5. Szliszka E, Czuba ZP, Jemas K, Krol W: **Dietary flavonoids sensitize Hela cells to tumor necrosis factor-related apoptosis-inducing ligand (TRAIL).** *Int J Mol Sci* 2008, **9:**56–64.
6. Fresco P, Borges F, Diniz C, Marques MPM: **New insights on the anticancer properties of dietary polyphenols.** *Med Res Rev* 2006, **26:**747–766.
7. Daneshrad A, Aynehchi Y: **Chemical studies of the oil from *Pistacia* nuts growing wild in Iran.** *J Am Oil Chem Soc* 1980, **57:**248–249.
8. Peksel A: **Antioxidative properties of decoction of *Pistacia atlantica Desf* leaves.** *Asian J Chem* 2008, **20:**681–693.
9. Fathi Rezaei P, Fouladdel S, Cristofanon S, Ghaffari SM, Amin GR, Azizi E: **Comparative cellular and molecular analysis of cytotoxicity and apoptosis induction by doxorubicin and *Baneh* in human breast cancer T47D cells.** *Cytotechnology* 2011, **63:**503–512.
10. Fathi Rezaei P, Fouladdel S, Hassani S, Yousefbeyk F, Ghaffari SM, Amin GR, Azizi E: **Induction of apoptosis and cell cycle arrest by pericarp polyphenol-rich extract of *Baneh* in human colon carcinoma HT29 cells.** *Food Chem Toxicol* 2012, **501:**1054–1059.
11. Abdolmohammadi MH, Fouladdel S, Shafiee A, Amin GR, Ghaffari SM, Azizi E: **Anticancer effects and cell cycle analysis on human breast cancer T47D cells treated with extracts of *Astrodaucus persicus (Boiss) Drude* in comparison to doxorubicin.** *Daru J Pharm Sci* 2008, **16:**112–118.
12. Fulda S, Sieverts H, Friesen C, Herr I, Debatin KM: **The CD95 (apo-1/fas) system mediates drug-induced apoptosis in neuroblastoma cells.** *Cancer Res* 1997, **57:**3823–3829.
13. He ML, Li A, Xu CS, Wang SL, Zhang ML, Gu H, Yang YQ, Tao HH: **Mechanisms of antiprostate cancer by gum mastic: NF-κB signal as target.** *Acta Pharmacol Sin* 2007, **28:**446–425.
14. He ML, Yuan HQ, Jiang AL, Gong AY, Chen WW, Zhang PJ, Young CYF, Zhang JY: **Gum mastic inhibits the expression and function of the androgen receptor in prostate cancer cells.** *Cancer* 2006, **106:**2547–2555.
15. Balan KV, Prince J, Han Z, Dimas K, Cladras M, Wyche JH, Sitaras NM, Pantazis P: **Antiproliferative activity and induction of apoptosis in human colon cancer cells treated in vitro with constituents of a product derived from *Pistacia lentiscus* L. *var. chia.*** *Phytomedicine* 2007, **14:**263–272.
16. Theys DL, Pottier L, Dufranse F, Neve J, Dubois J, Komienko A, Kiss R, Ingrassia L: **Natural polyphenols that display anticancer properties through inhibition of kinase activity.** *Curr Med Chem* 2010, **17:**812–825.
17. Yi W, Fischer J, Krewer G, Akoh CC: **Phenolic compounds from blueberries can inhibit colon cancer cell proliferation and induce apoptosis.** *J Agr food chem* 2005, **53:**7320–7329.y.
18. Wang YA, Johnson SK, Brown BL, McCarragher LM, Al-Sakkaf K, Royds JA, Dobson PR: **Enhanced anti-cancer effect of a phosphatidylinositol-3 kinase inhibitor and doxorubicin on human breast epithelial cell lines with different p53 and oestrogen receptor status.** *Int J Cancer* 2008, **123:**1536–1544.
19. Doisneau-Sixou SF, Sergio CM, Carroll JS, Hui R, Musgrove EA, Sutherland RL: **Estrogen and antiestrogen regulation of cell cycle progression in breast cancer cells.** *Endocr Relat Cancer* 2003, **10:**179–186.
20. Brunelli E, Piton G, Bellini P, Minassi A, Appendino G, Moro L: **Flavonoid-induced autophagy in hormone sensitive breast cancer cells.** *Fitoterapia* 2009, **80:**327–332.
21. Michalides R, Van Tinteren H, Balkenende A, Vermoken JB, Benraadt J, Huldij J, Diest PV: **Cyclin A is a prognostic indicator in early stage breast cancer with and without tamoxifen treatment.** *Br J Cancer* 2002, **86:**402–408.
22. Abdolmohammadi AH, Fouladdel S, Shafiee A, Amin GR, Ghaffari SM, Azizi E: **Antiproliferative and apoptotic effect of *Astrodaucus orientalis* (L.) *drude* on T47D human breast cancer cell line: potential mechanisms of action.** *Afr J Biotechnol* 2009, **8:**4265–4276.
23. Bukholm IK, Berner JM, Nesland JM, Borresen-Dale AL: **Expression of cyclin Ds in relation to p53 status in human breast carcinoma.** *Virchows Arch* 1998, **433:**223–228.
24. Berthet C, Kaldis P: **Cell-specific responses to loss of cyclin-dependent kinases.** *Oncogene* 2007, **26:**4469–4477.
25. Vayssade M, Haddada H, Faridoni-Laurens L, Tourpin S, Valent A, Benard J, Ahomadegbe JC: **p73 functionally replaces p53 in Adriamycin-treated p53-deficient breast cancer cells.** *Int J Cancer* 2005, **116:**860–869.
26. Hinz M, Krappmann D, Eichten A, Heder A, Scheidereit C, Strauss M: **NF-κB function in growth control: regulation of cyclin D1 and G0/G1-to-S phase transition.** *Mol Cell Biol* 2005, **19:**2690–2698.
27. Fu M, Wang C, Li Z, Sakamaki T, Pestell RG: **Minireview: Cyclin D1: Normal and abnormal functions.** *Endocrinol* 2004, **145:**5439–5447.
28. Mizutani H, Tada-Oikawa S, Hiraku Y, Kojima M, Kawanishi S: **Mechanism of apoptosis induced by doxorubicin through the generation of hydrogen peroxide.** *Life Sci* 2005, **76:**1439–1453.
29. Grzanka A, Zuryn A, Stycynski J, Grzanka AA, Wisniewska H: **The effect of doxorubicin on the expression of cyclin A in K-562 leukemia cell line.** *Neoplasma* 2005, **52:**489–493.
30. Ling YH, El-Naggar AK, Priebe W, Perez-Soler R: **Cell cycle-dependent cytotoxicity, G2/M phase arrest, and disruption of p34cdc2/cyclin B1 activity induced by doxorubicin in synchronized p388 cells.** *Mol Pharmacol* 1996, **49:**832–841.

12

The cytotoxic activities of 7-isopentenyloxycoumarin on 5637 cells via induction of apoptosis and cell cycle arrest in G2/M stage

Fereshteh Haghighi[1], Maryam M Matin[1,2*], Ahmad Reza Bahrami[1,2], Mehrdad Iranshahi[3], Fatemeh B Rassouli[1] and Azadeh Haghighitalab[1]

Abstract

Background: Bladder cancer is the second common malignancy of genitourinary tract, and transitional cell carcinomas (TCCs) account for 90% of all bladder cancers. Due to acquired resistance of TCC cells to a wide range of chemotherapeutic agents, there is always a need for search on new compounds for treatment of these cancers. Coumarins represent a group of natural compounds, which some of them have exerted valuable anti-tumor activities. The current study was designed to evaluate anti-tumor properties and mechanism of action of 7-isopentenyloxycoumarin, a prenyloxycoumarin, on 5637 cells (a TCC cell line).

Results: MTT results revealed that the cytotoxic effects of 7-isopentenyloxycoumarin on 5637 cancerous cells were more prominent in comparison to HDF-1 normal cells. This coumarin increased the amount of chromatin condensation and DNA damage in 5637 cells by 58 and 33%, respectively. The results also indicated that it can induce apoptosis most probably via activation of caspase-3 in these cells. Moreover, propidium iodide staining revealed that 7-isopentenyloxycoumarin induced cell cycle arrest at G2/M stage, after 24 h of treatment.

Conclusion: Our results indicated that 7-isopentenyloxycoumarin had selective toxic effects on this bladder cancer cell line and promoted its effects by apoptosis induction and cell cycle arrest. This coumarin can be considered for further studies to reveal its exact mechanism of action and also its anti-cancer effects *in vivo*.

Keywords: Bladder cancer, Cytotoxicity, 7-isopentenyloxycoumarin, Apoptosis, Cell cycle

Background

About 7 million people die from different types of cancer, which makes it the second cause of death worldwide every year [1]. Bladder cancer is the second most common genitourinary malignancy with a higher incidence in men. More than 90% of all bladder cancers are transitional cell carcinomas (TCCs). Although cisplatin-based combination chemotherapies like MVAC (methotrexate-vinblastine-adriamycin-cisplatin) are the standard treatments in patients with TCC, harnessing metastatic bladder cancer still remains one of the main challenges in urologic oncology [2,3]. The resistance of TCC cells to a wide range of chemotherapeutic agents is the main reason for the failure of such treatments [4].

Apoptosis, also known as programmed cell death, is a naturally occurring process that plays a central role in the normal development and homeostasis of all multi-cellular organisms [5]. Apoptosis is accompanied by cell shrinkage, reduction of cellular volume, nuclear fragmentation, chromatin condensation, plasma membrane blebbing and engulfment by phagocytes *in vivo* [6]. There are two main apoptotic pathways in mammals: the extrinsic or death receptor pathway and the intrinsic or mitochondrial pathway. Both mechanisms end at the point of execution phase, which is initiated by the cleavage of executioner caspases and results in the apoptotic morphology. Caspase-3 is one of the most important executioner caspases, which is activated in both extrinsic and intrinsic pathways [7].

* Correspondence: Matin@um.ac.ir
[1]Department of Biology, Faculty of Science, Ferdowsi University of Mashhad, Mashhad, Iran
[2]Cell and Molecular Biotechnology Research Group, Institute of Biotechnology, Ferdowsi University of Mashhad, Mashhad, Iran
Full list of author information is available at the end of the article

Coumarins are a large group of natural compounds that are mainly found in the plant families of Rutaceae, Apiaceae and Umbelliferae as well as some bacteria and fungi [8]. Biological properties of coumarins include anti-coagulant, anti-viral, anti-microbial, anti-inflammatory, anti-oxidant and anti-tumor activities [9-12]. Induction of cell cycle arrest by coumarins is also reported frequently [9-11]. Prenyloxycoumarins represent a class of secondary metabolites that based on the length of their carbon chains, are categorized in three groups; C5 (isopentenyl), C10 (geranyl) and C15 (linear, mono- or bicyclic sesquiterpenyl) [8]. One of these studied coumarins is 7-isopentenyloxycoumarin (7-IP) [13].

7-IP, a secondary metabolite with an isopentenyl chain fixed at C7 of the 1, 2-benzopyrone ring, exerts valuable and promising anti-microbial, anti-inflammatory and anti-cancer effects [14]. The chemopreventive [15], neuroprotective [16] and anti-genotoxic [17] properties of 7-IP have been shown previously. This coumarin was first isolated by Prokopenko from the fruit of *Libanotis intermedia* in 1966. In nature, 7-IP is biosynthesized from 7-hydroxycoumarin and dimethylallyl diphosphate [14] and is widespread in edible vegetables and fruits such as grapefruit, lemon, orange, mandarin and many other plants [18].

In this study, 7-IP was synthesized by a reaction between 7-hydroxycoumarin and its relevant prenyl bromide. Here, we evaluated its toxic effects on 5637 and HDF-1 cell lines by MTT assay. Since, there is no report on the mechanism of action of 7-IP, we report the effects of this coumarin in more details by DAPI staining, comet assay, caspase-3 activity and cell cycle analysis.

Methods

Chemical synthesis

7-IP (Figure 1A) was synthesized as described by Askari *et al.* [13]. Briefly, it was synthesized by a reaction between 7-hydroxycoumarin (Figure 1B) and isopentenyl bromide in the presence of DBU (1, 8-diazabicyclo [5.4.0]undec-7-ene), in acetone at room temperature. The purity and chemical structure of 7-IP was then assessed by ^{1}H- and ^{13}C-NMR spectroscopy (Additional file 1: Table S1 and Additional file 2: Table S2).

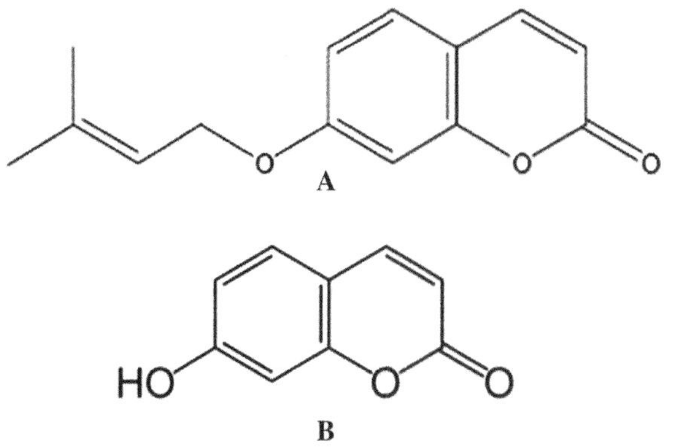

Figure 1 Chemical structure of coumarins. A) 7-IP and **B)** 7-hydroxycoumarin.

Preparation of different 7-IP concentrations

To prepare different concentrations of 7-IP (10 to 100 μg/ml), 2 mg of the powder was dissolved in 500 μl dimethyl sulfoxide (DMSO, Merck, Germany), and diluted with complete culture medium before experiments. Since the solvent has cytotoxic effects, the control treatments were run at the same time with equivalent solutions of DMSO.

Cell lines and cell culture

Human 5637 cells (a TCC subline) were obtained from Pasteur Institute (Tehran, Iran). These epithelial like cells were first derived in 1974 of a primary bladder carcinoma from a 68- year old Caucasian man. HDF-1 (human dermal fibroblast) cells, derived from human skin fibroblasts, were a generous gift from Royan Institute (Tehran, Iran). All cells were maintained in Dulbecco's modified Eagle's medium (DMEM, Gibco, Scotland) supplemented with 10% heat-inactivated fetal bovine serum (FBS, Gibco, Scotland) for 5367 cells, and 15% FBS for HDF-1 cells. 5637 and HDF-1 cells were grown at 37°C in a humisdified atmosphere of 10% and 5% CO_2 in air, respectively. To subculture the cells, they were washed with phosphate buffered saline (PBS) and incubated with 0.25% trypsin/ 1 mM ethylenediaminetetraacetic acid (EDTA) (Gibco, Scotland) for 5 min. Detached cells were resuspended in fresh serum-containing medium to inactivate the trypsin and transferred to new labeled flasks.

Cell viability assay

Cell viability was determined by MTT assay [19]. In this method, tetrazolium dye, 3-(4,5-Dimethyl-2-thiazolyl)-2,5-diphenyl-2*H*-tetrazolium bromide, is reduced by mitochondrial enzymes to insoluble purple formazan in living cells. The absorbance of the colored product (after dissolving in DMSO) can be determined by a spectrophotometer. Briefly, 5637 and HDF-1 cells were seeded at a density of 1.3×10^4 and 1.0×10^4 cells/well in 96-well tissue culture plates (Orange Scientific, France), respectively. The cells were allowed to attach and grow for 24 h. In order to identify the half maximal inhibitory concentration (IC_{50}) values of 7-IP, cells were treated with increasing concentrations (10 to 100 μg/ml) of the compound for 24, 48 and 72 h. To perform MTT assay, 5 mg MTT dye (Sigma Aldrich, Germany) was dissolved in 1 ml PBS, filtered through a 0.22 μm filter (Orange Scientific, France) and used freshly before each experiment. Then 20 μl MTT solution (500 μg/ml final concentration) was added to each well and plates were incubated at 37°C for 4 h. After this period, the remaining MTT solution was removed and 150 µl DMSO was added to each well to dissolve the formazan crystals. The absorbance of each well was then measured at 545 nm using an enzyme linked immunosorbent assay (ELISA) plate reader (Awareness, USA). The percentage of cell viability was calculated by dividing the mean absorbance of each treatment (7-IP) to the mean absorbance of its controls (DMSO) multiply by 100.

Morphological alterations

Cells treated with various concentrations of 7-IP were observed under a light inverted microscope (Olympus, Japan) for morphological changes after 24, 48 and 72 h of the treatments.

Apoptosis assay with DAPI staining

In order to evaluate the apoptotic effects of 7-IP semi-quantitatively, DAPI (4′, 6-diamidino-2-phenylindole dichloride) staining was performed. To do so, 5637 cells were grown to 80% confluency in 6-well tissue culture plates (Orange Scientific, France). Then the cells were treated with 65 µg/ml 7-IP and its equivalent amount of DMSO (1.625%) for 72 h. Cells were then washed gently with PBS and fixed with 4% paraformaldehyde (Sigma, Germany) for 10 min at room temperature. After that cells were washed with PBS, permeabilized with 0.1% Triton X-100 (Merck, Germany) and stained with 2 µg/ml DAPI (Merck, Germany) at 37°C for 10 min. Approximately, 700 cells from each treatment were visualized and counted under a fluorescent microscope (Olympus, Japan). Chromatin condensation was considered as a specific criterion for apoptotic morphology.

Alkaline comet assay

To investigate the DNA-damaging effects of 7-IP, the alkaline version of comet assay, which is a rapid, reliable and quantitative technique for detection of possible DNA lesions at the individual eukaryotic cells, was performed [20]. Briefly, untreated 5637 and HDF-1 cells, and cells treated for 72 h with 65 µg/ml 7-IP and its DMSO control were trypsinized and centrifuged at 1100 g for 10 min. The cell pellets were resuspended in 50 µl PBS and then mixed with 50 µl of 1.5% (w/v) low melting point agarose (LMA, Fermentas, Germany) and spread on glass slides precoated with 1% (w/v) normal melting point agarose (NMA, Helicon, Russia). Four slides were prepared for each treatment. The slides were kept for 20 min at 4°C to allow the agarose to solidify. After 20 min 100 µl of 0.75% (w/v) LMA was added to each slide, and kept for another 20 min at 4°C. When the gel was solidified, slides were submerged in freshly prepared lysing buffer (2.5 M NaCl, 100 mM Na_2EDTA, 10 mM Tris, 2% (v/v) Triton X-100, pH 10) for at least 4 h at 4°C. Then the slides were placed in an electrophoresis chamber filled with freshly prepared cold alkaline electrophoresis buffer (1 mM EDTA, 0.3 N NaOH, pH 13) and incubated for 30 min at 4°C. Electrophoresis was conducted at 300 mA and 25 V for 20 min at 4°C. Slides were then washed with ice-cold neutralizing buffer (0.4 M Tris–HCl, pH 7.5) for three times, dried with 96% ethanol and stained with ethidium bromide (20 µg/ml). The slides were viewed and analyzed with a fluorescent microscope (Olympus, Japan). One hundred cells per slide were evaluated and the mean of comet tail (a product of fraction of DNA in tail and tail length) was determined using TriTek Cometscore version 1.5 software. The DNA damage was expressed as % DNA in tail.

Caspase-3 activity assay

Caspase-3 activity was assessed using caspase-3 colorimetric assay kit (Abcam, USA) according to manufacturer's protocol. Briefly, 5637 cells were treated with 65 µg/ml of 7-IP and its equivalent amount of DMSO for 12 h. Cells treated with 15 µg/ml of cisplatin for 24 h were used as a positive control. After the period of treatments, cells were trypsinized and centrifuged at 1100 g for 10 min. Cell pellets were suspended in 1 ml cold PBS and centrifuged at 4000 g for 5 min at 4°C. In order to extract total protein, cell pellets were resuspended and lysed with 100 µl of chilled lysis buffer and incubated on ice for 10 min. Cell lysates were then centrifuged at 10000 g for 1 min at 4°C. The concentration of proteins was measured by Bradford assay. Then 50 µl of 2× reaction buffer containing 10 mM DTT and 5 µl of 4 mM caspase-3 substrate (DEVD-*p*NA) were added to 200 µg protein from each sample and incubated at 37°C for 4 h. The *p*-NA light emission was quantified using ELISA plate reader at 405 nm. Comparison of the absorbance of *p*-NA from an apoptotic sample with an uninduced control allowed determination of the fold increase in caspase-3 activity.

Cell cycle analysis

The cell cycle distribution was assayed by flow cytometry after DNA staining with propidium iodide (PI). 5637 cells were treated with 65 µg/ml 7-IP and its equivalent amount of DMSO. After 24 h of treatments, floated cells were harvested and attached cells were trypsinized, washed with a protein-containing buffer (PBS + 5% FBS) and centrifuged at 1100 g for 10 min. The cell pellets were resuspended in 500 µl PBS containing 5% FBS and centrifuged at 200 g for 7 min at 4°C. After that cells were stained with a solution containing 100 µg/ml PI (Sigma Aldrich, Germany), 0.1% Triton X-100, 0.1% sodium citrate (Merck, Germany) and RNase (100 µg/ml) (Merck, Germany) in ice cold PBS. The samples were then incubated at 4°C in dark for 1 h and flow cytometric analyses were performed using a FACSCalibur (BD

Biosciences, USA) instrument and WinMDI version 2.9 software.

Statistical analyses

Data generated from experiments were collected in a completely randomized design. All assays were carried out at least three times. Statistical procedures were performed using Microsoft Office Excel (2007) SPSS, version 16.0 (SPSS software Inc., Chicago, IL, USA) and SAS, version 9.1 (SAS Institute, Inc., Cary, N.C., USA) softwares. A one-way analysis of variance (ANOVA) according to general linear model procedure of SAS software was performed to evaluate possible differences among the treatments. The statistical significant differences among means between each group were determined by using Tukey's single-step multiple comparison test. Differences among treatment means were compared at *P*-value of < 0.001. Values are expressed as mean ± SD.

Results

IC_{50} value determination of 7-IP in 5637 and HDF-1 cell lines

The cytotoxic effects of 7-IP were assessed by MTT assay in 5637 and HDF-1 cells exposed to 10–100 μg/ml of this coumarin for three consecutive days. Cell survival analyses showed that 7-IP had a concentration and time-dependent inhibitory effect on the growth of 5637 cells (Figure 2A). By increasing the concentrations, cell viabilities were significantly different ($P < 0.001$) especially after 48 and 72 h of treatments. The IC_{50} values of this coumarin were calculated as 76, 76 and 65 μg/ml after 24, 48 and 72 h of treatments, respectively.

To assess the cytotoxic effects of 7-IP on normal cells, HDF-1 cells were used. As shown in Figure 2B, although this coumarin induced cell death in these non-cancerous cells, but its cytotoxic effects were not significant in comparison to 5637 cells. Statistical analysis revealed that the slight cytotoxic effects of 7-IP on HDF-1 cells were not dose-dependent except at higher concentrations.

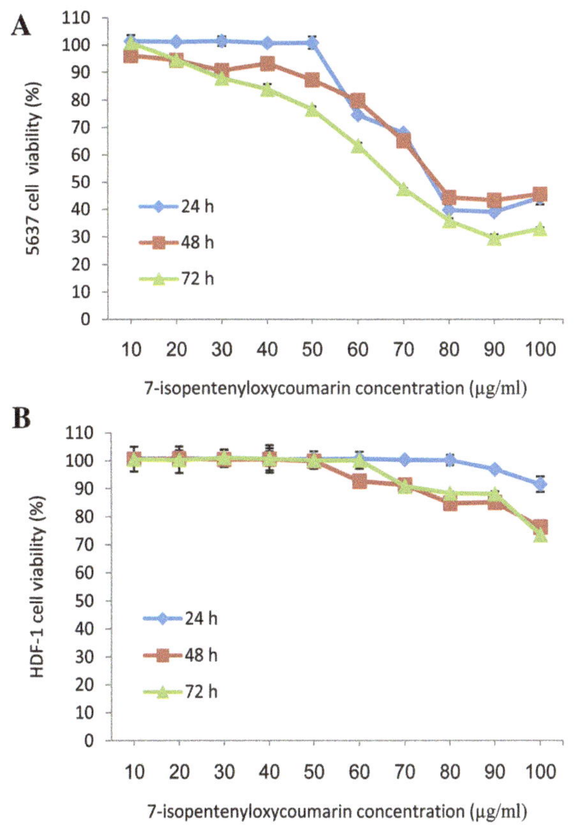

Figure 2 Time-based dose response curves of cancerous and normal cells. 5637 **(A)** and HDF-1 **(B)** cells treated with 7-IP during 24, 48 and 72 h. All the points represent results from three independent experiments performed in triplicate. Data are expressed as mean ± SD.

Morphological alterations

The cytotoxic effects of 7-IP were confirmed by morphological observations. As shown in Figure 3 (A-C), 5637 cells treated with 65 μg/ml 7-IP for 72 h, revealed prominent cytoplasmic granulation and cell number was significantly decreased as compared with control and untreated cultures. In the case of HDF-1 cells, there were no significant changes between cells treated with 100 μg/ml of 7-IP with control and untreated groups (Figure 3 D-F).

7-IP induces apoptosis in 5637 cells

To determine what kind of cell death has been induced by 7-IP, the chromatin condensation and DNA damage were assessed using DAPI staining and alkaline comet assay, respectively. Based on MTT results, 5637 cells were treated with 65 μg/ml 7-IP and equivalent amount of DMSO for 72 h. As shown in Figure 4 (A-C) cells treated with this compound, showed highly condensed chromatin and nuclear fragmentation in comparison to control and untreated cells. Quantitative results revealed that 89% of cells treated with 65 μg/ml 7-IP presented condensed chromatin, which was significantly ($P < 0.001$) higher than control (31%) and untreated (7.5%) cultures (Figure 4D).

Furthermore, detecting DNA damage inducing effects of 7-IP in 5637 cells by comet assay, showed comet tail in a high percentage of individual cells treated with this coumarin (Figure 5 A-C). Data analysis showed that 7-IP induced approximately 43% DNA damage, significantly ($P < 0.001$) higher than that induced by its DMSO control (11%, Figure 5G). In order to investigate the genotoxic effects of 7-IP in non-cancerous cells, comet assay was also performed in HDF-1 cells treated with the same amount of the compound. As shown in Figure 5 (D-F) the difference between comet tail in HDF-1 and 5637 cells

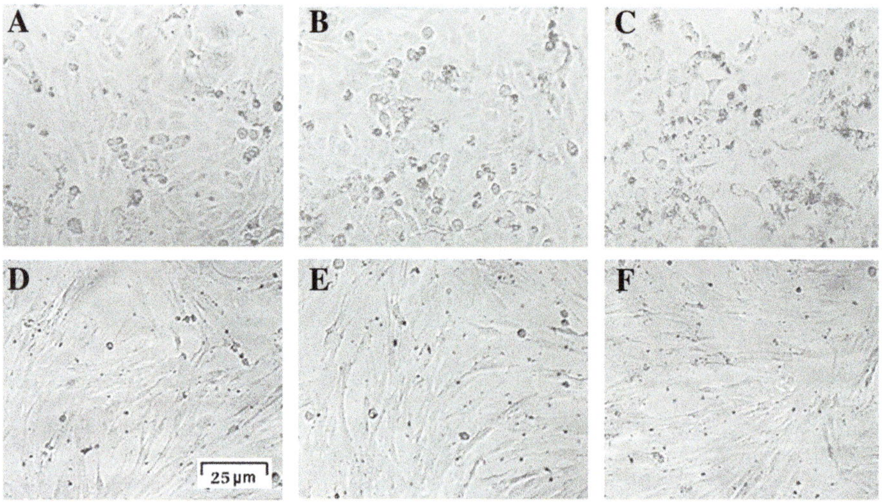

Figure 3 Light microscopic images of 5637 and HDF-1 cells. Untreated 5637 cells **(A)**. 5637 cells treated with 1.625% DMSO **(B)** represent little morphological changes as compared with untreated cells. 5637 cells treated with 65 μg/ml 7-IP **(C)** revealed prominent cytoplasmic granulation and cell death. Untreated HDF-1 cells **(D)**. HDF-1 cells treated with 2.5% DMSO **(E)**. HDF-1 cells treated with 100 μg/ml 7-IP after 72 h with little changes in their morphology **(F)**.

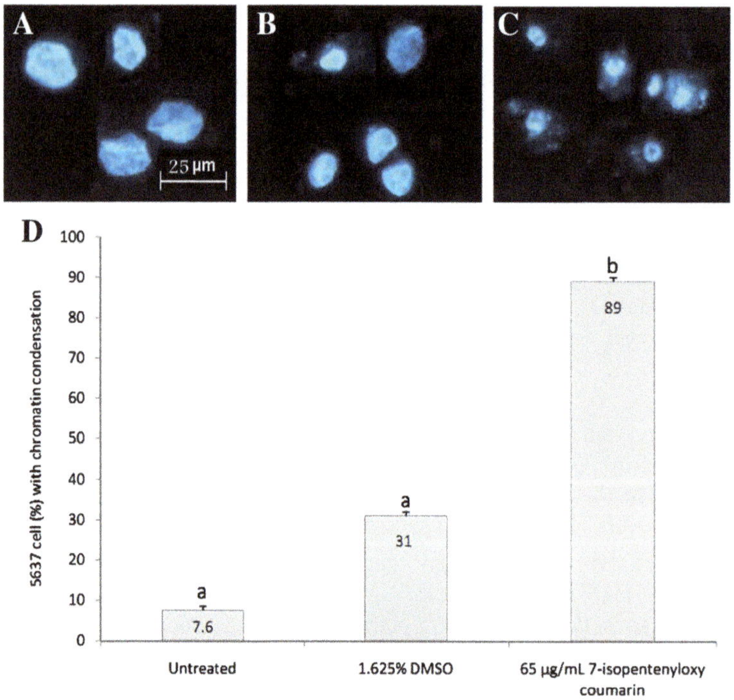

Figure 4 Investigating the apoptotic morphology of cells by DAPI staining. Chromatin condensation of 5637 cells without any treatment **(A)**, treated with 1.625% DMSO **(B)** and treated with 65 μg/ml 7-IP **(C)** for 72 h. The percentages of condensed chromatin, 72 h after treatments are compared with untreated and control groups **(D)**. Data are expressed as mean ± SD. The assay was done three times. Distinct letters indicate significant differences ($P < 0.001$) between cells treated with 65 μg/ml 7-IP and other cultures.

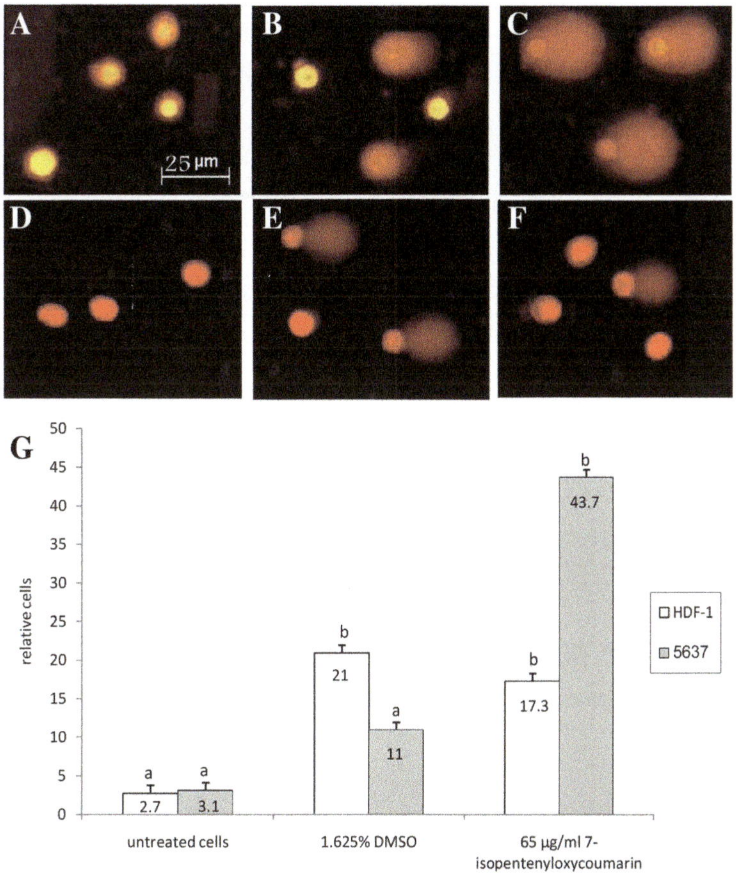

Figure 5 Evaluating the DNA damaging effects of 7-IP by comet assay. DNA damage of 5637 and HDF-1 cells without any treatment **(A and D)**, treated with 1.625% DMSO **(B and E)** and treated with 65 µg/ml 7-IP **(C and F)** for 72 h, respectively. The percentages of damaged DNA, 72 h after treatments are compared with untreated and control groups in both 5637 and HDF-1 cells **(G)**. Data are expressed as mean ± SD. The assay was repeated three times. Distinct letters show significant differences ($P < 0.001$) between different groups.

was obvious, treated HDF-1 cells represented a very small comet tail (Figure 5F). Statistical analysis revealed that the effect of 7-IP to induce DNA damage in HDF-1 cells (17%) is probably due to the presence of DMSO as a solvent since the DMSO control group induced the DNA damage by 21% (Figure 5G).

7-IP activates caspase-3

To confirm the apoptotic effects of 7-IP, the activity of caspase-3 enzyme was also analyzed. After 12 h of incubation, the caspase activity in 7-IP-treated 5637 cells was increased approximately 2.5 folds as compared with untreated culture (Figure 6), significantly ($P < 0.001$) higher than DMSO-treated group.

7-IP arrests 5637 cells at G2/M stage

To further study the anti-proliferative properties of 7-IP, its effects on cell cycle progression were evaluated by flow cytometry after PI staining. 5637 cells were treated with 65 µg/ml 7-IP and its equivalent amount of DMSO for 24 h. As shown in Figure 7, treatment with this compound caused an increase in the percentage of cells in G2/M correlating with decreased number of cells in G1 as compared with DMSO and untreated cultures. Thus, exposure to 7-IP led to cell cycle arrest at G2/M stage (Figure 7C). Percentages of cells at different stages of cell cycle are presented in Table 1.

Discussion

Cancer is a consequence of unregulated cell growth with high morbidity and mortality worldwide. Despite major advances in cancer therapy, its treatment is far from being satisfactory and more research on new compounds and strategies to fight this disease is urgently needed.

As mentioned before, coumarins represent a large class of natural compounds with various biological activities, among which prenyloxycoumarins exert valuable antitumor properties both *in vitro* and *in vivo* [8,12,21].

In search for anti-cancer agents to treat bladder cancer, 7-IP was tested for its cytotoxicity on 5637 and HDF-1 cells (as control) *in vitro*. This compound belongs to prenyloxycoumarins with various biological properties, which

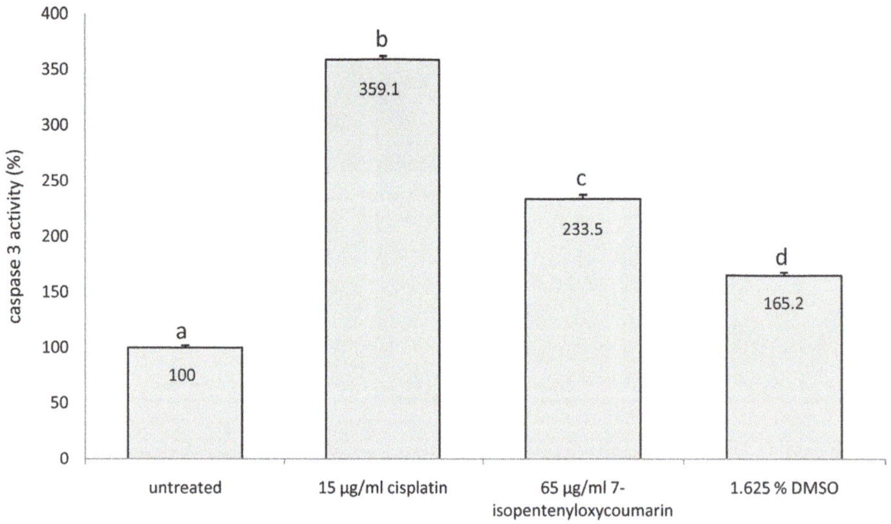

Figure 6 The effects of 7-IP on caspase-3 activity in 5637 cells as detected by colorimetric assay. 7-IP-treated cells show approximately 2.5 folds higher caspase activity than untreated cells. Cells treated with 15 µg/ml cisplatin showed elevated caspase-3 activity by approximately 3.5 folds. Data are expressed as mean ± SD. Results are from three independent experiments in triplicate. Distinct letters indicate significant differences ($P < 0.001$) between different groups.

can be synthesized both naturally and chemically [13]. Although this coumarin derivative exerts various biological properties, there is no report on its toxic effects and mechanism of action on bladder cancer cells in the literature. Our results revealed that the IC_{50} value of 7-IP in 5637 cells was 65 µg/ml (>100 µM) after 72 h of treatment, which is less than vinblastine but higher than vincristine and cisplatin [22]. Similar results were reported by Bruyere and coworkers who showed that 7-IP had IC_{50} values more than 100 µM in various human cancer cell lines [23]. Furthermore, Kawaii and colleagues determined low cytotoxicity of 7-IP on other cancers including lung, melanoma and leukemia [24]. On the other hand, Kofians and colleagues reported the ID_{50} values of 7-IP on KB and NSCLC-N6 cell lines, as 10.6 and 9.9 µg/ml, respectively [25]. Considering different reports on toxic effects of 7-IP, it can be concluded that depending on the cell line, the cytotoxicity of this coumarin would be different. High IC_{50} value of 7-IP in 5637 cells can be explained by the multi-drug resistance (MDR) of these cells [26,27]. Several ATP-binding cassette (ABC) transporters have been discovered, including multidrug resistance-associated proteins (MRPs) and P-glycoproteins, which play critical roles in MDR [28]. For instance, it has been reported that TCC cells over express MDR1 and MRP2 proteins, two members of MRP family [29]. Therefore, it is possible that 7-IP is exported from 5637 cells by these efflux pumps, so high amounts of this compound are required to be accumulated inside the cell, in order to induce cytotoxicity. To investigate the anti-cancer

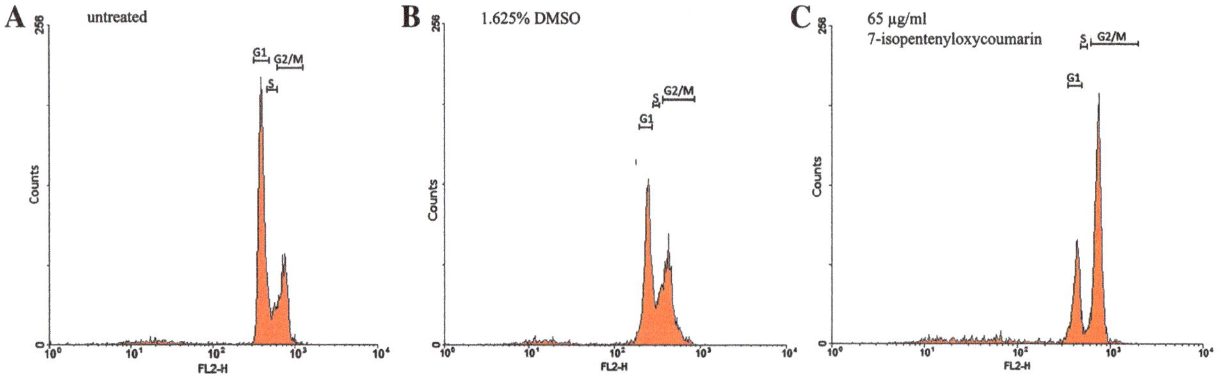

Figure 7 G2/M arrest of 5637 cells treated with 7-IP, 24 h after treatment. Cell cycle distribution of 5637 cells without any treatment **(A)**. Cells treated with 1.625% DMSO **(B)** do not show remarkable changes in cell cycle phases. Cells treated with 65 µg/ml 7-IP **(C)** show a marked cell cycle arrest at G2/M stage, 24 h after treatment.

Table 1 Effects of 7-IP on 5637 cell cycle distribution

Treatment	Percentage of cells		
	G1 (Mean ± SD)	S (Mean ± SD)	G2/M (Mean ± SD)
untreated	55.7 ± 6.16[a]	13.3 ± 1.20[a]	32.5 ± 0.88[a]
1.625% DMSO	43 ± 0.87[b]	12 ± 0.41[a]	36 ± 1.53[a]
65 μg/ml 7-IP	22.4 ± 1.63[c]	5.2 ± 1.47[b]	53.5 ± 2.54[b]

Percentages of cells in each stage of cell cycle is represented as mean ± SD. Results are from three independent experiments. Distinct letters in each column indicate statistical significant differences ($P < 0.001$) between groups.

properties of 7-IP, non-cancerous HDF-1 cells were treated with the same concentrations as 5637 cells and results revealed no significant growth-inhibitory effects of this coumarin in HDF-1 cells (Figure 2B). This confirms the selective activity of 7-IP in cancerous 5637 cells.

Results of DAPI staining and comet assay also revealed that, in comparison with control cultures, 65 μg/ml 7-IP significantly ($P < 0.001$) increased both chromatin condensation and DNA damage in 5637 cells, which were in agreement with morphological observations and MTT results and indicate that cells are undergoing apoptotic cell death [30,31]. Moreover, to evaluate genotoxic effects of 7-IP in HDF-1 cells, comet assay was also performed in these cells. Comet results revealed that the DNA damaging effects of 7-IP were due to its solvent DMSO and there was no significant difference ($P < 0.001$) between these two groups. Thus, 7-IP does not have any significant toxic or genotoxic effects on normal HDF-1 cells.

To confirm the type of cell death, caspase-3 activity (the executioner upon which many apoptotic pathways converge) was evaluated using caspase-3 colorimetric assay kit. As shown in Figure 6, caspase activity in 7-IP-treated 5637 cells was elevated. The relative caspase-3 activity was increased about 2.5 folds in cells treated with this compound in comparison to untreated cells; which was also significantly increased compared to cells treated with equivalent amount of DMSO ($P < 0.001$).

Cell cycle analysis was performed by flow cytometry after PI staining to investigate the effects of 7-IP in more details. It was shown that this compound arrested 5637 cells in G2/M stage of the cell cycle (Figure 7C), which is similar to the effects of other anti-cancer drugs like taxol, doxorubicin and vincristine [32-34]. It is well established that progression of cell cycle is a tightly ordered and regulated process involving multiple checkpoints. Upregulation of cyclin B1/Cdc2 kinase activity, which regulates the entry and progression of the mitotic phase in eukaryotic cells, is known to be involved in the G2/M stage transition of the cell cycle. On the other hand, cells are arrested in M stage when microtubule network is disrupted [35]. Since 7-IP arrests 5637 cells in G2/M stage of the cell cycle, it is possible that this compound may act on cell cycle checkpoints or acts like a microtubule inhibitor, preventing further cell division and subsequently initiates cell death by apoptosis. Our results are similar to other studies that determined the ability of different coumarins in caspase-3 activation and cell cycle arrest. For instance, Barthomeuf and colleagues showed that umbelliprenin (another prenyloxycoumarin with a farnesyl chain) markedly inhibited proliferation of M4Beu cells through induction of caspase-dependent apoptosis and cell-cycle arrest [9]. Another study by Chuang and his coworkers revealed that coumarin induced cell cycle arrest and caspase-3 dependent apoptosis in HeLa cells [10].

Conclusion

In summary, it can be concluded that 7-IP had toxic effects on 5637 cells. Exploring the anti-tumor activity of 7-IP showed that this coumarin has selective cytotoxic effects on 5637 cancerous cells in comparison to normal HDF-1 cells. Further studies in 5637 cells revealed that 7-IP induces chromatin condensation, DNA damage and apoptosis most probably via activation of caspase-3 and arrests the cell cycle at G2/M stage. Further studies are needed to determine its exact mechanism of action. For example, since antioxidants have different effects in cancer treatment [36], it is important to explore this property of 7-IP and its mechanism of action. Moreover, since *in vitro* conditions are very different from *in vivo* environments, in order to evaluate 7-IP effects on biological systems, an approved method on animal models is required [37].

Our study represents the first report describing 7-IP as an anti-tumor agent for bladder cancer cells *in vitro*. Although 7-IP was synthesized in this study, but considering the fact that it is widespread in edible vegetables and fruits, the present study could be regarded as a topic for future studies aiming to put in evidence dietary feeding chemopreventive effects on baldder cancer.

Additional files

Additional file 1: Table S1. 1H-NMR data for 7-isopentenyloxycoumarin (CDCl3, 500 MHz).

Additional file 2: Table S2. 13 C-NMR data for 7-isopentenyloxycoumarin (CDCl3, 125.7 MHz).

Abbreviations

DAPI: 4′, 6-diamidino-2-phenylindole dichloride; DMEM: Dulbecco's modified Eagle's medium; DMSO: Dimethyl sulfoxide; EDTA: Ethylenediaminetetraacetic acid; ELISA: Enzyme linked immunosorbent assay; FBS: Fetal bovine serum; HDF1: Human dermal fibroblast 1, IC_{50}: Half maximal inhibitory concentration; 7-IP: 7-isopentenyloxycoumarin; LMA: Low melting agarose; MTT: 3-(4,5-Dimethyl-2-thiazolyl)-2,5-diphenyl-2*H*-tetrazolium bromide; NMA: Normal melting agarose; NMR: Nuclear magnetic resonance; PBS: Phosphate buffered saline; PI: Propidium iodide; SD: Standard deviation; TCC: Transitional cell carcinoma.

Competing interests

The authors have no conflict of interests to declare.

Authors' contributions

MMM conceived the strategy of study and supervised the project. FH performed the experimental work and data interpretation. ARB gave consultation on designing the study, complemented the data. MI provided the compound and gave consultation. FBR and AH were involved in performing the experimental work and data interpretation. All authors read and approved the final manuscript.

Authors' information

Fereshteh Haghighi, M.Sc. in Cell and Molecular Biology; Maryam M. Matin, Ph.D. in Molecular Biotechnology and Associate Professor at Ferdowsi University of Mashhad; Ahmad Reza Bahrami, Ph.D. in Molecular Biotechnology, Head of Institute of Biotechnology and Professor at Ferdowsi University of Mashhad; Mehrdad Iranshahi, Ph.D. in Pharmacognosy and Associate Professor at Mashhad University of Medical Sciences, Fatemeh B. Rassouli, Ph.D. in Cell and Molecular Biology and Azadeh Haghighitalab, M.Sc. in Cell and Molecular Biology.

Acknowledgments

This work was supported by a grant from Ferdowsi University of Mashhad. The authors would like to thank Dr. Parsaee, Dr. Tayarani-Najjaran, Mrs. Saeinasab, Mr. Malaekeh-Nikouei and Mr. Nakhaei for their excellent support and technical help. We are also grateful to Dr. Sadeghi for his great support and statistical advice.

Author details

[1]Department of Biology, Faculty of Science, Ferdowsi University of Mashhad, Mashhad, Iran. [2]Cell and Molecular Biotechnology Research Group, Institute of Biotechnology, Ferdowsi University of Mashhad, Mashhad, Iran. [3]Biotechnology Research Center and School of Pharmacy, Mashhad University of Medical Sciences, Mashhad, Iran.

References

1. Coseri S: **Natural products and their analogues as efficient anticancer drugs.** *Mini Rev Med Chem* 2009, **9:**560–571.
2. Bolenz C, Becker A, Trojan L, Schaaf A, Cao Y, Weiss C, Alken P, Michel MS: **Optimizing chemotherapy for transitional cell carcinoma by application of bcl-2 and bcl-xL antisense oligodeoxynucleotides.** *Urol Oncol* 2007, **25:**476–482.
3. Nicholson BE, Frierson HF, Conaway MR, Seraj JM, Harding MA, Hampton GM, Theodorescu D: **Profiling the evolution of human metastatic bladder cancer.** *Cancer Res* 2004, **64:**7813–7821.
4. Behnam Rassouli F, Matin MM, Iranshahi M, Bahrami AR, Neshati V, Mollazadeh S, Neshati Z: **Mogoltacin enhances vincristine cytotoxicity in human transitional cell carcinoma (TCC) cell line.** *Phytomedicine* 2009, **16:**181–187.
5. Kannan K, Jain SK: **Oxidative stress and apoptosis.** *Pathophysiology* 2000, **7:**153–163.
6. Kroemer G, Galluzzi L, Vandenabeele P, Abrams J, Alnemri ES, Baehrecke EH, Blagosklonny MV, El-Deiry WS, Golstein P, Green DR, Hengartner M, Knight RA, Kumar S, Lipton SA, Malorni W, Nunez G, Peter ME, Tschopp J, Yuan J, Piacentini M, Zhivotovsky B, Melino G: **Classification of cell death: recommendations of the Nomenclature Committee on Cell Death 2009.** *Cell Death Differ* 2009, **16:**3–11.
7. Elmore S: **Apoptosis: a review of programmed cell death.** *Toxicol Pathol* 2007, **35:**495–516.
8. Curini M, Cravotto G, Epifano F, Giannone G: **Chemistry and biological activity of natural and synthetic prenyloxycoumarins.** *Curr Med Chem* 2006, **13:**199–222.
9. Barthomeuf C, Lim S, Iranshahi M, Chollet P: **Umbelliprenin from *Ferula szowitsiana* inhibits the growth of human M4Beu metastatic pigmented malignant melanoma cells through cell-cycle arrest in G1 and induction of caspase-dependent apoptosis.** *Phytomedicine* 2008, **15:**103–111.
10. Chuang JY, Huang YF, Lu HF, Ho HC, Yang JS, Li TM, Chang NW, Chung JG: **Coumarin induces cell cycle arrest and apoptosis in human cervical cancer HeLa cells through a mitochondria- and caspase-3 dependent mechanism and NF-kappaB down-regulation.** *In Vivo* 2007, **21:**1003–1009.
11. Lopez-Gonzalez JS, Prado-Garcia H, Aguilar-Cazares D, Molina-Guarneros JA, Morales-Fuentes J, Mandoki JJ: **Apoptosis and cell cycle disturbances induced by coumarin and 7-hydroxycoumarin on human lung carcinoma cell lines.** *Lung Cancer* 2004, **43:**275–283.
12. Riveiro ME, De Kimpe N, Moglioni A, Vazquez R, Monczor F, Shayo C, Davio C: **Coumarins: old compounds with novel promising therapeutic perspectives.** *Curr Med Chem* 2010, **17:**1325–1338.
13. Askari M, Sahebkar A, Iranshahi M: **Synthesis and purification of 7-prenyloxycoumarins and herniarin as bioactive natural coumarins.** *Iranian J Basic Med Sci* 2009, **12:**63–69.
14. Epifano F, Pelucchini C, Curini M, Genovese S: **Insights on novel biologically active natural products: 7-isopentenyloxycoumarin.** *Nat Prod Commun* 2009, **4:**1755–1760.
15. Baba M, Jin Y, Mizuno A, Suzuki H, Okada Y, Takasuka N, Tokuda H, Nishino H, Okuyama T: **Studies on cancer chemoprevention by traditional folk medicines XXIV. Inhibitory effect of a coumarin derivative, 7-isopentenyloxycoumarin, against tumor-promotion.** *Biol Pharm Bull* 2002, **25:**244–246.
16. Epifano F, Molinaro G, Genovese S, Ngomba RT, Nicoletti F, Curini M: **Neuroprotective effect of prenyloxycoumarins from edible vegetables.** *Neurosci Lett* 2008, **443:**57–60.
17. Rezaee R, Hashemzaie M, Iranshahi M, Behravan E, Behravan J, Soltani F: **Evaluation of antigenotoxic effect of 7-hydroxy coumarin and 7-isopentenyloxy coumarin on human peripheral lymphocytes exposed to oxidative stress.** *Toxicol Lett* 2011, **205:**108.
18. Epifano F, Curini M, Menghini L, Genovese S: **Natural coumarins as a novel class of neuroprotective agents.** *Mini Rev Med Chem* 2009, **9:**1262–1271.
19. van Meerloo J, Kaspers GJ, Cloos J: **Cell sensitivity assays: the MTT assay.** *Methods Mol Biol* 2011, **731:**237–245.
20. Collins AR: **The comet assay for DNA damage and repair: principles, applications, and limitations.** *Mol Biotechnol* 2004, **26:**249–261.
21. Epifano F, Genovese S, Menghini L, Curini M: **Chemistry and pharmacology of oxyprenylated secondary plant metabolites.** *Phytochemistry* 2007, **68:**939–953.
22. Rassouli FB, Matin MM, Iranshahi M, Bahrami AR: **Investigating the cytotoxic and apoptosis inducing effects of monoterpenoid stylosin *in vitro*.** *Fitoterapia* 2011, **82:**742–749.
23. Bruyere C, Genovese S, Lallemand B, Ionescu-Motatu A, Curini M, Kiss R, Epifano F: **Growth inhibitory activities of oxyprenylated and non-prenylated naturally occurring phenylpropanoids in cancer cell lines.** *Bioorg Med Chem Lett* 2011, **21:**4174–4179.
24. Kawaii S, Tomono Y, Ogawa K, Sugiura M, Yano M, Yoshizawa Y, Ito C, Furukawa H: **Antiproliferative effect of isopentenylated coumarins on several cancer cell lines.** *Anticancer Res* 2001, **21:**1905–1911.
25. Kofinas C, Chinou I, Loukis A, Harvala C, Roussakis C, Maillard M, Hostettmann K: **Cytotoxic coumarins from the aerial parts of *Tordylium apulum* and their effects on a non-small-cell bronchial carcinoma line.** *Planta Med* 1998, **64:**174–176.
26. Gottesman MM: **How cancer cells evade chemotherapy: sixteenth Richard and Hinda Rosenthal Foundation Award Lecture.** *Cancer Res* 1993, **53:**747–754.
27. Shoemaker RH, Curt GA, Carney DN: **Evidence for multidrug-resistant cells in human tumor cell populations.** *Cancer Treat Rep* 1983, **67:**883–888.
28. Choi CH: **ABC transporters as multidrug resistance mechanisms and the development of chemosensitizers for their reversal.** *Cancer Cell Int* 2005, **5:**30–35.
29. Wu C, Zhang W, Chang J, Zhao Z, Sun G, Han R: **MDR1/P-glycoprotein overexpression in bladder transitional cell carcinoma and its correlation with expression of survivin and Fas.** *Chin J Onco* 2006, **3:**191–195.
30. Hasegawa M, Yagi K, Iwakawa S, Hirai M: **Chitosan induces apoptosis via caspase-3 activation in bladder tumor cells.** *Jpn J Cancer Res* 2001, **92:**459–466.
31. Nguyen SM, Lieven CJ, Levin LA: **Simultaneous labeling of projecting neurons and apoptotic state.** *J Neurosci Methods* 2007, **161:**281–284.
32. Das GC, Holiday D, Gallardo R, Haas C: **Taxol-induced cell cycle arrest and apoptosis: dose–response relationship in lung cancer cells of different wild-type p53 status and under isogenic condition.** *Cancer Lett* 2001, **165:**147–153.

33. Ling YH, el-Naggar AK, Priebe W, Perez-Soler R: **Cell cycle-dependent cytotoxicity, G2/M phase arrest, and distruption of p34cdc2/cyclin B1 activity induced by doxorubicin in synchronized p388 cells.** *Mol Pharmacol* 2012, **81**:832–841.
34. Blajeski AL, Phan VA, Kottke TJ, Kaufmann SH: **G1 and G2 cell-cycle arrest following microtubule depolymerization in human breast cancer cells.** *J Clin Invest* 2002, **110**:91–99.
35. Dash BC, El-Deiry WS: **Phosphorylation of p21 in G/M promotes cyclin B -Cdc2 kinase activity.** *Mol Cell Biol* 2005, **25**:3364–3387.
36. Abdollahi M, Shetab-Boushehri SV: **Is it right to look for anti-cancer drugs amongst compounds having antioxidant effect?** *DARU* 2012, **20**:61.
37. Shetab-Boushehri SV, Abdollahi M: **Current concerns on the validity of *in vitro* models that use transformed neoplastic cells in pharmacology and toxicology.** *Int J Pharmacol* 2012, **8**:594–595.

13

Novel 9-(alkylthio)-Acenaphtho[1,2-e]-1,2,4-triazine derivatives: synthesis, cytotoxic activity and molecular docking studies on B-cell lymphoma 2 (Bcl-2)

Mohammad K Mohammadi[1], Omidreza Firuzi[2], Mehdi Khoshneviszadeh[2], Nima Razzaghi-Asl[3], Saghi Sepehri[4] and Ramin Miri[2,3*]

Abstract

Background and purpose of the study: Acenaphtho derivatives have been reported as antitumor agents. Due to this fact and also with the aim of developing the chemistry of potentially bioactive heterocyclic compounds via efficient reactions, a facile procedure for the synthesis of 9-(alkylthio)-acenaphtho[1,2-e]-1,2,4-triazines via two step condensation of thiosemicarbazide and acenaphtylene-9,10-quinone to form acenaphtho[1,2-e]-1,2,4-triazine-9(8H)-thiones and subsequent reaction with benzyl chloride derivatives is reported.

Methods: 9-(alkylthio) acenaphtho[1,2-e]-1,2,4-triazines were synthesized via the reaction of acenaphtho-9,10-quinone with thiosemicarbazide, and then with the benzyl chloride derivatives. Cytotoxicity of some prepared compounds was assessed through MTT assay on three different human cancerous cell lines (HL-60, MCF7, and MOLT-4 cells). Molecular docking studies were performed via AutoDock4.2 software in order to confirm an apoptosis-inducing activity of acenaphtho scaffolds via the Bcl-2 protein.

Results: Excellent yields of the products, short reaction times and simple work-up are attractive features of this synthetic protocol. The evaluated compounds exhibited moderate to good cytotoxic activities. Docking results on the active site of B-cell lymphoma 2 (Bcl-2) supported the experimental biological data and agreed well with previous *in silico* data for commonly used anti-cancer drugs. Moreover; results were analyzed considering binding efficiency indices.

Conclusions: The outcomes of the present study may be helpful in future targeting of Bcl-2 with the aim of developing apoptosis-inducing agents.

Keywords: Synthesis, Acenaphtho-9,10-quinone, Cytotoxic activity, Docking

Introduction

Economic generation of bioactive compounds has been a major concern in modern organic chemistry [1]. In this regard, development of novel compounds and especially diverse small molecule scaffolds caused higher attention of medicinal and biological chemists [2-4]. This can be attributed to the growing requirement in assembling libraries of structurally complex substances to be evaluated as hit/lead compounds in drug discovery projects.

Polycyclic aromatic hydrocarbon (PAH) heterocycles are highly important structural units in a variety of pharmacologically active substances [5-9]. At first glance, rigid polycyclic structures seem to have role in the development of antitumor agents owing to their ability in insertion between stacked base pairs of oligonucleotides and action as intercalator [10-12]. Particularly important is that when these planar polycyclic heterocycles bear appropriate side chains, further interactions with other important macromolecules might be envisaged [11,13].

* Correspondence: mirir@sums.ac.ir
[2]Medicinal and Natural Products Chemistry Research Center, Shiraz, University of Medical Sciences, PO Box 3288–71345, Shiraz, Iran
[3]Departments of Medicinal Chemistry, School of Pharmacy, Shiraz University of Medical Sciences, Shiraz, Iran
Full list of author information is available at the end of the article

In this view, privileged heterocyclic structures have been constructed around the acenaphtho core [14,15]. Some of the acenaphtho derivatives containing thiazole backbone have been reported as antitumor agents [16]. Recently in an attempt to develop protein-targeted instead of DNA-targeted antitumor agents, some derivatives of 8H-acenaphtho[1,2-b]pyrrole have been constructed [17].

The authors demonstrated that 8-oxo-3-thiomorpholin-4-yl-8H-acenaphtho[1,2-b]pyrrole-9-carbonitrile could serve as an apoptosis-inducing agent via interacting Bcl-2 protein [17]. It is well known that the Bcl-2 family of proteins is comprised of pro-apoptotic and anti-apoptotic proteins and all members of this family are not anti-apoptotic. Anti-apoptotic Bcl-2 family proteins, including Bcl-2, Bcl-XL, Bcl-w, Mcl-1 and A1, prevent cell death by binding and sequestering pro-apoptotic proteins so, inhibition of these anti-apoptotic proteins might be lethal to cancer cells.

Indeed, Bcl-2 proteins have been regarded as important targets for anti-neoplastic drug development and Bcl-2 gen has been identified as over expressed in various cancers. Bcl-2 is an anti-apoptotic protein possessing an important role in various types of cancers. Bcl-2 is the member of the Bcl-2 family of apoptosis regulator proteins which is encoded by the BCL2 gene [18,19].

Various reactions of acenaphthaquinone with nucleophiles, organic and inorganic reagents have been reviewed elsewhere [20,21]. In the framework of our program to develop the chemistry of potentially bioactive heterocyclic compounds [22] and in connection with our ongoing interests in this field [23-25], we represent here a facile procedure for the synthesis of 9-(alkylthio)-acenaphtho[1,2-e]-1,2,4-triazines via two step condensation of thiosemicarbazide and acenaphtylene-9,10-quinone to form acenaphtho[1,2-e]-1,2,4-triazine-9(8H)-thiones and subsequent reaction with benzyl chloride derivatives. Prepared compounds were subjected to cytotoxic assay in three different cancerous cell lines. Moreover; molecular docking was used to gain further insight into the binding mode and binding affinity of acenaphtho derivatives in the active site of Bcl-2.

Material and methods

All of the reagents were purchased from commercial sources and were freshly used after being purified by standard procedures. Melting points were determined on the Electro-thermal Melting Point apparatus and were uncorrected. Infrared spectra were recorded on the Shimadzu-420 infrared spectrophotometer. ^{1}H-NMR and^{13}C-NMR spectra were recorded in DMSO-d_6 or $CDCl_3$ on Brucker 300 MHz spectrometer (Chemical shifts are given in parts per million or ppm). Mass spectra were recorded on a MS model 5973 Network apparatus at ionization potential of 70 eV. Elemental analyses (C, H, N) were performed by the Microanalytical Unit.

General procedure for preparation of acenaphtho[1,2-e]-1,2,4-triazine-9(8H)-thione (3)

To the acenaphtylene-9,10-quinone (5 mmol) and thiosemicarbazide (5 mmol) in chloroform (30 mL), small amount of acetic acid was added as an catalyst. The reaction mixture was stirred under reflux condition. The progress of the reaction was monitored with TLC and at the completion of the reaction, The precipitated product was filtered off, washed with mixture of H_2O/EtOH, dried and recrystallized from ethanol to give yellow crystalline acenaphtho[1,2-e]-1,2,4-triazine-9(8H)-thione (Scheme 1).

General procedure for preparation of 9-(alkylthio)-acenaphtho[1,2-e]-1,2,4-triazines (5a-g)

To a well-stirred solution of acenaphtho[1,2-e]-1,2,4-triazine-9(8H)-thione (**3**) in 10 ml Chloroform was added triethylamine (3 mmol).

The solution was stirred and then the benzyl chloride derivatives, methyl iodide or ethyl iodide were added and the mixture was heated and stirred under reflux condition. After completion of the reactions, the precipitated residue was filtered, recrystallized in ethanol, filtered, washed with water (2 × 5 mL) and then completely dried in electrical oven (Scheme 1). All prepared compounds were characterized using FT-IR, ^{1}H NMR, ^{13}C NMR and mass spectroscopy (Additional file 1: Table S1).

Acenaphtho[1,2-e]-1,2,4-triazine-9(8H)-thione (3)

Yield 88%, m.p. 148-150°C. ^{1}HNMR (300 MHz, DMSO-d_6) δ: 7.81 (d, 2H, J = 7.5Hz, CH-aromatic), 7.65 (dd, 2H, J = 7.6, 5.9 Hz, CH-aromatic), 7.46 (d, 2H, J = 8Hz CH-aromatic), 3.21 (s, 1H, SH); IR (KBr, cm^{-1}): 3245, 3151, 2922, 1689, 1607, 777; ^{13}C-NMR (75 MHz, DMSO-d_6) δ: 163, 150, 131, 128, 126, 124, 123; MS: m/z (%) 255 (M^+, 51), 213 (100), 180 (75), 152 (49), 139 (44); Anal. Calcd for $C_{13}H_7N_3S$: C, 65.80; H, 2.97; N, 17.71. Found: C, 65.62; H, 2.98; N, 17.58.

9-(benzylthio)-acenaphtho[1,2-e]-1,2,4-triazine (5a)

Yield 94%, m.p. 151-153°C. ^{1}HNMR (300 MHz, DMSO-d_6) δ: 7.78 (d, 2H, J = 7.6Hz, CH-aromatic), 7.61 (dd, 2H, J = 7.6, 6.6 Hz, CH-aromatic), 7.46 (d, 2H, J = 8.5Hz, CH-aromatic), 7.05-7.19 (m, 5H, CH-phenyl), 3.26 (s, 2H, CH_2-benzylic); IR (KBr, cm^{-1}): 3153, 3050, 1694, 1606; ^{13}C-NMR (75 MHz, DMSO-d6) δ: 170.9, 139.7, 142.4, 138.9, 133.5, 128.5, 128.3, 128, 127.8, 127.7, 127.3, 127.2, 126.6, 124.5, 42.2; MS: m/z (%) 327 (M^+, 100), 294 (63), 208 (71), 164 (52), 91 (75); Anal. Calcd for $C_{20}H_{13}N_3S$: C, 73.37; H, 4.00; N, 12.83. Found: C, 73.62; H, 3.88; N, 12.58.

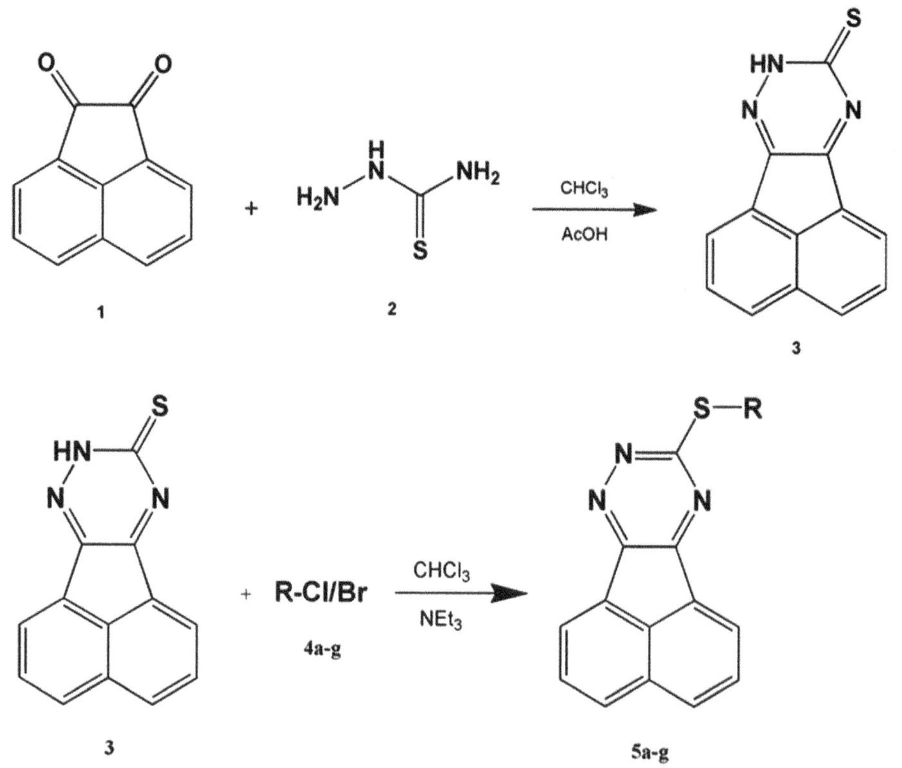

Scheme 1 Synthetic rout to acenaphtho[1,2-e]-1,2,4-triazine-9(8H)-thione and 9-(alkylthio)-acenaphtho[1,2-e]-1,2,4-triazines.

9-(4-nitro-benzylthio)-acenaphtho[1,2-e]-1,2,4-triazine (5b)

Yield 79%, m.p. 156-158°C. ^{1}HNMR (300 MHz, DMSO-d_6) δ: 8.08 (d, 2H, J = 7.5Hz, CH-phenyl), 7.83 (d, 2H, J = 7.6Hz, CH-aromatic), 7.75 (dd, 2H, J = 7.3, 6.6 Hz, CH-aromatic), 7.46 (d, 2H, J = 7.6Hz, CH-phenyl), 7.48 (d, 2H, CH-phenyl), 3.32 (s, 2H, CH_2-benzylic); IR (KBr, cm^{-1}): 3121, 3035, 1670, 1585, 1532, 1486, 937; ^{13}C-NMR (75 MHz, DMSO-d6) δ: 172.4, 149.8, 145.8, 142.4, 133.5, 131.7, 130.3, 127.6, 127.8, 127.3, 128.9, 128.5, 127.5, 124.1, 44.5; MS: m/z (%) 372 (M^+, 12), 255 (48), 213 (100), 180 (87), 152 (62); Anal. Calcd for $C_{20}H_{12}N_4O_2S$: C, 64.50; H, 3.25; N, 15.04. Found: C, 64.62; H, 3.18; N, 15.28.

9-(2,4-dichloro-benzylthio)-acenaphtho[1,2-e]-1,2,4-triazine (5c)

Yield 83%, m.p. 187-188°C. ^{1}HNMR (300 MHz, DMSO-d_6) δ: 7.79 (d, 2H, J = 7.5Hz, CH-aromatic), 7.60 (dd, 2H, J = 7.5, 6.1 Hz, CH-aromatic), 7.46 (d, 2H, J = 8.3Hz CH-aromatic), 7.19 (s, 1H, CH-phenyl), 7.09 (d, 1H, J = 7.3Hz, CH-phenyl), 6.98 (d, 1H, J = 7.3Hz, CH-phenyl), 3.33 (s, 2H, CH_2-benzylic); IR (KBr, cm^{-1}): 3175, 3095, 1656, 1578, 951, 875, 839; ^{13}C-NMR (75 MHz, DMSO-d6) δ: 171.8, 145.4, 134.5, 134.1, 133.5, 131.4, 130.8, 130.4, 129.2, 128.6, 128.1, 127.9, 127.6, 127.3, 127.1, 125.6, 40.4; MS: m/z (%) 395 (M^+, 29), 360 (100), 208 (94), 164 (58); Anal. Calcd for $C_{20}H_{11}Cl_2N_3S$: C, 60.62; H, 2.80; N, 10.60. Found: C, 60.42; H, 2.91; N, 10.73.

9-(3,4-dichloro -benzylthio)-acenaphtho[1,2-e]-1,2,4-triazine (5d)

Yield 60%, m.p. 156-159°C. ^{1}HNMR (300 MHz, DMSO-d_6) δ: 7.80 (d, 2H, J = 7.5Hz, CH-aromatic), 7.52 (dd, 2H, J = 7.4, 6.2 Hz, CH-aromatic), 7.41 (d, 2H, J = 8.3Hz CH-aromatic), 7.18 (d, 1H, J = 7.3Hz, CH-phenyl), 7.08 (s, 1H, CH-phenyl), 6.93 (d, 1H, J = 7.4Hz, CH-phenyl), 3.29 (s, 2H, CH_2-benzylic); IR (KBr, cm^{-1}): 3106, 3019, 1686, 1557, 984, 854; ^{13}C-NMR (75 MHz, DMSO-d6) δ: 170.5, 143.4, 139.2, 133.8, 133.4, 131.8, 130.9, 129.5, 129, 128.6, 128.3, 128.1, 127.6, 127.1, 126.9, 126.5, 38.9; MS: m/z (%) 395 (M^+, 46), 362 (13), 255 (53), 213 (100), 180 (85), 152 (54), 86 (83); Anal. Calcd for $C_{20}H_{11}Cl_2N_3S$: C, 60.62; H, 2.80; N, 10.60. Found: C, 60.53; H, 2.99; N, 10.44.

9-(4-chloro-benzylthio)-acenaphtho[1,2-e]-1,2,4-triazine (5e)

Yield 84%, m.p. 153-156°C. ^{1}HNMR (300 MHz, DMSO-d_6) δ: 7.89 (d, 2H, J = 7.7Hz, CH-aromatic), 7.58 (dd, 2H, J = 7.5, 6.5 Hz, CH-aromatic), 7.42 (d, 2H, J = 8.6Hz CH-aromatic), 7.13 (d, 2H, J = 7.5Hz, CH-phenyl); 6.99 (d, 2H, J = 7.4Hz, CH-phenyl), 3.36 (s, 2H, CH_2-benzylic); IR (KBr, cm^{-1}): 3126, 3058, 1629, 1612, 1597, 1005, 917; ^{13}C-NMR (75 MHz, DMSO-d6) δ: 169.9, 142.4, 138.7, 137.8, 132.7, 133.5, 129.2, 128.9, 128.3, 128, 127.7, 127.3, 126.1, 125.5, 38.5; MS: m/z (%) 361 (M^+, 100), 328 (42), 208 (83), 180 (38), 164 (58), 125 (61); Anal. Calcd for $C_{20}H_{12}ClN_3S$: C, 66.39; H, 3.34; N, 11.61. Found: C, 66.62; H, 3.38; N, 11.40.

9-(methylthio)-acenaphtho[1,2-e]-1,2,4-triazine (5f)
Yield 31%, ^{1}HNMR (500 MHz, $CDCl_3$): 8.44-8.46 (m, 2H, CH-aromatic), 8.24 (m, 1H, CH-aromatic), 8.14 (d, 1H, J = 8.25 Hz, CH-aromatic), 7.86-7.90 (m, 2H, CH-aromatic), 2.84 (s, 3H, $-CH_3$); IR (KBr, cm $^{-1}$): 3150, 2923, 1615, 1416 and 1382; Anal. Calcd for $C_{14}H_9N_3S$: C, 66.91; H, 3.61; N, 16.72. Found: C, 66.82; H, 3.68; N, 16.59.

9-(ethylthio)-acenaphtho[1,2-e]-1,2,4-triazine (5g)
Yield 30%, ^{1}HNMR (500 MHz, DMSO-d_6): 8.38-8.44 (m, 3H, CH-aromatic), 8.29 (d, 1H, J = 8.1 Hz, CH-aromatic), 7.91-7.96 (m, 2H, CH-aromatic), 3.33 (q, 2H, CH_2-CH_3), 1.44-1.47 (t, 3H, J = 7.2 Hz, CH_2-CH_3); IR (KBr, cm $^{-1}$): 3148, 2944, 1617, 1420 and 1381; Anal. Calcd for $C_{15}H_{11}N_3S$: C, 67.90; H, 4.18; N, 15.84. Found: C, 68.06; H, 4.28; N, 15.73.

Cytotoxicity assay
RPMI 1640, fetal bovine serum (FBS), trypsin and phosphate buffered saline (PBS) were purchased from Biosera (Ringmer, UK). 3-(4,5-dimethylthiazol-2-yl)-2,5-diphenyltetrazolium bromide (MTT) was obtained from Sigma (Saint Louis, MO, USA) and penicillin/streptomycin was purchased from Invitrogen (San Diego, CA, USA). Doxorubicin and dimethyl sulphoxide were obtained from EBEWE Pharma (Unterach, Austria) and Merck (Darmstadt, Germany), respectively.

HL-60 (human promyelocytic leukemia), MCF-7 (human breast adenocarcinoma) and MOLT-4 (human acute lymphoblastic leukemia) cells were obtained from the National Cell Bank of Iran, Pasteur Institute, Tehran, Iran. All cell lines were maintained in RPMI 1640 supplemented with 10% FBS, and 100 units/mL penicillin-G and 100 μg/mL streptomycin. Cells were grown in monolayer cultures.

Cell viability following exposure to synthetic compounds was evaluated by using the MTT reduction assay. HL-60, MCF7, and MOLT-4 cells were plated in 96-well microplates at a density of 5×10^4 cells/ mL (100 μl per well). Positive control wells contained cisplatin and doxorubicin and blank wells contained only growth medium for background correction. After overnight incubation at 37°C, half of the growth medium was removed and 50 μL of medium supplemented with different concentrations of synthetic compounds dissolved in DMSO were added in quadruplicate. Maximum concentration of DMSO in the wells was 0.5% (The solution of 0.5% DMSO was also tested as a cytotoxicity control). Cells were further incubated for 72 h. At the end of the incubation time, the medium was removed and MTT was added to each well at a final concentration of 0.5 mg/mL and plates were incubated for another 4 h at 37°C. Then formazan crystals were solubilized in 200 μl DMSO. The optical density was measured at 570 nm with background correction at 655 nm using a Bio-Rad microplate reader (Model 680). The percentage of viability compared to control wells was calculated for each concentration of the compound and IC50 values were calculated with the software CurveExpert version 1.34 for Windows. Each experiment was repeated 3–4 times. Data are represented as mean ± S.E.M.

Molecular docking study
The ligand-flexible docking studies were performed using the widely distributed molecular docking software, AutoDock 4.2 [26]. Lamarckian Genetic Algorithm of the AutoDock 4.2 program was used to perform the flexible-ligand docking studies [27]. All the x-ray crystallographic *holo* structures of Bcl-2 were retrieved from the Brookhaven protein data bank (http://www.rcsb.org/). The protein structure was subjected to optimization step in order to minimize the crystallographic induced bond clashes using steepest descent method. All the preprocessing steps for receptor and ligand files were done by Auto-Dock Tools 1.5.4 (ADT) [28]. For the preparation of protein, Kollman united atom charges and polar hydrogen's were added to the receptor and crystallographic waters were removed. For docked ligands, Gasteiger charge was assigned, non-polar hydrogens were merged into the related carbon atoms of the receptor and torsions degrees of freedom were also allocated by ADT program.

Lamarckian genetic algorithm (LGA) was used to simulate the binding affinity and binding mode of acenaphtho derivatives in the active site of Bcl-2. 100 independent genetic algorithm (GA) runs were considered for each ligand under study. For Lamarckian GA; 27000 maximum generations; a gene mutation rate of 0.02; and

Table 1 Cell growth inhibitory activity of synthetic acenaphtho derivatives assessed by the MTT reduction assay

Comp. no.	IC_{50}[a] (μM)		
	HL-60 cells	MCF-7 cells	MOLT-4 cells
5a	48.4 ± 8.7	NA[b]	30.1 ± 5.6
5b	36.0 ± 5.4	NA	28.0 ± 4.6
5c	51.2 ± 7.6	NA	30.3 ± 8.2
5d	NA	NA	NA
5e	30.1 ± 3.6	NA	33.6 ± 2.9
5f	ND[c]	61.9 ± 20.6	65.5 ± 20.4
5g	ND	NA	NA
Cisplatin	3.0 ± 0.1	23.7 ± 6.8	3.0 ± 0.2
Doxorubicin	0.014 ± 0.002	0.221 ± 0.095	0.017 ± 0.002

[a]*Values represent mean ± S.E.M..*
[b]*NA: not active.*
[c]*ND: not determined.*

Table 2 Top ranked AutoDock scores based on the binding free energies (ΔG) of acenaphtho structures docked into the Bcl-2 active site (Isoform 1: 1G5M) along with interacted amino acids of Bcl-2

Comp. no.	ΔG_b (kcal/mol)	H-bonds		Amino acids in non-bonded contacts
		Amino acid	Distance (Å)	
5a	−7.03	Arg12	2.22	Glu13, Met16, Lys17, His20, Ala32, Asp35, Val36, Glu38, Asn39, Thr41
		Glu48	1.95	
5b	−9.29	Ser49	2.50	Asp10, Gly46, Glu50
		Lys17	1.73	
5c	−8.09	Arg12	1.96	Glu13, Met16, Ala32, Val36, Glu38, Asn39, Thr41
5d	−8.22	Arg12	2.20	Glu13, Met16, Ala32, Asp35, Val36, Glu38, Asn39, Thr41
5e	−7.73	Arg12	2.16	Glu13, Met16, Ala32, Asp35, Val36, Glu38, Asn39, Thr41

a crossover rate of 0.8 were applied. The grid maps of the protein were calculated using AutoGrid (part of the AutoDock package). The size of grid was set in a way to include not only the active site but also considerable portions of the surrounding surface. For this purpose, a grid of 60 × 60 × 60 points in x, y, and z directions was built centered on the center of mass of the catalytic site of Bcl-2 with a spacing of 0.375 Å. Cluster analysis was performed on the docked results using an Root mean square deviation (RMSD) tolerance of 2 Å.

Ligand-receptor interactions were all detected on the basis of docking results using LIGPLOT [29]. Molecular images were produced using VMD program [30].

Results and discussion

Chemistry

Some new acenaphtho derivatives were obtained by condensation of acenaphtylene-9,10-quinone and thiosemicarbazide followed by reaction with different benzyl chloride derivatives under mild conditions in chloroform solution (Scheme 1). The isolated compounds were then characterized by elemental analyses, FT-IR, MS and NMR spectroscopy. The applied synthetic method afforded all the 9-(alkylthio)-acenaphtho[1,2-e]-1,2,4-triazines in high yields and short reaction times except for 9-(methylthio) and 9-(ethylthio) derivatives that were produced in lower yields (Additional file 1: Table S1).

Cytotoxicity assay

The *in vitro* cytotoxic activities for prepared acenaphtho derivatives are shown in Table 1.

All the compounds under study exhibited medium cytotoxic activity on the evaluated cancerous cell lines except for 9-(methylthio) (5f) and 9-(ethylthio) (5 g) derivatives. Compound 5 g was inactive in MCF-7 and MOLT-4 cells. Compound 5b showed higher cytotoxicity in MOLT-4 cells. In HL-60 cells, compound 5e exhibited superior cytotoxic activity. The order of cytotoxic effects in HL-60 and MOLT-4 cell lines could be shown as 5e > 5b > 5a > 5c > 5d and 5b > 5a > 5c > 5e > 5f > 5d = 5 g. Variations of cytotoxic results were less pronounced for MOLT-4 cell lines. Moreover, all of the tested compounds were inactive on MCF-7 cells except for 5f which exhibited an IC_{50} value of 61.9 μM.

With the exception of compound **5e**, a common trend, might be deduced that the presence of electron withdrawing/hydrogen acceptor nitro group on the phenyl ring of 9-(alkylthio)-acenaphtho[1,2-e]-1,2,4-triazines afforded higher cytotoxic effects while halogenated compounds showed lower *in vitro* potencies. It was also revealed that acenaphtho derivatives bearing aralkyl substituents on their sulfur atom (5a-e) might exhibit better cytotoxicity profiles than acenaphtho derivatives bearing alkyl substituents (5f and 5 g). Further structure activity relationship developments is under investigation via preparing more diverse sets of these derivatives.

Table 3 Top ranked AutoDock scores based on the binding free energies (ΔG) of acenaphtho structures docked into the Bcl-2 active site (Isoform 2: 1GJH) along with interacted amino acids of Bcl-2

Comp. no.	ΔG_b (kcal/mol)	H-bonds		Amino acids in non-bonded contacts
		Amino acid	Distance (Å)	
5a	−6.78	Ser49	2.18	Thr7, Pro44, Gly46, Glu48, Glu50
5b	−9.13	Asp10	1.87	Thr7, Gly8, Tyr9, Glu13, Thr41, Glu42, Ala43, Pro44, Gly46, Ser49
5c	−8.11	Ala32	2.36	Glu13, Met16, His20, Trp30, Asp31, Gly33, Val36
5d	−7.74	-		Glu13, Met16, His20, Glu29, Trp30, Ala32
5e	−7.84	-		Glu13, Met16, His20, Glu29, Trp30, Ala32

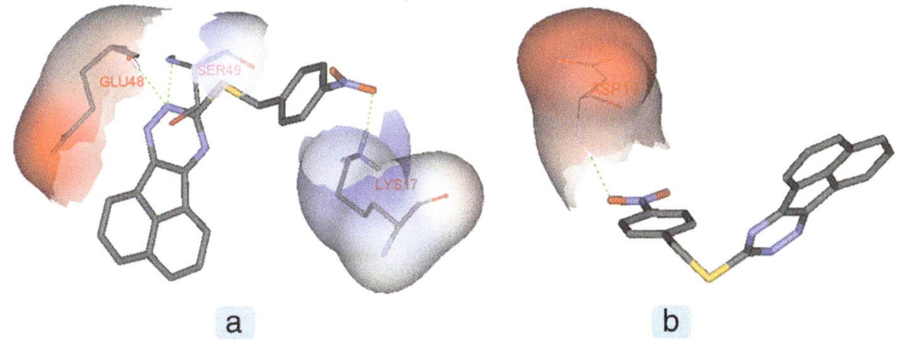

Figure 1 H-bond interactions of compound 5b in the active site of Bcl-2 isoforms a) PDB ID: 1G5M and b) PDB ID: 1GJH.

Molecular modeling studies

We decided to gain some information on binding modes of tested compounds on the Bcl-2 active site via molecular docking. Previous reports proposed that despite the similarity in the structures of two Bcl-2 isoforms, they behave differently in binding to the pro-apoptotic members of the Bcl-2 family [31]. For this purpose we decided to conduct our modeling studies on the structures of the two isoforms of Bcl-2 protein (isoforms 1: 1G5M and isoform 2: 1GJH).

Due to the lower cytotoxic activities of 9-(methylthio) and 9-(ethylthio) derivatives and also considering our main focus on 9-(Aralkylthio)-acenaphtho[1,2-e]-1,2,4-triazines rather than 9-(alkylthio)-acenaphtho[1,2-e]-1,2,4-triazines, all modeling studies were performed on 9-(benzylthio) derivatives.

Validation of molecular docking

A performance of a typical docking protocol can be checked via testing its ability in predicting predominant binding mode of a cognate (co-crystallographic) ligand. This procedure is performed via extracting the structure of a cognate ligand and re-docking it into its receptor (self-docking). RMSD of the Cartesian coordinates of the atoms of the ligand in the docked and crystallographic conformations will be the criterion of the docking validation (RMSD ≤ 2 Å).

Various PDB derived Bcl-2 structures were subjected to docking validation procedure. PDB structures were chosen on the basis of crystallographic resolutions. Regarding RMSD values and also conformation population in the top-ranked cluster of AutoDock output file, 1G5M and 1GJH were selected as the most appropriate crystallographic structure for further modeling studies.

Docking simulation of acenaphtho derivatives

Considering the well obtained *in vitro* results, it was thought worthy to perform molecular docking studies, hence considering both *in silico* and *in vitro* results. Owing to the potential apoptosis-inducing activity of acenaphtho scaffolds via the Bcl-2 protein [17], we decided to model the binding interactions of assayed 9-(alkylthio)-acenaphtho[1,2-e]-1,2,4-triazines in the active site of Bcl-2 via docking simulation. For this purpose, 9-(alkylthio)-acenaphtho[1,2-e]-1,2,4-triazines were all docked into the active site of selected receptors *i.e.* various isoforms of Bcl-2 (1G5M and 1GJH) which differed in two amino acids [31].

Docking results with isoforms 1 (PDB code: 1G5M) and 2 (PDB code: 1GJH) are summarized in Tables 2 and 3, respectively. Top ranked binding energies (kcal/mol) in AutoDock dlg output files were considered as the best docking result in each case. It should be noted that all top ranked clusters were supported by high conformation populations. This observation could be expected since literature evidence implied that docking studies with compounds bearing less active torsions can significantly promote the docking success rates due to the limited conformational degrees of freedom [32].

In silico results revealed that synthesized molecules showed relatively good binding energies toward Bcl-2 active site ranging from −7.03 to −9.29 kcal/mol in isoform1 (1G5M) and −6.78 to −9.13 kcal/mol in isoform 2 (1GJH). Estimated binding energies were in the order of 5b > 5d > 5c > 5e > 5a in the active site of isoform 1 and 5b > 5c > 5d > 5e > 5a in the active site of isoform 2. The trends may also highlight slight conformational differences for two Bcl-2 isoforms [31].

Molecular docking study revealed that 9-(alkylthio)-acenaphtho[1,2-e]-1,2,4-triazine derivatives (5a-e) may inhibit Bcl-2 protein via H-bond and hydrophobic interactions (Tables 2 and 3). Compound 5b exhibited the best docking score (Tables 2 and 3) while being most potent in human MOLT-4 cells (Table 1). It seemed that the presence of *para*-nitro substituent on phenyl ring of 5b might be responsible for additional H-bonds with the active site of the receptor. This H-bond acceptor site would potentially support one key H-bond interactions with NH of Lys17 in isoform 1 and NH of Asp10 in isoform 2 through oxygen atom of a nitro substituent (Figure 1). The profile of interaction in 5b (Figure 1) further announced us that *para* nitro substituent in *9-(4-nitro-alkylthio)-acenaphtho[1,2-e]-1,2,4-triazine* (5b) might have some directional effect on the active site oriented conformation of the ligand. This rationale could be shown in Figure 2 in which different orientation of acenaphtho cycle in 5b compared to other compounds is obviously detectable. This new orientation would relocate a triazine ring in a position to make H-bond interactions with Ser49 and Glu48 via polar hydrogen of N15 atom (Figures 1 and 3). From another aspect of view, docking simulation could be applied to find the binding mode and mechanism of less active derivatives.

To add more, it seemed that H-bond connections contributed more significantly in complex stabilization in the case of 5b and Bcl-2 isoform 1 (1G5M) rather than isoform 2 (1GJH). Compounds 5a, 5c, 5d and 5e all participated in key H-bonds with nitrogen atoms of a triazine ring (Figure 2). We found that Arg12 interacted via its guanine side chain (NH1; Figure 2) with nitrogen

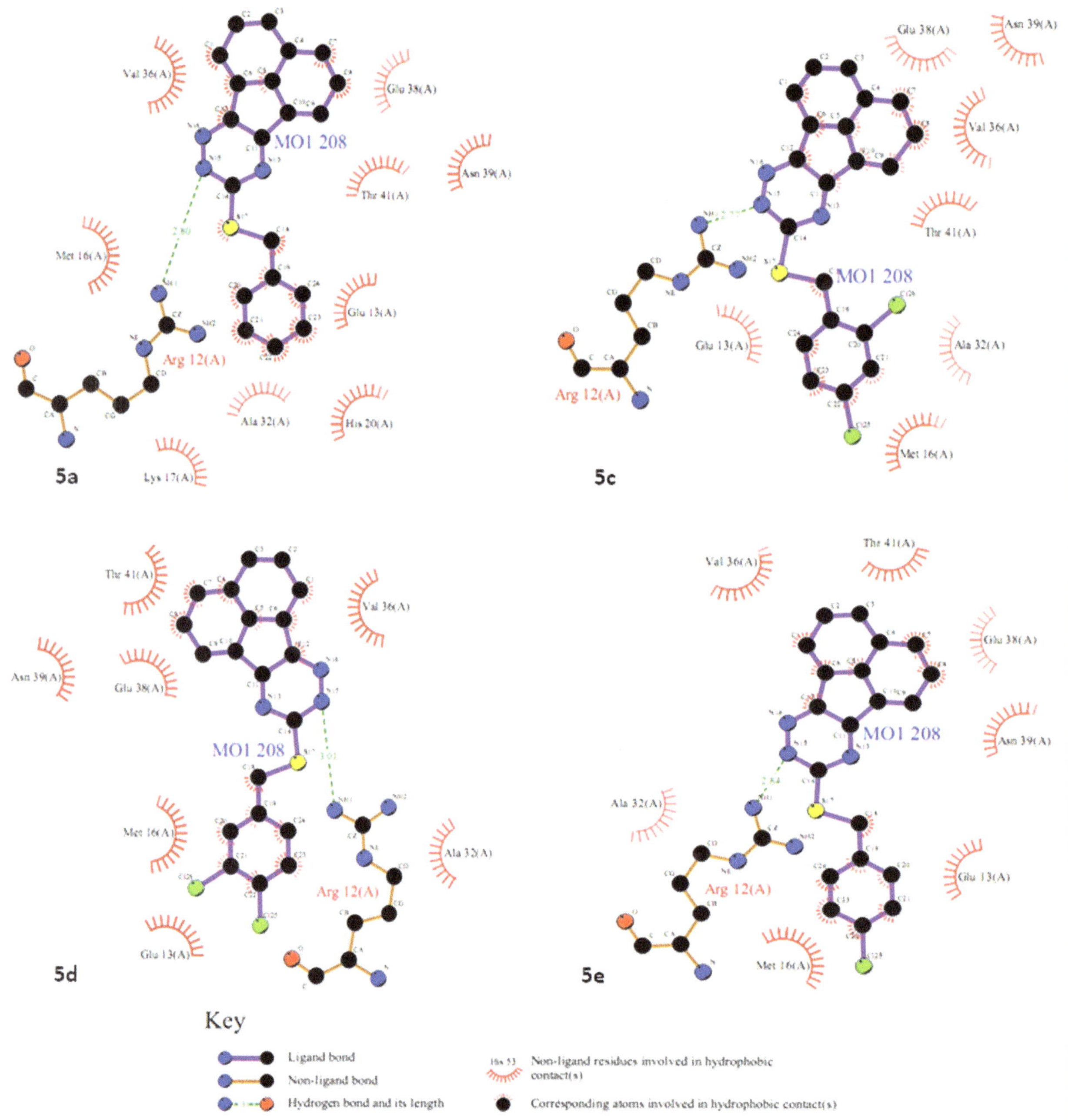

Figure 2 H-bond interactions between acenaphtho derivatives (5a, 5c, 5d and 5e) and active site residues in isoform 1 of Bcl-2.

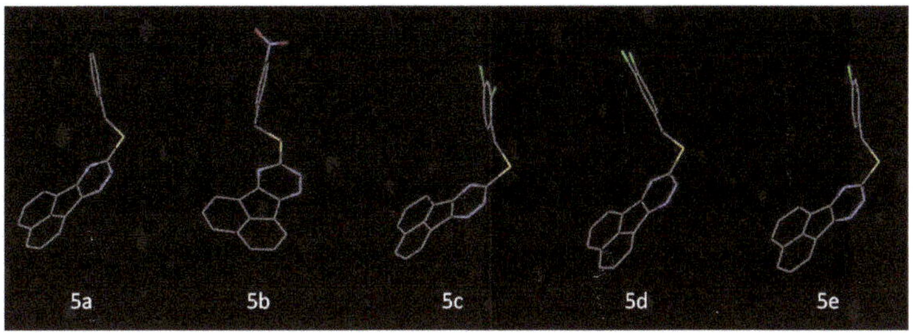

Figure 3 Different active site oriented conformations for docked acenaphtho derivatives (5a, 5b, 5c, 5d and 5e) in the active site of Bcl-2 isoform 1.

atom of a triazine ring in acenaphtho derivatives (N15; Figure 2).

Docking of commonly used neoplastic drugs *i.e.* Geftinib, Cisplatin, 5-FU, Gemcitabine and Vinorelbine into the active site of Bcl-2 (isoform 1; 15GM) has been reported elsewhere [6]. It was revealed that Asp10, Glu13, Lys17, Glu42 and Ser49 contributed to H-bond formation with the docked drugs [6]. Same residues were found to be key H-bond/non-bonded participants for inhibitor recognition in our study. Docking results showed that Glu13 contributed to non-bonded contacts with 5a, 5b, 5c and 5d (Table 1) while Asp10 participated in non-bonded contacts with 5b. Moreover; H-bond network in the case of Cisplatin (Asp10, Lys17 and Ser49) was very similar to that of 5b (Lys17, Glu48 and Ser49). The residue atoms involved in the binding pattern were the same for cisplatin and 5b in the case of Lys17 (quaternary NH of side chain; Figure 1) while for Ser49, cisplatin interacted with hydroxyl group of the Ser49 side chain but compound 5b made hydrogen bond via Ser49 backbone NH (Figure 1). Lys17 has also been reported to be involved in efficient H-bonds with Geftinib, Gemcitabine and Vinorelbine while stabilizing H-bonds were detected in the case of Glu13 for Gemcitabine and Vinorelbine [6].

Literature data revealed the effect of position of substituent(s) on phenyl moiety in comparison to our results [33]. It has been discussed that considering substituent groups being attached to the *para* or *meta*-position, the hydrophobic pocket of Bcl-2 exhibited varied tolerability. This further identified the size of the hydrophobic pocket of Bcl-2 to be limited. *Meta* or *para*-halogen atoms on phenyl ring induce different conformations leading to decreased interactions with hydrophobic pocket of Bcl-2 (compounds 5d and 5f) (Figure 4).

Molecular docking on human anti-apoptotic Bcl-2 further supported the biological data. Regarding the obtained results, compound 5b could serve as an appropriate starting point for designing new chemical entities as potent Bcl-2 inhibitors.

Binding efficiency indices

Another criterion which has recently absorbed much attention in ligand-receptor interaction studies is the ligand efficiency (LE) parameter. Nowadays LE indices are regarded as undeniable tools in modern drug discovery projects [34]. The model of analyzing ligand binding in terms of the free energy per heavy atom (heavy atom count; HAC) was first introduced by Andrews [35]. Concept of the binding energy per atom or binding efficiency of a ligand could be a useful parameter in the selection of lead compounds, considering the real potency of a compound and hence might consider optimized fragments [36]. Generally speaking, molecules achieving a desirable potency with fewer HACs are by definition

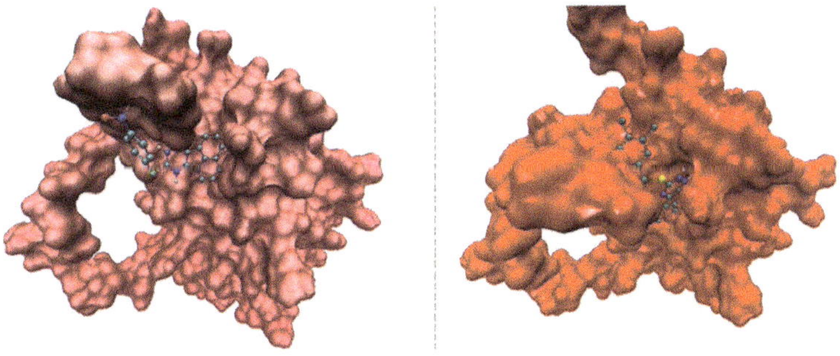

Figure 4 Compounds 5b (left) and 5d (right) in the active site of Bcl-2.

Table 4 Experimental/theoretical binding/ligand efficiency indices for 9-(benzylthio)-acenaphtho[1,2-e]-1,2,4-triazine derivatives (Bcl-2, isoforms 1 & 2, PDB IDs: 1G5M & 1GJH)

HL-60 cells								MOLT-4 cells							
Molecule no.	Related PDB code	IC50 (μM)	pIC50	Experimental LE[a]	Estimated LE[b] ($kcal.mol^{-1}.HAC^{-1}$)	Experimental BEI [c]	Estimated BEI ($kcal.mol^{-1}.kDa^{-1}$)	Molecule no.	Related PDB code	IC50 (μM)	pIC50	Experimental LE	Estimated LE ($kcal.mol^{-1}.HAC^{-1}$)	Experimental BEI	Estimated BEI ($kcal.mol^{-1}.kDa^{-1}$)
5a	1G5M	48.4	4.32	0.179	0.208	13.20	15.77	**5a**	1G5M	30.1	4.52	0.188	0.208	13.83	15.77
5b	1G5M	36.0	4.44	0.114	0.134	11.95	14.36	**5b**	1G5M	28.0	4.55	0.190	0.134	12.24	14.36
5c	1G5M	51.2	4.29	0.165	0.228	10.86	15.01	**5c**	1G5M	30.3	4.52	0.188	0.228	11.44	15.01
5d	1G5M	-	-	-	0.218	-	15.26	**5d**	1G5M	-	-	-	0.218	-	15.26
5e	1G5M	30.1	4.52	0.170	0.219	12.52	15.69	**5e**	1G5M	33.6	4.47	0.186	0.219	12.39	15.69
5a	1GJH	48.4	4.31	0.179	0.214	13.20	15.24	**5a**	1GJH	30.1	4.52	0.188	0.214	13.83	15.24
5b	1GJH	36.0	4.44	0.114	0.137	11.95	14.05	**5b**	1GJH	28.0	4.55	0.190	0.137	12.24	14.05
5c	1GJH	51.2	4.29	0.165	0.228	10.86	15.04	**5c**	1GJH	30.3	4.52	0.188	0.228	11.44	15.04
5d	1GJH	-	-	-	0.232	-	14.36	**5d**	1GJH	-	-	-	0.232	-	14.36
5e	1GJH	30.1	4.52	0.170	0.237	12.52	15.18	**5e**	1GJH	33.6	4.47	0.186	0.237	12.39	15.18

[a] *LE values are defined in the range of 0–1* [34].
[b] *Estimated LEs were calculated according to equation (2).*
[c] *Reference value for BEI is 27* [35].

more efficient. LE index can be simply calculated using the equations (1) or (2):

$$LE = -\frac{\Delta G_b}{HAC} \quad (1)$$

$$LE = -\frac{pK_i;\ pK_d;\ or\ pIC50}{HAC} \quad (2)$$

Regarding the ligand efficiencies, it was postulated that molecular weights are prior to the HACs in considering the contribution of heteroatoms from different rows of the periodic table [37]. Thus a modified efficiency value was suggested as binding efficiency index (BEI). The importance of BEI can be emphasized regarding an increase in molecular weight at the clinical candidate step, which is regarded as an undeniable paradox with a common trend towards lower MWs and better pharmacokinetic profiles in marketable drugs [38]. BEI could be easily estimated from equation (3):

$$BEI = -\frac{pK_i;\ or\ pIC50}{MW\ (kDa)} \quad (3)$$

Accordingly, assayed acenaphtho derivatives were re-evaluated on the basis of their experimental and theoretical BEI/LE values (Table 4).

Regarding the summarized data in Table 4, following rationales might be pointed out:

- In our calculations, estimated LEs in terms of pKi values (equation 2) produced results more compatible to the experimental LEs (cellular assays) when compared to the LEs in terms of ΔG_b values (equation 1; the related data are not shown in the Table).
- Compound 5b is the top ranked bioactive molecule in docking results and also MOLT-4 based cellular assay. But this compound achieved relatively lower scores in terms of experimental/theoretical efficiency indices. The observed paradox demonstrated that larger bioactive compounds may require special attention in their design toward efficiency indices [25].
- Efficient bioactive molecules may be better categorized considering estimated BEIs rather than LEs. In some cases, especially for molecules bearing larger atoms, incorporating molecular weights rather than number of heavy atoms in the calculation of efficiency indices produced less biased results.
- The application of theoretical ligand/binding efficiency indices in the cell –based cytotoxicity protocols should be considered with care due to the multi-target nature of the cytotoxic agents. For example, compound 5d which is the structural isomer of compound 5c, was inactive in MTT assays.

Conclusion

Various studies have demonstrated that chemical structures bearing sulfur atom(s) may possibly induce apoptosis [39,40]. On the basis of results from this study, corresponding 9-(benzylthio) acenaphtho[1,2-e]-1,2,4-triazines might be regarded as valuable cytotoxic polycyclic heterocycles and potential candidates for additional molecular modifications with the aim of developing potent cytotoxic agents. Experimental and modeling studies confirmed the previous reports on acenaphtho derivatives and moreover; the docking results agreed well with the observed *in silico* data for commonly used anticancer drugs. Despite the closeness of docking scores, relatively different binding profiles for acenaphtho derivatives might confirm the previous results on conformational difference between two Bcl-2 isoforms. Concept of binding efficiency as a common and well–approached tool in modern drug discovery strategies was reviewed in our study. Confirming previous reports, it was demonstrated that bioactive molecular design on the basis of potency alone or binding efficiency values might be considered as different strategies leading to dissimilar results in lead/drug development campaigns. However several literature reports demonstrated that lead/drug discovery projects on the basis of binding efficiency indices would afford bioactive compounds with better pharmacokinetic outcomes. Extended cytotoxicity assays on diverse sets of acenaphtho-based scaffolds with the aim of establishing more rational structure activity relationships are under investigation.

Additional file

Additional file 1: Table S1. Physical and analytical data of 9-(alkylthio)-acenaphtho[1,2-e]-1,2,4-triazines 5a-h.

Competing interests
The authors declare that they have no competing interests.

Authors' contributions
MKM: Synthesis of some target compounds. OF: Supervision of biological tests. MKH: Design of target compounds and collaboration in manuscript preparation. NR-A: Performed the molecular docking study and collaboration in manuscript preparation. SS: Performed the molecular docking study. RM: supervision of the design, synthetic and pharmacological parts. All authors read and approved the final manuscript.

Acknowledgement
Financial supports of this project by Vice-chancellor Research of Shiraz University of Medical Sciences are acknowledged.

Author details
[1]Faculty of sciences, Ahvaz Branch, Islamic Azad University, Ahvaz, Iran. [2]Medicinal and Natural Products Chemistry Research Center, Shiraz, University of Medical Sciences, PO Box 3288-71345, Shiraz, Iran. [3]Departments of Medicinal Chemistry, School of Pharmacy, Shiraz University of Medical Sciences, Shiraz, Iran. [4]Departments of Medicinal Chemistry, Faculty of Pharmacy, Isfahan University of Medical Sciences, Isfahan, Iran.

References

1. Weber L, Illgen K, Almstetter M: **Discovery of new multi component reactions with combinatorial methods.** *Synlett* 1999, **3**:366–374.
2. Tietze LF, Modi A: **Multicomponent domino reactions for the synthesis of biologically active natural products and drugs.** *Med Res Rev* 2000, **20**:304–322.
3. Ganem B: **Strategies for innovation in multicomponent reaction design.** *Acc Chem Res* 2009, **42**:463–472.
4. Marcaurelle LA, Johannes CW: **Application of natural product-inspired diversity-oriented synthesis to drug discovery.** *Prog Drug Res* 2008, **66**:187–216.
5. Ulaczyk-Lesanko A, Hall DG: **Wanted: New multicomponent reactions for generating libraries of polycyclic natural products.** *Curr Opin Chem Biol* 2005, **9**:266–276.
6. Ahmed A, Daneshtalab M: **Polycyclic quinolones (part 1)-thieno[2,3-b] benzo[h]-quinoline derivatives: design, synthesis, preliminary in vitro and in silico studies.** *Heterocycles* 2012, **85**:103–122.
7. Kock I, Heber D, Weide M, Wolschendorf U, Clement B: **Synthesis and biological evaluation of 11-substituted 6-aminobenzo [c] phenanthridine derivatives, a new class of antitumor agents.** *J Med Chem* 2005, **48**:2772–2777.
8. Khan IA, Kulkarni MV, Gopal M, Shahabuddin MS, Sun CM: **Synthesis and biological evaluation of novel angularly fused polycyclic coumarins.** *Bioorg Med Chem Lett* 2005, **15**:3584–3587.
9. Noushini S, Emami S, Safavi M, Ardestani SK, Gohari AR, Shafiee A, Foroumadi A: **Synthesis and cytotoxic properties of novel (E)-3-benzylidene-7-methoxychroman-4-one derivatives.** *DARU J Pharm Sci* 2013, **21**:31.
10. Rescifina A, Zagni C, Romeo G, Sortino S: **Synthesis and biological activity of novel bifunctional isoxazolidinyl polycyclic aromatic hydrocarbons.** *Bioorg Med Chem* 2012, **20**:4978–4984.
11. Banik BK, Becker FF: **Polycyclic aromatic compounds as anticancer agents: structure-activity relationships of chrysene and pyrene derivatives.** *Bioorg Med Chem* 2001, **9**:593–605.
12. Madakar Sobhani A, Rasoul Amini S, Tyndall JDA, Azizi E, Daneshtalab M, Khalaj A: **A theory of mode of action of azolylalkylquinolines as DNA binding agents using automated flexible ligand docking.** *J Mol Graph Model* 2006, **25**:459–469.
13. Lee CH, Jiang M, Cowart M, Gfesser G, Perner R, Kim KH, Gu YG, Williams M, Jarvis MF, Kowaluk EA: **Discovery of 4-amino-5-(3-bromophenyl)-7-(6-morpholino-pyridin-3-yl) pyrido [2, 3-d] pyrimidine, an orally active, non-nucleoside adenosine kinase inhibitor.** *J Med Chem* 2001, **44**:2133–2138.
14. Jellimann C, Mathe-Allainmat M, Andrieux J, Kloubert S, Boutin JA, Nicolas JP, Bennejean C, Delagrange P, Langlois M: **Synthesis of phenalene and acenaphtho derivatives as new conformationally restricted ligands for melatonin receptors.** *J Med Chem* 2000, **43**:4051–4062.
15. Kozlov NS, Shmanai GS, Tai DN: **Synthesis and spectral characteristics of acenaphtho derivatives of benzo [f] quinoline.** *Chem Heterocyc Compd* 1986, **22**:894–898.
16. Xie YM, Deng Y, Dai XY, Liu J, Ouyang L, Wei YQ, Zhao YL: **Synthesis and biological evaluation of novel acenaphtho derivatives as potential antitumor agents.** *Molecules* 2011, **16**:2519–2526.
17. Zhang Z, Jin L, Qian X, Wei M, Wang Y, Wang J, Yang Y, Xu Q, Xu Y, Liu F: **Novel Bcl-2 inhibitors: discovery and mechanism study of small organic apoptosis-inducing agents.** *Chembiochem* 2007, **8**:113–121.
18. Tsujimoto Y, Finger LR, Yunis J, Nowell PC, Croce CM: **Cloning of the chromosome breakpoint of neoplastic B cells with the t (14; 18) chromosome translocation.** *Science* 1984, **226**:1097–1099.
19. Cleary ML, Smith SD, Sklar J: **Cloning and structural analysis of cDNAs for bcl-2 and a hybrid bcl-2/immunoglobulin transcript resulting from the t(14;18) translocation.** *Cell* 1986, **47**:19–28.
20. El Ashry ESH, Abdel HH, Shoukry M: **Synthesis and reaction of acenaphthoquinones. part-1. A review.** *Ind J Heterocycl Chem* 1998, **7**:313–320.
21. El Ashry ESH, Hamid HA, Kassem AA, Shoukry M: **Synthesis and reactions of acenaphthoquinones-part-2. The reactions of acenaphthoquinones.** *Mol* 2002, **7**:155–188.
22. Vosooghi M, Yahyavi H, Divsalar K, Shamsa H, Kheirollahi A, Safavi M, Ardestani SK, Sadeghi-Neshat S, Mohammadhosseini N, Edraki N, Khoshneviszadeh M, Shafiee A, Foroumadi A: **Synthesis and in vitrocytotoxic activity evaluation of (E)-16-(substituted benzylidene) derivatives of dehydroepiandrosterone.** *DARU J Pharm Sci* 2013, **21**:34.
23. Miri R, Firuzi O, Peymani P, Zamani M, Mehdipour AR, Heydari Z, Masteri Farahani M, Shafiee A: **Synthesis, cytotoxicity, and QSAR study of new aza-cyclopenta [b] fluorene1, 9-dione derivatives.** *Chem Biol Drug Des* 2012, **79**:68–75.
24. Azizian J, Mohammadi MK, Firuzi O, Mirza B, Miri R: **Microwave-assisted solvent-free synthesis of bis(dihydropyrimidinone)benzenes and evaluation of their cytotoxic activity.** *Chem Biol Drug Des* 2010, **75**:375–380.
25. Azizian J, Mohammadi MK, Firuzi O, Razzaghi-asl N, Miri R: **Synthesis, biological activity and docking study of some new isatin Schiff base derivatives.** *Med Chem Res* 2012, **21**:3730–3740.
26. Morris GM, Huey R, Lindstrom W, Sanner MF, Belew RK, Goodsell DS, Olson AJ: **AutoDock4 and AutoDockTools4: automated docking with selective receptor flexibility.** *J Comput Chem* 2009, **30**:2785–2791.
27. Morris GM, Goodsell DS, Halliday RS, Huey R, Hart WE, Belew RK, Olson AJ: **Automated docking using a Lamarckian genetic algorithm and an empirical binding free energy function.** *J Comput Chem* 1998, **19**:1639–1662.
28. Morris GM, Huey R, Olson AJ: **Using AutoDock for ligand-receptor docking.** *Curr Protoc Bioinformatics* 2008, **11**:34–37.
29. Wallace AC, Laskowski RA, Thornton JM: **LIGPLOT: a program to generate schematic diagrams of protein-ligand interactions.** *Protein Eng* 1995, **8**:127–134.
30. Humphrey W, Dalke A, Schulten K: **VMD: visual molecular dynamics.** *J Mol Graphics* 1996, **14**:33–38.
31. Petros AM, Medek A, Nettesheim DG, Kim DH, Yoon HS, Swift K, Matayoshi ED, Oltersdorf T, Fesik SW: **Solution structure of the antiapoptotic protein bcl-2.** *Proc Natl Acad Sci* 2001, **98**:3012–3017.
32. Erickson JA, Jalaie M, Robertson DH, Lewis RA, Vieth M: **Lessons in molecular recognition: the effects of ligand and protein flexibility on molecular docking accuracy.** *J Med Chem* 2004, **47**:45–55.
33. Zhang Z, Yang H, Wu G, Li Z, Song T: **Probing the difference between BH3 groove of Mcl-1 and Bcl-2 protein: implications for dual inhibitors design.** *Eur J Med Chem* 2011, **46**:3909–3916.
34. Tanaka D, Tsuda Y, Shiyama T, Nishimura T, Chiyo N, Tominaga Y, Sawada N, Mimoto T, Kusunose N: **A practical use of ligand efficiency indices out of the fragment-based approach: Ligand efficiency-guided lead identification of soluble epoxide hydrolase inhibitors.** *J Med Chem* 2011, **54**:851–857.
35. Andrews PR, Craik DJ, Martin JL: **Functional group contributions to drug-receptor interactions.** *J Med Chem* 1984, **27**:1648–1657.
36. Hopkins AL, Groom CR, Alex A: **Ligand efficiency: a useful metric for lead selection.** *Drug Discov Today* 2004, **9**:430.
37. Abad-Zapatero C, Metz JT: **Ligand efficiency indices as guideposts for drug discovery.** *Drug Discov Today* 2005, **10**:464–469.
38. Wenlock MC, Austin RP, Barton P, Davis AM, Leeson PD: **A comparison of physiochemical property profiles of development and marketed oral drugs.** *J Med Chem* 2003, **46**:1250–1256.
39. Becattini B, Sareth S, Zhai D, Crowell KJ, Leone M, Reed JC, Pellecchia M: **Targeting apoptosis via chemical design: inhibition of bid-induced cell death by small organic molecules.** *Chem Biol* 2004, **11**:1107–1117.
40. Rahman MA, Dhar DK, Masunaga R, Yamanoi A, Kohno H, Nagasue N: **Sulindac and exisulind exhibit a significant antiproliferative effect and induce apoptosis in human hepatocellular carcinoma cell lines.** *Cancer Res* 2000, **60**:2085–2089.

New aspects of *Saccharomyces cerevisiae* as a novel carrier for berberine

Roshanak Salari[1], BiBi Sedigheh Fazly Bazzaz[1,2], Omid Rajabi[1,3] and Zahra Khashyarmanesh[1*]

Abstract

Background: Berberine was encapsulated in yeast cells of *Saccharomyces cerevisiae* as novel carriers to be used in different food and drug industries. The microcapsules were characterized by differential scanning calorimetry (DSC), fourier transform infra red spectroscopy (FT-IR) and fluorescence microscopy. The encapsulation factors such as plasmolysis of yeast cells which affects the % encapsulation yield were studied.

Results: Fluorescence microscopy showed the yeast cells became fluorescent after encapsulation process. DSC diagram was representing of new peak for microcapsule which was not the same as berberine and the empty yeast cells peaks, separately. FTIR spectrums of microcapsules and yeast cells were almost the same. The plasmolysed and non plasmolysed microcapsules were loaded with berberine up to about $40.2 \pm 0.2\%$ w/w.

Conclusion: Analytical methods proved that berberine was encapsulated in the yeast cells. Fluorescence microscopy and FTIR results showed the entrance of berberine inside the yeasts. DSC diagram indicated the appearance of new peak which is due to the synthesis of new product. Although plasmolysis caused changes in yeast cell structure and properties, it did not enhance berberine loading in the cells. The results confirmed that *Saccharomyces cerevisiae* could be an efficient and safe carrier for active materials.

Keywords: Berberine, Encapsulation, *Saccharomyces cerevisiae* yeast cells

Background

Microencapsulation is a process that nowadays developed in many industries. Encapsulation has a lot of advantages. The encapsulated compound can be released in a controlled way in different systems. Besides, it stabilizes the active materials against oxygen or other molecules by wall material as a physical barrier [1]. The stability and release properties of microcapsules are dependent on cell wall properties [2,3]. However, the new or novel coatings are needed due to the cost and legal limits in the food industries [4].

Saccharomyces cerevisiae yeast cell can be mentioned as an ideal carrier due to its food-grade and low cost characteristics. Unlike other carriers, it does not depend on active ingredients for its synthesis. We could culture this kind of carriers as much as needed without any excess expenses. Besides, its membrane phospholipids act like liposome structure and have been used for encapsulation of different molecules, hydrophobic and hydrophilic, like resveratrol [5-8].

It possesses the external thick cell wall which composes of a beta glucan network and a small amount of chitin associated with a mannoprotein layer [9]. These cell wall properties make *S. cerevisiae* such a kind of sustained release drug delivery system. The mechanical characteristics of the yeasts structure allow them to load different molecules.

Barberry (*Berberis vulgaris* L. family Berberidaceae) grows in Asia and Europe. The plant is famous worldwide for its medicinal properties [10]. Berberine is the most significant alkaloid of this plant which is responsible for its beneficial effects. Berberine is mostly accumulated in the root. Berberine as an isoquinoline alkaloid is a member of protoberberines class [11]. Berberine shows a lot of pharmacological effects [12].

Berberine shows antiplatelet effects and it is also used in treatment of congestive heart failure (CHF) [13-16]. Extracts are used to cure various inflammatory diseases such as lumbago and rheumatism and to reduce fever [17]. The reports represented immunosuppressive effect

* Correspondence: khashaiarmaneshz@mums.ac.ir
[1]Department of Drug and Food Control, School of Pharmacy, Mashhad University of Medical Sciences, Mashhad, Iran
Full list of author information is available at the end of the article

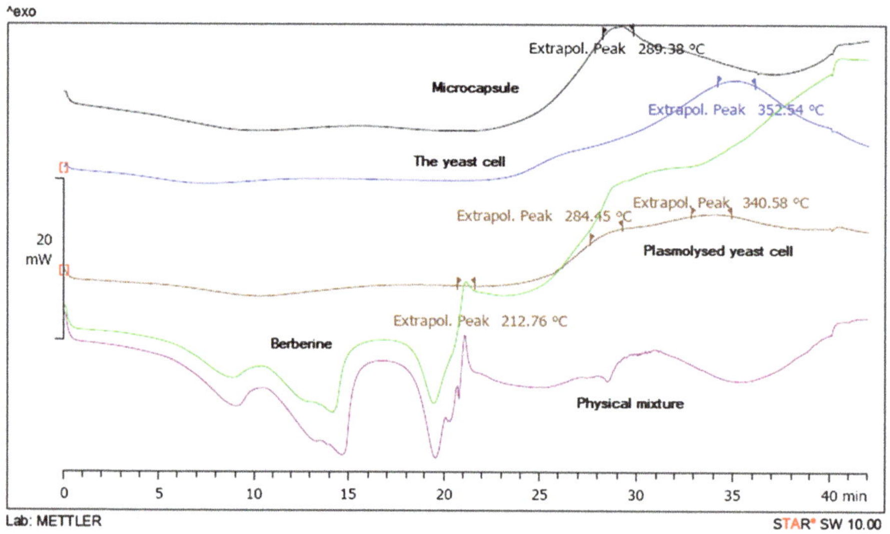

Figure 1 DSC thermograms of microcapsules, *Saccharomyces cerevisiae* yeast cell, berberine, plasmolysed yeast cells and physical mixture of berberine and yeast cells.

of berberine in the tubulointerstitial nephritis model. Peng et al. showed the antianxiety properties of berberine [11]. Berberine can be mentioned as an expectorant due to its ability to increase mucin release [18].

Berberine has been used to treat infectious diarrhea and gastroenteritis in China in the past [19]. Berberine is defined as an effective drug to cure acute diarrhea which is due to *Escherichia coli* or *Vibrio cholerae* [20,21]. Berberine shows significant antibacterial and antifungal activity against broad spectrum of microorganisms [22-28].

Berberine's poor water solubility and susceptibility to environmental conditions prevent its application in many industries. The goal of this study was to evaluate the new aspect of yeast cells of *S. cerevisiae* as an encapsulation carrier for berberine. Moreover, the berberine microcapsules were studied by different analytical methods such as fluorescence microscopy, (DSC) and (FT-IR).

Methods

Preparation of plasmolysed yeast cells, non plasmolysed yeast cells and berberine microcapsules

The yeast cells (commercially Bakers *S. cerevisiae)* were cultured in soybean casein digest broth medium (Himedia, India) for 10 hours [29] in shaker incubator (20 rpm) (JTSL 20, Iran). The medium was centrifuged and the yeast cells were washed for three times with deionised water. The final cells were classified in two groups. First group as non plasmolysed cells was directly freeze dried. The second one as plasmolysed cells was plasmolysed in different concentration of sodium chloride solutions. The yeast cells suspensions were provided in three different flasks. Each flask contained 10%, 20%, 30% w/w NaCl solutions, respectively. Then the flasks were stirred at 200 rpm for 72 h. The plasmolysed cells were centrifuged and washed three times with deionised water to remove impurities. At last, they have been freeze-dried. The freeze-dried plasmolysed and non plasmolysed yeast cells were studied as carriers [30].

Two kinds of freeze dried cells (plasmolysed and non plasmolysed) (100 mg) were suspended in two flasks containing 50 ml berberine solutions (500 mM). Berberine hydrochloride was obtained from China (XI AN Rongsheng biotechnology CO., LTD). The flasks were stirred at 200 rpm for 72 h and then centrifuged (6000 rpm, 20 min). The precipitants were washed three times to remove the free berberine. Then the berberine loaded microcapsules were freeze dried.

Analytical methods for confirmation of berberine encapsulation

Three methods were performed for confirmation of encapsulation process including fluorescence microscopy (color CCTV camera, model No.MV-CP470/G), fourier-transform Infrared Spectroscopy (FT-IR) (model. Spectrum two) and differential scanning calorimetry (DSC) (Mettler Toledo).

Fluorescence microscopy images were obtained from empty freeze-dried yeast cells and the yeast cells which encapsulated berberine. Besides Fluorescence microscopy, DSC and FT-IR studies were carried out to confirm the encapsulation of berberine in yeast cells.

In DSC studies, five types of freeze-dried samples were studied: empty yeast cells, berberine powder,physical mixture of berberine and empty cells, cells loaded with berberine (microcapsules) and plasmolysed empty yeast cells. To prepare a DSC sample, a definite amount of

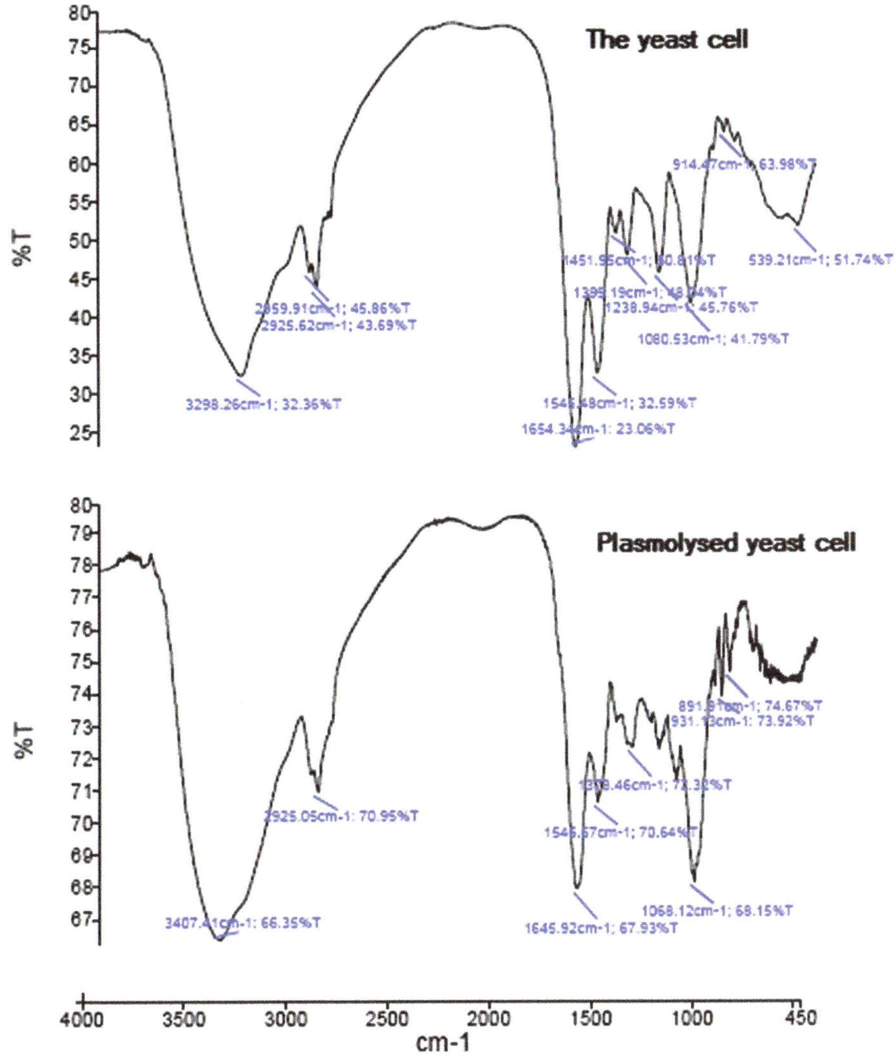

Figure 2 FTIR spectra of *Saccharomyces cerevisiae* yeast cell and plasmolysed yeast cells.

each sample was placed in 50 μl closed aluminium pans. The scan rate was 10°C/min between 0 and 400°C. The IR spectra (KBr disc method) of all the above mentioned samples were also obtained using an FT-IR spectrophotometer [8,10].

To determine the encapsulation yield (% EY), berberine was extracted from two kinds of microcapsules. In extraction process, each sample (50 mg) was suspended in deionised water and ethanol by ratio of 1:4. Then the suspensions were stirred for 48 h in room temperature. Each cell suspension was then centrifuged. Berberine in the supernatant was then quantified by UV/Visible spectroscopy. Then the (% EY) was calculated [28]:

$$(\%EY) = Mass\ of\ encapsulated\ berberine \div Mass\ of\ the\ resulted\ microcapsule \times 100$$

Results and discussion

Analytical studies of freeze-dried plasmolysed and non plasmolysed yeast cells

The DSC thermograms are showed in Figure 1. DSC thermograms indicate the heat capacity changes of a product based on temperature or time. Besides, we can prove the formation of a new product by omitting or obtaining of new peaks. The DSC thermogram shows an exothermic peak with maximum occurrence at 352°C for freeze-dried non plasmolysed yeast (Figure 1). This peak is originated from the phase transition temperature (Tm) of yeasts' phospholipid bilayer and at 352°C the hydrocarbon tail melted [30]. Tm is influenced by membrane structure so the DSC thermogram of the freeze-dried yeasts cells that had been plasmolysed in 20% w/w NaCl solution showed exothermic peaks with maximum occurrence at 284 and 340°C. It confirms that plasmolysis process causes

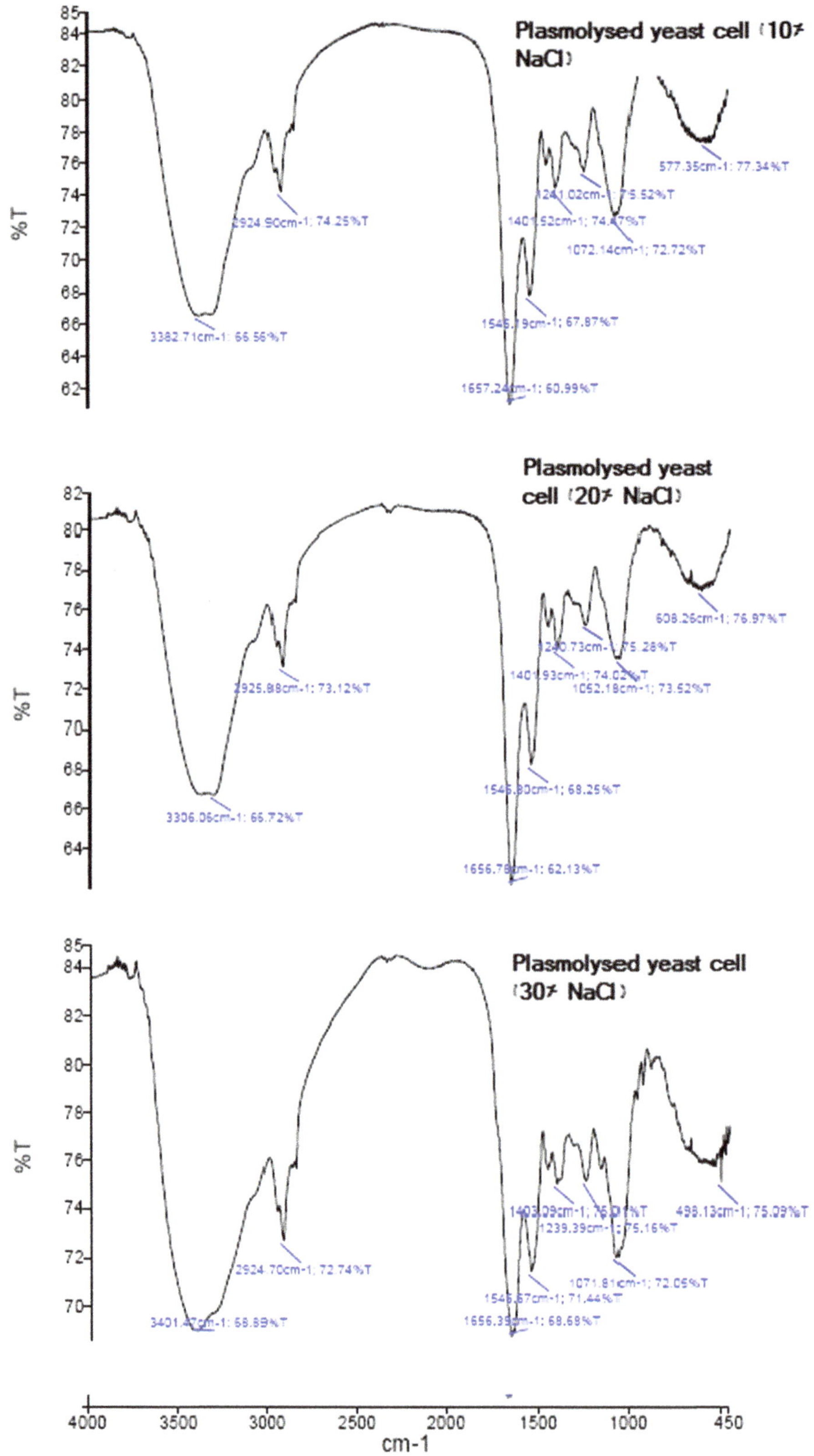

Figure 3 FTIR spectra of 10%, 20% and 30% plasmolysed *Saccharomyces cerevisiae* yeast cells.

changes in lipid composition of membrane and shows different maximum occurrence in comparison with non plasmolysed yeast cells [31]. Tm also depends on different parameters such as strain of *S. cerevisiae*, so we observed different Tm in different studies.

FT-IR was also used to study changes in the cells structure as a result of yeast cell plasmolysis. The IR spectra of both plasmolysed and non plasmolysed freeze-dried yeast cells are shown in Figure 2. The spectra of different plasmolysed yeast cells with 10%, 20% and 30% w/w NaCl solutions (Figure 3) show no significant differences among each other but in comparison with the spectra of non plasmolysed yeast cells (Figure 2), we could see characteristic changes that they represent the effects of plasmolysis on cell wall or membrane compositions such as proteins, carbohydrates, lipids and even nucleic acids.

The contributions of hydroxyl vibrations of carbohydrates and NH vibrations of proteins can be observed in a band at 3750–3000 cm^{-1} in IR spectra [31].

Region 3050–2700 cm^{-1} shows us the information about lipid composition of yeast cells. Plasmolysed yeast cells indicated a minor increase of their absorption intensities due to the changes in the length of membrane lipid chains in comparison with non plasmolysed yeast cells absorption peaks in 2959 and 2925 cm^{-1} (Figure 2) [32]. These two peaks are due to the vibrations of methyl and methylene groups. Plasmolysis effects on cell wall and membrane proteins could be seen in different regions. According to protein degradation by plasmolysis, we faced some changes in peak intensities in the region 1700–1550 cm^{-1}. After plasmolysis, some changes happened in the absorption bands at 1659 and 1553 cm^{-1}, which referred to protein amide I and amide II and carbon-nitrogen vibrations of yeast cells due to the shift of the degradated proteins to an unfolded state. Degradation of one part of yeast proteins in the cell membrane and the cell wall could be detected in the band region from 1530 to 1385 cm^{-1}.

Plasmolysis caused the cell wall polysaccharides degradation which could be detected by changes in the IR region from 1156 to 768 cm^{-1} (Figure 2).

Hypophosphite vibrations are originated from nucleic acid molecules, so we could find the effect of plasmolysis on nucleic acids degradation as the 1240 cm^{-1}. Nucleic acid molecules are placed inside the cell so the presence of their IR spectra are indicative of cells which are not completely emptied by plasmolysis (Figure 2).

Finally the results show us that plasmolysis causes disorganisation to the cell plasma membrane and thickness of cell wall but higher concentrations of NaCl solutions showed no additional disruptions in the yeast cell.

Plasmolysis enhances the intracellular space so it improves the capacity of carriers for encapsulation process [33]. Nowadays, yeast cells plasmolysis with NaCl [7] were mainly used for the encapsulation of different active materials.

The results indicated that the %encapsulation yield values were statistically similar ($p > 0.05$) amongst plasmolysed and non plasmolysed cells which confirms other researches results [30]. The average %encapsulation yield was 40.2±0.2%. No differences were observed in the %encapsulation yield amongst plasmolysed yeast cells when exposed to 10%, 20% or 30% w/w NaCl.

Analytical studies for confirmation of berberine encapsulation

In the fluorescence micrographs, empty yeast cells could not emit fluorescence (Figure 4b). But the yeast cells loaded with berberine emitted fluorescence due to the presence of berberine which shows fluorescence properties (Figure 4a). This event proved the interaction of berberine with yeast cells. Further analyses were carried out using DSC and FT IR to find out the effect of plasmolysis on cells structure.

Figure 1 showed the DSC thermograms of non-plasmolysed yeast cells, berberine, physical mixture of berberine and

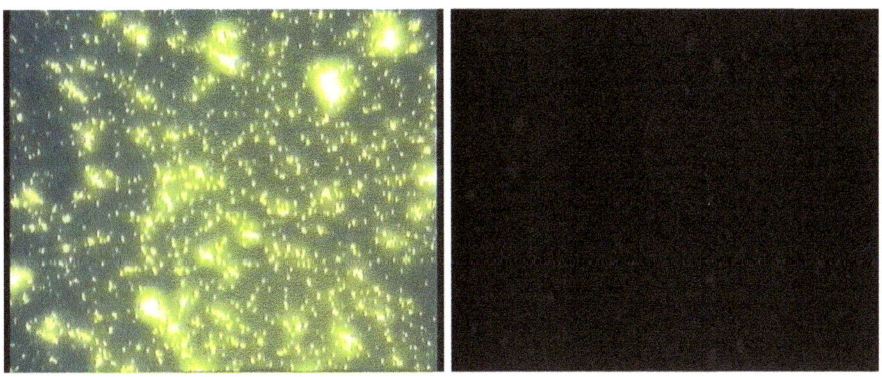

(a) (b)

Figure 4 Fluorescence micrographs of berberine yeast microcapsules (a) and empty *Saccharomyces cerevisiae* yeast cells (b).

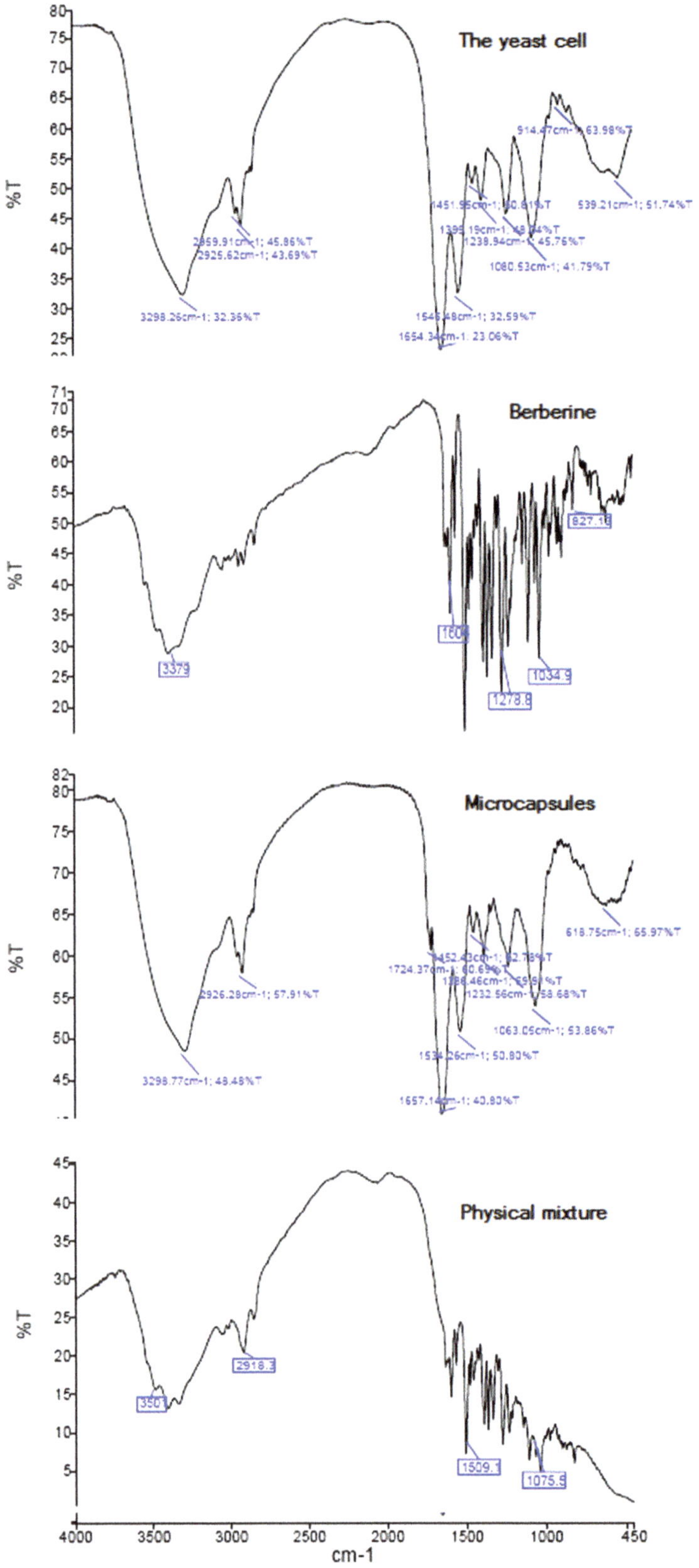

Figure 5 FTIR spectra of *Saccharomyces cerevisiae* yeast cells, berberine, berberine microcapsules and physical mixture.

yeast cells as well as berberine microcapsules and plasmolysed yeast cells.

The new peak that appeared at 289°C which differed from the peak of empty yeast cells and physical mixture showed that the new product was produced. This Tm variation was due to decrease of Van der Waals interactions happened to membrane as a result of berberine's integration. On the other hand, berberine influenced the bilayer organization by interaction of its polar groups with membrane polar groups. So the membrane became more fluid and Tm of microcapsules was lowered in comparison with empty yeast cells.

The samples were studied with FTIR spectroscopy too and their spectra are showed in Figure 5. The interaction of berberine with yeast cell would alter the intensity of yeast cell absorption bands and causes shifts of characteristic bands.

The characteristic absorption bands of berberine are shown in Figure 5. The IR spectra of empty yeast cells are explained before. The 3298 and 1654 cm^{-1} bands are due to the phenolic and carbonyl groups, respectively. The absorption peak at 1545 cm^{-1} shows us the carbonyl and carbon-carbon vibration. The peak at 1451 cm^{-1} refered to carbon-hydrogen vibration. The absorption peak at 1238 cm^{-1} is indicative of phenolic vibration. The methoxy groups are responsible for the 1080 cm^{-1} band. The aromatic carbon-hydrogen group vibrates at 914 cm^{-1} [34].

The IR spectrum of the physical mixture of berberine and yeast cells was a combination of the IR spectra of empty yeast cells and berberine, separately. The IR spectra of the microcapsules was relatively the same as the spectrum of the empty yeast cells. These spectra could prove the fact that berberine was placed inside the yeast cells. This observation confirmed Shi et al. [5,7] studies. However we had some peak disappearances at 914 cm^{-1} and variation in the absorption bands of 1654 and 1545 cm^{-1} as a result of berberine-protein interactions in microcapsules spectra.

Conclusions

In this study, *S. cerevisiae* were introduced as a novel carrier for berberine as a model. It has shown that yeast microcapsules were loaded with berberine up to $40.2 \pm 0.2\%$ w/w. Three analytic methods indicated that berberine located inside the cells mainly by hydrophobic interactions with the yeast cell membrane and cell wall.

Competing interests

The authors declare that they have no competing interests.

Authors' contributions

RS participated in project design, carried out analytic experiments and participated in drafting the manuscript. BS FB supervised the whole project, supported the culture of microorganism, and participated in drafting the manuscript. OR participated in project design and drafting the manuscript. ZK contribution in analytical methods, commented the analytical results and participated in drafting the manuscript. All authors read and approved the final manuscript.

Acknowledgement

This work was supported by a grant from Mashhad University of Medical Sciences Research Council, Mashhad, Iran. The authors wish to thank the authorities in Mashhad University of Medical Sciences, Biotechnology Research center and School of Pharmacy for their support. This project was part of Ph.D student thesis in School of Pharmacy. The authors have no conflicts of interest that are directly relevant to the content of this manuscript.

Author details

[1]Department of Drug and Food Control, School of Pharmacy, Mashhad University of Medical Sciences, Mashhad, Iran. [2]Biotechnology Research Centre, School of Pharmacy, Mashhad University of Medical Sciences, Mashhad, Iran. [3]Targetted Drug Delivery Research Centre, School of Pharmacy, Mashhad University of Medical Sciences, Mashhad, Iran.

References

1. Madene A, Jacquot M, Scher J, Desobry S: **Flavour encapsulation and controlled release: a review.** *Int J Food Sci Tech* 2006, **41**:1–21.
2. Gibbs BF, Kermasha S, Alli I, Mulligan N: **Encapsulation in the food industry: a review.** *Int J Food Sci Nutr* 1999, **50**:213–224.
3. Khodaverdi E, Khalili N, Zangiabadi F, Homayouni A: **Preparation, characterization and stability studies of glassy solid dispersions of indomethacin using PVP and isomalt as carriers.** *Iran J Basic Med Sci* 2012, **15**(3):820–32.
4. Gouin S: **Microencapsulation: industrial appraisal of existing technologies and trends.** *Trends Food Sci Tech* 2004, **15**:330–347.
5. Shi G, Rao L, Yu H, Xiang H, Yang H, Ji R: **Stabilization of photosensitive resveratrol within yeast cell.** *Int J Pharmaceut* 2008, **349**:83–93.
6. Bishop JRP, Nelson G, Lamb J: **Microencapsulation in yeast cells.** *J Microencapsul* 1998, **15**(6):761–773.
7. Shi G, Rao L, Yu H, Xiang H, Pen G, Long S, *et al*: **Yeast-cell based microencapsulation of chlorogenic acid as a water-soluble antioxidant.** *J Food Eng* 2007, **80**:1060–1067.
8. Chow C, Palecet P: **Enzyme encapsulation in permeabilized *Saccharomyces cerevisiae* cells.** *Biotechnol Progr* 2004, **20**:449–456.
9. De Nobel JG, Klis FM, Munnik T, Priem J, Van Den Ende H: **An assay of the relative cell wall porosity of *Saccharomyces cerevisiae, Kluveromyces lactis* and *Schizosaccharomyces pombe*.** *Yeast* 1990, **6**:483–490.
10. Shamsa F, Ahmadiani A, Khosrokhavar R: **Antihistaminic and anticholinergic activity of barberry fruit (Berberis vulgaris) in the guinea-pig ileum.** *J Ethnopharmacol* 1999, **64**:161–166.
11. Mazzini S, Bellucci MC, Mondelli R: **Mode of binding of the cytotoxic alkaloid berberine with the double helix oligonucleotide D (AAGAATTCTT).** *Bioorg Med Chem* 2003, **11**:505–514.
12. Imanshahid M, Hosseinzadeh H: **Pharmacological and therapeutic effects of berberis vulgaris and its active constituent, berberine.** *Phytother Res* 2008, **22**:999–1012.
13. Fatehi-Hassanabad Z, Jafarzadeh M, Tarhini A, Fatehi M: **The antihypertensive and vasodilator effects of aqueous extract from Berberis vulgaris fruit on hypertensive rats.** *Phytother Res* 2005, **19**:222–225.
14. DerMaderosian A: *The Review of Natural Products.* St. Louis, Missouri: Facts and Comparisons; 2001.
15. Chiou WF, Chen J, Chen CF: **Relaxation of corpus cavernosum and raised intracavernous pressure by berberine in rabbit.** *Br J Pharmacol* 1998, **125**:1677–1684.
16. Zeng XH, Zeng XJ, Li YY: **Efficacy and safety of berberine for congestive heart failure secondary to ischemic or idiopathic dilated cardiomyopathy.** *Am J Cardiol* 2003, **92**:173–176.
17. Yesılada E, Kupeli E, Berberis crataegina DC: **Root exhibits potent anti-inflammatory, analgesic and febri-fuge effects in mice and rats.** *J Ethnopharmacol* 2002, **79**:237–248.
18. Lee CJ, Lee JH, Seok JH, *et al*: **Effects of baicalein, berberine, curcumin and hesperidin on mucin release from airway goblet cells.** *Planta Med* 2003, **69**:523–526.
19. Lin SS, Chung JG, Lin JP, *et al*: **Berberine inhibits arylamine N-acetyltransferase activity and gene expression in mouse leukemia L 1210 cells.** *Phytomedicine* 2005, **12**:351–358.

20. Rabbani GH, Butler T, Knight J, Sanyal SC, Alam K: **Randomized controlled trial of berberine sulfate therapy for diarrhea due to enterotoxigenic *Escherichia coli* and *Vibrio cholerae*.** *J Infect Dis* 1987, **155**:979–984.
21. Rabbani GH: **Mechanism and treatment of diarrhoea due to *Vibrio cholerae* and *Escherichia coli*: roles of drugs and prostaglandins.** *Dan Med Bull* 1996, **43**:173–185.
22. Birdsall TC, Kelly GS: **Berberine: therapeutic potential of an alkaloid found in several medicinal plants.** *Altern Med Rev* 1997, **2**:94–103.
23. Khosla PK, Neeraj VI, Gupta SK, Satpathy G: **Berberine, a potential drug for trachoma.** *Rev Int Trach Pathol Ocul Trop* 1992, **69**:147–165.
24. Freile ML, Giannini F, Pucci G, *et al*: **Antimicrobial activity of aqueous extracts and of berberine isolated from Berberis heterophylla.** *Fitoterapia* 2003, **74**:702–705.
25. Kaneda Y, Torii M, Tanaka T, Aikawa M: **In vitro effects of berberine sulphate on the growth and structure of *Entamoeba histolytica*, *Giardia lamblia* and *Trichomonas vaginalis*.** *Ann Trop Med Parasitol* 1991, **85**:417–425.
26. Mahady GB, Pendland SL, Stoia A, Chadwick LR: **In vitro susceptibility of *Helicobacter pylori* to isoquinoline alkaloids from sanguinaria canadensis and Hydrastis Canadensis.** *Phytother Res* 2003, **17**:217–221.
27. Ghosh AK, Bhattacharya FK, Ghosh DK: ***Leishmania donovani*: Amastigote inhibition and mode of action of berberine.** *Exp Parasitol* 1985, **60**:404–413.
28. Seki T, Morohashi M: **Effect of some alkaloids, flavonoids and triterpenoids, contents of Japanese-Chinese traditional herbal medicines, on the lipogenesis of sebaceous glands.** *Skin Pharmacol* 1993, **6**:56–60.
29. Lord PG, Wheals AE: **Variability in individual cell cycles of *Saccharomyces cerevisiae*.** *J. Cell Sci* 1981, **50**:361–376.
30. Paramera EI, Konteles SJ, Karathanos VT: **Microencapsulation of curcumin in cells of *Saccharomyces cerevisiae*.** *Food Chem* 2010, **125**:892–902.
31. Laroche C, Gervais P: **Achievement of rapid dehydration at specific temperatures could maintain high *Sacharomyces cerevisiae* viability.** *Appl Microbiol Biot* 2003, **60**:743–747.
32. Burattini E, Cavanga M, Dell Anna R, Malvezzi Campeggi F, Monti F, Rossi F, *et al*: **An FT-IR microspectroscopy study of autolysis in cells of the wine yeast *Saccharomyces cerevisiae*.** *Vib Spectrosc* 2008, **47**:139–147.
33. Korber DR, Choi A, Wolfaardt GM, Caldwell DE: **Bacterial plasmolysis as a physical indicator of viability.** *Appl Environ Microb* 1996, **62**(11):3939–3947.
34. Barik A, Mishra B, Shen L, Mohan H, Kadam RM, Dutta S, *et al*: **Evaluation of a new copper (II)–curcumin complex as superoxide dismutase mimic and its free radical reactions.** *Free Radical Bio Med* 2005, **39**:811–822.

Cost-effectiveness of different interferon beta products for relapsing-remitting and secondary progressive multiple sclerosis: Decision analysis based on long-term clinical data and switchable treatments

Shekoufeh Nikfar[1,2], Abbas Kebriaeezadeh[1], Rassoul Dinarvand[1], Mohammad Abdollahi[1,3], Mohammad-Ali Sahraian[4], David Henry[5] and Ali Akbari Sari[1,6*]

Abstract

Background: Multiple sclerosis (MS) is a highly debilitating immune mediated disorder and the second most common cause of neurological disability in young and middle-aged adults. Iran is amongst high MS prevalence countries (50/100,000). Economic burden of MS is a topic of important deliberation in economic evaluations study. Therefore determining of cost-effectiveness interferon beta (INF β) and their copied biopharmaceuticals (CBPs) and biosimilars products is significant issue for assessment of affordability in Lower-middle-income countries (LMICs).

Methods: A literature-based Markov model was developed to assess the cost-effectiveness of three INF βs products compared with placebo for managing a hypothetical cohort of patients diagnosed with relapsing remitting MS (RRMS) in Iran from a societal perspective. Health states were based on the Kurtzke Expanded Disability Status Scale (EDSS). Disease progression transition probabilities for symptom management and INF β therapies were obtained from natural history studies and multicenter randomized controlled trials and their long term follow up for RRMS and secondary progressive MS (SPMS). A cross sectional study has been developed to evaluate cost and utility. Transitions among health states occurred in 2-years cycles for fifteen cycles and switching to other therapies was allowed. Calculations of costs and utilities were established by attachment of decision trees to the overall model. The incremental cost effectiveness ratio (ICER) of cost/quality adjusted life year (QALY) for all available INF β products (brands, biosimilars and CBPs) were considered. Both costs and utilities were discounted. Sensitivity analyses were done to assess robustness of model.

Results: ICER for Avonex, Rebif and Betaferon was 18712, 11832, 15768 US Dollars ($) respectively when utility attained from literature review has been considered. ICER for available CBPs and biosimilars in Iran was $847, $6964 and $11913.

(Continued on next page)

* Correspondence: akbarisari@tums.ac.ir
[1]Department of Pharmacoeconomics and Pharmaceutical Administration, Faculty of Pharmacy, Tehran University of Medical Sciences, Tehran, Iran
[6]Department of Health Management and Economics, School of Public Health, Tehran University of Medical Sciences, Tehran, Iran
Full list of author information is available at the end of the article

(Continued from previous page)

Conclusions: The Markov pharmacoeconomics model determined that according to suggested threshold for developing countries by world health organization, all brand INF β products are cost effective in Iran except Avonex. The best strategy among INF β therapies is CBP intramuscular INF β-1a (Cinnovex). Results showed that a policy of encouraging accessibility to CBPs and biosimilars could make even high technology products cost-effective in LMICs.

Keywords: Cost-Effectiveness, Decision analysis, Economic evaluation, Interferon beta, Markov model, Modeling, Switching

Multiple sclerosis (MS) is a highly debilitating immune mediated disorder of the central nervous system [1]. Since MS is a complicated illness to diagnose accurately, the worldwide variation in prevalence and incidence is not precisely known. The best estimate is that around 2.5 million people in the world suffer from MS [2]. The range of prevalence estimates of MS in different countries and regions differs from 5 to 189 per 100,000 [3,4]. In a report published in 2000, Iran as a Middle Eastern country was listed among low to medium zone incidence of MS based on the theory of geographical epidemiology [4]. The prevalence rate of MS is estimated to be 50 per 100,000, translating to around 35,000 cases (Table 1) [5-17]. Therefore, Iran can be considered to be amongst high MS prevalence countries [4]. The onset of MS usually occurs during early adulthood (age 15–45 years) [18] making MS the second most common cause of neurological disability in young and middle-aged adults [19]. In Iran, the mean age for incidence and prevalence of MS are 27 and 32, respectively with a 2.8 times higher incidence in women than that of men. The most recent census of the Iranian population (2011) shows a youth bulge in the age range of 20 to 29 years old [20]. This means that health providers have to be ready to face the MS burden and its economic consequences.

Several immunomodulatory treatments including interferon beta (INF β), glatiramer acetate and natalizumab and one immunosuppressive treatment (mitoxantrone) have been approved for MS patients with a relapsing course [21]. Three preparations of recombinant IFN β have been approved for use in MS, subcutaneous IFN β-1a (SC IFN β-1a), intramuscular IFN β-1a (IM IFN β-1a), and subcutaneous IFN β-1b (SC IFN β-1b). IFN β is indicated for the treatment of relapsing-remitting form of MS to reduce the frequency of clinical exacerbations and delay the development of physical disability [22]. According to a previous meta-analysis, INF β's effectiveness in MS varies with the different kinds of INF β and the types of MS. Generally, IFN β can control remission in MS but its effectiveness in secondary progressive multiple sclerosis (SPMS) and relapsing remitting multiple sclerosis (RRMS) is questionable [22,23]. On other hand, the use of the immunomodulatory therapies in clinical practice has been a topic of substantial debate concerning clinical and cost-effectiveness. Although interferon has not been recommended formally by The National Institute for Clinical Excellence (NICE) in the UK many clinical practice guidelines have recommended the immunomodulatory therapies for the treatment of MS [18].

Based on the experience of using INF β in treatment of patients with MS for about 20 years in the Europe and United States, it is considered expensive but modestly effective in terms of reduction of morbidity and improving the quality of life [24-26]. However, it is a challenge for most countries to afford new expensive therapies for MS within limited public resources [27]. Although studies have shown considerable differences between high-income and low- or middle-income countries in capacity to afford the flow of costly new therapies, INFs β have been in use in Iran since 1995, starting with SC INF β-1b and there has been an exponential increase in use. Since 2009, the 'copied biopharmaceuticals' (CBPs) and biosimilars versions of INF β with lower and more affordable prices have been registered and have become accessible in Iran [28,29].

Iran as an Asian country located in the Eastern Mediterranean region and a middle-income country has some specific demographic, economic and health indicators that are presented in Table 2 [30]. Iran is one of the oldest countries in the region that adopted a National Drug Policy (NDP) many years ago [31]. On the basis of the NDP, a specific National Drug List was established to regulate strategies and to ensure registration of only high-quality effective drugs for Iranian citizens at the lowest possible price, mostly by use of subsidization [32,33]. To implement this goal, the Iranian Food and Drug Organization has the mission to control the price of medicines and balance their usage on the basis of the established NDP [34] by considering cost efficacy and equity of access [35].

Cost-effectiveness and cost-utility analyses (CEA/CUAs) have been used increasingly in the last two decades by funders to judge the balance between the added expenses of new drugs and their incremental benefits (e.g., improved patient outcomes). The majority of published CEA/CUA reports on INF β therapies for MS

Table 1 Epidemiologic details of published studies of multiple sclerosis (MS) in Iran

Study	Number of patients	Location	Prevalence/ 100000	Incidence rate/ 100000	Female/ Male ratio	Age (mean ± SD)	Age of onset (mean ± SD)	Education (High school graduated & University education %)	Occupational State (Employed %)
Yousefi Pour et al., 2002 [5]	142	Fars	5.3	-	1.2:1	32.7±6.5	-	-	-
Kalani et al., 2003 [6]	200	Tehran, (Loghman hospital)	-	-	2.5:1	-	27±7.4	95%	-
Saadatnia et al., 2007 [7]	1718	Isfahan	43.8	3.64	-	-	25.36±8.6	-	-
Hashemilar et al., 2011 [8]	1000	East Azarbayjan	27.7	-	2.7:1	33.4	-	-	-
Abedini et al., 2008 [9]	582	Mazandaran	20.1	-	2.6:1	34.4±9.4	26.9±8.3	-	24.6%
Milo and Kahana, 2010 [10]	-	Iran	44	-	-	-	-	-	-
Sahraian et al., 2010 [11]	8146	Tehran	51.9	-	2.6:1	-	27.74±8.32	-	-
Etemadifar et al., 2006 [12]	1391	Isfahan	-	-	3.6:1	32.5	-	50.9%	30.8%
Elhami et al., 2011 [13]	7896	Tehran	50.57	2.93	3.11:1	-	-	-	-
Nabavi et al., 2006 [14]	203	Tehran (Shahid Mostafa Khomeini hospital)	-	-	1.5:1	35.6	-	-	30.2%
Ghandehari et al., 2010 [15]	800	Khorasan (Razavi, Northern, Southern)	9.86	-	1.6:1	-	-	-	-
Ghabaae et al., 2007 [16]	70	Tehran (Emam Khomeini hospital)	-	-	2:1	32.58±10.24	27.55±10.42	39.2%	-
Ale-Yasin et al., 2002 [17]	318	Iran	-	-	1.52	35.4±9.6	26.6±8.1	73.2%	

Table 2 Demographic, economic and health indicators of Iran

Total Population	73,974,000
Gross national income per capita (PPP) ($)	11,490
GDP/capita ($)	5810
Life expectancy at birth male/female(years)	70/75
Total expenditure on health per capita ($, 2010)	836
Total expenditure on health as % of GDP (2010)	6.8
Distribution of years of life lost by causes (2008)	
Communicable/Noncommunicable/Injuries	% 28/49/23

$: International Dollars.

come from studies carried out in high income countries [18,19,36-41]. Economic evaluations based on decision analytic modeling are an alternative to trial-based economic evaluations. The use of decision analytic models in economic evaluations is the only framework that has the potential to meet all the requirements for economic evaluation for decision making and to ensure their applicability in countries of varying national wealth [42]. Markov models are particularly useful when the clinical setting involves a risk that is ongoing over time.

The cost-effectiveness of INF β treatments has been estimated by Markov models in previous studies, but these have ignored differences of effectiveness and tolerability of different INF β products. Previous studies done by us have highlighted the varying efficacy of different kinds of INF β in RRMS or SPMS [22,23]. When there is a probability of switching to other drugs in a decision analysis model, overhead costing may affect results and decision-making processes [35]. Thus in this study we consider results due to switching to other drugs.

The main goal of this study was to perform CEA/CUA evaluations using a decision analysis model of INF β therapies for MS from the perspective of a low-middle-income countries (LMICs). We examined the cost-effectiveness of 4 treatment strategies in patients diagnosed with RRMS (symptom management alone and in combination with IM IFN β-1a, SC IFN β-1a, or SC IFN β-1b).

Methods

Description of the model

A new Markov model was set up to assess the cost-effectiveness of 4 treatment strategies to manage a hypothetical cohort of patients diagnosed with RRMS in Iran. A decision analysis approach was used to model the effects of switching treatments (Figure 1). The incremental cost-effectiveness analysis was the main analytical plan for the study, combining cumulative measures of costs over time with a cumulative measure of effectiveness. This approach evaluates the incremental costs per clinical benefit gained (expressed as cost per QALY gained). The analysis was performed for a hypothetical cohort of 30-year-old patients. The inclusion criteria used in the randomized controlled trials (RCTs) of INF β was taken into account and the effectiveness was noted as QALYs. The model embraced patterns of resource utilization in both outpatient and inpatient care. Also, both direct non-medical and indirect costs were included.

The treatment strategies were management of diseases symptoms alone and in combination with one of the following medicines: IM IFN β-1a, SC IFN β-1a, or SC IFN β-1b. The clinical course of RRMS (e.g., disease progression and transition to SPMS) was modeled in terms of the Kurtzke expanded disability status scale (EDSS) and withdrawal from treatment [43]. Specifically, 7 health states were modeled (Figure 1):

1. RRMS-EDSS 1–3.5: no or few limitations in mobility
2. RRMS-EDSS 4–6: moderate limitations in mobility

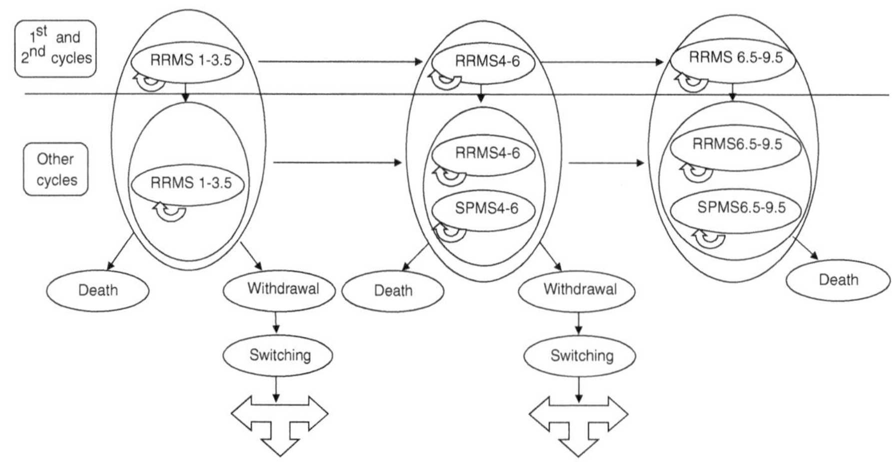

Figure 1 Schematic Representation of the Markov Model and decision tree for evaluation of INF β cost-effectiveness in MS.

3. RRMS-EDSS 6.5-9.5: walking aid or wheelchair required and restricted to bed
4. SPMS-EDSS 4–6: moderate limitations in mobility
5. SPMS-EDSS 6.5-9.5: walking aid or wheelchair required and restricted to bed
6. Death (natural causes or EDSS 10)
7. Withdrawal due to side effects and perceived lack of efficacy or other causes like pregnancy and financial problems

Transitions among the health states occurred in 2-years cycles. A 2-years cycle time was used, because this interval closely approximates the follow-up period of the IFN β RCTs for preventive treatment in RRMS. Most of information for SPMS was reported in 3 year intervals; thus they were calculated for 2 years to input to the model. The baseline time horizon of the model was assumed to be a lifetime in order to capture the full benefits of immunomodulatory therapy, which was assumed to be around 30 years after onset of the disease (15 cycles). Costs and outcomes were estimated from the societal perspective and were discounted at 7.2% per annum for cost [44] and 3% for quality of life [45]. The costs and QALYs were discounted from the end of first year. All the costs were reported in 2012 U.S. dollars and exchange rates of IRR to U.S. dollars of 12260. Data were obtained from literature covering RCTs of IFN β, official prices, and tariff lists (see below for details). To validate the methodology (model structure and assumptions), four expert opinion leaders were consulted.

The model calculated the following outcomes: numbers of patients remaining in lower EDSS; numbers of patients remaining in RRMS; numbers of patients remaining relapse free; QALYs; total costs and costs by component (i.e., IFN β therapy cost, MS-related medical costs [e.g., drugs for symptom management], and lost worker productivity costs; direct non-medical costs and incremental cost-effectiveness ratios (ICER) comparing symptom management alone with symptom management combined with each of the 3 IFN β therapies. Given that there is no accurate threshold calculated for Iran, the cost/QALY ICERs were compared with multiples of the gross domestic product (GDP) per capita according to recommendations of the World Health Organization (WHO) [46]. According to the WHO the treatments of MS with different IFN β would be considered "highly cost effective" if the cost/QALY is less than GDP per capita, "cost-effective" if the cost/QALY was between one to three times of GDP per capita and "not cost-effective" if it was more than three times of GDP per capita. The GDP per capita of Iran was considered as 5810 USD [30]. Model parameters were varied in sensitivity analyses.

A number of underlying assumptions were adopted for the base-case model:

1. In the model, all patients start in the health state stage of EDSS 1–3.5.
2. The point at which patients transitioned from RRMS to SPMS was assumed to be in the third cycle (approximately 5 years after diagnosis of illness) and the model assumed that this took place between EDSS 4–6 and EDSS 6.5-9.5 [47]. Corresponding to this assumption, the model assumed that relapses occurred in patients didn't change the state of EDSS [48].
3. The model assumed that as per product labeling and off-labeled prescriptions, only RRMS and SPMS patients in EDSS of 1–6 were eligible for and received IFN β therapies.
4. Switching among the IFN β therapies was permitted once in the model. Patients who withdrew IFN β therapy during the first three cycles were assigned the transition probabilities for relapse and disease progression used in the symptom management arm or other two IFN β arms. Patients who discontinued therapy were not permitted to reinitiate therapy. Switching between IFN β was acceptable within brands or biosimilar and CBPs only.
5. In case of withdrawal from IFN β therapy in cycles of 4 to 15, patients were allocated to the transition probabilities for relapse and disease progression used in the symptom management arm.
6. It was presumed that there was no variation in mortality between patients with or without preventive treatment [22] and there was no sex-related mortality risk factor in RRMS and SPMS [49].
7. Other direct medical and non-medical costs and indirect costs were calculated according to utilization in different status and stages of disease and the cycle of Markov model.
8. Medicinal treatments and laboratory tests for management of MS morbidity in different groups were deemed according to results of our previous meta-analysis [22]. Cost of antidepressants, anti-spasmodics, anti-fatigues, pain killers, and NSAIDs were considered in our model.
9. Weighted mean costs were considered for other medicines consumed by MS patients in both generic or brand forms. Frequency of use was based on survey data [28].
10. Calculations were performed for cost of hospitalization, physicians' visits, laboratory tests, imaging, psychotherapy and physiotherapy according to percentages of patients using governmental and private facilities or outpatient admission to daycare clinics.

Clinical and economic outcomes

The effectiveness measurement was based on the concept of utility, which measures the QALYs [50].

The cost assessment was based on the assignment of costs to the health states and interventions.

Data sources

Three different types of data can be distinguished in modeling studies:

1. Probabilities of clinical events: progress of disease, chance of an acute exacerbation, withdrawal, and death.
2. Utilities of different Markov health states.
3. Costing information derived from estimates of the units of resource utilization and their prices/tariffs (product of unit and price).
4. Probabilities of switching to other INF β or symptomatic treatments.

To design the strategy of retrieving data from PubMed, Scopus, Web of Science, and the Cochrane library, Iranmedex, SID, and MagIran were searched for studies reporting efficacy and/or tolerability of IFN β in multiple sclerosis, and epidemiology, natural history and costs of MS. Data were collected from 1966 to 2012 (up to December). The search terms were: "multiple sclerosis" or "MS" and "IFN beta" or "Interferon beta"; "multiple sclerosis" or "MS" and "Iran"; "multiple sclerosis" or "MS" and "IFN beta" or "Interferon beta" and "modeling" or "decision analysis", "cost". The language was restricted to English and Persian. The reference lists from retrieved articles were also reviewed to avoid missing any relevant studies (Figure 2).

The probabilities of clinical events, including disease progression, probability of an acute exacerbation, and withdrawal were based on IFN β clinical trial data and their long term data. A cross sectional study has been developed to evaluate cost and utility. An approved questionnaire was adopted and validated. Two-hundred MS patients were recruited consecutively in a random manner from three referral hospitals of two different cities and three private offices of MS specialists and members of Iranian society of MS through society's office in

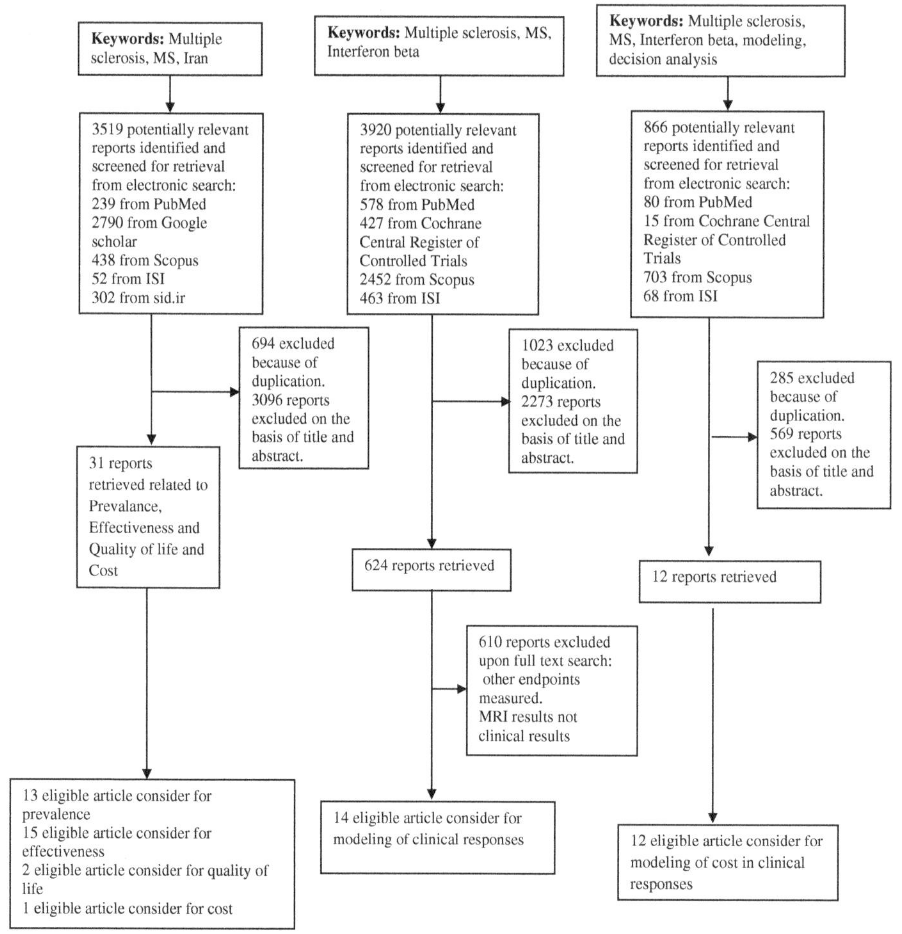

Figure 2 Search diagram for Multiple sclerosis (MS), Interferon beta (INF β) and Iran.

Table 3 Baseline characteristics of patients recruited to evaluate quality adjusted life years QALYs and Cost for multiple sclerosis (MS) in Iran (n = 200)

	Total recruited MS patients	RRMS			SPMS		Unknown or PPMS
		EDSS			EDSS		
		1-3.5	4-6	>6	4-6	>6	
Numbers of Patients	200	104	29	12	24	4	PPMS: 19 Unknown: 8
Age (mean±SD)	33.8±9.1	29±7.7	36±7.2	36.6±9.2	42.4±6.7	46±3.7	PPMS: 41.8±6.3 Unknown: 34.5±8.2
Sex (Female/Male)	148/52	80/24	24/5	10/2	16/8	2/2	PPMS:10/9 Unknown: 6/2
Urban/Rural	174/26	93/11	25/4	12/0	20/4	4/0	PPMS: 13/6 Unknown 4/4
Education (High school graduated & University education %)	83%	83%	79%	83%	83%	100%	PPMS: 53% Unknown: 75%
Occupational State (Employed %)	31%	37%	48%	0%	29%	0%	PPMS: 0% Unknown: 13%

MS multiple sclerosis, *RRMS* relapsing remitting multiple sclerosis, *SPMS* secondary progressive multiple sclerosis, *PPMS* primary progressive multiple sclerosis, *EDSS* expanded disability status scale.

Tehran and Arak and patients' email [51]. Evaluation of recruitment showed no bias (p>0.05) according to feature of MS retrieved through systematic review (Table 3). ANOVA statistical test for normal numerical variables was used to detect differences in the groups retrieved from literature search and recruited group corrected by Bonferroni post hoc test.

Age and sex-specific mortality rates assumed that MS alters life expectancy and increases the rate of death threefold across the different age or sex groups (Table 4) [49]. Age and sex-specific population mortality rates were derived from national statistics data [52].

Probabilities were derived from published literature (Table 5): Relapse and disease progression transition probabilities within the symptom management arm were obtained from published natural history studies [47,53,54].

Treatment Effects of the IFN β treatment effects were obtained from RCTs (IM IFN β-1a, SC IFN β-1a, SC IFN β-1b) and long-term follow-up studies [55-65].

The QALYs for the different health states were derived from a cross-sectional study as shown in Table 6. Utility estimates were based on direct elicitation methods of visual analogue scale (VAS) and generic preference-based measures of the EuroQol (EQ-5D) and the Health Utilities Index 3 (HUI3) by in-house translated and validated questionnaires. We also derived utility loss per EDSS and relapse from literatures [19,66,67].

Other necessary information were obtained indirectly by calculations that were done on the basis of long-term follow up data, hazard rate, variances of Kaplan–Meier curves [68,69] and/or by solving multiple-step equations.

Probabilities of switching to other INF βs or no treatment in case of withdrawal due to side effects or lack of perceived efficacy were derived from the cross sectional study.

Table 4 Age and sex adjusted mortality rate for multiple sclerosis (MS) patients

Age (range)	30-35	36-40	41-45	46-50	51-55	56-60	61-65	66-70
Mortality rate (%)	7.69	7.61	8.29	10.17	12.71	14.19	16.2	18.9

Costs

Data on costs were derived from cross sectional study (Table 7).

We used a backward-looking approach in which resource utilization and clinical data were gathered at a single point in time and covered the one-year period prior to the dates of inclusion. The cost of care of MS was calculated for patients in current clinical practice in Iran in 2012 for each state of disease. The costs due to relapses derived from the cost-of-care study in same cross sectional study and evaluating of patients files archived in the hospitals. All prices were extracted from official list of tariffs [70,71]. The friction cost method was used to evaluate workday's loss by on the go patients [72]. By use of this method, the significance of productivity loss was assumed to be 80% of the ordinary rate of employee's productivity during the "friction period." Thereafter, it was assumed that sick employees could be replaced. Time lost by inactive patients was considered as leisure time lost and was valued at 40% of the average wage, productivity and friction period in Iran [20,73,74].

Sensitivity analysis

Elementary effects sensitivity analyses were done according to basic clinical and economic assumptions and their changes in the clinical-outcome model. This was used to test the stability of the suppositions of the analysis over a range of assumptions, probability estimates, and value judgments. The first sensitivity analysis was performed to assess

Table 5 Probability of related outcomes to multiple sclerosis (MS) and interferon beta (INF β) therapy

	Natural History		Interferon beta-1a (Avonex)		Interferon beta-1a 44 Mcg/0.5 ml (Rebif)		Interferon beta-1b (Betaferon)	
Probability of EDSS progression within RRMS								
RRMS 1-3 to RRMS 3.5-6	0.4		0.219		0.193		0.2	
RRMS 3.5-6 to RRMS 6≤	0.27		0.11		0.115		0.15	
Probability of progression from RRMS to SPMS (the same EDSS)								
RRMS 3.5-6 to SPMS 3.5-6	0.43		0.43		0.197		0.433	
RRMS 6≤ to SPMS 6≤	0.31		0.31		0.31		0.31	
Probability of EDSS progression within SPMS								
SPMS 3.5-6 to SPMS 6≤	0.5		0.3		0.5		0.4	
Relapse rate								
RRMS	Cycle 1	2.54	Cycle 1	1.34	Cycle 1	1.73	Cycle 1	1.68
	Other cycles	2.04	Other cycles	1.31	Other cycles	1.18	Other cycles	1.01
SPMS	0.7		0.47		0.5		0.35	
Withdrawal								
RRMS 1-3	-		Cycles1 &2	0.04	Cycles1 &2	0.078	Cycles1 &2	0.086
			Other cycles	0.04	Other cycles	0.05	Other cycles	0.09
RRMS 3.5-6	-		Cycle 2	0.26	Cycle 2	0.42	Cycle 2	0.247
			Other cycles	0.04	Other cycles	0.05	Other cycles	0.09
SPMS 3.5-6	-		0.19		0.357		0.25	

RRMS relapsing remitting multiple sclerosis, *SPMS* secondary progressive multiple sclerosis, *EDSS* expanded disability status scale, *Mcg* microgram, ml milliliter.

the impact of CBPs and biosimilars on the analysis. We performed the second analysis to assess the sensitivity of the model to different ways of QALYs assessments obtained from questionnaires and literatures' searches-based QALYs. The third sensitivity analysis was performed to evaluate the sensitivity of analysis to discount cost and QALYs.

Consent

The study was approved in the Institute Review Board with code number 91-10-24:1–1. Additionally, the study was approved by Iranian Society of MS. Written informed consent was obtained from the patient for the publication of this report and any accompanying images.

Results

ICER of symptom management combined with IFN β comparing to symptom management alone

ICER of adding IM IFNβ-1a (Avonex) to symptom management based on evaluation of utility by literatures search, VAS, EQ-5D, and HUI3 as measurement tools of QALYs was $18712, $19954, $17398 and $20045. Not cost-effective intervention except while evaluated by EQ-5D.

Table 6 Utility scores related to multiple sclerosis (MS) type and expanded disability status scale (EDSS) states in cost-effectiveness model

State	Utility score: Literature review	Visual Analog Scale (VAS)	European Quality of Life-5 Dimensions (EQ-5D)	Health Utility Index 3 (HUI 3)
RRMS EDSS 1-3.5	0.68	0.79	0.76	0.68
RRMS EDSS 4-6	0.52	0.62	0.57	0.41
SPMS EDSS 4-6	0.52	0.58	0.52	0.18
RRMS EDSS 6<	0.17	0.38	0.18	0.08
SPMS EDSS 6<	0.17	0.18	0.02	0.06
Relapse (Utility loss)	0.5	0.42	0.42	0.42
Death	0	0	0	0

All utility scores have been obtained from cross section study based on questionnaire.

Table 7 Cost of multiple sclerosis disease (MS) and interferon beta (INF β) therapy

Cost per patient per year ($)		RRMS 1-3.5	RRMS 4-6	RRMS 6<	SPMS 4-6	SPMS 6<
		Total costs for other medications is related to" Interferons-beta" administration and duration, EDSS and type of disease				
Total medical direct cost (Medicines)						
Interferon beta-1a (Avonex)*		9861	9861	0	9861	0
Interferon beta-1a (Rebif)*		7106	7106	0	7106	0
Interferon beta-1b (Betaferon)*		9176	9176	0	9176	0
Interferon beta-1a IM (CBPs)*		3762	3762	0	3762	0
Interferon beta-1a SC (CBPs)*		5873	5873	0	5873	0
Interferon beta-1b (CBPs & BS)*		7969	7969	0	7969	0
Antidepressant medications	The first 3 cycles	2.3	2.7	3.2	2.7	3.2
	Other Cycles	1.5	1.8	2.2	1.8	2.2
Anti-spasm medications		11.65	11.65	11.65	11.65	11.65
Anti-fatigue medications		1.36	1.36	1.36	1.36	1.36
Pain killer medications		4.7	6.6	9.8	23.5	29.9
NSAIDs (control SE)	for Interferon beta-1a IM	0.15	0.15	0	0.15	0
	for Interferon beta-1a SC	0.42	0.42	0	0.42	0
	for Interferon beta-1b	0.53	0.53	0	0.53	0
Other medical direct cost (total)		**167**	**316**	**1543**	**316**	**1543**
Laboratory tests		13	13	0	13	0
Imaging		103	103	0	103	0
Physicians visits		45	32	14	32	14
Physiotherapy		0	15	326	15	326
Psychotherapy		6	64	0	64	0
Nursing		0	41	816	41	816
Cane, walker, wheelchair, Medical bed, Medical wave mattress		0	48	387	48	387
Non-medical direct cost (total)		**266**	**1841**	**3037**	**1841**	**3037**
Transport		266	373	40	373	40
House reconstructions		0	0	1529	0	1529
Car rebuilding		0	1468	1468	1468	1468
Indirect cost (total)		**90**	**130**	**616**	**379**	**740**
Absence from work		71	120	0	65	0
Unemployment or early retirement		7	0	616	308	740
Mortality		12	10	0	6	0
Cost per patient per relapse (total)		**33**	**33**	**33**	**54**	**54**
Medical treatment		27	27	27	45	45
Hospitalization		6	6	6	9	9

$ US Dollars 2012, *IM* intramuscular, *SC* subcutaneous, *NSAIDs* non steroid anti- inflammatory drugs, *Cost of injection is included for interferons beta; *CBPs* Copied biopharmaceuticals including IM IFNβ-1a (Cinnovex, Actovex), SC IFNβ-1a (Recigen, Actorif) and SC IFNβ-1b (Ziferon, Actoferon), *BS* biosimilar including SC IFNβ-1b (Extavia).

ICER of adding SC IFNβ-1a (Rebif) to symptom management based on evaluation of utility by literatures search, VAS, EQ-5D, and HUI3 was $11832, $11850, $10433 and $11437 (cost-effective intervention).

ICER of adding SC IFNβ-1b (Betaferon) to symptom management based on evaluation of utility by literatures search, VAS, EQ-5D, and HUI3 was $15768, $16864, $15030 and $16314 (cost-effective intervention).

ICER of adding CBPs IM IFNβ-1a (Cinnovex, Actovex with 98 and 2 percent of market share among CBPs IM IFNβ-1a) to symptom management based on evaluation of utility by literatures search, VAS, EQ-5D, and HUI3 as a measurement tools of QALYs was $847, $904, $788 and $908 (highly cost-effective intervention).

ICER of adding CBPs SC IFNβ-1a (Recigen, Actorif with 87.5 and 12.5 percent of market share among CBPs SC IFNβ-1a) to symptom management based on evaluation of utility by literatures search, VAS, EQ-5D, and HUI3 was $6964, $6975, $6140 and $6731 (cost-effective intervention).

ICER of adding CBPs SC IFNβ-1b (Ziferon, Actoferon with both 12.5 percent and (biosimilar); Extavia with 75 percent of market share among CBPs and biosimilar SC IFNβ-1b) to symptom management based on evaluation of utility by literatures search, VAS, EQ-5D, and HUI3 was $11913, $12740, $11355, and $12325 (cost-effective intervention). All results have been provided in Table 8.

Discounted ICER of symptom management combined with IFNβ comparing to symptom management alone

Discounted ICER of adding IM IFNβ-1a (Avonex) to symptom management based on evaluation of utility by literatures search, VAS, EQ-5D, and HUI3 as a measurement tools of QALYs was $18873, $20370, $18050, and $20104 (not cost-effective intervention).

Discounted ICER of adding SC IFNβ-1a (Rebif) to symptom management based on evaluation of utility by literatures search, VAS, EQ-5D, and HUI3 as a measurement tool of QALYs was $13482, $13885, $12347, and $13092 (cost-effective intervention).

Discounted ICER of adding SC IFNβ-1b (Betaferon) to symptom management based on evaluation of utility by literatures search, VAS, EQ-5D, and HUI3 was $15142, $16452, $14808, and $15663 (cost-effective intervention).

Discounted ICER of adding CBPs IM IFNβ-1a (Cinnovex, Actovex with 98 and 2 percent of market share among CBPs IM IFNβ-1a) to symptom management based on evaluation of utility by literatures search, VAS, EQ-5D, and HUI3 as a measurement tools of QALYs was $4026, $4345, $3850, and $4288(highly cost-effective intervention).

Discounted ICER of adding CBPs SC IFNβ-1a (Recigen, Actorif with 87.5 and 12.5 percent of market share among CBPs SC IFNβ-1a) to symptom management based on evaluation of utility by literatures search, VAS, EQ-5D, and HUI3 was $9553, $9838, $8749, and $9276 (cost-effective intervention).

Discounted ICER of adding CBPs SC IFNβ-1b (Ziferon, Actoferon with both 12.5 percent and (biosimilars) Extavia; with 75 percent of market share among CBPs and biosimilar SC IFNβ-1b) to symptom management based on evaluation of utility by literatures search, VAS, EQ-5D, and HUI3 was $11903, $12933, $11641 and $12312 (cost-effective intervention). All results have been provided in Table 9.

Table 8 ICER ($) of different Interferons-Beta in comparison to placebo therapy in MS patients according to different utility measurement methods

Therapy	Literature-based	VAS	EQ-5D	HUI 3
Interferon beta-1a (Intramuscular) (Avonex)	18712	19954	17398	20045
Interferon beta-1a (Subcutaneous) (Rebif)	11832	11850	10433	11437
Interferon beta-1b (Betaferon)	15768	16864	15030	16314
Interferon beta-1a (Intramuscular) (CBPs)	847	904	788	908
Interferon beta-1a (Subcutaneous) (CBPs)	6964	6975	6140	6731
Interferon beta-1b (CBPs and BS)	11913	12740	11355	12325

$ US dollars, *ICER* incremental cost effectiveness ratio, *VAS* visual analogue scale, *EQ-5D* EuroQol, *HUI3*: Health Utilities Index 3, *CBPs* Copied biopharmaceuticals including IM IFNβ-1a (Cinnovex, Actovex), SC IFNβ-1a (Recigen, Actorif) and SC IFNβ-1b (Ziferon, Actoferon), *BS* biosimilar including SC IFNβ-1b (Extavia).

Table 9 Discounted ICER ($) of different Interferons-Beta in comparison to placebo therapy in MS patients according to different utility measurement methods

Therapy	Literature-based	VAS	EQ-5D	HUI 3
Interferon beta-1a (Avonex)	18873	20370	18050	20104
Interferon beta-1a (Rebif)	13482	13885	12347	13092
Interferon beta-1b (Betaferon)	15142	16452	14808	15663
Interferon beta-1a (Intramuscular) (CBPs)	4026	4345	3850	4288
Interferon beta-1a (Subcutaneous) (CBPs)	9553	9838	8749	9276
Interferon beta-1b (CBPs & BS)	11903	12933	11641	12312

$ US dollars, *ICER* incremental cost effectiveness ratio, *VAS* visual analogue scale, *EQ-5D* EuroQol, *HUI 3* Health Utilities Index 3, *CBPs* Copied biopharmaceuticals including IM IFNβ-1a (Cinnovex, Actovex), SC IFNβ-1a (Recigen, Actorif) and SC IFNβ-1b (Ziferon, Actoferon), *BS* biosimilar including SC IFNβ-1b (Extavia).

Discussion

The results of these analysis showed that all kinds of available branded, CBPs or biosimilar IFN β in Iran are cost-effectiveness except Avonex. The analysis was based on Markov model and long-term data of effectiveness and tolerability and considering progress to SPMS. Switching is the noteworthy difference of this model that has been implemented for the first time for cost-effectiveness of IFN β in MS. WHO's recommendation about threshold of developing countries considers ICER less than triplet of GDP as a cost-effective intervention [46]. GDP of 2012 for Iran is 5810 USD, thus all ICER less than 17430 USD per QALYs could be considered cost-effective. Analysis showed ICER of 847 to 16864 USD per QALYs for CBPs and biosimilar of IM IFNβ-1a, SC IFNβ-1a and SC IFNβ-1b, Rebif and Betaferon. For Avonex, intervention is cost-effective only when EQ-5D has been applied for assessment of utility. The differences of QALYs assessment tools in calculation of utility in MS have been demonstrated before [75]. It seems that this difference happened because EQ-5D questionnaire is not capable to measure one of the important disutility of MS, cognition. However sensitivity analysis showed that our model was not sensitive to evaluation methods of utility or literature-based ones. The model is not sensitive to discounting either. Our model is sensitive to replacing CBPs and biosimilars that it is a dominated approach. Sensitivity in case of bivariate analysis of discounting and CBPs IM IFNβ-1a and SC IFNβ-1a have occurred. This may happen because of significant impact of IFN β in cost of MS treatment. Therefore, reducing the price of IFN β by replacement with CBPs will decrease the influence of this factor and may highlight other reasons that affect utility. It must be emphasized that the unit price of CBPs IM IFNβ-1a and SC IFNβ-1a are significantly lower than Avonex and Rebif in Iran. Overall sensitivity analysis in this study showed robustness of this model.

This is the first time that cost-effectiveness of IFN β have been analyzed in context of one of developing countries by applying decision analytic modeling. Markov model has been applied to assess the progression of disease and its prevention with adding IFN β to management protocol. Spreading on the concept of switching to other IFN β in case of withdrawal due to side effects or lack in perceived efficacy to model is novel. The idea for modifying the Markov model in case of switchable interventions has been established by Nikfar 2012 [35]. In case of probability of switching to other drugs in decision analysis model, overhead costing and utility may affect results and decision-making processes, thus, for the first time we consider switching to other IFN β in case of withdrawal from one of them. Therefore, to conclude the utility and cost of each intervention, decision tree model has been used as an additional decision analytic modeling. Additional analysis showed that without considering switching to other IFN β, ICER will be beyond threshold and intervention will not be cost-effective.

In our Markov model, the probability of transition to SPMS is one of the transition states. Nuijten and Hutton have also considered SPMS in their Markov model [19]. Their analysis revealed that IFN β were much more cost-effective compared with the results of other cost-effectiveness study performed in patients with RRMS only. They believe that reduction in the cost-effectiveness ratio of IFN β may be in line for a longer follow-up period and continuation of treatment with IFN β in SPMS.

Our designed model is based on thirty-year that is kind of life-long follow up complying with life expectancy of MS patients that is almost 10 years less than healthy population [49]. Considering the rate of mortality in MS patients rather than general population [18,19,41], the reliability of study is increased. Seeing IFN β act in MS patients differently is in contrast with modeling of Bell et al., and Nuijten and Hutton [18,19] and robust the results of current cost-effectiveness study and may help decision makers accurately. It should be emphasized that assuming tolerability as an essential part of drug therapy that interferes with health-related outcomes [76] is another advantage of this study. Withdrawal due to side effects of medicines or lack of effectiveness in long-term treatments may have a great impact in cost-effectiveness analysis [77]. Chilcott et al. [41] didn't consider withdrawal in their decision analysis model, although Nuijten and Hutton [19] and Bell and his colleagues [18] have used withdrawal data in their model. The withdrawal data was retrieved from short-term trials and only due to side effects [19] or lack of efficacy [18] and just for one cycle of model. To be closer to reality, withdrawal is considered in all long of intervention in recent model. Availability of long-term follow-up data (effectiveness and withdrawal) of patients initially enrolled in clinical trials [63-65] helped us to not repeating the mistake of previous studies in use of extrapolated data from short-term trials to assess effectiveness and discontinuation of therapy [19,41].

However, our model is much more improved but always the results of modeling need to be treated with some degree of caution from a health-economic perspective. Amongst is the data for probabilities of preventive effects for IFN β. All such kinds of data in this analysis have been retrieved from RCTs and their long-term follow up data. Therefore, the fact of controversy between real effectiveness and efficacy obtained from protocol-restricted RCTs will remain. Usually, conducting meta-analysis can solve this problem, but in case of rare diseases like MS due to lack of variety of available trials, this method is even unlikely. The indirect cost in developing countries may be affected by low productivity of such regions. Furthermore, Iran has adapted generic based pharmaceutical policy.

These two reasons may consequence underestimation of the cost in this model and the low ICER than other cost-effectiveness studies [18,19,41,78] that reported approximately 50000 USD per QALYs, for prevention effect of IFN β. The utilities in our model were derived from a cross-sectional study based on EDSS and disease conditions. Adverse effects of therapeutics medicines have not been considered in assessment of utilities and this may also modify the results of ICERs. There are specific health related quality of life (HRQOL) questionnaires for MS like Hamburg Quality of Life Questionnaire in Multiple Sclerosis (HAQUAMS) or multiple sclerosis quality of life with 54 questions (MSQOL-54), moreover quality of life in MS can be also determined by generic HRQOL like EQ-5D or HUI-3. The problem of specific HRQOL is measurement of utility or preference-based measures by them that is impossible; on the other hand, utility or preference-based measures have the advantage of leading to a single number that balances gains in one domain against losses in another. The best known utility or preference-based measures according to reliability, validity and feasibility for MS are the HUI-3 and the EQ-5D index [79,80]. There are varieties in concepts and scores of utility measurement tools. It seems that HUI3 with potential of scoring cognitive problems of MS patients could act better than other tools like EQ-5D or VAS. Nevertheless, sensitivity analysis in our model didn't show differences between utilities obtained from different forms and literature reviews. The characteristics of patients related to age, sex, educational and employment status were taken from 200 patients in cross sectional filled questionnaires. According to prevalence of different kind of MS and EDSS state, in some states like higher EDSS or SPMS there are too few recruited patients. This problem may underweight the results and considering equal and sufficient amount of patients for each state, in future studies is recommended to vigorous results. Our model with 50% progression to SPMS after 10 years and 90% after 25 years [47] and life expectancy of thirty after incidence of illness corresponds with natural history of MS [49].

Our results showed that prescribing of all kind of IFN β except Avonex in context of Iran is cost-effective. Due to the fact that there is no difference among IFN β as regards of effectiveness and safety, thus the choice of them depends on clinicians in many cases. However, it seems that price is an important factor for prescription. Therefore CBP of IM IFNβ-1a (Cinnovex) is prescribed more than 50% in Iran [28]. As a pharmaceutical regulatory rule, clinical data for brands and CBPs and biosimilar of IFN β in this study considered to be the same [28,81]. If by availability of post marketing surveillance, we reach the same conclusion about ranking for ICERs, the most efficient way is to choose the most cost-effective IFN β with respect of compliance.

The results of this study demonstrated that generic based NDP is one of the strength of each country's policy to make medicines more accessible.

Competing interests
The authors declare that they have no competing interests. Since MA is Editor-in-Chief of DARU, all review process of the submission was handled by one of Section Editors.

Authors' contributions
SN made design of the study, acquisition of data, analysis and interpretation of data, drafted the article and revising it critically for important intellectual content, AK and RD reviewed all data and supervised whole study, MA supervised whole study and revised the paper critically for important intellectual content, MAS contributed in acquisition of data and interpretation of data, DH contributed in design of the study, AAS reviewed all data and design of study and supervised whole study. All authors approved final version for submission.

Acknowledgment
Authors thank Iranian Society of multiple sclerosis for their kind assistance in collecting information of patients. This paper is the outcome of a PhD thesis of the first author and was supported by Faculty of Pharmacy, Tehran University of Medical Sciences.

Author details
[1]Department of Pharmacoeconomics and Pharmaceutical Administration, Faculty of Pharmacy, Tehran University of Medical Sciences, Tehran, Iran. [2]Food & Drug Organization, Ministry of Health & Medical Education, Tehran, Iran. [3]Faculty of Pharmacy, and Pharmaceutical Sciences Research Center, Tehran University of Medical Sciences, Tehran, Iran. [4]Department of Neurology, Sina Hospital, Tehran University of Medical Sciences, Tehran, Iran. [5]Institute for Clinical Evaluative Sciences, Toronto, Canada. [6]Department of Health Management and Economics, School of Public Health, Tehran University of Medical Sciences, Tehran, Iran.

References
1. Disanto G, Morahan JM, Ramagopalan SV: **Multiple sclerosis: risk factors and their interactions.** *CNS Neurol Disord Drug Targets* 2012, **11**(5):545–555.
2. *Multiple sclerosis International federation.* http://www.msif.org
3. Ahlgren C, Odén A, Lycke J: **High nationwide prevalence of multiple sclerosis in Sweden.** *Mult Scler* 2011, **17**(8):901–908.
4. Kurtzke JF: **Multiple sclerosis in time and space-geographic clues to cause.** *J Neurovirol* 2000, **6**(2):S134–S140.
5. Yousefi Pour GA, Ali Reza Rasekhi AR: **Multiple sclerosis: a risk factor analysis Iran.** *Arch Iran Med* 2002, **5**(3):191–193.
6. Kalanie H, Gharagozli K, Kalanie AR: **Multiple sclerosis: report on 200 cases from Iran.** *Mult Scler* 2003, **9**:36–38.
7. Saadatnia M, Etemadifar M, Maghzi AH: **Multiple sclerosis in Isfahan, Iran.** *Int Rev Neurobiol* 2007, **79**:357–375.
8. Hashemilar M, Savadi Ouskui D, Farhoudi M, Ayromlou H, Asadollahi A: **Multiple sclerosis in East-Azerbaijan, north west Iran.** *Neurol Asia* 2011, **16**(2):127–131.
9. Abedini M, Habibi Saravi R, Zarvani A, Farahmand A: **Epidemiology of Multiple sclerosis in Mazandaran in 2007 (in Persian).** *J Mazand Univ Med Sci* 2008, **18**(66):82–87.
10. Milo R, Kahana E: **Multiple sclerosis: Geoepidemiology, genetics and the environment.** *Autoimmun Rev* 2010, **9**:A387–A394.
11. Sahraian MA, Khorramnia S, Ebrahim MM, Moinfar Z, Lotfi J, Pakdaman H: **Multiple sclerosis in Iran: a demographic study of 8,000 patients and changes over time.** *Eur Neurol* 2010, **64**:331–336.
12. Etemadifar M, Janghorbani M, Shaygannejad V, Ashtari F: **Prevalence of multiple sclerosis in Isfahan, Iran.** *Neuroepidemiology* 2006, **27**:39–44.
13. Elhami SR, Mohammad K, Sahraian MA, Eftekhar H: **A 20-year incidence trend (1989–2008) and point prevalence (March 20, 2009) of multiple sclerosis in Tehran, Iran: a population-based study.** *Neuroepidemiology* 2011, **36**(3):141–147.

14. Nabavi M, Poorfarzam S, Ghasemi H: **Epidemiology, clinical trend and prognosis of multiple sclerosis in 203 patients of MS clinic in Shahid Mostafa Khomeini hospital in 2002 (in Persian).** *Tehran Univ Med J* 2006, **64**(7):90–97.
15. Ghandehari K, Riasi HR, Nourian A, Boroumand AR: **Prevalence of multiple sclerosis in north east of Iran.** *Mult Scler* 2010, **16**(12):1525–1526.
16. Ghabaae M, Qelichnia Omrani H, Roostaeizadeh M: **Epidemiology of multiple sclerosis in Tehran: a three year study.** *Tehran Univ Med J* 2007, **65**(5):74–77.
17. Ale-Yasin H, Sarai A, Alaeddini F, Ansarian E, Lotfi J, Sanati H: **Multiple sclerosis: a study of 318 cases.** *Arch Iran Med* 2002, **5**(1):24–27.
18. Bell C, Graham J, Earnshaw S, Oleen-Burkey M, Castelli-Haley J, Johnson K: **Cost-effectiveness of four immunomodulatory therapies for relapsing-remitting multiple sclerosis: a Markov model based on long-term clinical data.** *J Manag Care Pharm* 2007, **13**(3):245–261.
19. Nuijten MJ, Hutton J: **Cost-effectiveness analysis of interferon beta in multiple sclerosis: a Markov process analysis.** *Value Health* 2002, **5**(1):44–54.
20. *Statistical center of Iran.* http://www.amar.org.ir
21. Nikfar S, Rahimi R, Rezaie A, Abdollahi M: **A meta-analysis on the efficacy and tolerability of natalizumab in relapsing multiple sclerosis.** *Arch Med Sci* 2010, **6**(2):236–244.
22. Nikfar S, Rahimi R, Abdollahi M: **A meta-analysis of the efficacy and tolerability of interferon-β in multiple sclerosis, overall and by drug and disease type.** *Clin Ther* 2010, **2**(11):1871–1888.
23. Nikfar S, Rahimi R, Abdollahi M: **A systematic review on the efficacy of interferon beta in relapsing remitting multiple sclerosis; comparison of different formulations.** *Inter J Pharmacol* 2010, **6**(5):638–644.
24. Packer C, Simpson S, Stevens A: **International diffusion of new health technologies: a ten-country analysis of six health technologies.** *Int J Technol Assess Health Care* 2006, **22**(4):419–428.
25. *European medicines agency, EMEA.* http://www.ema.europa.eu/ema/index
26. *United States of America Food and drug administration, US-FDA.* http://www.accessdata.fda.gov/scripts/cder/drugsatfda/index
27. Palesh M, Jonsson PM, Jamshidi H, Wettermark B, Tomson G, Fredrikson S: **Diffusion of interferon beta in Iran and its utilization in Tehran.** *Pharmacoepidemiol Drug Saf* 2008, **17**(9):934–941.
28. *Iranian Food and Drug Organization.* http://fdo.behdasht.gov.ir
29. Cheraghali AM: **Biosimilars; a unique opportunity for Iran national health sector and national pharmaceutical industry.** *Daru* 2012, **20**(1):35.
30. World Health Organization, WHO (Ed): www.who.int
31. Nikfar S, Kebriaeezadeh A, Majdzadeh R, Abdollahi M: **Monitoring of National Drug Policy (NDP) and its standardized indicators; conformity to decisions of the national drug selecting committee in Iran.** *BMC Int Health Hum Rights* 2005, **5**(1):5.
32. Abdollahiasl A, Nikfar S, Kebriaeezadeh A, Dinarvand R, Abdollahi M: **A model for developing a decision support system to simulate national drug policy indicators.** *Arch Med Sci* 2011, **7**(5):744–746.
33. Cheraghali AM, Nikfar S, Behmanesh Y, Rahimi V, Habibipour F, Tirdad R, Asadi A, Bahrami A: **Evaluation of availability, accessibility and prescribing pattern of medicines in the Islamic Republic of Iran.** *East Mediterr Health J* 2004, **10**(3):406–415.
34. Nikfar S, Khatibi M, Abdollahiasl A, Abdollahi M: **Cost and utilization study of antidotes: An Iranian experience.** *Int J Pharmacol* 2011, **7**(1):46–49.
35. Nikfar S: **A new model for decision analysis in economic evaluations of switchable health interventions.** *J Med Hypotheses Ideas* 2012, **6**:12–15.
36. Kobelt G, Jonsson L, Fredrikson S: **Cost-utility of interferon beta1b in the treatment of patients with active relapsing-remitting or secondary progressive multiple sclerosis.** *Eur J Health Econ* 2003, **4**(1):50–59.
37. Iskedjian M, Walker JH, Gray T, Vicente C, Einarson TR, Gehshan A: **Economic evaluation of Avonex (interferon beta-1a) in patients following a single demyelinating event.** *Mult Scler* 2005, **11**(5):542–551.
38. Bose U, Ladkani D, Burrell A, Sharief M: **Cost-effectiveness analysis of glatiramer acetate in the treatment of relapsing-remitting multiple sclerosis: first estimates.** *J Med Econ* 2001, **4**:207–219.
39. Parkin D, McNamee P, Jacoby A, Miller P, Thomas S, Bates D: **A cost-utility analysis of interferon beta for multiple sclerosis.** *Health Technol Assess* 1998, **2**(4):iii–54.
40. Phillips CJ, Gilmour L, Gale R, Palmer M: **A cost utility model of beta-interferon in the treatment of relapsing-remitting multiple sclerosis.** *J Med Econ* 2001, **4**:35–50.
41. Chilcott J, McCabe C, Tappenden P, O'Hagan A, Cooper NJ, Abrams K, Claxton K, Miller DH, Cost Effectiveness of Multiple Sclerosis Therapies Study Group: **Modelling the cost effectiveness of interferon beta and glatiramer acetate in the management of multiple sclerosis. Commentary: evaluating disease modifying treatments in multiple sclerosis.** *BMJ* 2003, **326**(7388):522.
42. Briggs A, Claxton K, Sculpher M: **Decision modelling for health economic evaluation.** In *Handbooks in health economic evaluation.* vol. 1st edition. Oxford: Oxford University Press; 2006.
43. Kurtzke JF: **Rating neurologic impairment in multiple sclerosis: an expanded disability status scale (EDSS).** *Neurology* 1983, **33**(11):1444–1452.
44. Abdoli G: **Estimation of social discount rate for Iran.** *Eco Res Rev* 2009, **10**:135–156.
45. Robberstad B: **Estimation of private and social time preferences for health in northern Tanzania.** *Soc Sci Med* 2005, **61**(7):1597–1607.
46. Baltussen R, Adam T, Tan Torres T, Hutubessy R, Acharya A, Evans DB, Murray CJL: **Generalized cost-effectiveness analysis: a guide.** In *World Health Organization. Global programme on evidence for health policy.* Geneva: World Health Organization (WHO); 2002.
47. Weinshenker BG, Bass B, Rice GP, Noseworthy J, Carriere W, Baskerville J, Ebers GC: **The natural history of multiple sclerosis: a geographically-based study. I. Clinical course and disability.** *Brain* 1989, **112**:133–146.
48. Hirst C, Ingram G, Pearson O, Pickersgill T, Scolding N, Robertson N: **Contribution of relapses to disability in multiple sclerosis.** *J Neurol* 2008, **255**(2):280–287.
49. Hirst C, Swingler R, Compston DA, Ben-Shlomo Y, Robertson NP: **Survival and cause of death in multiple sclerosis: a prospective population-based study.** *J Neurol Neurosurg Psychiatry* 2008, **79**:1016–1021.
50. Whitehead SJ, Ali S: **Health outcomes in economic evaluation: the QALY and utilities.** *Br Med Bull* 2010, **96**:5–21.
51. Tappenden P, Chilcott JB, Eggington S, Oakley J, McCabe C: **Methods for expected value of information analysis in complex health economic models: developments on the health economics of interferon-β and glatiramer acetate for multiple sclerosis.** *Health Technol Assess* 2004, **8**(27). http://www.hta.ac.uk/fullmono/mon827.pdf
52. *National organization for civil registration: Survival data of Iran.* www.sabteahval.ir
53. Tremlett H, Zhao Y, Devonshire V: **Natural history of secondary-progressive multiple sclerosis.** *Mult Scler* 2008, **14**:314–324.
54. Tremlett H, Zhao Y, Devonshire V: **Natural history comparisons of primary and secondary progressive multiple sclerosis reveals differences and similarities.** *J Neurol* 2009, **256**:374–381.
55. European Study Group on interferon beta-1b in secondary progressive MS: **Placebo-controlled multicentre andomized trial of interferon beta-1b in treatment of secondary progressive multiple sclerosis.** *Lancet* 1998, **352**(9139):1491–1497.
56. Secondary Progressive Efficacy Clinical Trial of Recombinant Interferon-beta-1a in MS (SPECTRIMS) Study Group: **Randomized controlled trial of interferon-beta-1a in secondary progressive MS: clinical results.** *Clinical results. Neurology* 2001, **56**(11):1496–1504.
57. Jacobs LD, Cookfair DL, Rudick RA, Herndon RM, Richert JR, Salazar AM, Fischer JS, Goodkin DE, Granger CV, Simon JH, Alam JJ, Bartoszak DM, Bourdette DN, Braiman J, Brownscheidle CM, Coats ME, Cohan SL, Dougherty DS, Kinkel RP, Mass MK, Munschauer FE III, Priore RL, Pullicino PM, Scherokman BJ, Whitham RH, *et al*: **Intramuscular interferon beta-1a for disease progression in relapsing multiple sclerosis. The Multiple Sclerosis Collaborative Research Group (MSCRG).** *Ann Neurol* 1996, **39**(3):285–294.
58. Panitch H, Miller A, Paty D, Weinshenker B, North American Study Group on Interferon beta-1b in Secondary Progressive MS: **Interferon beta-1b in secondary progressive MS: results from a 3-year controlled study.** *Neurology* 2004, **63**(10):1788–1795.
59. PRISMS (Prevention of Relapses and Disability by Interferon beta-1a Subcutaneously in Multiple Sclerosis) Study Group: **Randomised double-blind placebo-controlled study of interferon beta-1a in relapsing/remitting multiple sclerosis.** *Lancet* 1998, **352**(9139):1498–1504.
60. Andersen O, Elovaara I, Färkkilä M, Hansen HJ, Mellgren SI, Myhr KM, Sandberg-Wollheim M, Soelberg Sørensen P: **Multicenter, randomized, double blind, placebo controlled, phase III study of weekly, low dose, subcutaneous interferon beta-1a in secondary progressive multiple sclerosis.** *J Neurol Neurosurg Psychiatry* 2004, **75**(5):706–710.
61. Leary SM, Miller DH, Stevenson VL, Brex PA, Chard DT, Thompson AJ: **Interferon beta-1a in primary progressive MS: an exploratory, randomized, controlled trial.** *Neurology* 2003, **60**(1):44–51.
62. The IFN, β Multiple Sclerosis Study Group: **Interferon beta-1b is effective in relapsing-remitting multiple sclerosis. I. Clinical results of a multicenter,**

randomized, double-blind, placebo-controlled trial. *Neurology* 1993, **43**(4):655–661.
63. Kappos L, Traboulsee A, Constantinescu C, Erälinna JP, Forrestal F, Jongen P, Pollard J, Sandberg-Wollheim M, Sindic C, Stubinski B, Uitdehaag B, Li D: **Long-term subcutaneous interferon beta-1a therapy in patients with relapsing-remitting MS.** *Neurology* 2006, **67**:944–953.
64. Ebers GC, Traboulsee A, Li D, Langdon D, Reder AT, Goodin DS, Bogumil T, Beckmann K, Wolf C, Konieczny A, Investigators of the 16-year Long-Term Follow-Up Study: **Analysis of clinical outcomes according to original treatment groups 16 years after the pivotal IFNB-1b trial.** *J Neurol Neurosurg Psychiatry* 2010, **81**:907–912.
65. Rudick RA, Lee JC, Cutter GR, Miller DM, Bourdette D, Weinstock-Guttman B, Hyde R, Zhang H, You X: **Disability progression in a clinical trial of relapsing-remitting multiple sclerosis: eight-year follow-up.** *Arch Neurol* 2010, **67**(11):1329–1335.
66. Phillips CJ: **The cost of multiple sclerosis and the cost effectiveness of disease-modifying agents in its treatment.** *CNS Drugs* 2004, **18**(9):561–574.
67. O'Brien B: *Multiple sclerosis.* London: Office of Health Economics; 1987.
68. Tappenden P, Chilcott J, O'Hagan A, McCabe C: **Cost effectiveness of beta interferons and glatiramer acetate in the management of multiple sclerosis.** In *Final Report to the National Institute for Clinical Excellence.* London: National Institute for Clinical Excellence (NICE); 2001.
69. Gani R, Giovannoni G, Bates D, Kemball B, Hughes S, Kerrigan J: **Cost-effectiveness analyses of natalizumab (Tysabri®) compared with other disease-modifying therapies for people with highly active relapsing-remitting multiple sclerosis in the UK.** *PharmacoEconomics* 2008, **26**(7):617–627.
70. Iran ministry of health and medical education: *Tariff of healthcare services in public and private sectors in Iran (2012).* Tehran: Iran ministry of health and medical education press; 2012.
71. *National Organization of Transportation.* http://upto.ir
72. Koopmanschap MA, Rutten FFH, Van Ineveld BM, Van Roijen L: **The friction cost method for measuring indirect costs of disease.** *J Health Econ* 1995, **14**:171–189.
73. Ganjali M, Baghfalaki T: **Bayesian analysis of unemployment duration data in presence of right and interval censoring.** *JRSS* 2012, **5**(1):17–32.
74. Asian Productivity Organization: *APO productivity data book 2012.* Tokyo: Keio university press INC; 2012.
75. Fisk JD, Brown MG, Sketris IS, Metz LM, Murray TJ, Stadnyk KJ: **A comparison of health utility measures for the evaluation of multiple sclerosis treatments.** *J Neurol Neurosurg Psychiatry* 2005, **76**:58–63.
76. Strom BL, Kimmel SE: *Textbook of pharmacoepidemiology.* Chichester, West Sussex: John Willey & Sons; 2006.
77. Bobes J, Cañas F, Rejas J, Mackell J: **Economic consequences of the adverse reactions related with antipsychotics: an economic model comparing tolerability of ziprasidone, olanzapine, risperidone, and haloperidol in Spain.** *Prog Neuropsychopharmacol Biol Psychiatry* 2004, **28**:1287–1297.
78. Goldberg LD, Edwards NC, Fincher C, Doan QV, Al-Sabbagh A, Meletiche DM: **Comparing the cost-effectiveness of disease-modifying drugs for the first-line treatment of relapsing-remitting multiple sclerosis.** *J Manag Care Pharm* 2009, **15**(7):543–555.
79. Fisk JD, Brown MG, Sketris IS, Metz LM, Murray TJ, Stadnyk KJ: **A comparison of health utility measures for the evaluation of multiple sclerosis treatments.** *J Neurol Neurosurg Psychiatry* 2005, **76**(1):58–63.
80. Kuspinar A, Rodriguez AM, Mayo NE: **The effects of clinical interventions on health-related quality of life in multiple sclerosis: a meta-analysis.** *Mult Scler* 2012, **18**(12):1686–1704.
81. European Medicines Agency (EMEA): EMEA Guideline on Similar Biological Medicinal Products, CHMP/437/04. [http://www.emea.europa.eu/docs/en_GB/document_library/Scientific_guideline/2009/09/WC500003517.pdf]

Assessment of the vaccine industry in Iran in context of accession to WTO: a survey study

Amir Hashemi Meshkini[1], Abbas Kebriaeezadeh[1*], Rasoul Dinarvand[1,2], Shekoufeh Nikfar[1,3], MohammadGafar Habibzadeh[4] and Iman Vazirian[2]

Abstract

Background: The vaccine industry is one of the most important health-related industries. It can be affected by accession to the World Trade Organization (WTO) because of probable dramatic changes in the business environment. Iran has already initiated accession negotiations.

Purpose of the study: In this paper, we investigate the position of, challenges to, and opportunities for vaccine manufacturing in Iran with regard to accession to the WTO.

Methods: This is a qualitative and cross sectional study. To collect information, we designed a questionnaire and interviewed some of the vaccine industry's key opinion leaders in Iran. Before the interviews were conducted, the questionnaires were sent to these individuals by email.

Results: According to the interviewees, the country's main challenges with regard to accession to the WTO are the lack of firm internal intellectual property (IP) rules, not being recognized as pre-qualified by the World Health Organization (WHO), the use of old equipment, and a lack of cooperation with global vaccine companies.

Major conclusions: Iran's local vaccine industry, with a long history and international reputation that could be used as an advantage, is faced with several challenges, such as problems with keeping up with Current Good Manufacturing Practice (cGMP), a lack of adequate and meaningful investment in research and development (R&D), and limitations on private sector participation in the production of vaccines.
Gradual privatization of the industry, improved international relations, utilization of the R&D power of small hi-tech companies, consistent education of human resources, and modernization of infrastructures and equipment are among the suggested solutions.

Keywords: Vaccine, WTO, Iran, WHO

Introduction

Globalization could be defined as the process of making nationalization irrelevant in markets, laws, and politics in the production of common goods, based on comparative advantages [1].

Today, most countries have joined the World Trade Organization (WTO) and some are observer members waiting to start negotiations in the accession process [2]. Iran (the Islamic Republic of Iran) was accepted into this organization in 2005 as an observer member. The Iranian trade regime report was sent to the WTO in 2009, and currently, the first level of negotiation is on the table.

Accession to the WTO most probably affects many aspects of various industries; being familiar with these effects can provide organizations opportunities to deal with the potential challenges that lie ahead. Among these industries, those related to public health, such as the pharmaceutical and vaccine industries, are extremely vulnerable and sensitive: "vulnerable" because they are faced with competition from big international companies inside and outside of the country, and "sensitive" because these industries are related to one of the most important aspects of people's life—their health—especially in developing countries where accessibility to medicines and vaccines has been improved by domestic manufacturing.

* Correspondence: Kebriaee@tums.ac.ir
[1]Department of Pharmacoeconomics and Pharmaceutical administration, Faculty of pharmacy, Tehran University of Medical Sciences, 16th Azar st, Keshavarz Blvd, Tehran, Iran
Full list of author information is available at the end of the article

The vaccine industry in Iran has a long history. The Razi Serum and Vaccine Research Institute started manufacturing veterinary vaccines in 1929, and soon after, added human products to its agenda [3]. The Institute Pasteur of Iran is the second vaccine manufacturer in Iran. It started in 1920 with the cooperation of the Institute Pasteur of France [4].

With regard to human vaccines, Razi produces measles, polio, MMR, MR, trivalent vaccines, and divalent vaccines. The Institute Pasteur produces BCG and Hepatitis B vaccines.

These two vaccine producers experienced glorious periods in the past. To ensure continued success, the Iran vaccine industry needs to determine its weaknesses and strengths as well as the obstacles and opportunities that lie ahead with regard to WTO accession.

The aim of this study is to assess the probable impacts of WTO accession on the vaccine industry in Iran.

Method

This is a qualitative cross sectional study to investigate the current situation as well as the upcoming issues affecting the vaccine industry in Iran. To collect data and information, we interviewed some of the key opinion leaders in the Iranian vaccine industry. This group of experts was comprised of representatives from both local vaccine manufacturers and the Ministry of Health. We designed an open questionnaire, including 13 questions that were asked orally.

The questions were classified in 6 groups in terms of the subject:

1- The need for vaccines in Iran in terms of the current health conditions.
2- The vaccine supply in Iran.
3- The effect of international relationships on the vaccine supply in Iran.
4- The vaccine production capacity in Iran in case of crises.
5- The introduction of model countries to the Iranian vaccine industry.
6- The importance of international cooperation in the vaccine industry and Iran's current status.
7- The current technology level in Iran's vaccine industry.
8- The current human resources situation in Iran's vaccine industry.
9- The current situation regarding R&D investment in Iran's vaccine industry.
10- Public and private sector partnerships in the Iranian vaccine industry.
11- The probable challenges in WTO accession.
12- Iran's ability to compete in the international vaccine market.
13- Suggested solutions.

In the first question, our aim was to collect information about Iran's domestic vaccine market and immunization trends in Iran.

In questions 2, 3, and 4, we asked the experts about the capabilities of Iran's production of necessary vaccines in routine situations and in the event of a crisis.

In questions 5 and 6, we asked about the country's vaccine manufacturers' international cooperation and their visions and patterns for the future.

In questions 7, 8, and 9, we were searching for an evaluation of three important factors—the level of technology, human resources, and R&D—in the Iranian vaccine industry.

In question 10, we asked about possession and ownership issues in the vaccine industry in Iran.

Questions 11, 12, and 13 reflect an international market perspective and Iran's ability to penetrate these markets after WTO accession. We wanted to know about the challenges ahead and the experts' suggested solutions for overcoming them.

The questionnaires were sent to the interviewees before the interviews.

Among the 16 respondents selected, 11 of the key opinion leaders opted to answer the questions orally. Some of these interviewees only answered some of the questions. Two interviewees preferred to communicate through email, and one of these answered only half of the questions.

Results

The need for vaccines in Iran in terms of the current health conditions

The interviewees believed that, regarding routine and traditional vaccines, the immunization coverage in terms of the health conditions (polio has been eradicated, and some diseases, like measles, are expected to be eradicated soon) is adequate. However, the young population and the geographic position of Iran, which neighbors poor countries like Iraq and Afghanistan in terms of health conditions, and illegal immigrants coming from these countries makes Iran vulnerable to the transmission of diseases coming from outside of its borders. Additionally, the large number of foreign trips embarked upon by Iranian citizens, like the Hajj pilgrimage, and communication with people from poor-health-conditioned countries, such as some African countries, are threats to the current domestic situation.

Two of the interviewees believed that the need for vaccines is independent of the prevailing health conditions and is almost constant and contingent upon the population. Another interviewee highlighted the increasing need for vaccines in Iran because of the young population, illegal immigration from neighboring countries (without powerful governments and health systems), and the existence of remote rural areas without adequate health care in some parts of Iran.

The vaccine supply in Iran, the effect of international relationships, and the vaccine production capacity in Iran in case of crises

Only 9 out of 11 interviewees answered the first question about the vaccine supply in Iran. All of them believed that most of Iran's vaccine supply is supported by two local manufacturers and, each year, shortages are compensated by import. We were not able to access accurate information about the vaccine market value and market share of Iranian manufacturers, but an estimation by the drug office of the Food and Drug Organization (FDO) from the Health Deputy's orders for vaccines shows that sales have been 250 to 400 billion Rials annually for the past five years, depending on the year's requirements. No separate data was available about the value and volume of domestic and imported vaccines.

Ten interviewees answered the second question regarding the effects of international relationships on the vaccine supply. Two respondents thought that international relationships were important and one thought that international relationships would greatly affect the vaccine supply. The other respondents went into detail regarding their opinions: they felt that the main effects of international relationships are on the transfer of technology and access to modern equipment, and that the vaccine supply is not greatly influenced by political issues.

Ten out of 11 interviewees answered the question about Iranian manufacturers' capacity to supply the needed vaccines in the event of crises. Seven respondents said that, with concentration on the vaccine industry, Iran would be able to cover its domestic needs in crises and extraordinary situations.

The introduction of model countries and the importance of international cooperation in the vaccine industry

Eleven persons expressed their thoughts on model countries for the Iranian vaccine industry. They listed various countries among their answers: Turkey, Pakistan, Jordan, Egypt, the USA, Canada, India, the European countries, Japan, South Korea, Indonesia, Cuba, and Thailand. Out of these countries, India (seven persons), Indonesia (six persons), and Cuba (four persons) were the most mentioned. Four out of the 11 key opinion leaders believed that developed countries like the USA, Japan, and Canada should be used as models, while the others emphasized the significance of economic similarity between Iran and the model countries. They selected their models from developing countries with WHO prequalification.

Regarding the importance of international cooperation between vaccine companies and the current situation in Iran, 9 out of the 10 persons who answered this question pointed to the importance of this relationship with certainty. Seven out of 11 interviewees found Iran's current situation undesirable and two of them did not respond.

The current situation in Iran's vaccine industry regarding technology, human resources, and R&D

Regarding the level of technology, 10 out of 11 respondents mentioned difficulties in accessing new equipment. Three of them found that the position of the Institute Pasteur was superior to the Razi Institute because it has newer facilities. Regarding the level of technology in vaccine manufacturing, two out of seven respondents said that Iranian methods of vaccine production are current and are based on international protocols, and the only problem is accessing new equipment; however, four of these seven felt that the vaccine technology level is undesirable and that Iran is not in a good global position. Nine respondents believed that Iran has achieved significant improvements in biotechnology in recent years but that these achievements have not yet been fully exploited. All of those with positive outlooks regarding the level of technology were representatives from Iranian vaccine manufacturers.

Four out of 10 interviewees who answered the question regarding the human resource situation called it satisfactory and the others mentioned some weaknesses, like the shortage of well-educated persons and experts in the industry, the lack of industry skills in university graduates, problems in consistent education within the industry, and the lack of cooperation between Iranian and foreign vaccine makers in the field of human resources enhancement.

Nine persons responded to the question about R&D. All of them called the investment of local Iranian manufacturers in R&D negligible in comparison with international norms. Five persons believed that the Institute Pasteur's investment in R&D is superior to that of the Razi Institute. Low levels of investment, non-applicable and non-targeted research, and problems in R&D management were the main issues presented by the interviewees.

Public and private sector partnerships

All 11 persons who responded to this question stated that the private sector does not have a role in vaccine production in Iran. Three pointed out the tendency of the private sector to engage in vaccine production. The extent of private sector participation in vaccine development and production in Iran is very small and limited to a few companies that import vaccines ordered by the government. One interviewee believed that the only route of entry into this market is focusing on exportation and foreign markets. Some of the experts believed that most of the problems in Iran's vaccine industry are related to its public structure.

Iran's ability to compete in the international market, the probable challenges to WTO accession, and suggested solutions

For the question about Iran's ability to compete in the international vaccine market, two experts responded positively and three believed that it is not possible for Iran to compete. The others believed there is a provisional possibility. Four interviewees stated that this ability depends on obtaining WHO prequalification and one person stated that this ability depends on using current capacities and expanding upon them.

Ten out of 11 interviewees commented on the probable challenges to the vaccine industry during WTO accession. One of them believed that joining the WTO would be detrimental to the vaccine industry in Iran, but he did not provide any support for his opinion. Another respondent believed that IP issues are the main challenges. Other challenges mentioned included outdated equipment and political challenges, like sanctions and lack of international cooperation. Not being prequalified (one person) and weaknesses in state-run industries (one person) were the other ideas. Two believed there are no challenges, as the country is able to overcome any obstacles by using WTO flexibilities.

These key opinion leaders believed in the effectiveness of the following solutions: privatization of the industry (four persons), consistent education for employees (three persons), allowing private sector involvement along with the government in production (two persons), using the capacity of small science-based companies in R&D and related areas (two persons), the improvement of international cooperation in the vaccine industry (one person), the resolution of political challenges (one person), and determination and implementation of IP rights in Iran with the help of foreign consultants (one person).

Discussion

Need for vaccines in Iran in terms of the current health conditions

Vaccines needed for immunization programs in Iran (EPI) include BCG, DTP, HepB, polio, and MCV (see Table 1). The influenza, rabies and HPV vaccines (all imported from other countries) are available on the market but not in the EPI and there is still a clear lack of availability of Haemophilus influenza type B (Hib) and rotavirus vaccines in EPI. According to an internal study, the prevalence of Hib carriers is 7.6%, similar to other developing countries, yet this vaccine is still not part of the program [5]. The government intends to include these two vaccines in the program; this is dependent both on adding them to the Iranian drug list and the ability of vaccine producers to produce them, which has not been the case so far. It should be emphasized that Iran has already adopted a National Drug List (NDL), which is selected by the Iran Drug Selecting Committee (IDSC). All drug supply management process, including registration, procurement, inspection, quality control, and post marketing control, can be handled by the IDSC for a drug that is accepted for inclusion on the NDL [6].

Table 1 Immunization schedule of expanded program of immunization program in Iran, 2010

Age of vaccination	Type of vaccine
At birth	BCG, OPV, Hep B
2 month	OPV, DTwP, HepB
4 month	OPV, DTwP
6 month	OPV, DTwP, Hep B
12 month	MMR
18 month	OPV, DTwP, MMR
6 years	OPV, DTwP

The vaccine supply in Iran, the effect of international relationships, and the vaccine production capacity in Iran in case of crises

It seems there is no clear vision in Iran regarding the vaccine supply in the future. The world's approach toward combo vaccines and changes in the type of vaccines, such as the expanded use of inactivated polio vaccine (IPV) instead of oral polio vaccine (OPV) and the probable eradication of some diseases within the country in the coming years, could significantly affect Iran's vaccine industry.

With the advent of new diseases and phenomena like bioterrorism, the capacity for vaccine production has become increasingly important. Some developed countries, such as the United Kingdom [7] and the United States [8] have invested in this sector to assure their ability to control such threats. The Iranian vaccine industry has illustrated its abilities to supply domestic need in crises; the main example of this is its performance during the imposed war with Iraq. As most key opinion leaders stated, they are not concerned about crises, however, the country must continually increase its capacity.

The introduction of model countries and the importance of international cooperation in the vaccine industry

There was general agreement among those interviewed regarding international cooperation for growth in this industry. Today, the importance of collaboration by vaccine makers in developing countries has become clear. The LG Company in Korea, which has obtained WHO prequalification, is establishing strategic cooperation in the field of R&D with large vaccine companies [9].

According to reports published by the local government, such cooperation by the Institute Pasteur for production of pentavalent vaccine and other biotechnology products with countries such as Cuba, India, Malaysia, and France has already been enacted [10], although most of the interviewees found these partnerships to be very limited, especially in the case of the Razi Institute.

The current situation of Iran's vaccine industry regarding technology, human resources, and R&D

According to the interviewees, there are lesser problems in access to technology for traditional and well-established vaccines; however, because of the current and upcoming changes in the methods of producing these vaccines, Iran's vaccine industry needs to be updated by acquiring new technologies for surviving international competition. In the field of newer vaccines, access to equipment and devices, especially access to technology, is influenced dramatically by political issues.

It seems that despite highly educated professionals in this industry, the human resources situation in Iran is far from ideal because of the lack of regular targeted training and the need for updated knowledge and information, which could be because of governmental structure and political problems and challenges.

The best source for R&D work on the diseases of developing countries is the countries where the diseases are endemic. The Commission on Health Research for Development in 1990 showed that only 10% of investment in health research is allocated to 90% of the diseases and health problems of the world. This is called the 10/90 gap. Children in developing countries do not benefit from advances in the field of vaccines in richer countries [11]. Iran could recognize the vaccine market in developing and less developed countries and manage research and development investments toward their needs to be able to use these opportunities in the future. By following the current approach in the management of R&D in Iran, the vaccine industry will not be able to participate in global markets or even cover domestic needs. According to an internal report by the Razi Institute [12], the rate of capital invested by the Razi Institute in R&D in the annual budget is only 2%; in light of the large areas of activity in this institute in the field of vaccines and serums (human and animal), this seems to be a very limited amount.

Public and private sector partnerships

The Ministry of Health is responsible for supplying the needed vaccines and planning the vaccination programs. In Iran, the government is involved in both producing and supplying vaccines. The Institute Pasteur is under supervision of the Ministry of Health and the Razi Institute operates under the Ministry of Agriculture. However, because of being regarded as a strategic industry for Iran in the area of national security, the possible privatization of these two vaccine makers is not imminent. As previously stated, it seems that the presence of the private sector along with the public sector would help the vaccine industry to overcome many problems, such as efficiently maintaining and strengthening human resources, managing and optimizing targeted areas of R&D capacities, and the provision on opportunities to establish a presence in international markets. Several factors impede the private sector from becoming involved in vaccine production. The only purchaser for the EPI vaccine is the government and because both vaccine manufacturers belong to the government, there is not an opportunity for the private sector to become involved in such a market. The government prefers to have complete authority in vaccine production and supply so that it can assure a consistent supply regardless of gain or loss (which is the main incentive for the private sector) at different times and in different situations.

Iran's ability to compete in international markets, the probable challenges to WTO accession, and suggested solutions

Most expert interviewees feel that the first step in moving toward international market status is obtaining WHO prequalification for the country's vaccines. Today, many countries are faced with several problems in supplying essential vaccines. Concerns in this regard increased after the implementation of IP rules and discussions related to world trade [13]. But some vaccine-related agencies, such as the United Nations Children's Fund (UNICEF) and the Pan American Health Organization (PAHO), and government–private cooperatives, like the Global Alliance for Vaccines and Immunization (the GAVI Alliance), are working to help these countries. GAVI, for example, aims to increase the economic attractiveness of the market by stimulating vaccine demand in developing countries, as well as strengthening infrastructure and ensuring their ability to procure such products [14]. UNICEF also purchases about 55% of the world's vaccines [15]. The World Health Organization grants prequalification to ensure that UN agencies buy quality, safe, and efficacious vaccines. According to internal news, Iran's National Regulatory Authority (NRA) recently gained WHO prequalification, but many problems concerning cGMP compliance still require resolution. Unfortunately, due to lack of sufficient investment, it is not possible to upgrade the facilities and equipment at the Razi Institute to comply with the principles of cGMP. However, most interviewees believed that it will be easier to obtain these standards by the Institute Pasteur's new facility (where the Hep B vaccine is manufactured).

The future of the vaccine industry after accession is very important because it is directly related to the country's public health. Therefore, it is necessary to understand the WTO rules affecting this industry. Three agreements— "Trade Related Aspects of Intellectual Property Rights (TRIPs)," "Subsidies and Compensatory Measures," and "Government Procurement Agreement (GPA)"—could be associated with this industry and must be carefully considered. Here, we review one of the most important agreements: TRIPS.TRIPs: Intellectual property right is considered as an asset by companies which could be seen as patents, distinctive signs, copyright, industrial designs and trade secrets [16]. In pharmaceuticals, patent rights cause a monopoly for patent holders by preventing others from using a particular invention for a specified period of time [17]. Nevertheless, to resolve the concerns of developing countries [18], the TRIPs agreement offers some flexibility for governments in providing their social goals. Transition periods, compulsory licenses, and parallel importation are from such flexibilities [19]. But in terms of being influenced by TRIPs, there are some differences between vaccines and other pharmaceutical products. The most important difference is the complexity of the processes used to manufacture biological products like vaccines. There are considerable scientific techniques and secrets (know-how) in the manufacturing processes of such products that companies prefer to maintain in-house as trade secrets and which will not be disclosed; therefore, compulsory licenses would not be all that useful [20]. Another issue is that it has become usual to patent one or more of the vaccine components, such as adjutants [21]. In a study conducted in 2005, the World Health Organization showed that most suppliers of vaccines in developing countries have not considered that IP plays an important role in vaccine R&D [22]. Iranian drug policy makers should also ensure efficacy, quality, and safety measures by full adherence to Iranian national drug policy rules [23]. These issues should be paid adequate attention before proceeding to WTO accession.

Conclusions

Both strengths and weaknesses were found in the Iranian vaccine industry, although the weaknesses outweigh the strong points. Considering the fact that it is a large market in relation to its young population and large area as well as its specific geographical location (associated with the war-torn countries without strong health systems and appropriate levels of health), Iran is experiencing an ever-increasing need to supply vaccines; the increasing need and market could be an opportunity for this industry, even on a domestic level. The long history and reputation of Iran's local vaccine industry could be considered advantages. However, this industry is faced with some weaknesses, such as non-compliance with cGMP, a lack of adequate and meaningful investment in R&D, a lack of mutual reliance of the government on the private sector in vaccine production, and the problems and political challenges that have hindered the development of this industry. According to most of the key opinion leaders, the most significant problem in Iran's vaccine industry has roots in its government ownership, which cannot be quickly solved.

Some useful solutions for improving the position of this industry in international competition include: a) privatization of current vaccine manufacturers (in the long-term) and relying on private vaccine producers to come into the field, b) improving international relations and cooperation with the large vaccine manufacturers in the world, c) utilizing small knowledge-oriented companies with the aim of fueling R&D, d) consistent education for employees, e) investment in order to modernize the old infrastructure of the Razi Institute regarding compliance with the principles of cGMP to achieve international quality standards to facilitate WHO prequalification. For the implementation of these strategies and to minimize the negative effects of implementing WTO agreements like GPA, TRIPs, and subsidies and compensatory measures, the role of negotiation teams in the accession process is extremely crucial. These teams should be familiar with the status of the vaccine industry. Achieving agreement among the industry's key opinion leaders about the future of this industry in the process of WTO accession can facilitate the negotiations. It is obvious, then, that recruiting professional experts in this field is necessary for this purpose.

Competing interest

The authors declare that they have no competing interests.

Author's contribution

AHM: literature review, designing the questionnaire and conducting interviews. AK: Designing the study method, selection of interviewees and monitoring the various stages of study. RD: Selection of interviewees, monitoring various stages of study. SN: Interpreting the results and final revision of the manuscript. MGH: providing advices in legal issues. IV: Participation in literature review and designing the questionnaire. All authors read and approved the final manuscript.

Acknowledgment

The authors would like to appreciate all experts and key opinion leaders of Iranian vaccine industry and ministry of Health who participated in this study and helped us by their invaluable information. This study was the outcome of Pharm.D thesis and supported by Tehran University of Medical Sciences.

Author details

[1]Department of Pharmacoeconomics and Pharmaceutical administration, Faculty of pharmacy, Tehran University of Medical Sciences, 16th Azar st, Keshavarz Blvd, Tehran, Iran. [2]Department of Pharmaceutics, Faculty of Pharmacy, Tehran University of Medical Sciences, 16th Azar st, Keshavarz Blvd, Tehran, Iran. [3]Food & Drug Laboratory Research Center, Food & Drug Organization, Ministry of Health & Medical Education, Tehran 1314715311, Iran. [4]The Department of Law, human science faculty of Tarbiat Modarres University, Kargar Street, Tehran, Iran.

References

1. Delbruck J: **Globalization of law, politics and Markets: Implication for Domestic law.** *IJGLS* 1993, **1**:9–36.
2. Understanding WTO: *Basic*. Geneva: World Trade Organization; Available from: http://www.wto.org/english/thewto_e/whatis_e/tif_e/fact1_e.htm (accessed: Sep 2009).
3. *Introduction to Razi vaccine and serum research institute*. Tehran: Razi vaccine and serum research institute; Available from: http://www.rvsri.ir/Portal/Home/Default.aspx?CategoryID=b3c873dc-b7b9-40c7-8480-e8751c8f524a (accessed: Sep 2009).
4. *The History of Iranian Pasteur institute*. Tehran: Iranian Pasteur institute; Available from: http://www.pasteur.ac.ir/History.htm (accessed: June 2009).
5. Karimi A, Alborzi A, Fahimzad A: **Prevalence of oropharyngeal colonization by Haemophilus influenza type b in Iranian children.** *East Mediterr Health J* 2009, **15**(3):544–548.
6. Nikfar S, Kebriaeezadeh A, Majdzadeh R, Abdollahi M: **Monitoring of National Drug Policy (NDP) and its standardized indicators; conformity to decisions of the national drug selecting committee in Iran.** *BMC Int Health Hum Rights* 2005, **5**(1):5.
7. Duggan JM, Brooks TJG: **A strategic vaccine facility for the UK.** *Vaccine* 2005, **23**:2090–2094.
8. Santoli JM, Peter G, Arvin AM, *et al*: **Strengthening the supply of routinely recommended vaccines in the United States: recommendations from the National Vaccine Advisory Committee.** *JAMA* 2003, **290**(23):3122–8.
9. Business insights: *The top 10 Biosimilar players, positioning, performance and SWOT analysis*. London: Business insights Ltd; 2009.
10. Iranian Ministry of Health and Medical Education: *The achievement in Health subjects*. secondth edition. Tehran: MOH pubic relation: the government's report; 2009.
11. Milstein JB, Kaddar M: **Managing the effect of TRIPS on availability of priority vaccines.** *Bull World Health Organ* 2006, **84**:360–365.
12. *Introduction to Razi vaccine & serum institute (the Development and Reinstruction Plan*. Tehran: Ministry of agriculture, Deputy of Research & Education; 2000.
13. Martin JF: **Vaccine in the developing world: looking for new solution.** *Vaccine* 1999, **17**:113–115.
14. WHO/EDM/PAR: *The world medicines situation*. Geneva: World Health Organization; 2004.
15. WHO, UNICEF, World Bank: *State of the world's vaccines and immunization*. 3rd edition. Geneva: World Health Organization; 2009.
16. *IP Rights*. Geneva: World Intellectual Property Organization; Available from: http://www.wipo.int/sme/en/ip_rights.html (accessed: March 2012).
17. World Health Organization: *Access to medicines and vaccines: implications of intellectual property protection and trade agreement*. Sri Lanka: Proceeding of 23rd Meeting of Health Ministers of Countries of SEAR Colombo; 2005.
18. Fergusson Ian F: *The WTO, Intellectual property right, and Access to medicines controversy*. Congressional Research Services: CRS Report for Congress; 2003.
19. WTO OMC Fact sheet: *Trips and pharmaceutical patents*. Geneva: World Trade Organization; 2006.
20. WTO agreement and public health: *a joint study by WHO and WTO secretariat*. Geneva: World Health Organization; 2004.
21. Berndt NR, Denoncourt NR, Warner AC: *US Markets for vaccines: Characteristics, Case studies and Controversies,: The EPI Press (American Enterprise Institute)*. D.C.: Washington; 2009:12–16.
22. Global Vaccine Supply: *the Changing Role of Suppliers*. Paris, France: Project summary of 16th GAVI Board meeting; 2005.
23. Abdollahiasl A, Nikfar S, Kebriaeezadeh A, Dinarvand R, Abdollahi M: **A model for developing a decision support system to simulate national drug policy indicators.** *Arch Med Sci* 2011, **7**(5):744–6.

17

Financial perspective of private pharmacies in Tehran (Iran); is it a lucrative business?

Khosro Keshavarz[1], Abbas Kebriaeezadeh[1*], Amir Hashemi Meshkini[1], Shekoufeh Nikfar[1,2], Iman Mirian[3] and Hasan Khoonsari[4]

Abstract

Background and purpose of the study: Pharmacies as direct providers of medicine and pharmaceutical services to patients have an important role in the health status of a society. The assessment of their financial situations by healthcare policy makers is necessary to prevent any negative effects on population's health. In this study we aim to analyze the financial status of pharmacies in Tehran, Iran.

Methods: This study is a cross-sectional study based on a survey. Two-hundred and eighty-eight private community daytime pharmacies in Tehran were selected by random sampling. We used two questionnaires to collect data regarding cost, expense and income factors of private pharmacies and the significance of each of them from these selected pharmacies. The data was collected in 2011 from Tehran pharmacies. Profitability of pharmacies in Tehran, Iran was calculated in its current situation and then estimated for three defined scenarios: 1. The dispensing fee is omitted (ceteris paribus), 2. Pharmacies are prohibited from selling hygienic & cosmetic products (ceteris paribus), 3. Scenarios 1 and 2 together (ceteris paribus). These data were analyzed by using SPSS and descriptive-analytic statistics.

Results: About 68% of interviewees responded to our questionnaires. Our analysis indicated that the average annual costs (and expenses), income and profits of pharmacies are 73,181; 106,301; and 33,120 United States Dollar (USD), respectively. The analysis indicated that omission of dispensing fee (scenario 1) and prohibition of pharmacies from selling hygienic & cosmetic products (scenario 2) would decrease income of pharmacies to 18438 and 14034 USD/year, respectively. According to respondents, the cost (or expense) of properties and buildings, energy, taxes, delays in reimbursement by insurance companies, and renting the place of pharmacy could be considered as cost factors and prescription medicines, OTC medicines, dispensing fees, hygienic & cosmetic products, and long-term payment to pharmaceutical distribution companies as income factors, which have significant effects on a pharmacy's economy.

Major conclusions: According to the results of this study, regarding the pharmacies' cost (and expenses) and incomes, the omission of dispensing fees for prescriptions has considerable negative effects on the profitability of pharmacies and likely on society's health.

Keywords: Pharmacy, Income, Cost and expense, Profitability, Dispensing fee, Iran

* Correspondence: Kebriaee@tums.ac.ir
[1]Department of Pharmacoeconomics and Pharmaceutical administration, Faculty of pharmacy, Tehran University of Medical Sciences, Tehran, Iran
Full list of author information is available at the end of the article

Introduction

Different countries use a variety of methods to organize their health systems. In these systems, the position of the pharmaceuticals is especially critical [1]. Pharmacies as direct providers of medicines and pharmaceutical services as well as potential centers for research in health services are one of the most important components of a health system [2]. Existence of private pharmacies in distribution network of medicines could provide good accessibility for medicines within the country [3,4]. Regarding to Iranian National Drug Policy (NDP) Private pharmacies belong to pharmacists who are allowed to establish their pharmacy under district regulation and legislation of Ministry of Health (MOH). They are responsible to provide medicines of National Drug List (NDL) for all patients and provide appropriated information according use of medicines [4]. Chain pharmacies and investment in multiple pharmacies are not allowed in Iran.

Nowadays, a wide range of services are provided by pharmacists, the results of which are an improvement in the overall health of a society. Studies have shown that the services provided by practical pharmacists create considerable improvement in health outcomes of society [5]. In addition, numerous studies show the role of pharmacists in diagnosing medical errors, medical interactions, and inappropriate prescribing [6-10]. Therefore, pharmacists have an important role in choosing the most appropriate, optimal and effective method of treatment [11].

In recent years, there has been controversy between policy makers and pharmacies regarding the omission of dispensing fees in Iran. Dispensing fee is a payment by patient to pharmacist after receiving prescription medicines to compensate pharmacy services including consultation, education on medicine usage and etc. The opposing sides have two different approaches. To solve the high amount of out-of-pocket payments by patients in Iran, some policymakers' approach is to omit the dispensing fee, given that it is not covered by most insurance companies. This approach is supported by some views in society regarding the extraordinary profit of pharmacies. In the second approach, pharmacists believe that the present situation of implemented policies in pricing areas, public pharmacy monopolies, internal inflation, etc. have caused many hardships, and the omission of the dispensing fee would lead to bankruptcy. Dispensing fee in Iran has two level: for prescriptions that their price are more than 0.8 USD it is about 0.75 USD and for prescription price under 0.8 USD it is 0.4 USD.

Currently in Iran, community pharmacies are divided into two types: public and private. According to the latest statistics from the Iranian Food and Drug Organization (2011), there are about 8,400 active pharmacies in Iran. Of these, 88% are privately owned and the rest are affiliated with public organizations or institutions. Although there are very few public pharmacies in Iran, they still have a large market share for many reasons, such as a monopoly in providing scarce and expensive medicines [12]. The pharmaceutical market has been extended by growth in GDP and health budgets but this extension had a small effect on health indicators [13]. Paying attention to the incentives for health service providers including pharmacies could improve health indicators.

Regarding the important role of pharmacies and their potential effects on the health of society, especially in low- and middle-income countries [14-17], all financial and non-financial incentives and disincentives regarding their role have to be monitored, and before any decisions are made the impacts of that policy on pharmacies' business has to be exactly analyzed.

In this study, we aim to analyze the financial situation and factors that affect the financial flow of private pharmacies and also attitudes of pharmacy owners regarding these factors to render a more clear understanding of the business aspects of pharmacies for policy makers.

Method

This research is a cross-sectional study based on a survey, which was conducted in 2011 in two steps. In the first step, we tried to calculate the average profitability of private community pharmacies in Tehran based on data collected through questionnaires filled out by pharmacy owners. In this step, the profitability of a pharmacy was recalculated in three predefined scenarios to predict the situation of pharmacies after implementing such policies.

1. The dispensing fee is omitted (*ceteris paribus*)
2. Pharmacies are prohibited from selling hygienic & cosmetic products (*ceteris paribus*), [approximately all pharmacies in Iran provide hygienic & cosmetic products].
3. Scenarios 1 and 2 together (*ceteris paribus*)

In the second step, we aimed to achieve a general knowledge about the attitude of respondents toward the factors affecting the cost, expense and income components of pharmacies. The results of this step and the previous step were combined to suggest solutions for the current problems that face pharmacies and patients.

Data collection measures

To evaluate the cost (and expense) and income information of pharmacies, the factors that affect the costs, expenses and income, and the importance of each factor from the pharmacy owners' point of view, two questionnaires were designed after a comprehensive literature review. The first was an open-ended and self-administered questionnaire in order to collect data from the pharmacy owners about costs, expenses and incomes of pharmacies. The second was a Likert-scaled questionnaire to collect information about the attitude of pharmacy managers toward the factors that affect the financial flow of a pharmacy. In both steps the data collection was designed to be through direct interviews. The validity and reliability of each questionnaire were checked by combination of expert opinion, pilot data collection from 10 pharmacies based on likert scale, and test-retest methods (r=0.83).

The respondents were free to refuse to answer these questionnaires, and they were assured before the interview that their identity would remain private.

Sampling

Our population of interest included all of the private community pharmacies in Tehran (capital of Iran). According to Iranian Pharmacists' Association statistics (2011), there are 1,176 private pharmacies in Tehran, including 1,115 daytime pharmacies and 61 pharmacies open 24/7. As a sample, 228 pharmacies were selected by a random sampling method. Daytime pharmacies were only included in our study. For random selection we used random number table after assigning to all daytime pharmacies a number.

The respondents to the questionnaires were the pharmacy managers, whether they were pharmacists or not.

Analysis

The analysis was conducted based on a typical daytime pharmacy, which was extracted from questionnaires. We used nonparametric techniques, including chi-square test by SPSS 18 software to analyze the data of study. To exchange IR Rial to US Dollar the official exchange rate declared by central bank (12260 IR Rials) was used.

The method of study was reviewed and approved by Institutional Review Board (IRB) of Tehran University of Medical Sciences (code of project: 900410216512).

Results

About 68% of interviewees responded to our questionnaires. The results of our analysis is presented below.

Part 1: Profitability of pharmacies

In Table 1, the general information regarding the number of pharmacies, margins and other needed data are collected. Knowing these data help Tables 2 and 3 to be better understood.

Table 1 General information about Iran pharmaceutical market[12]

Total number of pharmacies	8393[a]
profit margin of selling domestic drugs (2011)	20%
profit margin of selling imported drugs (2011)	10-15%
The average profit gained from distribution companies discount	3%
percentage of expired drugs in pharmacies	1%

In Table 2, all the detailed information about the cost (and expense) components of pharmacies are presented. It shows that an average cost and expense of a daytime pharmacy is 73,181 USD/year. Of this, 52% of expenses relate to manpower, 26.8% relate to renting the pharmacy building, and the remainder (21.2%) relate to other expenses.

In Table 3, all income components of a typical pharmacy are presented. The table shows that an average annual income of a pharmacy equals 106,301 USD. This income relates to prescription medicines (26.1%), over-the-counter (OTC) drugs (17.5%), hygienic & cosmetic products and orthopedics (18%), and dispensing fees (13.8%). The results of Tables 2 and 3 show that the average profit of a pharmacy equals 33,120 USD annually and 2,760 USD monthly. This monthly amount varies from 1631.3 (Min) to 4894 (Max).

Scenario 1. The dispensing fee is omitted (ceteris paribus)

The results of the tables show that if the dispensing fee is omitted, the average pharmacy income would be decreased to 91,619 USD/year. If we deduct the costs and expenses of pharmacy from this amount, the net income of a pharmacy equals 18,438 USD in a year and 1,536.5 USD in a month (44% reduction).

Scenario 2. Pharmacies are prohibited from selling hygienic & cosmetic products (ceteris paribus)

If the dispensing fee exists but the sale of hygienic & cosmetic products is omitted, the pharmacy income would be decreased to 87,215 USD/year. If we deduct costs and expenses of pharmacy from this amount, the net income of a pharmacy equals 14,034 USD per year and 1,169.5 USD per month (58% reduction).

Scenario 3. Scenarios 1 and 2 together (ceteris paribus)

If both the dispensing fees and hygienic & cosmetic products are omitted and only the income of medicine sales is calculated, then the pharmacy would generate an income of 72533 USD, resulting in a net income of 648 USD and 54 USD lost annually and monthly, respectively (98% reduction).

Table 2 The cost and expense components of pharmacies in 2011

Cost and Expense items		Amount (USD)	Min & Max (USD)	Details (according to questionnaire information and experts attitude
Fixed	The average of depreciation expense of properties[b]	1697	(821 and 2049)	The average, Min and Max properties price is obtained from questionnaire information and market price
Variable	The average manpower expense	38203	(31593 and 44814)	The average is based on four personnel: pharmacist, pharmacy technician, cashier, hygienic salesman. Max: 5 and Min: 3 personnel are included
	The average expense of renting pharmacy location	19576	(9788 and 48940)	The average of monthly renting expense is 1631 USD (Max: 4078 USD and Min: 816 USD)
	The average expense of consumed energy (electricity, gas, water, telephone)	1958	(1468 and 2936)	The average of monthly consumed energy expense is 163 USD (Max: 245 USD and Min: 122 USD)
	The average expense of consumables	1468	(979 and 1958)	The averageexpense of monthly consumablesis 122 USD/year (Max: 163 and Min: 82 USD/year)
	Annual tax expense	2447	(1631 and 3263)	The average expense of yearly tax is 2447 USD/year (Max: 3263 USD/year and Min: 1631 USD/year)
	The average of imposed expenses and costs during activities (insurance deductions, drug expiration, drug waste)	1958	(979 and 2936)	The average expense of monthly imposed is 163 USD/year (Max: 245 USD/year and Min: 82 USD/year)
	The average expenses of delays in insurance companies reimbursements	3467	(2600 and 4333)	It is calculated based on %17 bank profits. The average delay is considered as 4 months (Max: 5 months and Min: 3 months)
	The average expense of entering prescription data on computer	1918	(343 and 3837)	To register each prescription .07 USD/year and 24.5 days in a month is calculated. The average 100 prescriptions in a day are included (Max 200 and Min 70 prescriptions
	The average of other expenses (advertisement, repair and maintenance, internet, personnel food, software updates, transportation)	489	(294 and 979)	the average is 408 USD/year (Max: 979 USD/year and Min 82 USD/year)
	The average total expense of a pharmacy (2011)	**73181**		

Part 2: The factors affecting the cost, expense and income components of pharmacy business

In this part, the results of responders' attitude toward the significance of effective factors on a pharmacy's economic improvement are shown.

1. Factors affecting pharmacy costs: To answer this question, two fixed factors and nine variable factors were defined. In Table 4, the results of the statistical analysis are presented to answer this question.
   As Table 4 shows, according to respondents' views, the most significant factors affecting a pharmacy's costs and expenses are the properties and building (as fixed costs); the manpower, consumed energy, tax, and delays in reimbursement by insurance companies to pharmacies (most of insurance organization reimburse pharmacies after several months from providing medicines to patient); and renting the pharmacy location. However, the consumed materials, insurance deductions, drug expiration, and entering prescription data into a computer program (some pharmacies doesn't have in-time prescription data entering in system and have to pay for that) do not have a significant effect on pharmacy costs and expenses.
2. Factors affecting pharmacies' income: To answer this question, seven factors are defined. In Table 5, statistical analysis results are presented to answer this question.
   As the results in Table 5 show, according to responders' views, the income earned from the sale of prescription medicines, OTC medicines, dispensing fees, hygienic & cosmetic products and long-term payment of purchasing from distribution

Table 3 The income components of pharmacies in 2011

Income items	Amount (USD/year)	Max & Min (USD/year)	Details (according to questionnaire information and experts attitude)
The average net income gained from selling prescription medicines	27732	(11093 and 55465)	The net income is calculated based on averagely 17% margin
The average net income gained from selling OTC drugs	18597	(14682 and 36705)	The net income is calculated based on averagely 19% margin
The average net income gained from selling hygienic & cosmetic products	19086	(14682 and 36705)	The net income is calculated based on averagely 18% averagely margin
The average net income gained from dispensing fees	14682	(12235 and 23246)	It is calculated based on averagely 49 USD/year
The average net income gained from discounts and distribution companies prizes	13051	(979 and 19576)	It is calculated based on 5% discounts
The average net income gained from purchases with long-term payments	5200	(1733 and 8666)	It is calculated based on average reimbursement of 3 months (Max: 5months and Min: 1 month). Also bank profit in 2011 supposed to be 17%
The average net income gained from increase of drug prices	7953	(3670 and 12235)	It is calculated based on the average stock of 122349 USD/year and 3%-10% increase in prices
The average total income of a pharmacy (2011)	**106301**		

companies have a significant effect on pharmacies' income ($p < 0.01$), but other factors, such as the income gained from pharmaceutical company discounts and increases in drug prices, do not have significant effects on pharmacies' income ($p > 0.05$).

3. Solutions to improve pharmacies' economy: To answer this question, nine factors were defined. In Table 6, the statistical analysis results are presented to answer this question.
   As Table 6 shows, according to responders' views, tax exemption, selling of hygienic & cosmetic products, scarce and exclusive medicine (in Iran some medicines like opioids, and very expensive anti cancers and etc. are only available in public pharmacies), medicine margin, insurance coverage of medicines, quick insurance reimbursement, dispensing fees, and financial support ($p < 0.01$) are the most effective methods of pharmacies' financial improvement. However, the increase in share of insurance from drug costs is not effective on pharmacies' financial improvement ($p > 0.05$), from the pharmacy owners' points of view.

Discussion

According to the results, our study showed that the average profit of a typical pharmacy in Tehran is 2,760

Table 4 the results of statistical analysis (the attitude of pharmacists about the factors relating the expenses of pharmacy)

Variables		Responders attitude					Degree of freedom (df)	chi square (X^2)	Significance
		Strongly agree	agree	neutral	disagree	Strongly disagree			
Fixed	properties	63	164	38	12	11	4	277.521	0
	building	113	130	23	14	8	4	240.785	0
Variable	manpower	156	85	24	14	9	4	274.743	0
	consumables	45	66	62	55	60	4	4.535	0.338
	consumed energy	61	78	61	41	47	4	14.361	0.006
	renting location	65	74	62	41	46	4	13.076	0.011
	tax	38	93	60	49	48	4	31.41	0
	insurance deductions	50	71	62	50	55	4	5.576	0.233
	drug expiration	47	75	62	49	55	4	8.944	0.063
	delay in reimbursement	70	83	58	42	35	4	26.965	0
	description registration	44	60	72	60	52	4	7.556	0.109

Table 5 the results of statistical analysis (attitude of pharmacists about the factors relating the income of pharmacies)

Variables	Responders attitude					Degree of freedom (df)	chi square (X^2)	Significance (sig)
	Strongly agree	agree	neutral	disagree	Strongly disagree			
Description	173	70	22	13	10	4	329.743	0
OTC	82	162	28	9	7	4	33.229	0
dispensing fee	171	85	19	7	6	4	352.833	0
cosmetic hygienic products	103	142	21	14	8	4	258.424	0
company discounts	40	56	72	62	58	4	9.361	0.053
increase in drug prices	44	65	67	53	59	4	6.097	0.192
A	78	162	32	9	7	4	293.285	0

USD per month. Also, our analysis in the second part showed that some factors—including tax exemptions, sale of hygienic & cosmetic products, coverage of medicines by insurance companies, quick insurance reimbursement, dispensing fees, and appropriate financial incentives—have a greater effect on offering pharmaceutical services and also pharmacy income.

This is the first comprehensive study about business-related issues of pharmacies in Iran, which encompasses most of the expense (and cost) and income components of pharmacies as well as the effective factors on the profitability of pharmacies from pharmacists' and pharmacy owners' points of view. Similar studies from other countries were also not found.

Our research seems to be consistent with Pourheidari's study (2010) in which the pharmacy income was only slightly more than its costs and expenses [18]. This result is also in conflict with some policymakers' views about the extraordinary profitability of pharmacies. It also should be mentioned that to establish a pharmacy and enter the market, a large amount of investment is needed in advance (an average investment to establish a pharmacy in Tehran is estimated to be 264698 USD). In this study, however, only the active pharmacies were taken into account in order to calculate their fixed and variable costs and expenses, so we neglected establishment costs. On the other hand, regarding the social responsibility and important role of pharmacies, the difference between cost and income does not seem to be appropriate because this calculated profit encompasses some nonprofessional service provision, including sale of hygienic & cosmetic products. If pharmacies were prohibited from providing such services, their profitability would likely decrease, as the scenarios showed. From this aspect, our study is similar to a study by Mohammadzade (2010), indicated that pharmacies are not profitable but even disadvantageous if they only provide medicines [19].

The evidence showed that pharmacy margins have an important role in whether or not pharmacists convince patients to use brand or generic medicines [20]. Therefore, it must be mentioned by policymakers that decreasing pharmacies' profitability by cost containment or any other strategy may lead the pharmacies to compensate their profit through other ways, either legal or illegal, including selling non-OTC medicines without prescription,

Table 6 the results of statistical analysis (the ways to improve business of pharmacy)

Variables	Responders attitude					Degree of freedom (df)	chi square (X^2)	Significance (sig)
	Strongly agree	agree	neutral	disagree	Strongly disagree			
tax exemption	82	169	21	9	7	4	334.5	0
exclusive selling of some cosmetic-hygienic products	64	169	30	13	12	4	33.021	0
elimination of monopolies regarding providing medicines	93	156	21	11	7	4	295.264	0
drug margin increase	88	161	23	9	7	4	307.903	0
coverage of drug items	64	162	37	13	12	4	267.938	0
increasing the share of insurance companies	40	56	72	62	58	4	9.361	.053
quick insurance reimbursements	80	164	27	12	5	4	305.646	0
dispensing fee	68	165	32	13	10	4	287.382	0
loans	93	149	28	10	8	4	264.049	0

imposing unnecessary costs to patients, etc., that can offset those policies and sometimes threaten the society's health. A study regarding European Union (EU) countries' pharmaceutical policies after the economic crisis indicated that pharmacies, as one of the important stakeholders in the healthcare system, were taken into consideration in designing such cost-controlling policies [21]. We must note that our results were concluded regardless of the appropriateness or weaknesses of the current implemented policies, including dispensing fees, and they must be evaluated in term of equity, efficiency, patient satisfaction, and other issues in further studies.

Another point is about the effect of insurance coverage level on pharmacies' business. However, the coverage of medicines by insurance, probably because of its effect of increasing demand, was considered as an effective factor on profitability of pharmacies from the pharmacy owners' point of view, but the increase in share of insurance from pharmaceutical costs was not identified by them as a significantly effective factor. This could be justified by reasons including the irrational delays by insurance in reimbursement to pharmacies. The studies also showed that the profitability of prescription medicines has decreased [22]; a primary reason could be the increasing contribution of insurance on prescription price [11, 22].

Limitations

In this study we were faced with limited access to data, given that most pharmacists and pharmacy owners were reluctant to disclose their business-related data. The expense (and cost) and income data were collected in a self-reported way, and the validity of their claims could not be evaluated.

Conclusion

It can be concluded that there is a gap in the current financial situation of pharmacies in Tehran of optimal status in terms of profitability. This situation would be worse, however, if the considered scenarios (omission of dispensing fees and sales of hygienic & cosmetic products) are implemented.

Endnotes

[a] According to Food and Drug Organization about 95% of them have private ownership and only 5% are public

[b] The Straight-line depreciation method was used to compute depreciation of assets in pharmacies

Competing interests

One of the authors, H. Khoonsari is a pharmacist and pharmacy owner.

Authors' contributions

AK: designing the research method, final approval of results. KK: data collection, analyzing collected data, contribution in designing research method. AHM: data collection, analyzing collected data, revising the manuscript. SN: designing the research method. IM: analyzing the collected data, drafting the manuscript. HK: data collection, contribution in designing research method. All authors read and approved the final manuscript.

Acknowledgment

The authors would like to thank Knowledge Utilization Research Center, Tehran University of Medical Sciences (KURC) for supporting this study and also Hadi Gholami (Pharm D), Gholamreza Keshavarz for their kindly cooperation in this study.

Author details

[1]Department of Pharmacoeconomics and Pharmaceutical administration, Faculty of pharmacy, Tehran University of Medical Sciences, Tehran, Iran. [2]Food & Drug Laboratory Research Center, Food & Drug Organization, Ministry of Health & Medical Education, Tehran, Iran. [3]Department of Public Health, Faculty of Public Health, Hormozqan University of Medical Sciences, Bandar abbas, Iran. [4]Department of Clinical Pharmacy, Faculty of Pharmacy, Tehran University of Medical Sciences, Tehran, Iran.

References

1. Moen E, Toverud EL, Grund J, Brinchmann S: **Pricing and reimbursement of pharmaceuticals. A new culture for the community pharmacist.** *Pharm World Sci* 1998, **20**(3):107–12.
2. Sabzghabaee AM, Etebari M, Sajadi H, Badri S, Hosseini-Biuki SM, Sheikhabumasudi R: **Financial performance of the teaching pharmacies in Isfahan: an economic evaluation.** *Res pharm sci* 2009, **4**(2):99–104.
3. Cheraghali AM, Nikfar S, Behmanesh Y, Rahimi V, Habibipour F, Tirdad R, Asadi A, Bahrami A: **Evaluation of availability, accessibility and prescribing pattern of medicines in the Islamic Republic of Iran.** *East Mediterr Health J* 2004, **10**(3):406–15.
4. Nikfar S, Kebriaeezadeh A, Majdzadeh R, Abdollahi M: **Monitoring of national drug policy (NDP) and its standardized indicators; conformity to decisions of the national drug selecting committee in Iran.** *BMC Int Health Hum Rights* 2005, **5**:5.
5. Bero LA, Mays NB, Barjesteh K, Bond C: **Expanding the roles of outpatient pharmacists; effects on health services utilization, costs, and patient outcomes.** *Cochrane Database Syst Rev* 2000, (2):CD000336.
6. Zhan C, Sangl J, Bierman AS, *et al*: **Potentially inappropriate medication use in the community-dwelling elderly.** *JAMA* 2001, **286**(22):2823–9.
7. Aparasu RR, Mort JR: **Inappropriate prescribing for the elderly: Beers criteria-based review.** *Ann Pharmacother* 2000, **34**(3):338–46.
8. The US: **Pharmacopoeia drug utilization review advisory panel. Drug utilization review. mechanisms to improve its effectiveness and broaden its scope.** *J Am Pharm Assoc* 2000, **40**(4):538–45.
9. Erah PO: **The changing roles of pharmacists in hospital and community pharmacy practice in Nigeria.** *Trop J Pharm Res* 2003, **2**(2):195–196.
10. Barber N, Smith F, Anderson S: **Improving quality of health care: the role of pharmacists.** *Qual Health Care* 1994, **3**(3):153–158.
11. Carroll NV, Miederhoff PA, Water LW: **Profitability, third-party reimbursement, and access to community pharmacies.** *Clin Ther* 1996, **18**(4):703–15.
12. Ministry of health, Food and drug organization, the affair of pharmacies:, Tehran, Iran; 2012.
13. Abdollahiasl A, Nikfar S, Abdollahi M: **Pharmaceutical market and health system in the Middle Eastern and Central Asian countries: Time for innovations and changes in policies and actions.** *Arch Med Sci* 2011, **7**(3):365–7.
14. World Health Organization: *The role of the pharmacist in the health care system*. Geneva: WHO; 1994. http://whqlibdoc.who.int/hq/1994/WHO_PHARM_94.569.pdf. Accessed 25 Feb 2009.
15. World Health Organization: *Good Pharmacy Practice; Guidelines in community and hospital settings*. Geneva: WHO; 1996. http://whqlibdoc.who.int/hq/1996/WHO_PHARM_DAP_96.1.pdf. Accessed 25 Feb 2009.
16. International Pharmaceutical Federation. Standards for quality of pharmacy services:; 1993. Available at http://www.fip.ul/www/uploads/?page=statements. Accessed 25 Feb 2009.

17. World Health Organization: *The role of the pharmacist in selfcare and self-medication*. Geneva: WHO; 1998. http://whqlibdoc.who.int/hq/1998/WHO_DAP_98.13.pdf. Accessed 25 Feb 2009.
18. Pourheidari H: *The overview of Iranian pharmacies' economy in 2010*. Tehran: Iranian pharmacist association magazine. No 20; 2010.
19. Mohammadzadeh M: *The study of profitability of drugstores in Iran's pharmaceutical system*. (Isfahan, Iran): IJPS; 2010:209–216.
20. Brekke KR, Holmas TH, Straume OR: *Margins and market shares: pharmacy incentives for generic substitution*. Braga, Portugal: NIPE Working Papers; 2010.
21. Vogler S, Zimmermann N, Leopold C, Joncheere KD: **Pharmaceutical policies in European countries in response to the global financial crisis.** *Southern Med Rev* 2011, **4**(2):22–32.
22. Hargis JR: **Lilly Digest 1992**. In *Survey of 1991 operational Data*. 60th edition. Indianapolis, Ind: Eli lilly and company; 1992.

18

Assessing the effectiveness and cost-effectiveness of audit and feedback on physician's prescribing indicators: study protocol of a randomized controlled trial with economic evaluation

Fatemeh Soleymani[1,2], Arash Rashidian[1,3,4,8*], Rassoul Dinarvand[1,5], Abbas Kebriaeezade[1,6], Mostafa Hosseini[7] and Mohammad Abdollahi[1,6]

Abstract

Background: Physician prescribing is the most frequent medical intervention with a highest impact on healthcare costs and outcomes. Therefore improving and promoting rational drug use is a great interest. We aimed to assess the effectiveness and cost-effectiveness of two forms of conducting prescribing audit and feedback interventions and a printed educational material intervention in improving physician prescribing.

Method/design: A four-arm randomized trial with economic evaluation will be conducted in Tehran. Three interventions (routine feedback, revised feedback, and printed educational material) and a no intervention control arm will be compared. Physicians working in outpatient practices are randomly allocated to one of the four arms using stratified randomized sampling. The interventions are developed based on a review of literature, physician interviews, current experiences in Iran and with theoretical insights from the Theory of Planned Behavior. Effects of the interventions on improving antibiotics and corticosteroids prescribing will be assessed in regression analyses. Cost data will be assessed from a health care provider's perspective and incremental cost-effectiveness ratios will be calculated.

Discussion: This study will determine the effectiveness and cost-effectiveness of three interventions and allow us to determine the most effective interventions in improving prescribing pattern. If the interventions are cost-effective, they will likely be applied nationwide.

Trial registration: Iranian Registry of Clinical Trials Registration Number: IRCT201106086740N1Pharmaceutical Sciences Research Center of TUMS Ethics Committee Registration Number: 90-02-27-07

Keywords: Intervention study, Rational drug use, Audit and feedback, Printed educational material, Iran

Background

Over the past decades, new generations of antibiotics, analgesics, corticosteroids and other medicines have been introduced to the pharmaceuticals market. At the same time, health care systems are confronted with a continuing pressure to provide high-quality care in the face of increasing costs and limited financial resources.

Due to the rising pharmaceutical expenditures in the world, governments are struggling to keep costs under control [1-3]. There are valid concerns about the rationality of use of medicines, mostly as a result of inappropriate physician prescribing. Physicians' prescribing is the most common medical intervention with a high impact on health care costs [4]. Improving and promoting rational use of medicines contributes to a more efficient use of meager health care resources, as well as ensuring better population health outcomes.

* Correspondence: arashidian@tums.ac.ir
[1]Department of Pharmacoeconomics and Pharmaceutical Management, Faculty of Pharmacy, Tehran University of Medical Sciences (TUMS), Tehran, Iran
[3]Department of Health Management and Economic, School of Public Health, TUMS, Tehran, Iran
Full list of author information is available at the end of the article

Changing prescriber behavior is difficult and may require complex multilayered interventions [5]. Such interventions may include using audit and feedbacks, dissemination of printed educational materials, educational outreach visits, reminders, and opinion leaders among others [6,7]. Implementing the multilayered intervention is more costly and resource intensive. Hence, it is important to identify easy to implement an effective intervention to improve physicians' prescribing. Several studies have been conducted to develop interventions and strategies to improve prescribing [8-13] but most of them have been carried out in high-income countries, sometimes with conflicting results [14]. Only limited high quality studies exist from low and middle-income countries.

According to a Cochrane Review, audit and feedback is defined as a summary of health care performance over a specified period of time with or without recommendations for a clinical action [15]. Evidence from 118 randomized controlled trials indicated that audit and feedback resulted in a modest improvement in care [15]. Grimshaw and colleagues [16] undertook a comprehensive review of the effects of using different strategies for implementing guidelines. They found that audit and feedback alone or combined with educational meetings and materials result in a modest improvement in the implementation of guidelines in comparison to no intervention group. Furthermore the studies on assessing the effectiveness of printed educational materials indicated only a small impact on practice, but there was no reliable assessment of the cost effectiveness of such programs. As the small benefits from dissemination of printed educational materials are achieved at relatively low costs, they may still be worthwhile interventions [17,18].

In Iran for many years, the problems of irrational drug use have been investigated by academic members of several universities [19-24]. In 1996, the National Committee of Rational Use of Drug (NCRUD) was established and a formal process of assessing physician prescribing started in the country. To make this possible, different data sources were developed that included a central data warehouse as well as access to insurance organization prescription datasets. Also different interventions including audit and feedbacks, dissemination of printed educational materials, public education and workshops and conferences were employed. Although these national plans were not subjected to formal evaluations, descriptive assessments suggest that they may have resulted in improving prescribing behavior, including a descending trend in the mean medicine items per prescription as an important indicator for rational drug use [25,26]. So far, no systematic and scientific evaluation has been conducted to determine the effectiveness and cost effectiveness of audit and feedback interventions in Iran. This trial is designed to test three different interventions for improving rational drug use indicators of general physicians, pediatricians and infectious disease specialists.

The main objectives of the study are:

1) Does the routinely conducted prescribing audit and feedback intervention influence general physicians, pediatricians and infectious disease specialists prescribing behavior in comparison to printed educational materials and no intervention?
2) Does a revised audit and feedback intervention improve prescribing behavior compared to the routinely conducted prescribing audit and feedback, printed educational materials and no intervention? At the same time, we evaluated cost-effectiveness of the interventions compared to the control groups.

Methods

Study design

The study design is a four- armed randomized controlled trial with economic evaluation. It includes three different intervention arms and one control arm: routinely conducted audit and feedback, revised audit and feedback, printed educational materials (pamphlets), and a no intervention control group (see Trial Flow in Figure 1).

Population and setting

The target population included general physicians, pediatricians and infectious disease specialists who have an outpatient practice in Tehran, and have a current contract with at least one of the two main social health insurance organizations.

Details of the interventions

Routinely conducted audit and feedback involves a three-page summary of prescriptions indicators based on the analysis of insured prescriptions. The summary reports the prescribing indicators for each physician in comparison with their peer groups in the same area in a given time period (annual and quarterly). The first page is cover letter signed by the Secretary of the RUD committee in the region, consisting of general points about the common problems especially in the area which they practice. The second page includes physician's profile such as name, specialty, medical council number, office address, the evaluation period and the insurance organization that have provided prescription data. Then, the prescription amount of main indicators will be listed in comparative tables that include the following:

1. Average medicine items per prescription

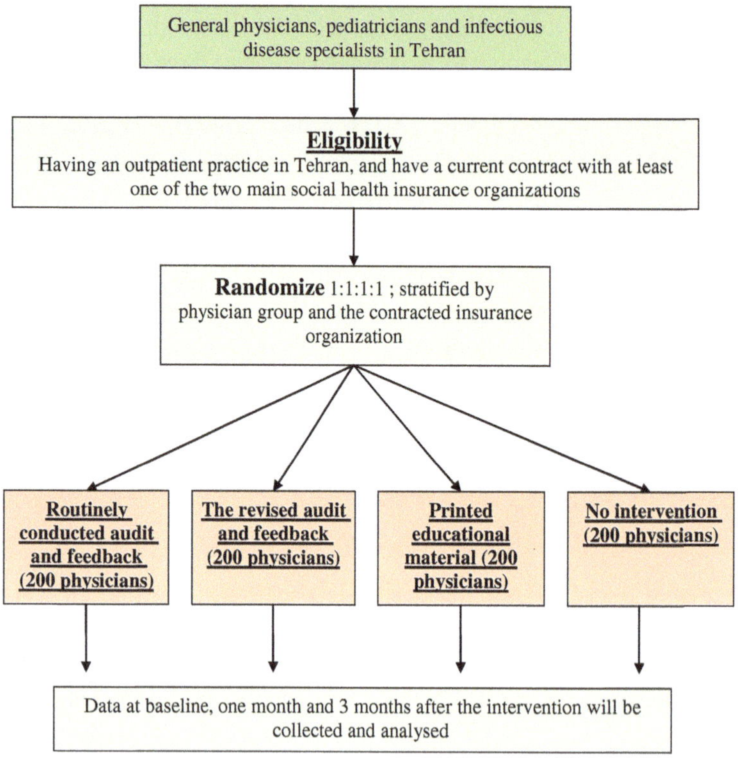

Figure 1 Trial flow proposed physicians enrollment and randomization procedures.

2. Average price per prescription (IR Rials)
3. Proportion of prescriptions including one medicine item (%)
4. Proportion of prescriptions including four or more medicine items (%)
5. Maximum medicine items in a prescription
6. Proportion of injectable medicine items per all prescribed items (%)
7. Proportion of prescriptions that includes at least one injectable medicine item (%)

Consequently, the prescription indicators for important drug groups such as antibiotics, corticosteroids and NSAIDs will be reported. These groups will be chosen based upon common prescribing problems in any given area. Moreover, the list of 10 most-prescribed drugs and 10 first most expensive drugs are reported in separate tables. Finally, 10 important drug interactions with high severity and intensity in the physician's prescriptions are reported [27].

The revised audit and feedback has been developed for this trial based on current drug use problems in Iran. We developed our intervention based on four inputs: the current audit and feedback, a literature review, interviews with physicians, and the theoretical justifications acquired from the Theory of Planned Behavior (TPB).

We conducted a literature review to obtain feedback' samples from other countries [28] and identifying current and important drug prescribing problems in our country [25,26]. Face-to-face interviews were conducted with16 physicians.

The TPB [29] is a social cognition theory to provide a theoretical basis for explaining volitional behavior. The theory has important merits in explaining and understanding physician behavior, including prescribing [30-33]. The TPB suggests that individuals' intention to perform behaviors is determined by their attitudes, perceived social or peer pressures (subjective norms) and perceived behavioral control [Figure 2].

The revised feedback form consisted of three pages. The form uses traffic light colors for reporting the prescribing indicators by physicians. Based on the findings from interviews, the revised feedback form was designed to look less crowded than the routinely conducted feedback and to ensure physicians' attention was attracted towards important messages in the feedback. The indicators were also selected more objectively. The first page expresses the purpose of providing feedback and interpreting the colors used in the report and the importance of improving the situation of irrational prescribing signed by secretary of the committee. If dexamethasone and ceftriaxone injectable forms and an oral form of cefixime are at the beginning of the list of 10 most prescribed drugs, notice will be given. The revised feedback includes the following indicators on the first page:

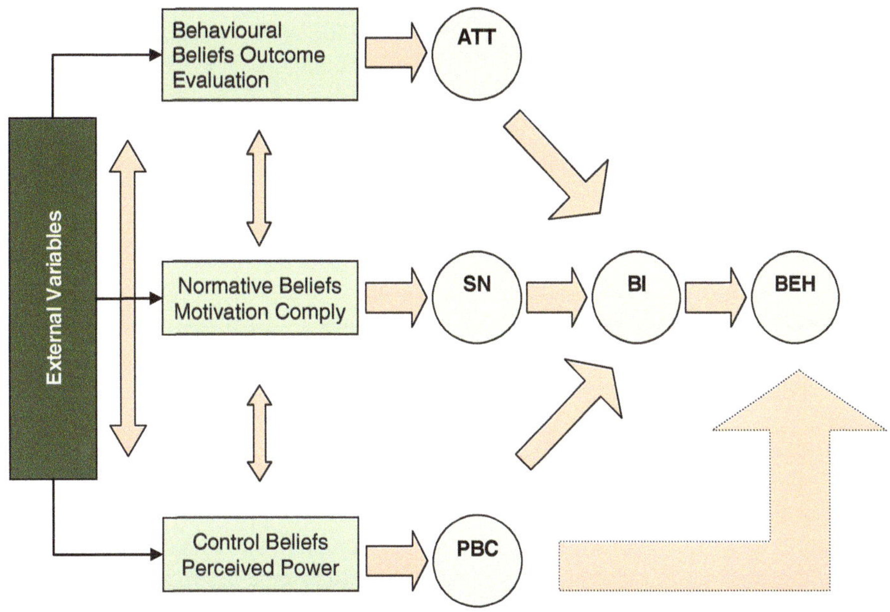

Figure 2 Theory of Planned Behavior [6].

1. Average medicine items per prescription
2. Average price per prescription (IR Rials)
3. Proportion of prescriptions including four or more medicine items (%)
4. Proportion of prescriptions that includes at least one injectable medicine item (%)
5. Proportion of prescriptions that includes at least one antibiotic medicine item (%)
6. Proportion of prescriptions that includes at least one corticosteroid medicine item (%)

In the second page, table of the most prescribed antibiotics in the country as prescribed by each physician are reported. Then, a graph reports all antibiotics prescribed by a physician and his/her peer group according to differentiate seasons. At the bottom of the second page, two important practice points related to prescribing antibiotics are presented.

Table of prescription amount of most prescribed systemic corticosteroids in the country as prescribed by the physician are presented on the third page. Then, a graph reports all injectable forms of medicines prescribed by the physician and compares it with his/her peer group. At the bottom of the third page, two important practice points related to prescription of injectable forms of medicines and corticosteroids are presented.

Printed educational material (pamphlet)

The educational material was also developed using literature review, interviews with physicians, with theoretical attentions based on the TPB. Most physicians participating in the interviews emphasized on the usefulness of a concise pamphlet with a practical training content. Hence, a 4-page A5 size pamphlet was designed. The pamphlet provides practical tips on prescribing antibiotics, corticosteroids and injectable dosage forms and the current status of utilization of these medicines in the country. It also documents examples of serious adverse effects reported from inappropriate usage of ceftriaxone injections and serious complications after dexamethasone injections.

Study setting and participants

The study is conducted in Tehran. All general physicians, pediatricians and infectious disease specialists who have an outpatient practice in Tehran, issue a minimum of 100 prescriptions per month, and have a current contract with at least one of the two main social health insurance organizations are eligible for inclusion in the study.

Sample size calculation and allocation to the intervention arms

Considering that about 14% of outpatient prescriptions in Tehran contain dexamethasone injections and expecting that the intervention may reduce such prescriptions by 10%, we aimed to recruit 200 participants in each study arm (i.e. a total 800 participants).

As the interventions will be delivered to all the physicians allocated to the study arms (effectiveness trial) and that we used routinely collected data to assess the effects, the prospect of loss to follow was low.

To allocate the participants to the study arms, we first prepare a list of all eligible physicians working in Tehran (about 6000 physicians). The physicians will be grouped into the three physician groups (i.e. general physicians, pediatricians, infectious disease specialists). Within each group we will randomly select the required number of physicians, proportional to the size of each group. Using a random number generator, the participants will be allocated to the study arms, and use the physician group and the contracted insurance organization as the stratifying factors. As a result we will have, in each study arm, 175 general physicians, 24 pediatricians, and four infectious disease specialists (totaling 203 physicians in each arm). Random numbers will be generated by a member of the team who is not involved in the delivery of the interventions.

Outcome measures

The main outcome measures for assessing the effectiveness of the interventions, the percentage of change in the proportion of dexamethasone injectable form, oral form of cefixime and amoxicillin which prescribed by general physicians, pediatricians and infectious disease specialists will be considered.

Costs are assessed from a health care provider perspective. We include all identifiable costs related to the implementation of the interventions. Our analysis therefore focuses on the incremental costs of developing and implementing audit and feedback and printed educational material interventions. Recurring and non-recurring costs are considered. Nonrecurring costs include revising the computer software and designing the new format of the feedback, and the pamphlet. Recurring costs include printing materials, travel costs, postage costs and other administrative tasks.

Study procedures and data collection

Data at baseline, one month and 3 months after the intervention will be collected.

Statistical and cost-effectiveness analyses

Demographic and baseline analyses will be conducted to ensure random allocation procedure has been effective in producing comparable study arms. Chi-square, *t*-test, repeated measure ANOVA and logistic regression analyses will be the primary modes of analyzing the results. As the primary outcomes, we will assess the effects of the study arms on the proportion of prescriptions containing each of the target prescribed medicines. We will also assess the effects of the interventions on the mean cost per prescription, and the mean number of items prescribed per prescription. Appropriate interaction analyses will be conducted to assess the interactions between the selected variables and the interventions. A fixed-effect two-level analysis approach will be followed in which prescriptions will be used as the first level and the physicians as the second level of data.

Cost data will be assessed using the actual costs incurred in the study, from a health care provider view point. Incremental cost-effectiveness ratios will be calculated and sensitivity analyses will be also conducted to assess the effects of changes in important variables in the cost-effectiveness of the interventions.

Intention-to-treat analyses will be carried out with physicians as the primary analysis approach. We will also conduct a per protocol analysis as a sensitivity analysis.

Ethical considerations

These data have been extracted from the Health Insurance Organization claims database and are provided confidentially for each physician for personal review. This study was approved by the Ethics Committee of Pharmaceutical Sciences Research Center of TUMS and has been registered with the Center for International Registration of Clinical Trial.

Discussion

A thorough evaluation of the intervention for improving and promoting rational drug use may bring important benefits, whereas inappropriate prescribing may lead to undesirable consequences. We see this trial as a necessary prerequisite for the development and implementation of a cost-effective intervention that will improve and promote rational drug use in Iran.

This study will determine the effectiveness of the three interventions, and allow us to determine what kind of intervention will be the most effective in improving prescribing pattern. This work will be the first to assess the effectiveness and cost-effectiveness of the routinely conducted audit and feedback that has been widely used in the country.

The risk of contamination between the study arms is a potential limitation of the study. However as the study sample is selected from a large number of physicians working in Tehran, the risk of contamination should be small. Additional potential limitation of the study may arise due to concurrent interventions that might happen by the responsible authorities within the Ministry of Health and Medical Education, as well as the universities in charge of health care in Tehran. We will follow such activities throughout the study, and will assess their potential impacts on the study findings, if they occur.

We believe that the current proposal may have other benefits. We expect that it will lead to the development of focused interventions that could greatly promote rational drug use. Changing physician's behavior is challenging and involves attention to the views and concerns of practicing physicians. We attended to the physicians' views while developing our interventions. In addition, this trial shall establish whether the design of targeted feedback can be used as a novel format of interventions for promoting rational drug use. We hope that, if our interventions are cost-effective, they shall be widely applied nationwide. The interventions may also be of use in middle income countries with appropriate infrastructures.

Competing interests

Authors have no conflict of interest. Since MA is Editor-in-Chief of DARU, all the review process is handled by one of Section Editors.

Authors' contributions

AR, FS designed the study with contributions from RD, AK, MH, and MA. FS collected data, registered the study and wrote the first draft of the manuscript. FS and AR revised the manuscript based on comments from the other authors. All the authors approved the final manuscript.

Acknowledgement

We thank the assistance of Ahmadali Mostoufi for his technical support in designing the presentational formats of the interventions.

Funding sources

The study is the PhD thesis of the first author and has been supported by the Faculty of Pharmacy and in the meantime as a project in TUMS with number of 90-03-33-14661.

Author details

[1]Department of Pharmacoeconomics and Pharmaceutical Management, Faculty of Pharmacy, Tehran University of Medical Sciences (TUMS), Tehran, Iran. [2]National Committee on Rational Drug Use, Food and Drug Organization, Ministry of Health and Medical Education, Tehran, Iran. [3]Department of Health Management and Economic, School of Public Health, TUMS, Tehran, Iran. [4]Knowledge Utilization Research Center, TUMS, Tehran, Iran. [5]Department of Pharmaceutics, Faculty of Pharmacy and Nanotechnology Research Center, TUMS, Tehran, Iran. [6]Department of Toxicology and Pharmacology, Faculty of Pharmacy and Pharmaceutical Sciences Research Center, TUMS, Tehran, Iran. [7]Department of Epidemiology and Biostatistics, School of Public Health, TUMS, Tehran, Iran. [8]National Institute of Health Research, Tehran University of Medical Sciences, No 78, Italia Ave, Tehran, Iran.

References

1. Lexchin J: **Improving the appropriateness of physician prescribing.** *Int J Health Serv* 1998, **28:**253–267.
2. Bloor K, Freemantle N: **Lessons from international experience in controlling pharmaceutical expenditure. II: influencing doctors.** *BMJ* 1996, **312:**1525–1527.
3. Beilby JJ, Silagy CA: **Trials of providing costing information to general practitioners: a systematic review.** *Med J Aust* 1997, **167**(2):89–92.
4. Lopez Bastida J, Mossialos E: **Pharmaceutical expenditure in Spain: cost and control.** *Int J Health Serv* 2000, **30:**597–616.
5. Madridejos-Mora R, Amado-Guirado E, Teresa Pe'rez-Rodrı'guez M: **Effectiveness of the combination of feedback and educational recommendations for improving drug prescription in general practice.** *Med Care* 2004, **42:**643–648.
6. Grimshaw JM, Thomas RE, MacLennan G, Fraser C, Ramsay CR, Vale L, *et al*: **Effectiveness and efficiency of guideline dissemination and implementation strategies.** *Health Technol Assess* 2004, **8:**1–72.
7. Wensing M, van der Weijden T, Grol R: **Implementing guidelines and innovations in general practice: which interventions are effective?** *Br J Gen Pract* 1998, **48:**991–997.
8. Psaty BM, Smith NL, Siscovicd DS, Koepsell TD, Weiss NS, Heckbert SR, *et al*: **Health outcome associated with antihypertensive therapies used as first-line agents: a systematic review and meta-analysis.** *JAMA* 1997, **277:**739–745.
9. Wright JM, Lee C-H Chimbers GK: **Systematic review of antihypertensive therapies: does the evidvnce assist in choosing a first-line drug.** *CMAJ* 1999, **161:**25–32.
10. Messerku FH, Grossman E, Goldbourt U: **Are betablockers efficacious as first-line therapy hypertension in the elderly? A systematic review.** *JAMA* 1998, **279:**1903–1907.
11. Packer M, Bristow MR, Cohn JN, Colucci WS, Fowler MB, Gilbert EM, *et al*: **The effect of carvedilol on morbidity and mortality in patients with chronic heart failure. US Carvedilol Heart Failure Study Group.** *NEJM* 1996, **334:**1349–1355.
12. Scandinavian Simvastatin Survival Study Group: **Randomised trial of cholesterol lowering in 4444 patients with coronary heart disease: the Scandinavian Simvastatin Survival Study (4S).** *Lancet* 1994, **344:**1383–1389.
13. Shepherd J, Cobbe SM, Ford I, Isles CG, Lorimer AR, MacFarlane PW, *et al*: **Prevention of coronary heart disease with pravastatin in men with hypercholesterolemia. West of Scotland coronary prevention study group.** *NEJM* 1995, **333:**1301–1307.
14. Hogerzeil HV: **Promoting rational prescribing: an international perspective.** *Br J Clin Pharmacol* 1995, **39:**1–6.
15. Jamtvedt G, Young JM, Kristoffersen DT, O'Brien MA, Oxman AD: **Audit and feedback: effects on professional practice and healthcare outcomes.** *Cochrane Database Syst Rev* 2006, **3:**CD000259.
16. Grimshaw JM, *et al*: **Effectiveness and efficiency of guideline dissemination and implementation strategies.** *Health Technol Assess* 2004, **8**(6):1–72. iii–iv.
17. Freemantle N, Harvey EL, Wolf F, Grimshaw JM, Grilli R, Bero LA: **Printed educational materials: effects on professional practice and health care outcomes.** *Cochrane Database Syst Rev* 2000, **2:**CD000172.
18. Giguère A, Légaré F, Grimshaw J, Turcotte S, Fiander M, Grudniewicz A, Makosso-Kallyth S, Wolf FM, Farmer AP, Gagnon MP: **Printed educational materials: effects on professional practice and healthcare outcomes.** *Cochrane Database Syst Rev* 2012. doi:10.1002/14651858.CD004398.pub3. Issue 10. Art. No.: CD004398.
19. Cheraghali AM, Soleymani F, Behmanesh Y, Hbibipour F, Ismaeilzadeh A, Nikfar S, Rahimi W: **Physicians' Attitude toward Injectable Medicines.** *J Pharmacol Toxicol* 2006, **1**(1):33–39.
20. Nikfar S, Kebriaeezadeh A, Majdzadeh R, Abdollahi M: **Monitoring of National Drug Policy (NDP) and its standardized indicators; conformity to decisions of the national drug selecting committee in Iran.** *BMC Int Health Hum Rights* 2005, **5:**5–5.
21. Garjani A, Salimnejad M, Shamsmohamadi M, Baghchevan V, Vahidi RG, Maleki-Dijazi N, Rezazadeh H: **Effect of interactive group discussion among physicians to promote rational prescribing.** *East Mediterr Health J* 2009, **15**(2):408–415.
22. Cheraghali AM, Nikfar S, Behmanesh Y, Rahimi V, Habibipour F, Tirdad R, Asadi A, Bahrami A: **Evaluation of availability, accessibility and prescribing pattern of medicines in the Islamic Republic of Iran.** *East Mediterr Health J* 2004, **10**(3):406–415.
23. Sepehri G, Meimandi MS: **The quality of prescribing in general practice in Kerman, Iran.** *Int J Health Care Qual Assur* 2005, **18**(5):353–360.
24. Cheraghali AM, Soleymani F, Shalviri G: **Promoting rational use activities in Iran: a successful trend.** *Essential Drugs Monitor* 2003, **33:**10–11.
25. Soleymani F, Valadkhani M, Dinarvand R: **Challenges and achievements of promoting Rational Use of Drug in Iran.** *Iran J Public Health* 2009, **38**(Suppl 1):166–168.
26. Soleymani F, Abdollahi M: **Management information system in promoting rational drug use.** *Intl J Pharmacol* 2012, **8**(6):586–589.
27. Wickersham RM, Novak KK: *managing eds: Drug Facts and Comparisons.* St. Louis MO: Wolters Kluwer Health press; 2005.
28. Canadian Agency for Drugs and Technologies in Health 2008: *Audit and feedback on prescribing practices: a guide for decision makers in Canada.* Ottawa: CADTH; 2008.
29. Ajzen I: **The theory of planned behavior.** *Organ Behav Hum Decis Process* 1991, **50:**179–211.
30. Rashidian A, Miles J, Russell D, Russell I: **Sample size for regression analyses of theory of planned behavior studies: case of prescribing in general practice.** *Brit J Health Psychol* 2006, **11**(4):581–593.
31. Rashidian A, Russell I: **Intentions and statins prescribing: can the Theory of Planned Behavior explain physician behavior in following guideline recommendations?** *J Eval Clin Pract* 2011, **17:**749–757.

32. Rashidian A, Russell I: **General practitioners' intentions and prescribing for asthma: using the Theory of Planned Behavior to explain guideline implementation.** *Int J Prev Med* 2012, **3**(1):17–28.
33. Rashidian A, Eccles Martin P, Russell I: **Falling on stony ground? A qualitative study of implementation of clinical guidelines' prescribing recommendations in primary care.** *Health Policy* 2008, **85**(2):148–161.

19

5,6-Dimethoxybenzofuran-3-one derivatives: a novel series of dual Acetylcholinesterase/Butyrylcholinesterase inhibitors bearing benzyl pyridinium moiety

Hamid Nadri[1], Morteza Pirali-Hamedani[2], Alireza Moradi[1], Amirhossein Sakhteman[1], Alireza Vahidi[3], Vahid Sheibani[4], Ali Asadipour[4], Nouraddin Hosseinzadeh[5], Mohammad Abdollahi[2], Abbas Shafiee[2] and Alireza Foroumadi[4,5*]

Abstract

Background: Several studies have been focused on design and synthesis of multi-target anti Alzheimer compounds. Utilizing of the dual Acetylcholinesterase/Butyrylcholinesterase inhibitors has gained more interest to treat the Alzheimer's disease. As a part of a research program to find a novel drug for treating Alzheimer disease, we have previously reported 6-alkoxybenzofuranone derivatives as potent acetylcholinesterase inhibitors. In continuation of our work, we would like to report the synthesis of 5,6-dimethoxy benzofuranone derivatives bearing a benzyl pyridinium moiety as dual Acetylcholinesterase/Butyrylcholinesterase inhibitors.

Methods: The synthesis of target compounds was carried out using a conventional method. Bayer-Villiger oxidation of 3,4-dimethoxybenzaldehyde furnished 3,4-dimethoxyphenol. The reaction of 3,4-dimethoxyphenol with chloroacetonitrile followed by treatment with HCl solution and then ring closure yielded the 5,6-dimethoxy benzofuranone. Condensation of the later compound with pyridine-4-carboxaldehyde and subsequent reaction with different benzyl halides afforded target compounds. The biological activity was measured using standard Ellman's method. Docking studies were performed to get better insight into interaction of compounds with receptor.

Results: The in vitro anti acetylcholinesterase/butyrylcholinesterase activity of compounds revealed that, all of the target compounds have good inhibitory activity against both Acetylcholinesterase/Butyrylcholinesterase enzymes in which compound 5b (IC50 = 52 ± 6.38nM) was the most active compound against acetylcholinesterase. The same binding mode and interactions were observed for the reference drug donepezil and compound 5b in docking study.

Conclusions: In this study, we presented a new series of benzofuranone-based derivatives having pyridinium moiety as potent dual acting Acetylcholinesterase/Butyrylcholinesterase inhibitors.

* Correspondence: aforoumadi@yahoo.com
[4]Neuroscience Research Center, Kerman University of Medical Sciences, Kerman, Iran
[5]Drug design & Development Research Center, Tehran University of Medical Sciences, Tehran, Iran
Full list of author information is available at the end of the article

Introduction

Alzheimer's disease (AD) is a progressive and age-dependent neurodegenerative brain disorder that leads to dementia, cognitive impairment, and memory loss [1,2]. The main cause of Alzheimer's disease etiology is not completely known however, many diverse factors such as hippocampal acetylcholine (Ach) decrease, β-amyloid (Aβ) aggregation and τ-protein deposits seem to play significant roles in initiation and progression of the disease [3-5]. Based on these findings three hypotheses was established: cholinergic, β-amyloid and tau hypothesis.

Regarding cholinergic hypothesis one of the most useful approaches for improving AD's symptoms is to design new agents that raise the acetylcholine in the cholinergic system [6]. Acetylcholinesterase (AChE) is responsible for hydrolysis of acetylcholine in the synaptic cleft, therefore; employing the AChE inhibitors could be a helpful strategy to increase the level of acetylcholine in the damaged cholinergic neurons [7]. Several compounds have been previously synthesized as AChE inhibitors and successfully used to treat AD, such as Donepezil, Galantamine and Rivastigmine (Figure 1) [8].

Moreover, it has been demonstrated that the inhibition of AChE may lead to an increase in Butyrylcholinesterase (BuChE) activity in the hippocampus that causes hydrolysis of AChE by a new way. Therefore, the maintenance of AChE/BuChE activity ratio in the hippocampus as seen in the healthy brain, could improve the signs and symptoms of AD [9]. As a result, design and synthesis of dual AChE/BuChE inhibitors should be considered to find more potent agents against AD [10].

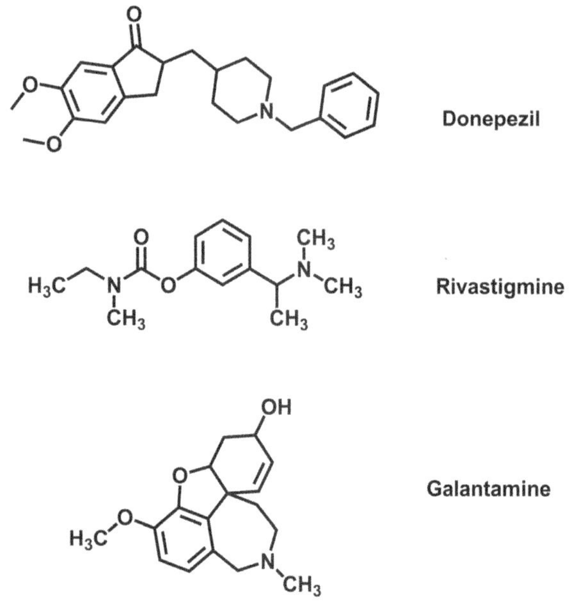

Figure 1 Donepezil, Rivastigmine and Galantamine three well-known AChE inhibitors.

In an earlier report, we have presented the preparation and evaluation of some new (*Z*)-1-benzyl-4-((6-alkoxy-3-oxobenzofuran-2(3*H*)-ylidene) methyl)pyridinium (Figure 2) as AChE inhibitors [11]. Most of these compounds proved to be potent AChE inhibitors in vitro, among which compounds bearing methoxy group on position 6 of benzofuran ring showed the most activity. Furthermore, it was reported that 5,6-dimethoxy benzofuranone structure is important to show more affinity toward the enzyme in some aurone-based AChE inhibitors [12,13]. Following these reasons and in pursuit of our previous study a series of new 5,6-dimethoxy benzofuran derivatives were designed, synthesized and evaluated for AChE/BuChE inhibitory activities. In this study, we decided to investigate the possible increase in the enzyme inhibitory activity by replacing the less hydrophilic 6-alkoxy benzofuranone scaffold with a more polar 5,6-dimethoxy benzofuranone motif. The final compounds have been tested for their ability to inhibit both AChE and BuChE using Ellman's method [14].

Materials and methods

Chemistry

All chemicals were obtained from Merck AG, Aldrich and Acros Chemicals. Thin layer chromatography (TLC) was carried out on Merck pre-coated silica gel F254 plates with various mobile phase systems, to check reaction progress and product mixtures. The Separating column chromatography and flash chromatography were done with silica gel (70-230 mesh). The ^1H nuclear magnetic resonance (NMR) spectra were recorded in DMSO-d_6 and/or $CDCl_3$ on a Bruker FT-500 MHz spectrometer with tetramethylsilane (TMS) as the internal standard. Coupling constants were reported in Hertz (Hz) and chemical shifts are given as δ value (ppm) relative to TMS as internal standard. To express spin multiplicities, s (singlet), d (doublet), t (triplet), q (quartet), dd (double doublet) and m (multiplet) were used. Mass spectra were obtained at 70 eV in a Finigan TSQ-70 spectrometer. Infrared (IR) spectra were determined using

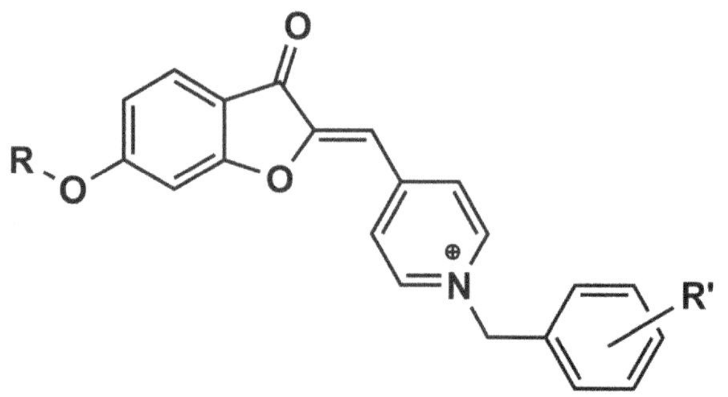

Figure 2 Previously reported (*Z*)-1-benzyl-4-((6-alkoxy-3-oxobenzofuran-2(3*H*)-ylidene) methyl)pyridinium derivatives as potent inhibitors of AChE.

a Nicolet FT-IR Magna 550 spectrophotometer. All melting points were determined using Kofler hot stage apparatus and are uncorrected.Elemental microanalyses were done on a Perkin–Elmer 240-C apparatus for C, H, and N. For better understanding of spectral data, the general structure and atom numbering of final compounds are depicted in Figure 3.

Synthesis of 3,4-dimethoxyphenol (1)

A mixture of *m*-chloro-peroxybenzoic acid (*m*-CPBA) (7 g, 32.5 mmol) in the dry dichloromethane (DCM) (40 ml) was prepared at 0°C and vigorously stirred. Then a solution of 3,4-dimethoxybenzaldehyde (5 g, 30 mmol) in the dry DCM (10 ml) was added dropwise during 1 hour. The resulting mixture was kept at room temperature and then refluxed for 16 hours. After cooling, the mixture was washed with aqueous solution of saturated sodium hydrogen carbonate (3 × 20 ml) followed by washing with sodium thiosulfate 10% (25 ml) to neutralize excess amount of *m*-CPBA. The solvent was then evaporated under reduced pressure and the resulting crude material was dissolved in methanol. The solution was stirred for 4 - hours with excess amount of sodium hydroxide 10% solution at room temperature. The pH of solution was adjusted to 1 using HCl 6 N solution. The solution was then extracted with DCM (3 × 25 ml) washed with brine and dried using anhydrous Na_2SO_4. The solvent was removed to yield brown syrup, which was purified with column chromatography using petroleum ether and ethyl acetate (1:1) as eluent to give compound 1. White brown solid, m. p. 74–78°C, 84% yield [15].

Synthesis of 2-chloro-1-(2-hydroxy-4,5-dimethoxyphenyl) ethanone (2)

To a mixture of 3,4-dimethoxyphenol (1) (4.93 g, 32 mmol) and chloroacetonitrile (2.4 g, 32 mmol) in dry ether (150 ml) was added anhydrous $ZnCl_2$ (1.44 g, 10.6 mmol). The mixture was cooled to 0°C and HCl gas was bubbled through the reaction for 2.5 hours. The mixture was left in the room temperature overnight and then cooled to 0°C. The precipitated iminium was filtered off and washed three times with ether. The imine was dissolved in 160 ml of 1 N HCl and refluxed for 90 min. The resulting mixture was extracted with DCM (3 × 100 ml) and the solvent was removed under reduced pressure to give 2.88 g white brown solid 40% yield (no further purification was needed).

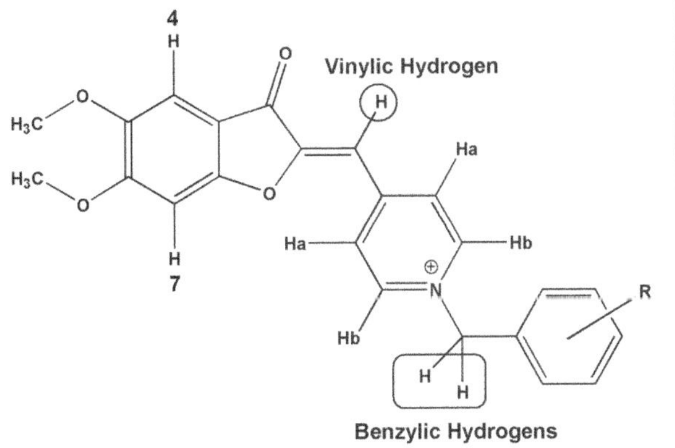

Figure 3 General structure and atom numbering of final compounds.

Synthesis of 5,6-dimethoxybenzofuran-3(2H)-one (3)

The crude extract of 2-chloro-1-(2-hydroxy-4,5-dimethoxyphenyl)ethanone (2) (1.15 g, 5 mmol) was dissolved in 10 ml ethanol and then refluxed for 10 min under argon. Sodium acetate trihydrate (700 mg) was added thereto and refluxed for 10 min again. The resulting mixture was cooled immediately and then filtered off. The solvent was evaporated and compound 3 was yielded by re-crystallization from ethanol. White needle crystals, m.p. 163–165, 470 mg, 48%. IR ν_{max}/cm^{-1} (KBr) : 1708 (C = O), ^1H NMR ($CDCl_3$, 80 MHz), 7.02 (s, 1H, $H_{4\text{-aromatic}}$) 6.59 (s, 1H, $H_{7\text{-aromatic}}$) 4.61 (s, 2H, $H_{2\text{-aliphatic}}$) 3.97 (s, 3H, -OCH_3) 3.87 (s, 3H, -OCH_3), EI-MS *m/z* (%) 194 (M^+, 100), 165 (45), 135 (88), 34 (57).

Synthesis of (Z)-5,6-dimethoxy-2-(pyridin-4-ylmethylene) benzofuran-3(2H)-one (4)

5,6-dimethoxybenzofuran-3(2*H*)-one 3 (388 mg, 2 mmol), pyridine-4-carbaldehyde (308 mg, 2.88 mmol) and PTSA (548 mg, 3.18 mmol) were suspended in the dry toluene (25 ml) and refluxed using Dean-Stark apparatus for 2 - hours. After cooling the resulting mixture, the precipitated solid was filtered off. The wet solid was suspended in aqueous 10% $NaHCO_3$ solution (50 ml) and stirred for 60 - minutes at room temperature. The filtered resulting solid was washed with water (50 ml) and then air dried. The crude solid was purified by re-crystallization from acetonitrile to yield compound 4. 400 mg, 70% yield, m.p. 265–268°C, IR ν_{max}/cm^{-1} (KBr) : 1705 (C = O), 1635 (C = C alkene), ^1H NMR ($CDCl_3$, 80 MHz), 8.69 (dd, 2H, $H_{a\text{-pyridine}}$, $J = 4.5$ Hz, $J = 2$ Hz), 7.70 (dd, 2H, $H_{b\text{-pyridine}}$, $J = 5$ Hz, $J = 1.5$ Hz), 7.17 (s, 1H, H_4), 6.83 (s, 1H, H_7), 6.69 (s, 1H, $H_{vinylic}$), 4.03 (s, 3H, -OCH_3), 3.91 (s, 3H, -OCH_3), EI-MS *m/z* (%) 284 ((M^+ + 1), 100), 224 (90), 33 (65).

General procedure for the synthesis of 1-benzyl-4-((5,6-dimethoxy-3-oxobenzofuran-2(3H)-ylidene)methyl) pyridinium halide derivatives (5a-g)

(*Z*)-5,6-Dimethoxy-2-(pyridin-4-ylmethylene) benzofuran-3(2*H*)-one (4) (1 equiv.), was suspended in 7 ml dry acetonitrile and heated under reflux condition. Afterwards different substituted benzyl halides (1.2 equiv.) were added thereto. The mixture was refluxed for 2–3 hours followed by cooling to room temperature. After that the solvent was evaporated and 15 ml n-hexane was added to the residue. The resulting mixture was filtered off and the precipitated crystals were separated, washed with n-hexane and dried. Flash chromatography of the crystals using the chloroform-methanol (99–1) as the mobile phase, furnished the final compounds 5a-g.

(Z)-1-Benzyl-4-((5,6-dimethoxy-3-oxobenzofuran-2(3H)-ylidene) methyl) pyridinium bromide (5a)

Starting from (*Z*)-5,6-dimethoxy-2-(pyridin-4-ylmethylene) benzofuran-3(2*H*)-one (1 mmol, 0.283 g) and benzyl bromide (1.2 mmol, 0.205 g), compound 5a was obtained, quantitative yield, mp over 300°C, IR ν_{max}/cm^{-1} (KBr) : 1689 (C = O), 1607 (C = C alkene), ^{1}H NMR (DMSO-d$_6$, 500 MHz), 9.20 (d, 2H, $H_{a\text{-Pyridine}}$, *J* = 6.7 Hz), 8.51 (d, 2H, $H_{b\text{-pyridine}}$, *J* = 6.7 Hz), 7.55-7.46 (m, 5H, H_{phenyl}), 7.27 (s, 1H, $H_{4\text{-benzofuranone}}$), 7.25 (s, 1H, $H_{7\text{-benzofuranone}}$), 7.04 (s, 1H, $H_{vinylic}$), 5.85 (s, 2H, $H_{benzylic}$), 3.98 (s, 3H, -OCH$_3$), 3.83(s, 3H, -OCH$_3$), EI-MS *m/z* (%) 283 (10), 91 (100), 77 (15), 43 (38), Anal. Calcd.for $C_{23}H_{20}BrNO_4$: C, 60.81; H, 4.44; N, 3.08 Found: C, 60.68; H, 4.72; N, 3.24.

(Z)-1-(4-Fluorobenzyl)-4-((5,6-dimethoxy-3-oxobenzofuran-2 (3H)-ylidene) methyl) pyridinium bromide (5b)

Starting from (*Z*)-5,6-dimethoxy-2-(pyridin-4-ylmethylene) benzofuran-3(2*H*)-one (1 mmol, 0.283 g) and 4-fluoro-benzyl bromide (1.2 mmol, 0.226 g), compound 5b was obtained, quantitative yield, mp 276–279°C, IR ν_{max}/cm^{-1} (KBr): 1687 (C = O), 1608 (C = C alkene), ^{1}H NMR (DMSO-d$_6$, 500 MHz), 9.22 (d, 2H, $H_{a\text{-pyridine}}$, *J* = 6.7 Hz), 8.52 (d, 2H, $H_{b\text{-pyridine}}$, *J* = 6.75 Hz), 7.67-7.64 (m, 2H, H_{phenyl}), 7.32-7.28 (m, 2H, H_{phenyl}), 7.25 (s, 1H, $H_{4\text{-benzofuranone}}$), 7.23 (s, 1H, $H_{7\text{-benzofuranone}}$), 7.04 (s, 1H, $H_{vinylic}$), 5.86 (s, 2H, $H_{benzylic}$), 3.97 (s, 3H, -OCH$_3$), 3.82(s, 3H, -OCH$_3$), EI-MS *m/z* (%) 283 (12), 109 (100), 95 (18), 43 (40), Anal. Calcd.for $C_{23}H_{19}BrFNO_4$: C, 58.49; H, 4.05; N, 2.97 Found: C, 58.85; H, 4.17; N, 2.74.

(Z)-1-(3-Methylbenzyl)-4-((5,6-dimethoxy-3-oxobenzofuran-2 (3H)-ylidene) methyl) pyridinium chloride (5c)

Starting from (*Z*)-5,6-dimethoxy-2-(pyridin-4-ylmethylene) benzofuran-3(2*H*)-one (1 mmol, 0.283 g) and 3-methyl-benzyl chloride (1.2 mmol, 0.169 g), compound 5c was obtained, quantitative yield, mp 293–295°C, IR ν_{max}/cm^{-1} (KBr) : 1694 (C = O), 1605 (C = C alkene), ^{1}H NMR (DMSO-d$_6$, 500 MHz), 9.25 (d, 2H, $H_{a\text{-pyridine}}$, *J* = 6.4 Hz), 8.51 (d, 2H, $H_{b\text{-pyridine}}$, *J* = 6.45 Hz), 7.48-7.41 (m, 3H, H_{phenyl}), 7.33 (s, 1H, H_{phenyl}), 7.26 (s, 1H, $H_{4\text{-benzofuranone}}$), 7.24 (s, 1H, $H_{7\text{-benzofuranone}}$), 7.03 (s, 1H, $H_{vinylic}$), 5.83 (s, 2H, $H_{benzylic}$), 3.94 (s, 3H, –OCH$_3$), 3.80 (s, 3H, –OCH$_3$), 2.3 (s, 3H, H –$CH_{3phenyl}$), EI-MS *m/z* (%) 283 (12), 105 (100), 91 (16), 43 (38), Anal. Calcd.for $C_{24}H_{22}ClNO_4$: C, 68.00; H, 5.23; N, 3.30 Found: C, 68.34; H, 5.05; N, 3.42.

(Z)-1-(2-Fluorobenzyl)-4-((5,6-dimethoxy-3-oxobenzofuran-2 (3H)-ylidene) methyl) pyridinium chloride (5d)

Starting from (*Z*)-5,6-dimethoxy-2-(pyridin-4-ylmethylene) benzofuran-3(2*H*)-one (1 mmol, 0.283 g) and 2-fluorobenzyl chloride (1.2 mmol, 0.173 g), compound 5d was obtained, quantitative yield, mp over 300°C, IR ν_{max}/cm^{-1} (KBr) : 1701 (C = O), 1608 (C = C alkene), ^{1}H NMR (DMSO-d$_6$, 500 MHz), 9.19 (d, 2H, $H_{a\text{-pyridine}}$, *J* = 5.8 Hz), 8.53 (d, 2H, $H_{b\text{-pyridine}}$, *J* = 5.95 Hz), 7.65-7.62 (m, 1H, H_{phenyl}), 7.54-7.52 (m, 1H, H_{phenyl}), 7.34-7.31 (m, 2H, H_{phenyl}), 7.26 (s, 1H, $H_{4\text{-benzofuranone}}$), 7.23 (s, 1H, $H_{7\text{-benzofuranone}}$), 7.05 (s, 1H, $H_{vinylic}$), 5.94 (s, 2H, $H_{benzylic}$), 3.95 (s, 3H, –OCH$_3$), 3.80 (s, 3H, –OCH$_3$), EI-MS *m/z* (%) 283 (16), 109 (100), 95 (18), 43 (35), Anal. Calcd.for $C_{24}H_{22}ClNO_4$: C, 68.00; H, 5.23; N, 3.30 Found: C, 68.12; H, 5.32; N, 3.37.

(Z)-1-(3-Fluorobenzyl)-4-((5,6-dimethoxy-3-oxobenzofuran-2 (3H)-ylidene) methyl) pyridinium chloride (5e)

Starting from (*Z*)-5,6-dimethoxy-2-(pyridin-4-ylmethylene) benzofuran-3(2*H*)-one (1 mmol, 0.283 g) and 3-fluorobenzyl chloride (1.2 mmol, 0.173 g), compound 5e was obtained, quantitative yield, mp 291–294°C, IR ν_{max}/cm^{-1} (KBr) : 1690 (C = O), 1611 (C = C alkene), ^{1}H NMR (DMSO-d$_6$, 500 MHz), 9.29 (d, 2H, $H_{a\text{-pyridine}}$, *J* = 6 Hz), 8.52 (d, 2H, $H_{b\text{-pyridine}}$, *J* = 6.2 Hz), 7.51-7.50 (m, 2H, H_{phenyl}), 7.43-7.41 (m, 1H, H_{phenyl}), 7.30-7.27 (m, 1H, H_{phenyl}), 7.26 (s, 1H, $H_{4\text{-benzofuranone}}$), 7.23 (s, 1H, $H_{7\text{-benzofuranone}}$), 7.04 (s, 1H, $H_{vinylic}$), 5.9 (s, 2H, $H_{benzylic}$), 3.95 (s, 3H, –OCH$_3$), 3.8 (s, 3H, –OCH$_3$), EI-MS *m/z* (%) EI-MS *m/z* (%) 283 (19), 109 (100), 95 (15), 43 (32), Anal.Calcd.for $C_{23}H_{19}ClFNO_4$: C, 64.57; H, 4.48; N, 3.27 Found: C, 64.72; H, 4.23; N, 3.16.

(Z)-1-(2-Methylbenzyl)-4-((5,6-dimethoxy-3-oxobenzofuran-2 (3H)-ylidene) methyl) pyridinium chloride (5f)

Starting from (*Z*)-5,6-dimethoxy-2-(pyridin-4-ylmethylene) benzofuran-3(2*H*)-one (1 mmol, 0.283 g) and 2-methyl-benzyl chloride (1.2 mmol, 0.169 g), compound 5f was obtained, quantitative yield, mp 287–290°C, IR ν_{max}/cm^{-1} (KBr) : 1692 (C = O), 1607(C = C alkene), ^{1}H NMR (DMSO-d$_6$, 500 MHz), 9.08 (d, 2H, $H_{a\text{-pyridine}}$, *J* = 6.85 Hz), 8.52 (d, 2H, $H_{b\text{-pyridine}}$, *J* = 6.8 Hz), 7.81- 7.78 (m, 1H, H_{phenyl}), 7.45-7.38 (m, 1H, H_{phenyl}), 7.32-7.30 (m, 2H, H_{phenyl}), 7.29 (s, 1H, $H_{4\text{-benzofuranone}}$), 7.24 (s, 1H, $H_{7\text{-benzofuranone}}$), 6.99 (s, 1H, $H_{vinylic}$), 5.88 (s, 2H, $H_{benzylic}$), 3.99 (s, 3H, –OCH$_3$), 3.84 (s, 3H, –OCH$_3$), 2.35 (s, 3H, H $CH_{3phenyl}$) EI-MS *m/z* (%) 283 (21), 105 (100), 91 (18), 43 (40), Anal. Calcd.for $C_{24}H_{22}ClNO_4$: C, 68.00; H, 5.23; N, 3.30 Found: C, 68.26; H, 5.15; N, 3.25.

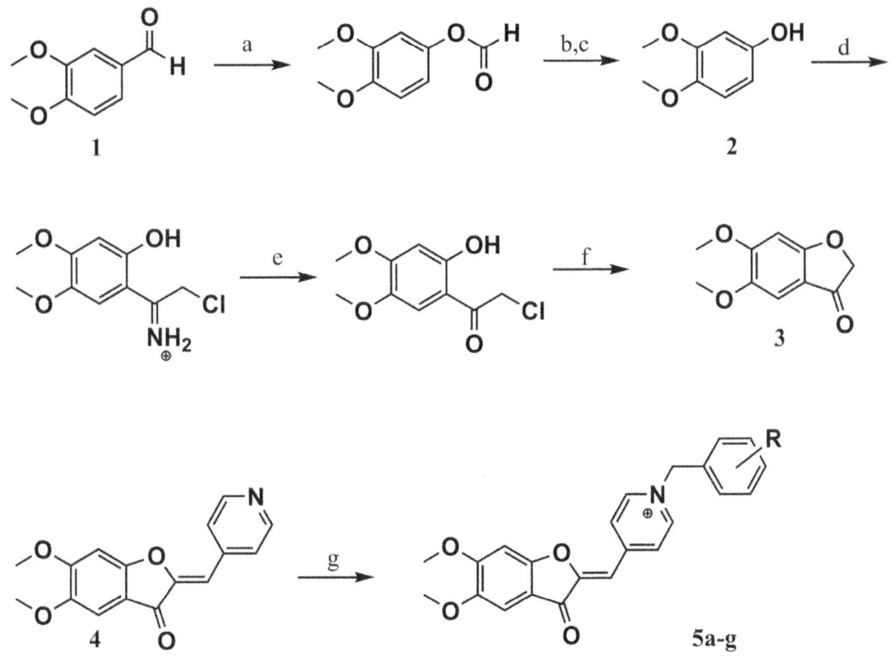

Scheme 1 Synthetic routes to final compounds 5a-g (a) *m*-CPBA, CH2Cl2, reflux 16 hrs; (b) NaOH 10%, r.t., stir., 4 hrs; (c) HCl 6 N; (d) ClCH2CN, HCl gas, ZnCl2, 0°C, 2.5 hrs, stir.; (e) HCl 1 N, reflux, 90 min; (f) Sodium acetate trihydrate, ethanol, reflux, 10 min; (g) Pyridine-4-carboxaldehyde, PTSA, toluene, reflux; (h) Substituted benzyl halide, CH3CN, reflux.

(Z)-1-(4-Methylbenzyl)-4-((5,6-dimethoxy-3-oxobenzofuran-2 (3H)-ylidene) methyl) pyridinium chloride (5g)

Starting from (*Z*)-5,6-dimethoxy-2-(pyridin-4-ylmethylene) benzofuran-3(*2H*)-one (1 mmol, 0.283 g) and 4-methylbenzyl chloride (1.2 mmol, 0.169 g), compound 5g was obtained, quantitative yield, mp 294–297°C, IR ν_{max}/cm^{-1} (KBr) : 1690 (C = O), 1606 (C = C alkene), ^{1}H NMR (DMSO-d_6, 500 MHz), 9.24 (d, 2H, $H_{a\text{-pyridine}}$, $J = 6.4$ Hz), 8.49 (d, 2H, $H_{b\text{-pyridine}}$, $J = 6.5$ Hz), 7.47 (d, 2H, $J = 6.3$ Hz, H_{phenyl}), 7.26 (d, 2H, $J = 6.4$ Hz, H_{phenyl}), 7.20 (s, 1H, $H_{4\text{-benzofuranone}}$), 7.17 (s, 1H, $H_{7\text{-benzofuranone}}$), 6.96 (s, 1H, $H_{vinylic}$), 5.80 (s, 2H, $H_{benzylic}$), 3.95 (s, 3H, $-OCH_3$), 380 (s, 3H, $-OCH_3$), 2.28 (s, 3H, H $-CH_{3phenyl}$), EI-MS *m/z* (%) 283 (17), 105 (100), 91 (22), 43 (31), Anal. Calcd.for $C_{24}H_{22}ClNO_4$: C, 68.00; H, 5.23; N, 3.30 Found: C, 67.76; H, 5.38; N, 3.19.

Biological activity

AChE (AChE, E.C. 3.1.1.7, Type V-S, lyophilized powder, from *electric eel,* 1000 unit), Cholinesterase from equine serum were purchased from Sigma–Aldrich (Steinheim, Germany). DTNB (5, 5′-Dithiobis-(2-nitrobenzoic acid)), KH_2PO_4, K_2HPO_4, KOH, $NaHCO_3$, BTChI (butyrylthiocholine iodide) and ATChI (acetylthiocholine iodide) were obtained from Fluka (Buchs, Switzerland). To afford an assay concentration range (10^{-4} to 10^{-9} M), the tested compounds were dissolved in a mixture of 20 ml distilled water and 5 ml methanol followed by dilution in 0.1 M KH_2PO_4/K_2HPO_4 buffer (pH 8.0) to obtain final concentration.

The colorimetric Ellman's method was applied to evaluate anti AChE/BuChE activity of tested compounds. The solutions temperature was adjusted to 25°C prior to use. Five different concentrations of each compound were tested to obtain 20% to 80% inhibition of AChE and/or BuChE activity. The assay medium contained 3 ml of 0.1 M phosphate buffer pH 8.0, 100 µl of 0.01 M 5, 5′-dithio-bis(2-nitrobenzoic acid), 100 µl of 2.5 unit/ mL enzyme solution (AChE, E.C. 3.1.1.7, Type V-S, lyophilized powder, from *electric eel* or BuChE from equine serum).

Then 100 µl of each tested compounds, were added to the assay medium and pre-incubated at 25°C for 15 min followed by adding 20 µl of substrate (acetylthiocholine iodide or butyrylthiocholine iodide). After that the rate of absorbance change was measured at 412 nm for 2 minutes. The blank reading solution was used to justify non-enzymatic hydrolysis of substrate during the assay. The blank solution contained 3 ml buffer, 200 µl water, 100 µl DTNB and 20 µl substrate. As a reference, an identical solution of the enzyme without the inhibitor is processed following the same protocol. The rate of the substrate enzymatic hydrolysis was calculated, and % inhibition of the tested compounds was calculated. Each concentration was evaluated in triplicate, and the

Table 1 AChE/BuChE inhibitory activity of compounds 5a-g compared with Donepezil hydrochloride (IC_{50} = Mean ± SD)

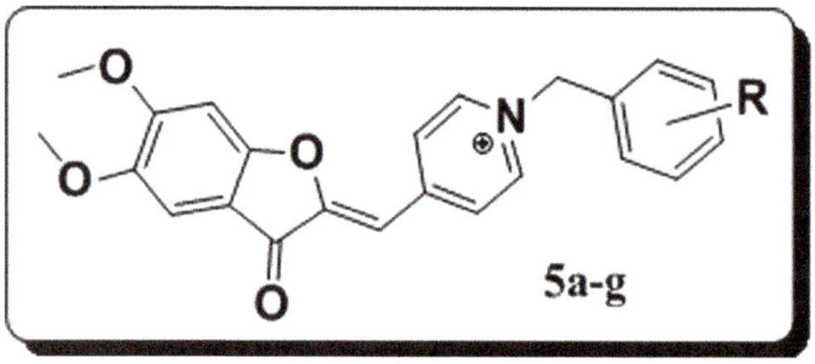

Compounds	R	AChE (IC_{50} ± SD)[a] (nM)	BuChE (IC_{50} ± SD)[a] (nM)	Selectivity for AChE[b] (S.I)
5a	H	86 ± 10.94	1400 ± 85	16.27
5b	2-F	52 ± 6.38	1620 ± 73	31.15
5c	3-F	115 ± 15.56	740 ± 23	6.43
5d	4-F	74 ± 11.32	960 ± 41	12.97
5e	2-CH_3	262 ± 27.49	3620 ± 84	13.81
5f	3-CH_3	208 ± 31.72	5310 ± 115	25.52
5g	4-CH_3	514 ± 29.53	7600 ± 260	14.78
Donepezil hydrochloride	-	31 ± 5.12	5400 ± 95	174.19

[a] Data are means ± standard deviation of three independent experiments.
[b] Selectivity Index (S.I): IC_{50} BuChE/ IC_{50} AChE.

IC_{50} values were determined from inhibition curves (% of inhibition versus log inhibitor's concentration) graphically. Kapková et al. reported more details of the procedure [16,17].

Docking study

Docking simulation studies were done using Autodock Vina 1.1.1 [18]. For this purpose, the pdb structure of acetylcholinesterase (1EVE) was retrieved from the Brookhaven protein database (RCSB)(http://www.rcsb.org) as a complex bound with inhibitor Donepezil. Subsequently, all water molecules and the co-crystallized ligand were removed from the pdb structure. Afterward the polar hydrogens were added to the receptor and pdbqt format of the receptor was created using Autodock Tools 1.5.4 [19]. The ligand coordinates were generated using Marvine-Sketch 5.8.3, 2012, ChemAxon (http://www.chemaxon.com). Then the structures were converted to pdbqt using Open babel 2.3.1 [20]. The docking site was defined by establishing a box at geometrical center of the native ligand present in the above mentioned PDB structure with the dimensions of 40, 40, and 40. The exhaustiveness parameter was set to 80 and the box center was set to the dimensions of x = 2.023, y = 63.295, z = 67.062. Finally, the lowest energy conformations between the AChE and inhibitor were selected for analyzing the interactions. The results were visualized using Chimera 1.6 [21].

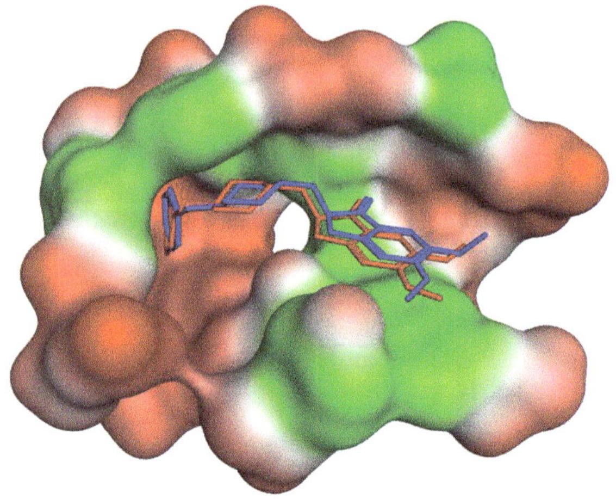

Figure 4 The superposition of the docked Donepezil (blue) and reference Donepezil (red) into the active site of the AChE.

Results and discussion

Chemistry

The target compounds (5a-g) were synthesized as illustrated in Scheme 1. The convenient Baeyer–Villiger oxidation of 3,4-dimethoxybenzaldehyde furnished 3,4-dimethoxyphenol (1) in a good yield [15]. Reaction of 3,4-dimethoxyphenol (1) with chloroacetonitrile using $ZnCl_2$ as Lewis acid yielded 2-chloro-1-(2-hydroxy-4,5-dimethoxyphenyl)ethane iminium as a key intermediate.

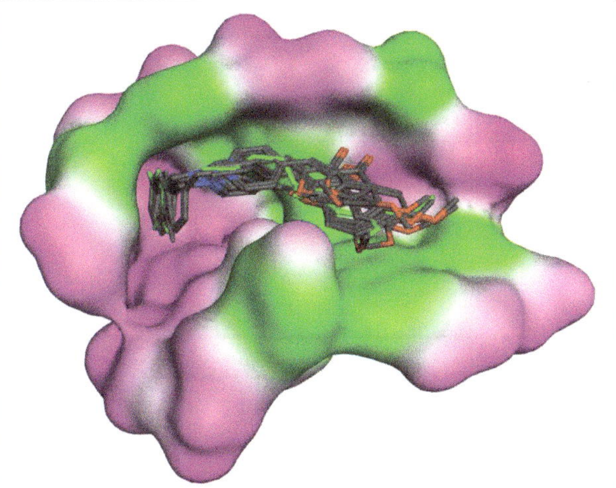

Figure 5 **The superposition of best docked poses of all target compounds (colored by element) as well as Donepezil (green) into the gorge of AChE.**

Afterwards, 2-chloro-1-(2-hydroxy-4,5-dimethoxyphenyl) ethanone (2) was prepared followed by treatment of iminium intermediate using hydrochloric acid. Intermolecular cyclization of compound (2) using sodium acetate resulted in formation of 5,6-dimethoxy-benzofuran-3(2*H*)-one (3) [22]. Condensation of 5,6-dimethoxybenzofuran-3 (2*H*)-one (3) with 4-formyl pyridine in the presence of PTSA gave (*Z*)-5,6-dimethoxy-2-(pyridin-4-ylmethylene) benzofuran-3(2*H*)-one (4). As previously reported, the configuration of exocyclic formed double bond was assigned as *Z* (*cis*) isomer [11]. Appropriate benzyl chloride or bromide derivatives were refluxed with compound (4) in dry acetonitrile to obtain final compounds (5a-g).

Biological activity

The new series of 5,6-dimethoxybenzofuranone derivatives bearing the benzyl pyridinium moiety was evaluated for AChE/BuChE activity using slightly modified Ellman's protocol.

The type and position of substituents on benzyl moiety could alter the electronic and steric properties of the phenyl ring. Therefore, the affinity of the target compounds toward the enzyme could be modified by changing the substituent on benzyl moiety.

The anti AChE/BuChE activity data of the target compounds were summarized in Table 1.

According to the data, all of the synthesized compounds have shown considerable anti AChE/BuChE activity however, did not reach the inhibition level of the reference compound (Donepezil hydrochloride $IC_{50} = 31 \pm 5.12$ nM).

As already shown in our previous study, the substitution on phenyl ring with small electron withdrawing group such as fluorine atom makes the compounds more active rather than their unsubstituted counterparts. In an opposite way the methyl phenyl substituted compounds proved to be less active than the unsubstituted compounds. In this study using the identical substitution on the ring, the anti cholinesterase activity of 5,6-dimethoxy-benzofuranone derivatives has changed in the same way. Regardless of the substitution on phenyl ring, the activity of more

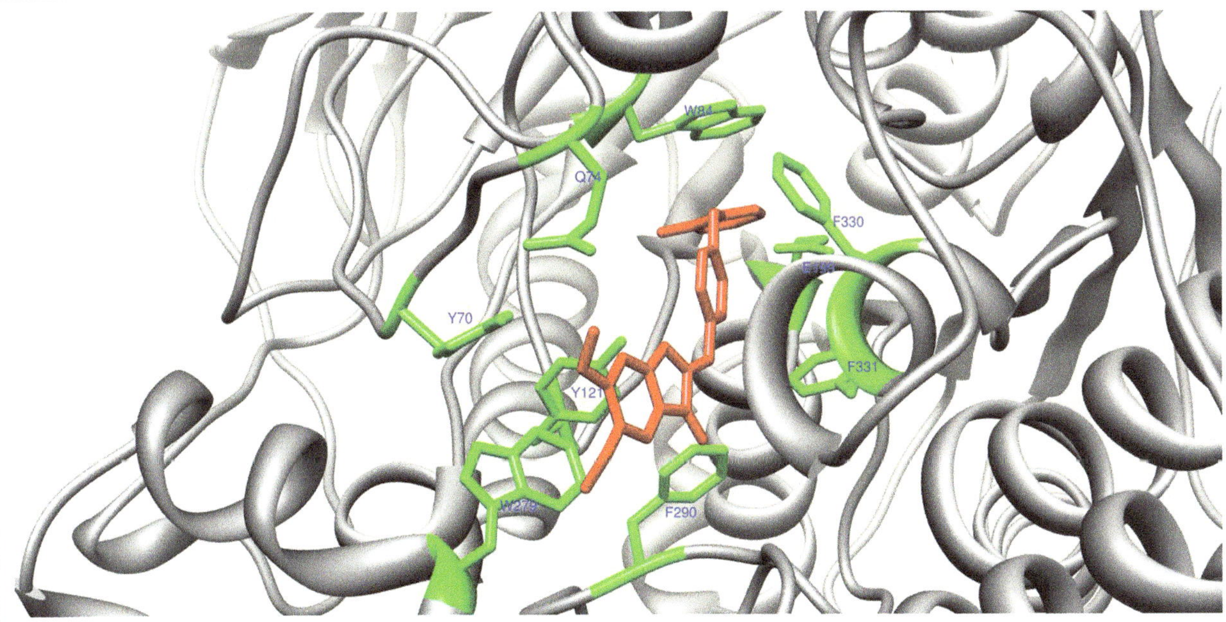

Figure 6 **The interacting mode of the most active compound 5b with the active site of AChE.**

polar 5,6-dimethoxybenzofuranone derivatives were slightly diminished, compared to 6-alkoxy benzofuranone derivatives that were previously reported [11].

As anticipated, the compound 5b (IC_{50} = 52 ± 6.38 nM) containing 2-F substituent exhibited the highest inhibitory activity toward the enzyme. However, its activity was less than its counterparts bearing 6-methoxy (IC_{50} = 10 ± 6.87 nM), 6-ethoxy (IC_{50} = 32 ± 7.75 nM) and 6-propoxy (IC_{50} = 50 ± 9.86) on benzofuranone.

Similarly, the 3 and 4-flouro phenyl compounds have shown lower activity in respect to corresponding 6-alkoxy benzofuranone series.

According to Table 1, changing the *ortho* position of fluorine to either *meta* or *para* decreased the activity as in compound (5c) with significantly diminished activity (IC_{50} = 115 ± 15.56).

Accordingly, methyl substituted compounds have exhibited the order of activity as follow: 5f > 5e > 5g. Insertion of methyl group on phenyl ring in any position reduced the activity in comparison with unsubstituted compound (5a).

In an accord to these findings, it was concluded that substitution on position 3 with F and position 4 with $-CH_3$ was not tolerated.

Docking simulation study

In order to investigate the binding mode for interaction of the target compounds with AChE, docking studies were performed. First the co-crystallized ligand was docked back into the binding site of the enzyme and superposed with the native ligand (Figure 4).

Being satisfied with the reasonable RMSD between the docked and native ligands (RMSD = 0.78 Å), the docking protocol was verified for further docking studies of the target compounds. The best docked poses of the synthesized compounds on the target were superposed and showed to be similarly docked in the gorge of AChE. As shown in Figure 5, this pattern of orientation resembled very much to that observed for donepezil.

In order to figure out the binding mode for interaction of the compounds, the most active compound (5b) was subjected to further analysis. As depicted in Figure 6, the 5,6-dimethoxybenzofuranone fragment of the ligand was well accommodated in the PAS (Peripheral Anionic Site) through a π–π stacking of the phenyl ring of benzofuranone and indole moiety of Trp279. This interaction was reinforced by a hydrogen bonding between the 6-methoxy of 5b and the hydroxyl group of Tyr70. In addition, the benzyl pyridinium part of the ligand was oriented towards the anionic site (AS) composed by Phe330, Trp84 and Glu199. The interactions responsible for stabilization of bezyl pyridinium in the active site included two π–π stacking and a π-cation interaction. The π-cation interaction was formed between Phe330 and the quaternary nitrogen of pyridine ring. Regarding the two π–π interactions, one was between 2-flouro substituted phenyl ring and Trp84 and the other between pyridine ring and Phe330. The same binding mode and interactions were also observed for the reference drug (Donepzil) [23].

Conclusions

In this study, we presented new benzofuranone-based derivatives of the pyridinium type. The inhibitory activity of new synthesized compounds were tested toward AChE using slightly modified Ellman's method and compared to those of other derivatives of this class synthesized earlier by our research group. Regarding the biological data, it was revealed that all tested compounds inhibited the AChE in nanomolar range concentration, in which compound 5b, was the most potent compound against AChE. Furthermore a same binding mode and interactions was observed for the reference drug Donepzil and compound 5b in docking study.

In conclusion, 5,6-dimethoxybenzofurane derivatives containing methylbenzyl substituent on pyridine ring demonstrated to be more potent than their corresponding 6-ethoxy and 6-propoxy benzofuranone derivatives [11].

Competing interests

The authors declare that they have no competing interests.

Authors' contributions

HN participated in the synthesis of compounds and performing biological assay. AF, Ash, AA and MP contributed in design of compounds, supervision of synthetic part, elucidation of the target compounds structure and manuscript preparation. AM, AS and AV performed the docking study and participated in manuscript preparation. NH partook in synthetic section. The biological assay part is supervised by VS and MA. All authors read and approved the final manuscript.

Acknowledgements

Molecular graphics and analyses were performed with the UCSF Chimera package. Chimera is developed by the 25 Resource for Biocomputing, Visualization, and Informatics at the University of California, San Francisco.

Author details

[1]Department of Medicinal Chemistry, Faculty of Pharmacy and Neurobiomedical Research Center, Shahid Sadoughi University of Medical Sciences, Yazd 8915173143, Iran. [2]Faculty of Pharmacy and Pharmaceutical Sciences Research Center, Tehran University of Medical Sciences, Tehran, Iran. [3]Herbal Medicine Center, Shahid Sadoughi University of Medical Sciences, Yazd 8915173143, Iran. [4]Neuroscience Research Center, Kerman University of Medical Sciences, Kerman, Iran. [5]Drug design & Development Research Center, Tehran University of Medical Sciences, Tehran, Iran.

References

1. Kung HF, Lee CW, Zhuang ZP, Kung MP, Hou C, Plossl K: **Novel stilbenes as probes for amyloid plaques.** *J Am Chem Soc* 2001, **123:**12740–12741.
2. Forstl H, Kurz A: **Clinical features of Alzheimer's disease.** *Eur Arch Psychiatry Clin Neurosci* 1999, **249:**288–290.
3. Fernandez-Bachiller MI, Perez C, Campillo NE, Paez JA, Gonzalez-Munoz GC, Usan P, Garcia-Palomero E, Lopez MG, Villarroya M, Garcia AG, Martinez A, Rodriguez-Franco MI: **Tacrine-melatonin hybrids as multifunctional agents for Alzheimer's disease, with cholinergic, antioxidant, and neuroprotective properties.** *ChemMedChem* 2009, **4:**828–841.

4. Yankner BA, Dawes LR, Fisher S, Villa-Komaroff L, Oster-Granite ML, Neve RL: **Neurotoxicity of a fragment of the amyloid precursor associated with Alzheimer's disease.** *Science* 1989, **245:**417–420.
5. Masters CL, Simms G, Weinman NA, Multhaup G, McDonald BL, Beyreuther K: **Amyloid plaque core protein in Alzheimer's disease and Down syndrome.** *Proc Natl Acad Sci U S A* 1985, **82:**4245–4249.
6. Bartus RT, Dean RL III, Beer B, Lippa AS: **The cholinergic hypothesis of geriatric memory dysfunction.** *Science* 1982, **217:**408–414.
7. Richman DP, Agius MA: **Treatment of autoimmune myasthenia gravis.** *Neurology* 2003, **61:**1652–1661.
8. Repantis D, Laisney O, Heuser I: **Acetylcholinesterase inhibitors and memantine for neuroenhancement in healthy individuals: a systematic review.** *Pharmacol Res* 2010, **61:**473–481.
9. Karlsson D, Fallarero A, Brunhofer G, Mayer C, Prakash O, Mohan CG, Vuorela P, Erker T: **The exploration of thienothiazines as selective butyrylcholinesterase inhibitors.** *Eur J Pharm Sci* 2012, **47:**190–205.
10. Musial A, Bajda M, Malawska B: **Recent developments in cholinesterases inhibitors for Alzheimer's disease treatment.** *Curr Med Chem* 2007, **14:**2654–2679.
11. Nadri H, Pirali-Hamedani M, Shekarchi M, Abdollahi M, Sheibani V, Amanlou M, Shafiee A, Foroumadi A: **Design, synthesis and anticholinesterase activity of a novel series of 1-benzyl-4-((6-alkoxy-3-oxobenzofuran-2(3H)-ylidene) methyl) pyridinium derivatives.** *Bioorg Med Chem* 2010, **18:**6360–6366.
12. Sheng R, Lin X, Zhang J, Chol KS, Huang W, Yang B, He Q, Hu Y: **Design, synthesis and evaluation of flavonoid derivatives as potent AChE inhibitors.** *Bioorg Med Chem* 2009, **17:**6692–6698.
13. Sheng R, Xu Y, Hu C, Zhang J, Lin X, Li J, Yang B, He Q, Hu Y: **Design, synthesis and AChE inhibitory activity of indanone and aurone derivatives.** *Eur J Med Chem* 2009, **44:**7–17.
14. Ellman GL, Courtney KD, Andres V Jr, Feather-Stone RM: **A new and rapid colorimetric determination of acetylcholinesterase activity.** *Biochem Pharmacol* 1961, **7:**88–95.
15. Li CC, Xie ZX, Zhang YD, Chen JH, Yang Z: **Total synthesis of wedelolactone.** *J Org Chem* 2003, **68:**8500–8504.
16. Kapkova P, Alptuzun V, Frey P, Erciyas E, Holzgrabe U: **Search for dual function inhibitors for Alzheimer's disease: synthesis and biological activity of acetylcholinesterase inhibitors of pyridinium-type and their Abeta fibril formation inhibition capacity.** *Bioorg Med Chem* 2006, **14:**472–478.
17. Alptuzun V, Kapkova P, Baumann K, Erciyas E, Holzgrabe U: **Synthesis and biological activity of pyridinium-type acetylcholinesterase inhibitors.** *J Pharm Pharmacol* 2003, **55:**1397–1404.
18. Trott O, Olson AJ: **AutoDock Vina: improving the speed and accuracy of docking with a new scoring function, efficient optimization, and multithreading.** *J Comput Chem* 2010, **31:**455–461.
19. Sanner MF: **Python: a programming language for software integration and development.** *J Mol Graph Model* 1999, **17:**57–61.
20. O'Boyle NM, Banck M, James CA, Morley C, Vandermeersch T, Hutchison GR: **Open Babel: an open chemical toolbox.** *J Cheminform* 2011, **3:**33.
21. Pettersen EF, Goddard TD, Huang CC, Couch GS, Greenblatt DM, Meng EC, Ferrin TE: **UCSF Chimera–a visualization system for exploratory research and analysis.** *J Comput Chem* 2004, **25:**1605–1612.
22. Lee CY, Chew EH, Go ML: **Functionalized aurones as inducers of NAD(P)H: quinone oxidoreductase 1 that activate AhR/XRE and Nrf2/ARE signaling pathways: synthesis, evaluation and SAR.** *Eur J Med Chem* 2010, **45:**2957–2971.
23. Sugimoto H, Iimura Y, Yamanishi Y, Yamatsu K: **Synthesis and structure-activity relationships of acetylcholinesterase inhibitors: 1-benzyl-4-[(5,6-dimethoxy-1-oxoindan-2-yl)methyl]piperidine hydrochloride and related compounds.** *J Med Chem* 1995, **38:**4821–4829.

Membrane stabilization as a mechanism of the anti-inflammatory activity of methanol extract of garden egg (*Solanum aethiopicum*)

Chioma A Anosike[1*], Onyechi Obidoa[2] and Lawrence US Ezeanyika[1]

Abstract

Background: Some observations and reports show that people with high consumption of *Solanum aethiopicum* (African garden egg) have relief in arthritic pains and swelling. We aimed at assessing the effect of methanol extract of *Solanum aethiopicum* in experimentally induced inflammation using leukocyte mobilization and vascular permeability tests in rats and human red blood cell (HRBC) membrane stabilization as studies.

Methods: Twenty five (25) adult Wistar rats of either sex (120 g – 200 g) divided into five groups of five rats each were used for each of the animal models. Groups 2, 3 and 4 were administered varied doses of the extract (100, 200 and 400 mg/kg), while groups 1 (vehicle control) and 5 (treatment control) received normal saline and indomethacin (50 mg/kg) respectively. Vascular permeability was induced by the intra-peritoneal injection of 1 ml of acetic acid and monitored using 0.5 ml intravenous injection of 1% Evans blue solution. Leukocyte mobilization was induced by the intra-peritoneal injection of 0.5 ml of 3% agar suspension in normal saline. Heat and hypotonicity induced heamolysis of HRBC membrane was used to assess membrane stabilization.

Results: The methanol extracts of garden egg significantly and dose dependently reduced ($p \leq 0.05$) the acetic acid induced vascular permeability and agar induced leukocyte mobilization in rats. The percentage inhibitions of induced vascular permeability were 21 ± 3.39, 25 ±1.92 and 60 ± 3.81 for the 100, 200 and 400 mg/kg of the extract while the inhibitions of the agar induced leucocyte migration were 23 ± 2.17, 26 ± 1.58 and 32 ± 1.58 for the 100, 200 and 400 mg/kg of the extract respectively. The extract also, at doses of 100, 200, 400, 600 and 800 μg/ml significantly inhibited heat induced lysis of the human red cell membrane with values of 66.46 ± 2.89, 65.14 ± 4.58, 46.53 ± 2.52, 61.88 ± 4.51and 86.67 ± 3.06 respectively.

Conclusions: These results show that methanol extract of *Solanum aethiopicum* has anti-inflammatory properties and can reduce inflammatory injury and tissue damage.

Keywords: Inflammation, Leucocyte migration, Vascular permeability, Human red cell membrane

Background

Inflammation is a complex biological response of vascular tissues to harmful stimuli. It is also a protective attempt by the organism to remove the injurious stimuli and initiate the healing process [1]. At the onset of an inflammation, the cells undergo activation and release inflammatory mediators. These mediators include histamine, serotonin, slow reacting substances of anaphylaxis (SRS-A), prostaglandins and some plasma enzyme systems such as the complement system, the clotting system, the fibrinolytic system and the kinin system [2]. These mediator molecules work collectively to cause increased vasodilatation and permeability of blood vessels. Thus, leading to increased blood flow, exudation of plasma proteins and fluids, and migration of leukocytes, mainly neutrophils, outside the blood vessels into the injured tissues [3]. Inflammation can be classified as either acute or chronic inflammation [1]. Acute inflammation is the initial response of the body to injurious stimuli and is achieved by increased movement of plasma

* Correspondence: chiomanos@yahoo.com
[1]Department of Biochemistry, University of Nigeria, Nsukka, Enugu State, Nigeria
Full list of author information is available at the end of the article

and leukocytes from the blood into the injured tissues. The process of acute inflammation is initiated by cells already present in the tissues. This is characterized by marked vascular changes, including vasodilatation and increased capillary permeability which are induced by the actions of the various inflammatory mediators [4]. Chronic inflammation is a prolonged inflammatory response that leads to a progressive shift in the type of cells present at the site of inflammation and is characterized by simultaneous destruction and healing of the tissues from the inflammatory process [5].

Solanum aethiopicum (African garden egg) is a fruiting plant of the genus *Solanum* and family Solanaceae. It is mostly found in Asia and tropical Africa, grows about 2.5m tall, and bears fruits varying in shapes and colours. Some West African species bear edible fruits; they include *S. aethiopicum*, *S. melogena*, *S. macrocarpon*, and *S. muricatum* [6]. The fruits of these species are awakening a growing interest in the speciality and exotic vegetable markets of the world. This is probably associated with the increase in the interest for African cuisine and with African immigration and the potentials of the fruits to improve nutrition [7]. The fruit has various shapes; oval and round, with different colours; white, stripped and green, and turns bright red when ripe (Figure 1). The fruits are usually harvested while still green before the skin becomes thick [8]. These fruits can be eaten fresh without cooking and have a long history of consumption in West Africa. Reports on the pharmacological activity of the garden egg show that it has purgative, sedative, anti-diabetic and anti-ulcerogenic properties [9-11]. The anti-inflammatory effect of the plant on egg albumin-induced oedema and cotton pellet induced granuloma in rats has also been reported [12].

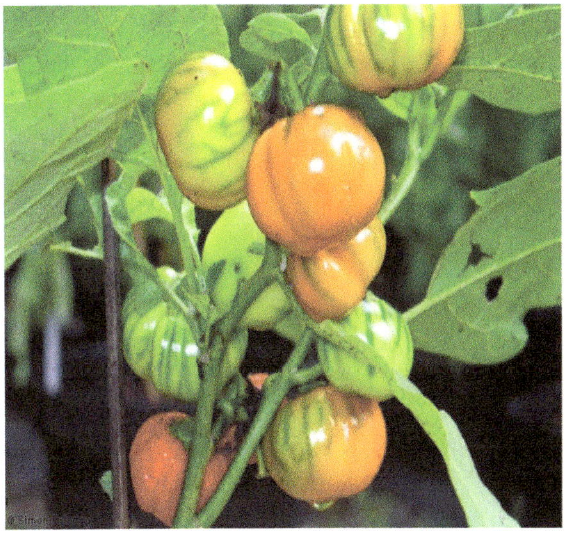

Figure 1 *Solanum aethiopicum* fruits.

This work was therefore aimed at further assessing the anti-inflammatory properties of the plant extract using experimentally induced vascular permeability and leucocyte mobilization in rats and HRBC membrane stabilization as inflammatory models.

Methods

Chemicals

All chemicals used in this study were of analytical grade. They were products of Sigma Aldrich, Germany.

Plant material

Fresh fruits of garden egg (*Solanum aethiopicum*) were obtained from the Agric Farm of the Faculty of Agricultural Sciences of the University of Nigeria, Nsukka and were identified by Mr. Ugwuozor, a taxonomist of Botany Department, University of Nigeria, Nsukka. A voucher specimen was deposited in the herbarium unit of the Department of Botany, University of Nigeria, Nsukka. The plant was chopped into tiny bits, air-dried for 2 weeks and milled with a mechanical grinder. The ground plant (500 g) was macerated in methanol for 24 hrs, filtered with a white cloth and the filtrate concentrated using a rotary evaporator (IKA, Germany) at an optimum temperature of 40–50°C.

Animals

Swiss albino mice (22–28 g) and adult Wistar rats (120–200 g) of both sexes obtained from the animal house of the Faculty of Biological Sciences, University of Nigeria, Nsukka were used. They were housed in metal steel cages and acclimatised in the laboratory for seven days before the experiments. They were given free access to water and fed with growers mash (Niger Feeds, Nigeria) bought from the local market. The research was conducted in accordance with the ethical rules and recommendations of the University of Nigeria committee on the care and use of laboratory animals and the revised National Institute of Health Guide for Care and Use of Laboratory Animal (Pub No.85-23, revised 1985).

Blood sample

Fresh whole blood (3 ml) was collected intravenously from healthy human volunteers into heparinised tubes to prevent coagulation.

Acute toxicity study

The acute toxicity test of the garden egg extract was carried out by the method of Lorke [13] with some modifications to define the range of lethal dose and safe dose for the extract. Eighteen Swiss albino mice starved of food for 18 hr but allowed access to water were used for the study. They were grouped into six (6) groups of three mice each and treated intraperitoneally (i.p.) with the plant extract at varied dose levels (100, 1000, 1500, 2000, 3000, and 5000 mg/kg). The animals were then observed for nervousness, dullness, in-coordination and or mortality for 24 h. Based on the results of the preliminary toxicity testing, the doses of the extract for further studies were decided to be 100, 200 and 400 mg/kg bodyweight of the rats.

Phytochemical analysis

The phytochemical analysis of the extract was carried out based on procedures outlined by Trease and Evans [14]. The phytochemicals assayed include alkaloid, glycosides, steroid, terpenoids, flavonoids, tannins, resins and saponinis.

Leukocyte mobilization test in rats

The effect of the methanol extract of *Solanum aethiopicum* on *in vivo* leukocyte mobilization induced by an inflammatory stimulus was evaluated in albino rats using the method of Rebeiro *et al.,* [15]. Twenty five (25) adult Wistar rats of either sex (120 g – 200 g) divided into five groups of five rats each were used for the test. Groups 2, 3 and 4 were administered varied doses of the extract (100, 200 and 400 mg/kg), while groups 1 (vehicle control) and 5 (treatment control) received normal saline and indomethacin (50 mg/kg) respectively. Three hours after oral administration of the extracts, normal saline or reference drug, each animal in the respective groups (n=5) received intraperitoneal injection (i. p) of 0.5 ml of 3% w/v agar suspension in normal saline. Four hours later, the animals were sacrificed and the peritoneal cavities washed with 5 ml of a 5% solution of EDTA in phosphate buffered saline (PBS). The peritoneal fluid was recovered and both total and differential leukocyte counts (TLC and DLC) were performed on the perfusates using a manual cell counter after staining with Wright's stain. The percent inhibition of leukoctye migration was calculated using the formula:

$$\% \text{ Leukocyte inhibition } (\%L.I) = \left(1 - \left(\frac{T}{C}\right)\right) \times 100$$

Where T and C represents the leukocyte count of the treated and control groups respectively.

Vascular permeability test in rats

The effect of the extract on acetic acid induced vascular permeability was assessed by a modified method of Whittles [16]. Twenty five (25) adult Wistar rats of either sex (120 g – 200 g) divided into five groups of five rats each were used. The animals were fasted for 10 hours prior to the experiment and were then administered with varied doses of the extract and drug as stated above.

Three hours later, each animal was given a 0.5 ml intravenous injection of 1% Evans blue solution. Vascular permeability was induced thirty minutes afterwards, by (i. p) injection of 1 ml of 0.6% acetic acid. The animals were sacrificed 20 minutes later, and their peritoneum washed with 10 ml of normal saline. The recovered peritoneal fluid was centrifuged and the absorbance of the supernatant measured at 610 nm using a spectrophotometer.

Preparation of erythrocyte suspension

Fresh whole blood (3 ml) collected from healthy volunteers into heparinised tubes was centrifuged at 3000 rpm for 10 min. A volume of normal saline equivalent to that of the supernatant was used to dissolve the red blood pellets. The volume of the dissolved red blood pellets obtained was measured and reconstituted as a 40% v/v suspension with isotonic buffer solution (10 mM sodium phosphate buffer, pH 7.4). The buffer solution contained 0.2 g of NaH_2PO_4, 1.15 g of Na_2HPO_4 and 9 g of NaCl in 1 litre of distilled water. The reconstituted red blood cells (resuspended supernatant) were used as such.

Assay of membrane stabilisation

The effects of the garden egg extract on haemolysis of HRBC induced by heat and distilled water was evaluated using the method of Shinde *et al.* [17] with some modifications.

Heat induced haemolysis

Samples of the extract used were dissolved in isotonic phosphate buffer solution. A set of 5 centrifuge tubes containing respectively, 5 ml graded doses of the extracts (100, 200, 400, 600 and 800 µg/ml) were arranged in quadruplicate sets (4 sets per dose). Two sets of control tubes contained 5 ml of the vehicle and 5 ml of 200 µg/ml of indomethacin respectively. HRBC suspension (0.1 ml) was added to each of the tubes and mixed gently. A pair of the tubes was incubated at 54°C for 20 minutes in a regulated water bath. The other pair was maintained at −10°C in a freezer for 20 minutes. Afterwards, the tubes were centrifuged at 1300 g for 3 min and the haemoglobin content of the supernatant was estimated using Spectronic 21D (Milton Roy) Spectrophotometer at 540 nm. The percent inhibition of haemolysis by the extract was calculated thus:

$$\% \text{ Inhibition of Haemolysis} = 1 - \left(\frac{OD_2 - OD_1}{OD_3 - OD_1}\right) \times 100$$

Where OD_1 = absorbance of test sample unheated
OD_2 = absorbance of test sample heated
OD_3 = absorbance of control sample heated.

Hypotonicity induced haemolysis

Samples of the extract used in this test were dissolved in distilled water (hypotonic solution). The hypotonic solution (5 ml) containing graded doses of the extracts

(100, 200, 400, 600 and 800 μg/ml) were put into duplicate pairs (per dose) of the centrifuge tubes. Isotonic solution (5 ml) containing graded doses of the extracts (100 – 800 μg/ml) were also put into duplicate pairs (per dose) of the centrifuge tubes. Control tubes contained 5 ml of the vehicle (distilled water) and 5 ml of 200 μg/ml of indomethacin respectively. Erythrocyte suspension (0.1 ml) was added to each of the tubes and mixed gently. The mixtures were incubated for 1 hr at room temperature (37°C), and afterwards, centrifuged for 3 min at 1300 g. Absorbance (OD) of the haemoglobin content of the supernatant was estimated at 540 nm using Spectronic 21D (Milton Roy) spectrophotometer. The percentage heamolysis was calculated by assuming the heamolysis produced in the presence of distilled water as 100%. The percent inhibition of haemolysis by the extract was calculated thus:

$$\% \text{ Inhibition of haemolysis} = 1 - \left(\frac{OD_2 - OD_1}{OD_3 - OD_1}\right) \times 100$$

Where OD_1 = absorbance of test sample in isotonic solution

OD_2 = absorbance of test sample in hypotonic solution

OD_3 = absorbance of control sample in hypotonic solution

Statistical analysis

Data obtained were analyzed using SPSS version 15.0 (SPSS Inc. Chicago, IL. USA). All values are expressed as mean ± SD. Data were analysed by one-way ANOVA and difference between means was assessed by Duncan's new multiple range. P<0.05 was considered statistically significant.

Results

Acute toxicity study

Result of acute toxicity study showed that there was no mortality or any significant change in the behaviour of the mice recorded up to the dose of 5000 mg/kg of the plant extract.

Phytochemical analysis of garden egg extract

The qualitative phytochemical composition of garden egg extract showed relatively high concentration of bioactive compounds such as alkaloids, glycosides, steroids, terpenoids, flavonoids and resins, with saponnins and acidic compounds being in trace amounts, while tannin was not detected (Table 1).

Effect of methanol extract of garden egg on agar induced leukocyte mobilization test in rats

Result obtained from the study showed that the methanol extract of garden egg (*S. aethiopicum*) caused a significant reduction ($p \leq 0.05$) in the *in vivo* leukocyte migration induced by agar. The percentage inhibitions of leukocyte migration were 23, 26 and 32% for 100, 200 and 400 mg/kg b.w respectively. Control group treated with indomethacin showed 40% inhibition. The proportion of neutrophils in the perfusate was higher than lymphocytes and other cells in all the groups (Table 2).

Table 1 Result of the phytochemical analysis of garden egg extract

Phytochemical	Garden egg
Alkaloid	++
Glycosides	+++
Steroids	+++
Terpenoids	+++
Flavonoids	+++
Tannins	-
Acidic compounds	+
Resins	++
Saponnins	+

Bioavailability Key
- = not present.
+ = present in low concentration.
++ = present in moderately high concentration.
+++ = present in very high concentration.

Effect of methanol extract of garden egg on acetic acid induced vascular permeability test in rats

Intraperitoneal injection of 0.6% acetic acid caused an increased vasodilation and permeability of the blood vessel of the animals. This was evidenced by the leakage of fluids including Evans blue across the blood vessel epithelial walls into the peritoneal cavity as shown by the bluish colouration of the peritoneal fluid. Data from Table 3 show that the garden egg extract caused a significant and dose dependent reduction ($p \leq 0.05$) in vascular permeability. This was evidenced by the reduced blue colouration and thus absorbance values of the peritoneal fluid of the animals treated with the garden egg extract when compared with the control animals.

Effect of *S. aethiopicum* extract on heat induced haemolysis of HRBCs

From data shown in Table 4, the garden egg extract at all the doses (100–800 μg/ml) protected the human erythrocyte membrane against lysis induced by heat as is shown by the high percentage inhibitions of haemolysis. The percentage inhibitions of lysis shown by the extract doses were lower than that obtained for 200 μg/ml of indomethacin.

Effect of *S. aethiopicum* extract on hypotonicity induced haemolysis of HRBCs

Data from Table 5 show that garden egg extracts significantly ($p \leq 0.05$) inhibited lysis induced by water. This is

Table 2 Effect of methanol extract of garden egg on agar induced *in vivo* leukocyte mobilization

Treatment	Dose (mg/kg)	TLC (X10^4)	% inhibition	Differential Leukocyte mobilization (%)				
				Neutrophils	Lymphocytes	Monocytes	Eosinophils	Basophils
Control		94.51 ± 7.93		62.75	34.75	1.0	0.75	0.75
Extract	100	72.62 ± 11.45**	23 ± 2.17	61	35	1.5	1.0	1.5
	200	70.25 ± 12.28**	26 ± 1.58	60	36	1.25	1.5	1.25
	400	64.00 ± 14.78**	32 ± 1.58	57	39	1.25	1.0	1.75
Indomethacin	50	56.7 5 ± 7.89***	40 ± 1.92	60.75	35	1.25	1. 5	1.5

Level of Significance ***= p<0.001, ** = p<0.01, * = p<0.05 Percent inhibition of migration was calculated relative to control.

shown by the high percentage inhibition of haemolysis (40.8, 53.3 and 50.8) obtained for doses of 400, 600 and 800 μg/ml respectively. The inhibition of haemolysis was found to be dose dependent, increasing with increased concentration of the extract in the medium and was comparable with that obtained for indomethacin (Table 5).

Discussion

In this study, the efficacy of garden egg extract against induced vascular permeability and infiltration of inflammatory cells to an injured area was carried out using acetic acid induced vascular permeability test and agar induced leukocyte migration. At the onset of an inflammation, the cells undergo activation and release inflammatory mediators that cause vasodilatation and increased permeability of blood vessels leading to the exudation of plasma proteins and fluids into the tissues; the vessel walls become engorged and dilated, allowing large numbers of neutrophils to extravasate and appear within the junctional epithelium and underlying connective tissue spaces [3]. In this study, intraperitoneal injection of 0.6% acetic acid caused an increased dilation and permeability of the blood vessels of the animals which was evidenced by the increased leakage of fluids, including Evans blue across the blood vessel epithelial walls. Administration of the garden egg extract caused a significant and dose dependent reduction in vascular permeability of the extract treated animals.

Table 3 Effect of methanol extract of garden egg on acetic acid induced vascular permeability test in rats

Treatment	Dose (mg/kg)	Absorbance	% inhibition
Control		0.82 ± 0.12	-
Extract	100	0. 65 ± 0.11*	21 ± 3.39
	200	0.59 ± 0.11*	25 ± 1.92
	400	0.32 ± 0.06**	60 ± 3.81
Indomethacin	50	0.26 ± 0.10**	68 ± 4.08

Level of Significance ***= p<0.001, ** = p<0.01, * = p<0.05 Percent inhibition of migration was calculated relative to control.

The extract also significantly (p≤0.05) reduced the migration of leukocytes in response to agar induced inflammatory stimulus. A number of different cells are recruited into an inflammatory area. These cells are responsible for the inactivation and removal of invading infectious agents and damaged tissues. Chemotactic movement of leukocytes towards the foreign body is the first and most important step in phagocytosis [18]. Leukocytes are found in tissues during acute inflammatory process and in the superficial surface aspects of a lesion during subacute or chronic inflammation. They function as phagocytes of bacteria, fungi and viruses, and detoxifiers of toxic proteins that may result from allergic reactions and cellular injury [19]. Eosinophils and basophils are predominant when inflammation is initiated by immediate allergic reactions or parasites [20]. In our result, neutrophils which engulf and eliminate microorganism were the most mobilized leukocytes. Generally, neutrophils are the first line of defense of the immunological system against pathogens. However, in an inflammatory disease such as rheumatoid arthritis, they represent a potential cause of tissue damage [21]. The interaction of recruited neutrophils in the site of inflammation with resident cells, local inflammatory mediators, and extracellular matrix may lead to the production of several other mediators, including cytokines, degrading enzymes, oxygen and nitrogen species that may further amplify the inflammatory response and injure surrounding tissues [22]. Increased infiltration and adhesion of leukocytes to endothelial cells, thus, increases the inflammatory process. The inhibition of leukocyte migration by garden egg extract therefore shows that garden egg could alter the action of the endogenous factors that are involved in the migration of these cells to the site of inflammation, thereby reducing the inflammatory process.

Garden egg extract at concentrations of 100–800 μg/ml protected the human erythrocyte membrane against lysis induced by hypotonic solution and heat. During inflammation, there are lyses of lysosomes which release their component enzymes that produce a variety of disorders. Non-steroidal anti-inflammatory drugs (NSAIDs) exert

Table 4 Effect of *S. aethiopicum* extract on heat induced haemolysis of HRBCs

Treatment	Conc. (μg/ml)	Mean absorbance ± SD		Percentage inhibition of haemolysis
		Heated solution	Unheated solution	
Control	-	0.67 ± 0.13	0.3 ± 0.01	
Extract	**100**	0.25 ± 0.04**	0.4 ± 0.01	66.46 ± 2.89
	200	0.28 ± 0.04**	0.08 ± 0.03	65.14 ± 4.58
	400	0.42 ± 0. 07**	0.12 ± 0.03	46.53 ± 2.52
	600	0.42 ± 0.06**	0.25 ± 0.06	61.88 ± 4.51
	800	0.43 ± 0.09**	0.38 ± 0.08	86.67 ± 3.06
Indomethacin	**200**	0.05 ± 0.01***	0.02 ± 0.00	95.32 ± 3.51

Level of Significance ***= p<0.001, ** = p<0.01, * = p<0.05. Percent inhibition of haemolysis was calculated relative to control.

their beneficial effects by either inhibiting the release of lysosomal enzymes or by stabilizing the lysosomal membranes [23]. Exposure of red blood cells (RBCs) to injurious substances such as hypotonic medium, heat, methyl salicylate or phenylhydrazine results in the lysis of the membranes, accompanied by haemolysis and oxidation of haemoglobin [24]. Since human red blood cell (HRBC) membranes are similar to lysosomal membrane components [23], the inhibition of hypotonicity and heat induced red blood cell membrane lysis was taken as a measure of the mechanism of anti-inflammatory activity of garden egg extract. The haemolytic effect of hypotonic solution is related to excessive accumulation of fluid within the cell resulting in the rupturing of its membrane. Injury to red cell membrane will render the cell more susceptible to secondary damage through free radical induced lipid peroxidation [25]. Membrane stabilization leads to the prevention of leakage of serum protein and fluids into the tissues during a period of increased permeability caused by inflammatory mediators [3]. Garden egg extract perhaps stabilized the red blood cell membrane by preventing the release of lytic enzymes and active mediators of inflammation.

Phytochemical results of this study showed that garden egg is abundantly rich in flavonoids, alkaloids, steroids and terpenoids. These phytochemicals occur in various parts of the plant. Many reports have shown that plant flavonoids possess potent anti-inflammatory and antioxidant properties [26-28]. Their anti-inflammatory activities are probably due to their inhibitory effect on enzymes involved in the production of the chemical mediators of inflammation and metabolism of arachidonic acid [29,30].

Conclusion

This study therefore shows that garden egg has modulatory effect on the vascular changes that occur during acute inflammation. Many anti-inflammatory plants and agents modify inflammatory responses by accelerating the destruction or antagonising the action of the mediators of inflammatory reaction. Foods and fruits rich in flavonoids and other phenolic compounds have been associated with decreased risk of developing inflammatory and other related diseases [31,32]. These reports, thus, suggest that the flavonoids in garden egg plant might be a major anti-inflammatory constituent in the plant.

We conclude that this study has shown that the methanolic extract of the fruits of garden egg (*Solanum aethiopicum*) have anti-inflammatory activity in the models studied.

Table 5 Effect of *S. aethiopicum* extract on hypotonicity induced haemolysis of HRBCs

Treatment	Conc. (μg/ml)	Mean absorbance ± SD		Percentage inhibition of haemolysis
		Hypotonic solution	Isotonic solution	
Control	-	0.65 ± 0.11	0.03 ± 0.01	
Extract	**100**	0.62 ± 0.1	0.04 ± 0.03	8.8 ± 1.76
	200	0.60 ± 0.12	0.07 ± 0.33	11.3 ± 4.16
	400	0.48 ± 0.07**	0.18 ± 0.06	40.8 ± 6.75
	600	0.5 ± 0.09**	0. 35 ± 0.15	53.3 ± 4.51
	800	0.49 ± 0.06**	0.32 ± 0.21	50.8 ± 3.75
Indomethacin	**200**	0.28 ± 0.02**	0.03 ± 0.01	61.47 ± 5.50

Level of Significance ***= p<0.001, ** = p<0.01, * = p<0.05. Percent inhibition of haemolysis was calculated relative to control.

Competing interests

The author(s) declare that they have no competing interests.

Authors' contributions

OO conceived of the study, and participated in its design and coordination. LUS participated in the coordination of the study. CA carried out the experimental studies and drafted the manuscript. All authors read and approved the final manuscript.

Acknowledgements

We wish to thank the technical staff of the Department of Biochemistry, and Mr, Ngene of the Faculty of Veterinary Medicine, University of Nigeria, Nsukka, for their assistance in the laboratory.

Author details

[1]Department of Biochemistry, University of Nigeria, Nsukka, Enugu State, Nigeria. [2]Department of Biochemistry, Kogi State University, Aiymgba, Kogi State, Nigeria.

References

1. Ferrero-Miliani L, Nielson OH, Andersen PS, Girardin SE: **Chronic inflammation: importance of NOD2 and NALP3 in interleukin-1β generation.** *Clin Exp Immunol* 2007, **147**(2):227–235.
2. Perianayagam JB, Sharma SK SK, Pillai SK: **Anti-inflammatory activity of *Trichodesma indicum* root extract in experimental animals.** *J Ethnopharmacol* 2006, **104**:410–414.
3. Chaitanya R, Sandhya S, David B, Vinod KR, Murali S: **HRBC Membrane Stabilizing Property of Roor, Stem and Leaf of *Glochidion velutinum*.** *Int J Res Pharmaceut Biomed Sci* 2011, **2**(1):256–259.
4. Okoli CO, Akah PA, Nwafor SV, Anisiobi AI, Ibegbunam IN, Erojikwe O: **Anti-inflammatory activity of hexane leaf extract of *Aspilia africana* C.D. Adams.** *J Ethnopharmacol* 2007, **109**(2):219–225.
5. Eming SA, Krieg J, Davidson JM: **Inflammation in wound repair. Molecular and cellular mechanisms.** *J Invest Dermatol* 2007, **127**(3):514–525.
6. Prohens J, Blanca JM, Neuz F: **Morphological and molecular variation in a collection of eggplant from a secondary centre of diversity: implications for conservation and breeding.** *J Am Soc Hortic Sci* 2005, **130**:54–63.
7. Gisbert C, Prohens J, Neuz F: **Efficient regeneration in two potential new cops for subtropical climates, the scarlet (*Solanum aethiopicum)* and gboma *(S. macrocarpon)* eggplants.** *New Zeal J Crop Hort Sci* 2006, **34**:55–62.
8. Lester RN, Thitai GNW: **Inheritance in *Solanum aethiopicum*, the scarlet eggplant.** *Euphtica* 1989, **40**:67–74.
9. Saba AB, Dina OA, Adedapo AA, Akhiromen IO: **Effect of aqueous leaf extract of *Solanum aethiopicum* on isolated guinea pig ileum.** *Afr J Biomed* 2003, **6**(3):146–147.
10. Ezeugwu CO, Okonta JM, Nwodo NJ: **Antidiabetic properties of ethanolic fruit extract of *Solanum aethiopicum* L.** *Res J. Pharmaceut Allied Sci* 2004, 2(2):251–254.
11. Anosike CA, Abonyi O, Ubaka CM: **Does the African garden egg offer protection against experimentally induced ulcers?** *Asian Pac J Trop Med* 2011, **4**(2):163–166.
12. Anosike CA, Obidoa O, Ezeanyika LUS: **The anti- inflammatory activity of garden egg (*Solanum aethiopicum*) on egg albumin-induced oedema and granuloma tissue formation in rats.** *Asian Pac J Trop Med* 2012, **5** (1):62–66.
13. Lorke D: **A new approach to practical acute toxicity testing.** *Arch of Toxicity* 1983, **54**:275–287.
14. Trease E, Evans WC: *Pharmacognosy*, Williams Charles Evans. 15th edition. London: Saunders Publishe; 2008.
15. Rebeiro RA, Flores CA, Cunha FQ, Ferreira SH: **IL-8 causes *in vivo* neutrophil migration by a cell dependent mechanism.** *Immunology* 1991, **73**:472–477.
16. Whittle BA: **The use of changes in capillary permeability in mice to distinguish between narcotic and nonnarcotic analgesics.** *Br J Pharmacol* 1964, **22**:246–253.
17. Shinde UA, Phadke AS, Nair AM, Mungantiwar AA, Dikshit VJ, Sarsf MN: **Membrane stabilization activity- a possible mechanism of action for the anti-inflammatory activity of Cedrus deodara wood oil.** *Fitoterapia* 1989, **70**:251–257.
18. Cunha TM, Verri WA Jr, Schivo IR, Napimoga MH, Parada CA, Poole S, Teixeira MM, Ferreira SH, Cunha FQ: **Crucial role of neutrophils in the development of mechanical inflammatory hypernociception.** *J Leukocyte Biol* 2008, **83**(4):824–832.
19. Ganachari MS, Kumar S, Bhat KG: **Effect of *Ziziphus jujuba* leaves extract on phagocytosis by human neutrophils.** *J Nat Remed* 2004, **4**:47–51.
20. Fehervari Z, Philips JM, Dunne DW, Cooke A: **Parasitic worms and inflammatory disease.** *Parasite Immunol* 2005, **28**(10):515–523.
21. Tanaka D, Kagari T, Doi H, Shimozato T: **Essential role of neutrophils in anti-type II collagen antibody and lipopolysaccharide-induced arthritis.** *Immunology* 2006, **119**:195–202.
22. Cunha TM, Verri WA Jr, Poole S, Parada CA, Cunha FQ, Ferreira SH: **Pain facilitation by proinflammatory cytokine actions at peripheral nerve terminals.** In *Immune and Glial Regulation of Pain*. Edited by Sorkin L, DeLeo J, Watkins LR. Seattle, WA, USA: IASP; 2007:67–83.
23. Mounnissamy VM, Kavimani S, Balu V, Drlin QS: **Evaluation of anti-inflammatory and membrane stabilizing properties of ethanol extract of *Canjera rehedi*.** *Iranian J Pharmacol Therapeut* 2008, **6**:235–237.
24. Feirrali M, Signormi C, Ciccolili L, Comporti M: **Iron release and membrane damage in erythrocytes exposed to oxidizing agents, phenylhydrazine, devicene and iso-uranil.** *Biochem Journal* 1992, **285**:295–301.
25. Halliwell B, Whiteman M: **Measuring reactive species and oxidative damage *in vivo* and in cell culture: how should you do it and what do the results mean?** *Br J Pharmacol* 2004, **142**(2):231–225.
26. Middleton E, Kandaswami C: **Effect of flavonoids on immune and inflammatory cell function.** *Biochem Pharmacol* 1992, **43**:1167–1179.
27. Read MA: **Flavonoids: naturally occurring anti-inflammatory agents.** *Amer J Pathol* 1995, **147**:235–237.
28. Halliwell B, Rafter J, Jenner A: **Health promotion by flavonoids, tocopherols, tocotrienols and other phenols: direct or indirect effects? Antioxidants or not?** *Am J Clin Nutr* 2005, **81**:268S–276S.
29. Oweyele B, Oloriegbe YY, Balaogun EA, Soladoye AO: **Analgesis and anti-inflammatory properties of *Nelsonia Canescens* leaf extract.** *J Ethnopharmacol* 2005, **99**:153–156.
30. Metowogo K, Agbonon A, Eklu-Gadegbeku K, Aklikokou AK, Gbeassor M: **Anti-ulcer and anti-inflammtory effects of Hydro-alcohol extract of *Aloe buettneri A. Berger* (Lilliaceae).** *Trop J Pharmaceut Res* 2008, **7**(1):907–912.
31. Sadik CD, Sies H, Schewe T: **Inhibition of 15-lipoxygenase by flavonoids: structure-activity relations and mode of action.** *Biochem Pharmacol* 2003, **65**:773–781.
32. Sies H, Schewe T, Heiss C, Kelm M: **Cocoa Polyphenols and inflammatory mediators.** *Am J Clin Nutr* 2005, **81**(1):304S–312S.

Study of the pharmacokinetic changes of Tramadol in diabetic rats

Hoda Lavasani[1], Behjat Sheikholeslami[1], Yalda H Ardakani[1], Mohammad Abdollahi[2,3], Lida Hakemi[1] and Mohammad-Reza Rouini[1,3*]

Abstract

Background: Besides the pathological states, diabetes mellitus may also alter the hepatic biotransformation of pharmaceutical agents. It is advantageous to understand the effect of diabetes on the pharmacokinetic of drugs. The objective of this study was to define the pharmacokinetic changes of tramadol and its main metabolites after *in vivo* intraperitoneal administration and *ex vivo* perfused liver study in diabetic rat model.
Tramadol (10 mg/kg) was administered to rats (diabetic and control groups of six) intraperitoneally and blood samples were collected at different time points up to 300 min. In a parallel study, isolated liver perfusion was done (in diabetic and control rats) by Krebs-Henseleit buffer (containing 500 ng/ml tramadol). Perfusate samples were collected at 10 min intervals up to 180 min. Concentration of tramadol and its metabolites were determined by HPLC.

Results: Tramadol reached higher concentrations after i.p. injection in diabetics (C_{max} of 1607.5 ± 335.9 ng/ml) compared with control group (C_{max} of 561.6 ± 111.4). M1 plasma concentrations were also higher in diabetic rats compared with control group. M2 showed also higher concentrations in diabetic rats. Comparing the concentration levels of M1 in diabetic and control perfused livers, showed that in contrast to intact animals, the metabolic ratios of M1 and M5 (M/T) were significantly higher in diabetic perfused liver compared to those of control group.

Conclusions: The pharmacokinetic of tramadol and its three metabolites are influenced by diabetes. As far as M1 is produced by Cyp2D6, its higher concentration in diabetic rats could be a result of induction in Cyp2D6 activity, while higher concentrations of tramadol can be explained by lower volume of distribution.

Introduction

The capacity of organisms to eliminate xenobiotics such as pharmaceutical drugs and environmental pollutants from their body is subject to change. One of the best-known effective factors is the genetic variation of drug metabolizing enzymes and transporters. Numerous genetic polymorphisms have been reported with cytochrome P450 (P450s) [1]. In addition to the genetic background, xenobiotic-induced transcriptional activation or deactivation (i.e. induction or inhibition) has been documented in large numbers and drawing many researchers' attention in order to avoid unfavorable drug–drug interactions and side effects of therapeutic drugs [2]. Physiological and pathophysiological conditions also affect the activity of P450s and other enzymes. Obesity and diabetes are worldwide concerns as risk factors for metabolic syndromes in the liver [3].

Diabetes mellitus, a disease with wide prevalence in humans, involves many complications including micro- and macro angiopathy as well as neuropathy, which in turn leads to increase the incidence of many diseases. Besides these pathological states, it is believed that possible diabetes-induced alterations in the hepatic biotransformation of pharmaceutical agents could also pose additional health risk because of dangerous side effects due to drug toxicity [4]. Considering the number of diabetic patients and their increased opportunities for drug therapy compared to healthy subjects, it is of great interest to understand the effect of this disease on drug metabolism.

Several chemicals have been used for induction of insulin-dependent diabetes mellitus in animal models, principally alloxan, streptozotocin and zinc chelators [5].

* Correspondence: rouini@tums.ac.ir
[1]Biopharmaceutics and Pharmacokinetics Division, Department of Pharmaceutics, Faculty of Pharmacy, Tehran University of Medical Sciences, 14155-6451, Tehran, Iran
[3]Pharmaceutical Sciences Research Centre, Faculty of Pharmacy, Tehran University of Medical Sciences, 14155-6451, Tehran, Iran
Full list of author information is available at the end of the article

According to the literature, streptozotocin causes structural alterations in pancreatic beta cells (total degranulation) within 48 h after administration and last up to 4 months [5].

In rat models of diabetes mellitus induced by streptozotocin (DMIS) some physiological changes including a decrease in bile flow rate [6], hepatotoxicity [7], impaired renal function [8,9], disorders of the gastrointestinal tract and reductions in protein binding of drugs due to elevated plasma fatty acid level and/or glycosylation of plasma proteins [9], have been reported. Glucuronidation and sulfation were also strongly affected in DMIS rats [10]. Recently, it was shown that the expression of CYP1A1, 2A1, 2B1, 2C12, 2E1, 3A4, 4A1 and/or 4A2 were apparently increased in DMIS rats [11-14]. However, CYP2C11, 2C13, 2A2 and 3A2 were suppressed [12].

Tramadol hydrochloride (T) is a centrally acting analgesic with efficacy and potency ranging between weak opioids and morphine. The drug is mostly eliminated via biotransformation in the liver in two main pathways including *O*-demethylation to *O*-desmethyltramadol (M1) (the pharmacologically active metabolite) by isoenzyme cytochrome P450 2D6 (CYP2D6) and *N*-demethylation to *N*-desmethyltramadol (M2) by cytochromes P450 2B6 (CYP2B6) and 3A4 (CYP3A4) [15]. These primary metabolites may be further metabolized to three additional secondary metabolites namely, *N, N*-didemethyltramadol (M3), *N, N, O*-tridesmethyltramadol (M4) and *N, O*-desmethyltramadol (M5). The *O*-desmethylated metabolites are then further conjugated with glucuronic acid and sulfate before excretion in urine [15].

Recently, tramadol was suggested as an effective oral medication to alleviate pain in diabetic painful neuropathy (DPN) [16,17] and the dose-dependent lowering effect of tramadol on the plasma glucose levels of DMIS rats was also reported by Cheng et al. [18]. Although tramadol is known to be effective for the symptomatic relief of DPN, little definitive data is available concerning the effects of diabetes on hepatic drug metabolism and pharmacokinetics of this compound. Moreover, the results of those studies are not equivocal and are often contradictory.

The objective of this study was to investigate the pharmacokinetic changes of tramadol and its main metabolites after *in vivo* intraperitoneal administration and *ex vivo* perfused liver study in the DMIS rat model.

Materials and methods

Materials

The pure substances of tramadol, M1, M2, M5 and cis-tramadol as internal standard (Figure 1) were kindly supplied by Grünenthal (Achen, Germany). All other chemicals were supplied by Merck (Darmstadt, Germany). Water used in all experiments was of Direct-Q® quality (Millipore, France).

Animals

Male Sprague–Dawley rats of 7 weeks old (weighing 250–300 g) were maintained in a clean room with 12 h light–dark cycle, controlled temperature environment between 20 and 23°C, a relative humidity of 50% and free access to standard laboratory chow and water. The study was approved by the Institutional Review Board of Pharmaceutical Research Centre of Tehran University of Medical Sciences. The animals were randomly divided into two experimental groups including control and DMIS rats.

Induction of diabetes

The animals were made diabetic with a single intravenous injection of streptozotocin (Sigma, USA). Freshly prepared streptozotocin (60 mg/kg) in 0.9% saline containing 0.01 M sodium citrate (pH adjusted to 4.5) was administered once to the overnight- fasted rats via the tail vein [19]. An equal volume of a citrate buffer of pH 4.5 (0.3 ml) was injected to the control rats. On day 7 after intravenous administration of streptozotocin (rat models of DMIS) or a citrate buffer (controls for rat model of DMIS), non-fasting blood glucose levels of rats were measured using the Accu-Chek Active® (Roche Diagnostics, Basel, Switzerland). The diabetic state was confirmed by glucose levels exceeding 200 mg/dl.

Intact diabetic rat study

At seventh day after the beginning of treatment with streptozotocin (DMIS rats), the femoral vein of one leg of DMIS and control rats were cannulated with previously heparinized intravenous 16–18 gauge catheter while each rat was under ketamine anesthesia using an intraperitoneal injection of xylazine/ketamine (15/75 mg/kg). Tramadol was administered intraperitoneally as 10 mg/kg, diluted in normal saline. The animals were kept under anesthesia until the end of the experiment. Approximately, 200 μl of venous blood samples were collected in heparinized tubes at: 0 (blank); 7.5, 15, 30, 45, 60, 90, 120, 165, 210, 255 and 300 min after tramadol administration. Blood samples were immediately centrifuged for 20 min at 1800 g and the plasma samples were stored at -80°C until HPLC analysis. A 250 μl of heparinized normal saline (15 units/ml) was used to flush the cannula to prevent blood clotting. At the end of the study, animals were sacrificed by cervical dislocation.

Isolated liver perfusion study

The isolated liver perfusion study was also conducted in the DMIS and control rats. Animals were anesthetized using an intraperitoneal injection of xylazine/ketamine (15/75 mg/kg). The portal vein and superior vena cava were catheterized with an intravenous 16–18 gauge catheter, respectively. 500 units of heparin were injected into the inferior vena cava. Freshly prepared Krebs-Henseleit

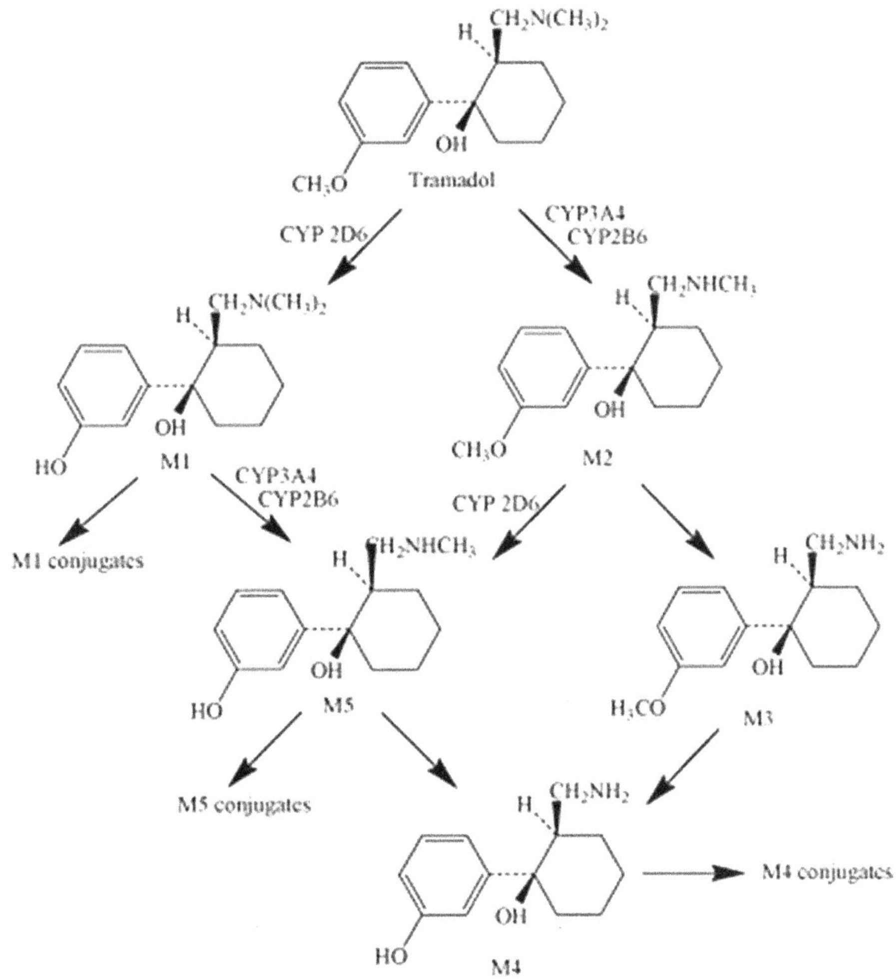

Figure 1 Metabolic pathway of tramadol.

buffer (118 mm NaCl, 4.5 mm KCl, 2.75 mm CaCl2, 1.19 mm KH2PO4, 1.18 mm MgSO4 and 25 mm Na HCO3, equilibrated with 95% O2/ 5% CO2, pH 7.4) (containing 500 ng/ml tramadol) was passed through the portal vein with a constant flow rate of 10 ml/min using a peristaltic pump. By this method, perfusion medium passed through the liver and then collected from the superior vena cava [20]. The total volume of the reservoir was 200 ml. The temperature (37°C), pH (7.4) and perfusion pressure (14 mmHg) were periodically monitored and kept unchanged through the study. Liver variability was proved by monitoring the liver enzymes activities (AST and ALT). Perfusate samples were collected at 10 min intervals up to 180 min.

Analytical method

Tramadol, M1, M2 and M5 concentration in rat plasma samples were determined by a previously described HPLC method [21]. Briefly, all analytes were extracted with ethylacetate and injected to a Knauer high-performance liquid chromatography (Berlin, Germany), equipped with a low-pressure gradient HPLC pump, a fluorescence detector, a Rheodyne injector with a 100 μL loop and an online degasser. Excitation and emission wavelength were 200 nm and 301 nm respectively. Separation was achieved by a Chromolith™ Performance RP-18e 100 × 4.6 mm column (Merck, Darmastadt, Germany) protected by a Chromolith™ guard cartridge RP-18e 5 × 4.6 mm. A methanol: water (adjusted to pH of 2.5 by phosphoric acid) mixture (19:81, v/v) at flow rate of 2 ml/min was used as mobile phase. Data acquisition was carried out by using ChromGate chromatography software (Knauer, Berlin, Germany).

Pharmacokinetic analysis

The pharmacokinetics of tramadol and its metabolites were determined by non-compartmental analysis using Microsoft® EXCEL under Windows XP in both intact animal and isolated rat liver studies. Maximum plasma and perfusate concentrations (C_{max}) of analytes and their

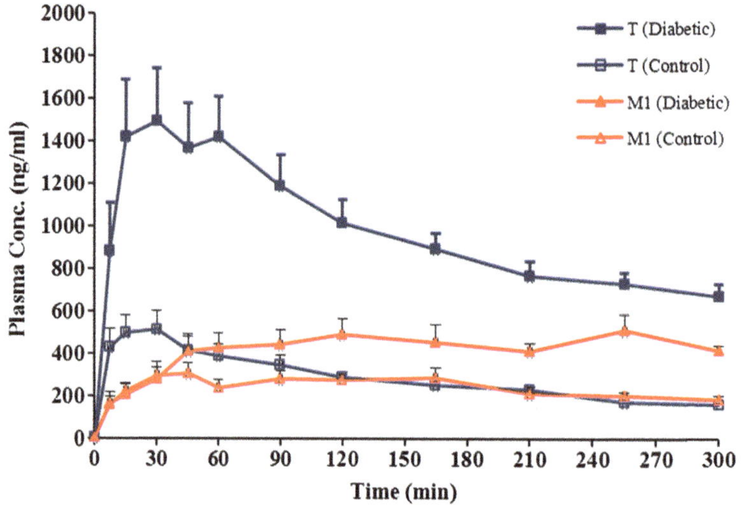

Figure 2 Plasma concentration-time profile of tramadol and M1 in intact control and diabetic rats after receiving a 10 mg/kg of tramadol intraperitoneally (n = 6 in each group, data are presented as mean ± SE).

corresponding times (Tmax) were recorded as observed. Elimination rate constant (β) was estimated as the absolute value of the slope of least-square linear regression of the terminal phase of the logarithmic concentration–time curves. The terminal half-life ($t_{1/2}$) was calculated as 0.693/β. The area under the concentration versus time curve was calculated by the trapezoidal rule for the duration of sampling or last quantifiable concentration and extrapolated from the last point to infinity with β. Plasma clearance for tramadol (CL/F) was calculated as Dose/$AUC_{0-\infty}$. Metabolic ratios for AUCs or concentrations were calculated by dividing the AUC_{0-t} or concentrations of the metabolite by that of tramadol for plasma and perfusate samples.

Statistical evaluation

Data was expressed as mean ± SD. To compare the pharmacokinetic parameters of tramadol and its metabolites in DMIS rats and control group, an unpaired t-test was used for all parameters except T*max*, with which a nonparametric Wilcoxon two-sample test was used. A p-value of less than 0.05 was considered to be statistically significant.

Results and discussion

Studies showed that pharmacokinetic parameters of drugs can change by diabetes mellitus [22,23]. It has been suggested that plasma protein binding of drugs may change because of change in plasma fatty acid levels [9]. Moreover, an intracellular dehydration has been observed in

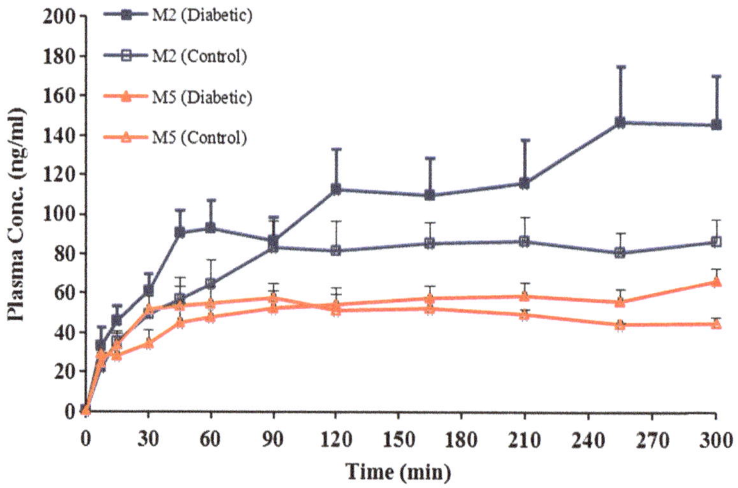

Figure 3 Plasma concentration-time profile of M2 and M5 in intact control and diabetic rats after receiving a 10 mg/kg of tramadol intraperitoneally (n = 6 in each group, data are presented as mean ± SE).

Table 1 Pharmacokinetic parameters of tramadol in diabetic and control rats

Parameter	$AUC_{0\text{-}300min}$ (ng.min/ml)		$AUC_{0\text{-}\infty}$ (ng.min/ml)		K_{el} (1/min)		App. Clearance (ml/min)	
	Control	Diabetic	Control	Diabetic	Control	Diabetic	Control	Diabetic
Mean	88879.2	292661.1	133344.4	548924.4	0.0036	0.0026	22.3	5.5
P Value	<0.05		<0.05		>0.05		<0.05	

male Sprague-Dawley DMIS rats [24]. Consequently both may affect the distribution of drugs in the body.

It has also been reported that cardiac index and the blood flow rate to the diaphragm, abdominal wall and kidney elevate in male Sprague-Dawley DMIS and Carworth Farms E (CFE) rats [25,26]. An increase in most cytochrome p450 isoenzymes activity has also been reported resulting in elevation of metabolites levels in diabetic rats [27].

Tramadol is quickly and almost entirely absorbed after an oral administration in human whereas its mean absolute bioavailability is reported to be only 65–70% as a result of the first-pass hepatic metabolism. The high total distribution volume of around 300 L after oral administration in human is caused by its high tissue affinity and distribution in fat tissues [28]. An enormous amount of tramadol is rapidly metabolized to three main metabolites in Liver. The principal metabolic pathways, *O*- and *N*-desmethylation, involve cytochrome P-450 isoenzyme 2D6, 2B6 and 3A4, respectively. The primary metabolites *O*-desmethyltramadol (M1) and *N*-desmethyltramadol (M2) may be further metabolized to *N, O*-didesmethyltramadol (M5). Ten to thirty percent of the parent drug is excreted unchanged in the urine. Tramadol and its metabolites are almost completely excreted via the kidneys and their biliary excretion is negligible [29].

Animal studies for diabetes especially in rats and mice have been commonly applied streptozocin to provide type 1 diabetes. It has been reported that intravenous administration of a dose ranging from 25 to 100 mg/kg STZ could successfully induce a dose dependent hyperglycemia in rats [30]. In this study, we used a single 60 mg/kg dose of STZ intravenously in order to induce the diabetes in rats.

Intact animals

Six rats completed the study in each group. Mean body weight of rats in two study groups were not statistically different at the beginning (285 ± 12 vs. 295 ± 16 grams in control and treatment groups respectively, $p > 0.05$). While rats in treatment group showed a significant decrease in their body weight during 7 days of diabetes induction (295 ± 16 vs. 235 ± 11 grams respectively, $p < 0.05$), no significant changes was observed in body weight of control group animals during this period. Plasma glucose concentrations measured 7 days from the beginning of the study were significantly increased in animals given streptozotocin, 388.4 ± 164.4 $mgdL^{-1}$ compared with the controls, 102.8 ± 31.1 $mgdL^{-1}$ ($P < 0.05$). Animal in treatment group had much higher water consumption in comparison to control group. Plasma concentration-time profiles of tramadol and M1 are presented in Figure 2 and those of M2 and M5 in Figure 3 respectively. Calculated pharmacokinetic parameters for Tramadol and metabolites are presented in Tables 1 and 2 respectively.

After i.p. injection in intact rats, tramadol was absorbed rapidly in both groups and reached much higher concentrations in diabetic in comparison to control group with a C_{max} of 561.6 ± 111.4 and 1607.5 ± 335.9 ng/ml in control and diabetic rats respectively ($p < 0.05$). However the time to C_{max} (T_{max}) was longer in diabetics compared to control group (36.1 ± 17.1 min vs. 18.2 ± 11.4 min in diabetic and control rats respectively). Much higher area under plasma-concentration-time curve was also observed in diabetics in comparison to control group (292661.1 ± 49048.2 vs. 88879.2 ± 14483.4 $ng.min.ml^{-1}$ respectively, $p < 0.05$). The terminal phase of tramadol plasma concentration-time profile in both groups showed no significant difference in elimination rate constant (0.0036 ± 0.0009 min^{-1} vs. 0.0026 ± 0.0008 min^{-1}) in control and diabetic groups respectively, ($p > 0.05$).

It has been assumed that tramadol is metabolized much more rapidly in animals than in humans, and M1, M2 and M5 are the main metabolites in all species [31]. Our study also confirms that M1, M2 and M5 are formed and M1 remains the major metabolite in rat. However it is not clear if the same enzymes in human and rat are responsible for metabolite formation in these two spices. In the present study, M1 remained the major metabolite of tramadol in both diabetic and non-diabetic intact rats.

Table 2 $AUC_{0\text{-}300min}$ (ng.min/ml) of tramadol metabolites; M1, M2, M5

Parameter	M1		M2		M5	
	Control	Diabetic	Control	Diabetic	Control	Diabetic
Mean	70835.2	124988.4	22447.3	31947.2	14486.2	15505.6
P Value	<0.05		>0.05		>0.05	

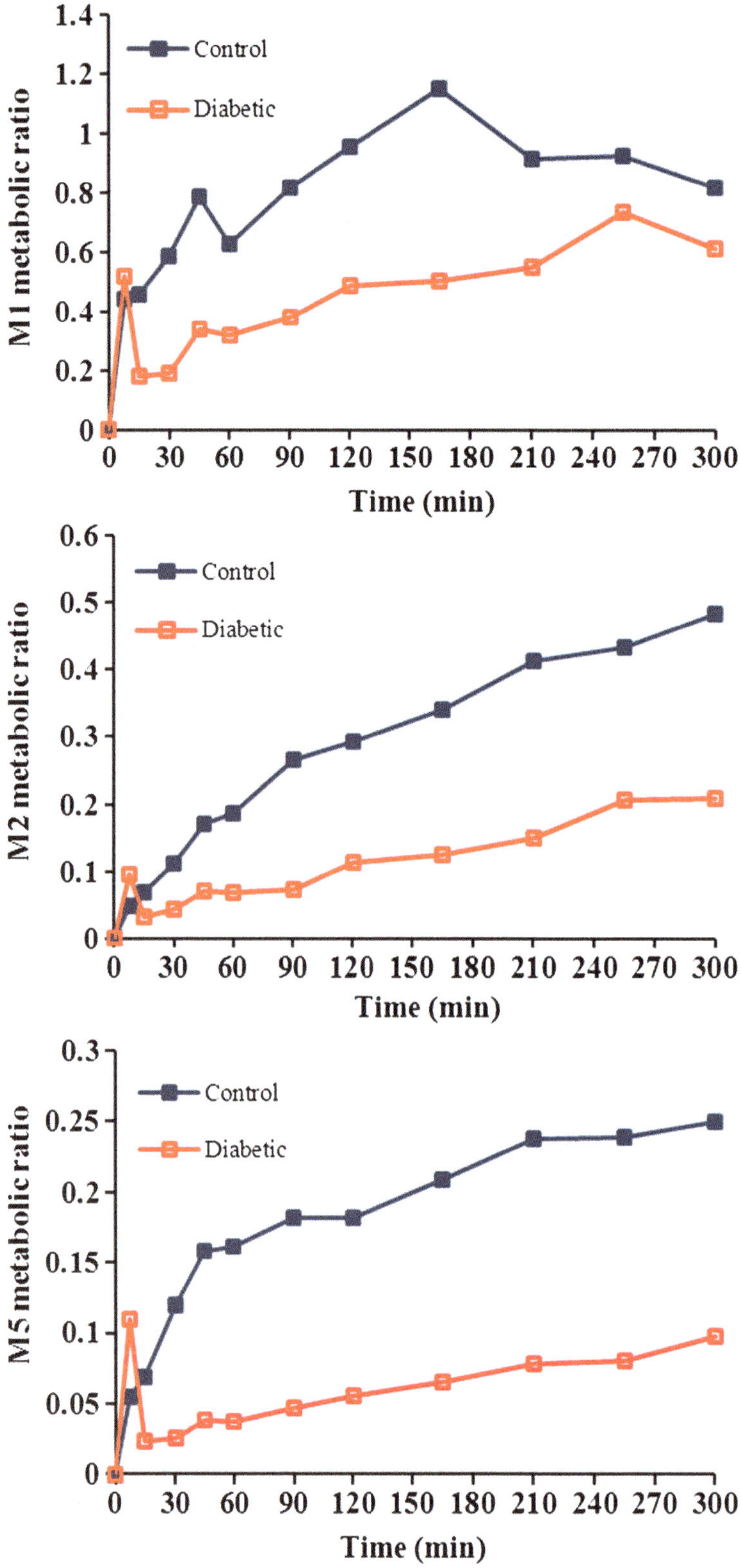

Figure 4 The metabolic ratio for M1, M2 and M5 in intact control and diabetic rats.

Similar to tramadol, the M1 plasma concentrations were higher in diabetic rats compared to control group which resulted in significantly higher AUCs in diabetics (124988.4 ± 33887.3 vs. 70835.2 ± 14341.5 ng.min.ml^{-1} in diabetic and control respectively). In both groups the concentration of M1 reached to an almost constant value in about 90 minutes after drug administration.

Similar to tramadol and M1, M2 showed higher concentrations in diabetics in comparison with control rats. The concentration of M2 in DMIS and control rats was increased up to last sampling point. However the increment trend in M2 concentration was much higher in diabetics resulted in marked increase in AUC of this metabolite in diabetics. As mentioned, diabetic group showed higher concentrations (almost 1.7 times in diabetic group after 300 min compared to control groups) and higher AUCs (31947.2 ± 9923.4 vs. 22447.3 ± 4871.6 ng.min.ml^{-1}) compared to control group. In contrast to M2 and similar to M1, the M5 concentrations reached to a plateau in both groups almost 60 minutes after drug administration and there was no significant differences between AUC of both groups (15505.6 ± 2433.2 vs. 14486.2 ± 2119.4 in diabetic and control respectively) ($p > 0.05$).

As it is clear from above explained data, the diabetes has markedly influenced pharmacokinetic of tramadol and its metabolites in rats. Figures 2 and 3 show that tramadol, M1 and M2 have higher concentrations in diabetic compared to control rats. Considering M1 as major metabolite and induction of its formation in diabetic rats, a reduction in plasma levels and AUC of tramadol

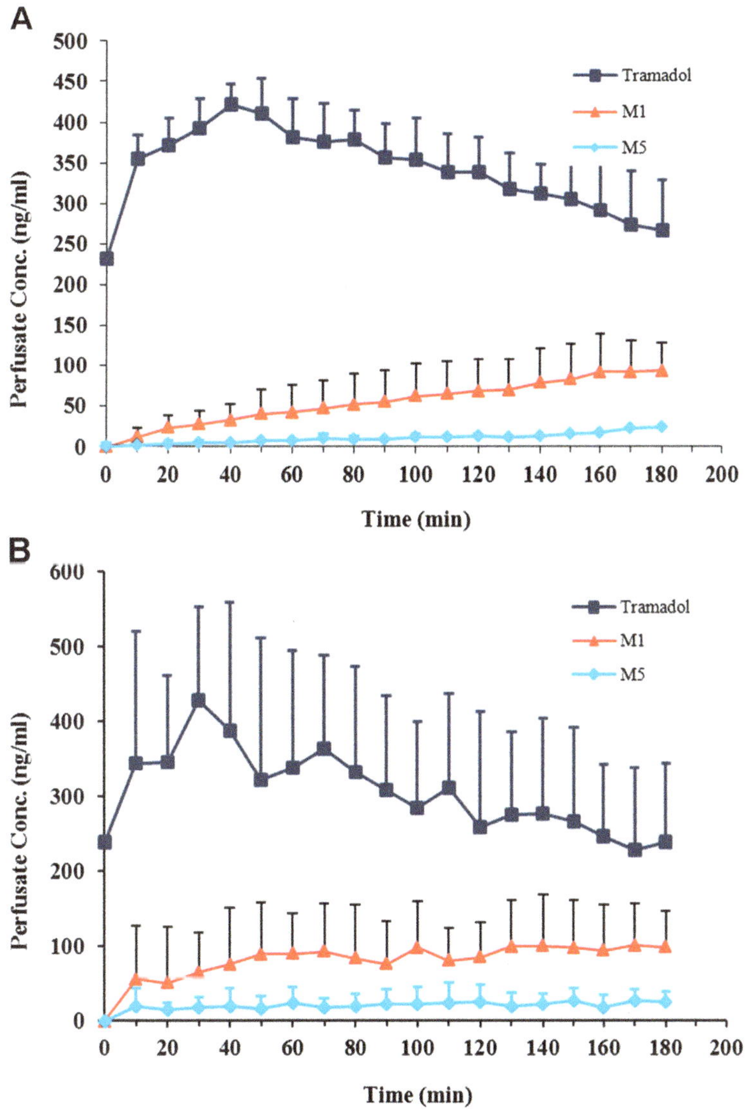

Figure 5 Perfusate concentration-time profile of tramadol, M1 and M5 in control (A) and diabetic (B) isolated rat liver (n = 6, data are presented as mean ± SE).

might be expected. Table 1 show that contrary to our expectation, both $AUC_{0\text{-}300min}$ and $AUC_{0\text{-}\infty}$ of tramadol are significantly higher in diabetic rats. To further pursue this argument, the metabolic ratios were studied for all three metabolites. Figure 4 shows that for all three metabolites, the metabolic ratio is higher in control in comparison to diabetic rats. These higher metabolic ratios in control rats may be caused by higher plasma levels of metabolites or lower tramadol plasma levels in control group. Lower plasma levels of tramadol could be resulted either from higher metabolism rate (contrary to our expectation) or higher distribution volume of the drug in control rats.

Diabetes may change the pattern of distribution of drugs in the body. Tramadol has a high volume of distribution in man [28]. Any reduction in fat tissue (which usually happens during diabetic state) may cause a reduction in volume of distribution of lipophilic drugs such as tramadol. Considering higher lipophilicity of tramadol compared to its metabolites and consequently higher distribution in fat tissue, such a phenomenon may also explain higher plasma concentration of tramadol in diabetic rats. In addition, the higher production level of alph1-acid glycoprotein, an acute-phase serum protein which is prominent in tramadol protein binding, in diabetic condition may further cause in decrease of volume of distribution and increase in plasma concentration of tramadol in diabetic rats. In isolated liver perfusion study, the metabolism of drugs could be investigated when to a high extent the effect of drug binding and distribution volume has been excluded. To further study the metabolic state of tramadol and clear the possible effect of distribution volume and protein binding on metabolite formation and metabolic ratios, an isolated rat liver study was performed in both normal and diabetic rat liver.

Isolated liver study

Six rats completed the study in each group. Similar to intact groups, the body weight and blood glucose levels between two groups were significantly different ($P < 0.05$). Perfusate sample concentrations of tramadol, M1 and M5 measured by HPLC in both groups. Similar to our previous study [20], M2 was not detected in isolated liver study samples. Figure 5 represents perfusate concentration-time profiles of tramadol, M1 and M5 in control and diabetic isolated livers respectively.

Similar to our previous study [20], M1 was the main metabolite formed in both diabetic and control livers and M2 metabolite was not seen (at least in concentrations higher than 2.5 ng/ml) in perfusion study. A comparison between concentration levels of M1 in diabetic and control livers showed that in contrast to intact animals, the metabolic ratios of M1 and M5 (M/T) are significantly higher in diabetic rats compared to those of control group (Figures 4 and 5). This higher metabolic ratio in diabetic livers is the consequence of higher metabolite (M1 and M5) production, a result that could not easily be concluded in intact animal data. So it could be fulfilled that higher metabolic ratios in intact control rats in comparison to intact diabetic rats could be resulted from lower plasma levels of tramadol itself in control group (instead of higher metabolite production) which most possibly has been resulted from higher volume of distribution and lower protein binding of tramadol. To confirm the exact role of distribution volume and even protein binding on tramadol concentration and their effects on metabolic ratios in control and diabetic rats, the PK study of tramadol after iv administration and calculation of exact volume of distribution and clearance (instead of apparent Vd and Cl) is recommended.

Conclusion

In conclusion, the results of this study show that the pharmacokinetic of tramadol and its three metabolites has been influenced by diabetic condition. The higher concentration of M1 could be a result of induction of tramadol to M1 formation pathway, while higher concentrations of tramadol itself can be explained by its lower volume of distribution in diabetic rats.

Competing interests

The authors declare that they have no competing interests.

Authors' contributions

M-RR, YHA , MA, BSH and HL conceived the study. HL, BSH, YHA and LH performed the experimental work. All authors were involved in data analysis and interpretation. HL, BSH and YHA prepared the manuscript. All authors read and approved the final version.

Acknowledgments

This study was supported by a grant from Pharmaceutical Sciences research centre, Tehran University of Medical Sciences. Authors wish to Thank Dr. Hadi Esmaeeli for his technical assistance.

Author details

[1]Biopharmaceutics and Pharmacokinetics Division, Department of Pharmaceutics, Faculty of Pharmacy, Tehran University of Medical Sciences, 14155-6451, Tehran, Iran. [2]Department of Pharmacology and Toxicology, Faculty of Pharmacy, Tehran University of Medical Sciences, 14155-6451, Tehran, Iran. [3]Pharmaceutical Sciences Research Centre, Faculty of Pharmacy, Tehran University of Medical Sciences, 14155-6451, Tehran, Iran.

References

1. Nagata K, Yamazoe Y: **Genetic polymorphism of human cytochrome p450 involved in drug metabolism.** *Drug Metab Pharmacokinet* 2002, **17**:167–189.
2. Waxman DJ: **P450 gene induction by structurally diverse xenochemicals: central role of nuclear receptors CAR, PXR, and PPAR.** *Arch Biochem Biophys* 1999, **369**:11–23.
3. Cheng PY, Morgan ET: **Hepatic cytochrome P450 regulation in disease states.** *Curr Drug Metab* 2001, **2**:165–183.
4. Gwilt PR, Nahhas RR, Tracewell WG: **The effects of diabetes mellitus on pharmacokinetics and pharmacodynamics in humans.** *Clin Pharmacokinet* 1991, **20**:477–490.
5. Pickup JC, Williams G: *Textbook of Diabetes. Volume 1.* Oxford: Blackwell Scientific Publications; 1991:151–155.

6. Carnovale CE, Marinelli RA, Rodríguez Garay EA: **Bile flow decrease and altered bile composition in streptozotocin-treated rats.** *Biochem Pharmacol* 1986, **35:**2625–2628.
7. Watkins JB 3rd, Sherman SE: **Long-term diabetes alters the hepatobiliary clearance of acetaminophen, bilirubin and digoxin.** *J Pharmacol Exp Ther* 1992, **260:**1337–1343.
8. Park JM, Moon CH, Lee MG: **Pharmacokinetic changes of methotrexate after intravenous administration to streptozotocin-induced diabetes mellitus rats.** *Res Commun Mol Pathol Pharmacol* 1996, **93:**343–352.
9. Nadai M, Yoshizumi H, Kuzuya T, Hasegawa T, Johno I, Kitazawa S: **Effect of diabetes on disposition and renal handling of cefazolin in rats.** *Drug Metab Dispos* 1990, **18:**565–570.
10. Price VF, Schulte JM, Spaethe SM, Jollow DJ: **Mechanism of fasting-induced suppression of acetaminophen glucuronidation in the rat.** *Adv Exp Med Biol* 1986, **197:**697–706.
11. Dong ZG, Hong JY, Ma QA, Li DC, Bullock J, Gonzalez FJ, Park SS, Gelboin HV, Yang CS: **Mechanism of induction of cytochrome P-450 ac (P-450j) in chemically induced and spontaneously diabetic rats.** *Arch Biochem Biophys* 1988, **263:**29–35.
12. Thummel KE, Schenkman JB: **Effects of testosterone and growth hormone treatment on hepatic microsomal P450 expression in the diabetic rat.** *Mol Pharmacol* 1990, **37:**119–129.
13. Raza H, Ahmed I, Lakhani MS, Sharma AK, Pallot D, Montague W: **Effect of bitter melon (Momordica charantia) fruit juice on the hepatic cytochrome P450-dependent monooxygenases and glutathione S-transferases in streptozotocin-induced diabetic rats.** *Biochem Pharmacol* 1996, **52:**1639–1642.
14. Raza H, Ahmed I, John A, Sharma AK: **Modulation of xenobiotic metabolism and oxidative stress in chronic streptozotocin-induced diabetic rats fed with Momordica charantia fruit extract.** *J Biochem Mol Toxicol* 2000, **14:**131–139.
15. Wu WN, McKown LA, Liao S: **Metabolism of the analgesic drug ULTRAM (Tramadol hydrochloride) in humans: API-MS and MS/MS characterization of metabolites.** *Xenobiotica* 2002, **32:**411–425.
16. Chong MS, Hester J: **Diabetic painful neuropathy: current and future treatment options.** *Drugs* 2007, **67:**569–585.
17. Freeman R, Raskin P, Hewitt DJ, Vorsanger GJ, Jordan DM, Xiang J, Rosenthal NR: **Randomized study of Tramadol/acetaminophen versus placebo in painful diabetic peripheral neuropathy.** *Curr Med Res Opin* 2007, **23:**147–161.
18. Cheng JT, Liu IM, Chi TC, Tzeng TF, Lu FH, Chang CJ: **Plasma glucose-lowering effect of Tramadol in streptozotocin-induced diabetic rats.** *Diabetes* 2001, **50:**2815–2821.
19. Park JH, Lee WI, Yoon WH, Park YD, Lee JS, Lee MG: **Pharmacokinetic and pharmacodynamic changes of furosemide after intravenous and oral administration to rats with alloxan-induced diabetes mellitus.** *Biopharm Drug Dispos* 1998, **19:**357–364.
20. Rouini MR, Ghazi-Khansari M, Ardakani YH, Dasian Z, Lavasani H: **A Disposition Kinetic Study in Rat perfused Liver.** *Biopharm Drug Dispos* 2008, **29:**231–235.
21. Ardakani YH, Rouini MR: **Improved liquid chromatographic method for the simultaneous determination of Tramadol and its three main metabolites in human plasma, urine and saliva.** *J Pharm Biomed Anal* 2007, **44:**1168–1173.
22. Chang FY, Lee SD, Yeh GH, Wang PS: **Hyperglycaemia is responsible for the Inhibited gastrointestinal transit in the early diabetic rat.** *Acta Physiol Scand* 1995, **155:**457–462.
23. Xie W, Xing D, Zhao Y, Su H, Meng Z, Chen Y, Du L: **A new tactic to treat postprandial hyperlipidemia in diabetic rats with gastroparesis by improving gastrointestinal transit.** *Eur J Pharmacol* 2005, **510:**113–120.
24. Anwana AB, Garland HO: **Intracellular dehydration in the rat made diabetic with streptozotocin: effects of infusion.** *J Endocrinol* 1991, **128:**333–337.
25. Hill MA, Larkins RG: **Alterations in distribution of cardiac output in experimental diabetes in rats.** *Am J Physiol* 1989, **257:**H571–H580.
26. Lucas PD, Foy JM: **Effects of experimental diabetes and genetic obesity on regional blood flow in the rat.** *Diabetes* 1977, **26:**786–792.
27. Lee JH, Yang SH, Oh JM, Lee MG: **Pharmacokinetics of drugs in rats with diabetes mellitus induced by alloxan or streptozocin: comparison with those in patients with type I diabetes mellitus.** *J Pharm Pharmacol* 2010, **62:**1–23.
28. Lewis KS, Han NH: **Tramadol: a new centrally acting analgesic.** *Am J Health Syst Pharm* 1999, **54:**643–652.
29. Budd K, Langford R: **Tramadol revisited.** *Br J Anaesth* 1999, **82:**493–495.
30. Hayashi K, Kojima R, Ito M: **Strain differences in the diabetogenic activity of streptozotocin in mice.** *Biol Pharmaceut Bull* 2006, **29:**1110–1119.
31. Lintz W, Erlacin S, Frankus E: **Biotransformation of Tramadol in man and animal.** *Arzneimittelforschung* 1981, **31:**1932–1943.

Determination of the role of calcium on instability of neurotoxic metabolite of ecstasy by HPTLC-mass

Bardia Jamali[1], Yalda Hosseinzadeh Ardakani[1], Mohammad-Reza Rouini[1], Alireza Foroumadi[2], Salimeh Amidi[3], Vahid Hossein Zadeh Aghdam[4] and Farzad Kobarfard[3*]

Abstract

Background: Ecstasy is one of the popular illicit drugs in the world and its usage has been recently increased in Iran. This compound can destroy the serotonergic neurons and produces cognitive and psychopathology diseases. 3,4-dihydroxymethamphetamine (HHMA) which is the main metabolite of this compound, seems to be responsible for this effect. However, no consensus has been reached among the researchers about its role. This disagreement between the researches may be due to failure in determination of HHMA as free form in physiological fluids. In this study, the stability of this crucial metabolite of ecstasy was examined in different mediums.

Methods: The stability of HHMA was studied in the perfusion medium and water at 100 and 10 ng/mL concentrations. Moreover, the effect of temperature (0–25°C), pH (3–10), calcium chloride (0–150 g/L) and ethylenediaminetetraacetic acid (EDTA) on the stability of HHMA was also examined.

Results: Our result suggested that the free form of HHMA could be degraded in the perfusion medium. The rate of this degradation has direct proportion to temperature (at 25°C = 0.037 min^{-1} and at 0°C = 0.002 min^{-1}). Calcium chloride and sodium bicarbonate are two responsible components in this instability. Moreover, the alkaline pHs and increasing the shaking time can accelerate this effect. Although, while degradation was prevented at pH=3, EDTA could only reduce this rate about 30%.

Conclusions: Calcium cation can act as an accelerator of HHMA degradation. Therefore, the perfusion medium should not contain Ca^{2+} and the pH of medium is better to be adjusted at acidic range. Since, the internal cellular source of calcium is endoplasmic reticulum system, it can be assumed that, this cation may change HHMA and dopamine to reactive compounds that can bind covalently to the cysteinyl group of biological compounds and damage cellular components.

Keywords: HHMA, HPTLC-MS, Stability, Calcium chloride, Neurotoxicity

Introduction

Ecstasy (3,4-methylenedioxymethamphetamine, MDMA) is one of the popular drugs of abuse among youths. The tendency toward this compound has increased since the last two decades [1,2]. In 2009, it was reported that 2.8 million of Americans over 12 years old have abused MDMA at least once [3]. The usage of this compound has been recently increased among Iranian youths as well [4,5].

MDMA is a releaser and reuptake inhibitor of serotonin and dopamine which can destroy serotonin axon terminal of brain and produces cognitive dysfunction and psychopathology diseases in humans. However, the mechanism behind this phenomenon is not clearly known [2,6,7]. It was reported that the intracranial administration of MDMA in animals does not produce any neurotoxic effects. However, the peripheral administration can do so [7]. This result and some other reports

* Correspondence: kobarfard@sbmu.ac.ir
[3]Department of Medicinal Chemistry, School of Pharmacy, Shahid Beheshti University of Medical Sciences, Tehran, Iran
Full list of author information is available at the end of the article

proposed that MDMA metabolites may have a role in its neurotoxic activity [7,8].

MDMA is metabolized via either O-demethylation or N-dealkylation in humans and rats. N-dealkylation pathways produce 3,4-methylenedioxyamphetamine (MDA) which is known as "Love drug" and has similar pharmacological effects to MDMA [1]. O-demethylation produces reactive catechol metabolite, i.e. 3,4-dihydroxymethamphetamine (HHMA) (Figure 1). HHMA is the main metabolite of MDMA in urine and plasma which exist in conjugated form (sulfate and glutathione) and there is no report for determination of its free form in biological fluids [2,7]. It has been reported that HHMA conjugated with glutathione could produce apoptosis on rat hipocampal neurons [8].

Over the years, different reports have been published about the neurotoxicity associated with MDMA metabolites. Some reports proposed that MDA is responsible for such an effect [6] and the others have introduced HHMA and thioether adducts as the toxic metabolite which cause apoptosis and damage in the cells [7,8]. This controversy may be due to the failure in determination of HHMA as a free form in brain after MDMA administration.

HHMA, due to its catecholamine structure, can display various properties. The catecholamine moiety is prone to oxidation and formation of ortho quinone-like structure. Oxidizing agents such as ClO^-, MnO_4^- and etc., alkaline pHs and light can trigger this reaction [9]. Moreover, MDA can also be O-demethylated and form another metabolite with catecholamine structure which can exert similar properties with HHMA [2]. To the best of our knowledge, there are no reports about HHMA stability in physiological fluids and there are only some reports regarding the stability of dopamine which has the closest structure to HHMA. These reports indicate that dopamine, in the presence of oxidizing agents like Mn^{3+} or $NaIO_4$, is converted to the reactive compounds such as aminochrome (AC), indole-5,6-quinone and 5,6-dihydroxyindole. These reactive compounds can bind covalently to the cysteinyl group of biological compounds in the body and damage cellular components such as DNA, proteins and lipids. The role of these reactive compounds in Alzheimer's and Parkinson's has been established (Figure 2) [10,11].

Due to the ethical and safety issues, studying the metabolism changes of illicit or toxic compounds at high concentration in human subjects is constrained. Therefore, the kinetic of these compounds is preferred to be studied in similar systems to human such as isolated animal organs. In these cases, the perfusion medium is used instead of plasma [12]. However, the stability of the compounds and their related metabolites in the perfusion medium is of important concern. Since MDMA is an illicit compound and can cause multi organ failure, especially liver damage and death at high concentrations [13], its metabolic transformation is preferred to be studied in intact animals or in in vitro perfused organs.

In the present study, stability of HHMA in perfusion medium was examined. The constituents of this medium appear in almost all of physiological fluids of human body. Determination of the possible effect of these constituents on the stability of HHMA free form could help researcher to determine the role of HHMA in MDMA neurotoxicity.

Materials and methods

Chemicals

Ultrapure water was obtained from Millipore Direct-Q system (France). HHMA was synthesized in four steps, from commercially available 3,4-dimethoxy-benzaldehyde and nitroethane, through procedures previously reported [8]. Dopamine was a gift from Caspian Tamin Pharmaceutical Company. HPLC (high performance

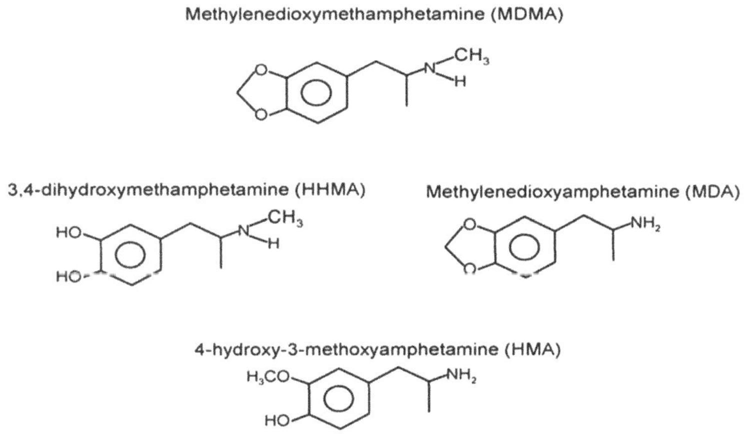

Figure 1 Structure of MDMA and its metabolites.

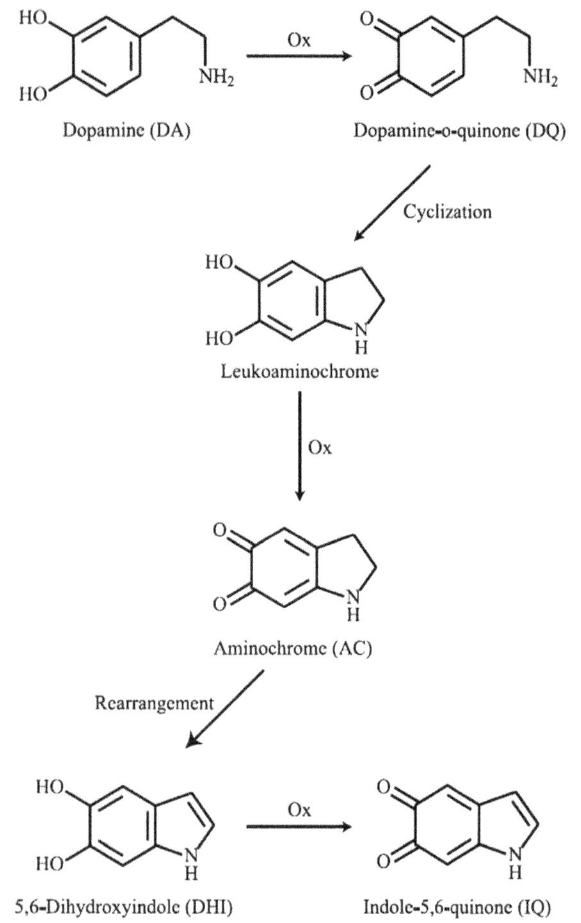

Figure 2 The oxidation pathway of dopamine [10].

liquid chromatography) grade methanol and all other chemicals of analytical grade were purchased from Merck (Darmstadt, Germany). The Krebs buffer (6.903 g/L NaCl, 0.335 g/L KCl, 0.162 g/L KH_2PO_4, 0.163 g/L $MgSO_4$, 0.305 g/L $CaCl_2$, 2.1 g/L $NaHCO_3$ and 1 g/L glucose, pH was adjusted to 7.2-7.4) was used as a perfusion medium.

Apparatuses and chromatographic conditions

The Knauer chromatographic system which was used, consisted of a pump model K-1001, a fluorescence detector (FL) model RF-10AXL, a photodiode array (PDA) detector model K-2800, a solvent degasser and a 100 μl loop injector. EZChrom Elite software was used for instrument control, data acquisition and analysis. The separation of analytes was performed at ambient temperature (25°C) on the Chromolith® Performance RP-18e (100 × 4.6 mm) column with Chromolith® RP-18e (5 × 4.6 mm) guard from Merck (Darmstadt, Germany). The FL detector wavelength was fixed at 285 nm for excitation and at 320 nm for emission and PDA wavelength was fixed at 285 nm. The mobile phase was 0.02 M potassium dihydrogen phosphate (KH_2PO_4) solution with pH = 3 (orthophosphoric acid was used for pH adjustment).

The Cecil UV spectrophotometer model CE9500 and Camag high performance thin layer chromatographic (HPTLC) system consisted of a Camag TLC Scanner 3, a TLC automatic developing chamber and a Camag automatic TLC Sampler 4 with a PDA and FL detectors, were used. In the HPTLC system, the separation was performed on HPTLC plates coated with silicagel 60 F_{254} (10 × 10 cm) from Merck (Darmstadt, Germany). A mixture of dioxane:methanol:chloroform:acid acetic (6:1:1:1,v/v/v/v) was used as the mobile phase. The instrument was controlled and the data were analyzed by winCATS planar chromatography manager software. TLC plates developed by HPTLC were subjected for TLC-Mass spectrometry using a 1200 Agilent HPLC pump coupled to a Agilent electrospray ionization (ESI) mass detector (6410 Triple Quadrupole) through a Camag TLC-MS interface. Methanol was used for elution of TLC spots to the mass detector. The mass detector was operated in positive mode (ESI+) and the fragmentor voltage was 60 V. Detection was performed in full scan mode.

Stability study

The stability of five replicate samples of HHMA at concentrations of 100 and 10 ng/mL, at ambient temperature (25°C) and 0°C, in both perfusion medium and water was examined for 24 hours. In the case of perfusion medium, the stability was checked at 0, 5, 15, 30, 60, 120 and 180 min, and in the case of water, samples were taken at 0, 5, 15, 30, 60, 120, 180, 240 min and 24 hours. These samples were analyzed by the HPLC/FL for the determination of HHMA residual in corresponding medium.

The impact of perfusion medium components on HHMA stability was examined separately on 5 replicate samples (at a concentration appeared in perfusion medium) of the 100 ng/mL aqueous solution of HHMA. Samples were analyzed immediately after dissolving the component by the HPLC/FL and were compared with the 100 ng/mL freshly prepared samples of HHMA in water. The influence of pH (3–10) and different concentration (up to saturated concentration) of ethylenediaminetetraacetic acid (EDTA) on the stability of HHMA in perfusion medium was also investigated.

Moreover, the stability of HHMA in water in the presence of calcium chloride ($CaCl_2$) (concentration 0–150 g/L) was studied. Samples were analyzed by HPLC/UV immediately after the changes were made and the results were compared with the results obtained for freshly prepared samples of HHMA in corresponding medium. This part was done on 5 replicate samples of 1 μg/mL solution of HHMA.

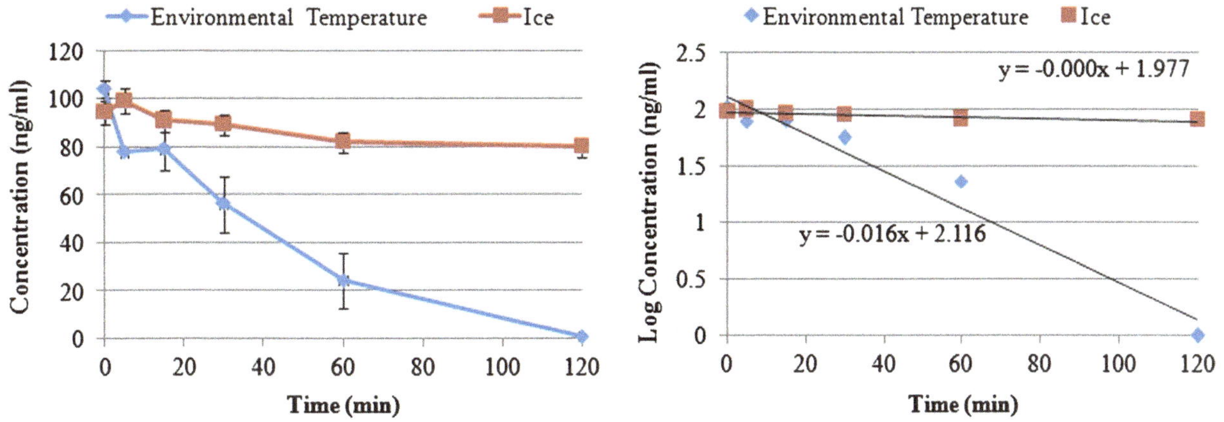

Figure 3 The degradation rate of 100 ng/mL solution of HHMA in perfusion medium at ambient temperature and 0°C. Points shown as mean ± SD, n=5.

The effect of $CaCl_2$ (150 g/L) on the stability of HHMA aqueous solution (1 µg/mL) was also examined by HPTLC system on 3 replicate samples.

In another part of the present study, those components which were supposed to be responsible for instability of HHMA in perfusion medium were also examined, for their impact on the stability of dopamine (1 µg/mL aqueous solutions).

Statistics

The t-independent test was used for determination of differences between means of groups ($P < 0.05$).

Results and discussion

The 100 and 10 ng/mL solutions of HHMA in water were stable at ambient temperature and 0°C for 24 hours. No significant differences between area under the curve (AUC) of peak of freshly prepared samples and tests were observed ($n = 5$, $P > 0.05$), whereas the 100 and 10 ng/mL solutions of HHMA in perfusion medium were unstable. After 2 hours, about 100% of the 100 ng/mL solution of HHMA was degraded at ambient temperature ($K_{degradation}$ = 0.037 min^{-1} (0.030-0.047) at 25°C) and a new small peak appeared in the HPLC/FL chromatogram. Reduction of the temperature to 0°C could reduce the rate of degradation, so that after 2 hours, only about 20% of the 100 ng/mL solution of HHMA was degraded ($K_{degradation}$ = 0.002 min^{-1} (0.0006-0.003) at 0°C) (Figure 3). In the case of 10 ng/mL solution of HHMA in perfusion medium, the similar pattern was observed.

While the reduction of pH to 3 could stop the degradation reaction, increasing the pH could accelerate degradation rate, in such a way that the corresponding peak to HHMA in HPLC/FL or HPLC/UV chromatograms disappeared rapidly after pH was reached to 9. The HHMA peak disappearance was permanent and by reducing the pH of the alkaline samples to 3, the HHMA peak did not appear again (Figure 4).

Our results were in accordance with Gouarne et al. report [14]. They reported that the degradation rate of

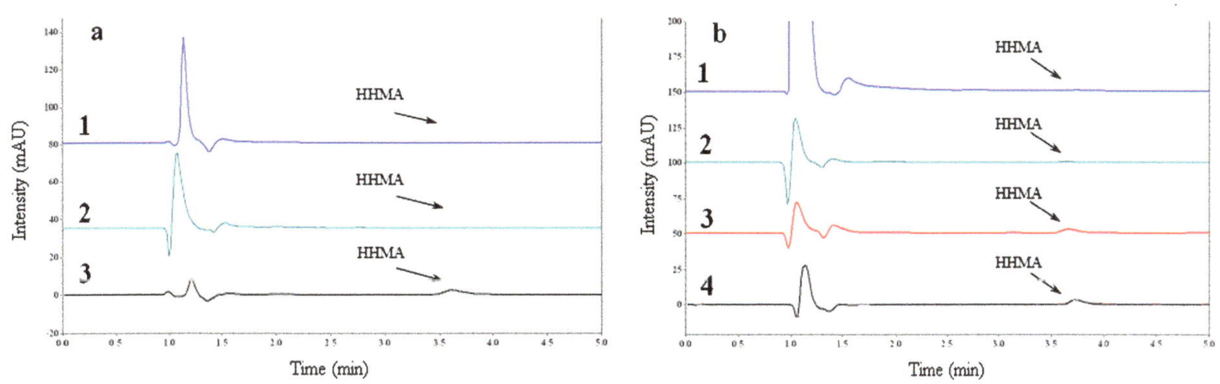

Figure 4 The effect of pH on degradation of HHMA (1 µg/mL) in water (a) and perfusion medium (b) at ambient temperature. a1: at pH=9; a2: changing the pH of alkaline sample to 3; a3: at pH=3; b1: at pH=9; b2: changing the pH of alkaline sample to 3; b3: at pH=3; b4: at pH=7.3.

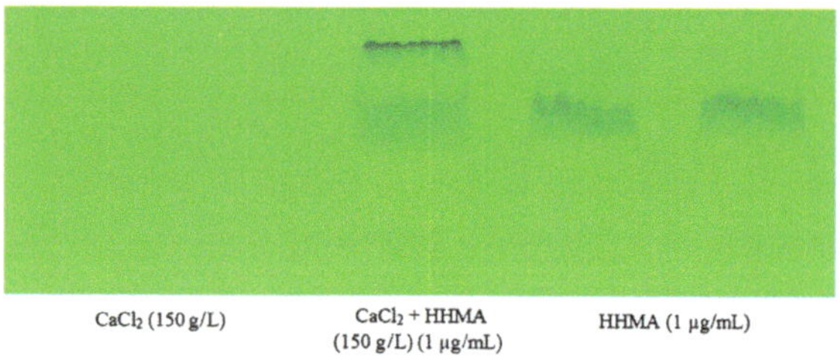

Figure 5 The HPTLC chromatogram of HHMA (1 µg/mL) in water and in the presence of $CaCl_2$ (150 g/L).

catecholamins is in direct proportion with pH of medium. The hydroxyl groups in the catecholamine structure deprotonate easier at pHs higher than 3 and form the corresponding quinone structure readily. At high pHs, quinine structures are susceptible to oxidation, cyclization and polymerization [10,11]. It should be mentioned that the pH of aqueous solutions of HHMA was about 3 and perhaps due to this reason, HHMA has been stable in these aqueous solutions.

Adding EDTA to the HHMA solution in perfusion medium, even at a saturated concentration could only reduce the rate of degradation about 30%. It has been reported that $MgCl_2$ and $CaCl_2$ enhances the oxidation of ascorbate [15]. EDTA, due to its chelating property, can reduce the rate of oxidation reaction by sequestering the Ca^{2+} and Mg^{2+}, but this chelator was not effective in inhibition of HHMA peak reduction.

In order to further investigate this phenomenon, the components of perfusion medium (at their concentrations in perfusion medium) were added to HHMA aqueous solution separately. Adding $MgSO_4$, NaCl, KCl, KH_2PO_4 or glucose did not affect the AUC of HHMA peak even after 2 hours. These results indicated that Mg^{2+}, which is a crucial cation in Catechol-O-methyltransferase (COMT, an enzymes that play a role in catecholamine degradation) activity [16] and can bind to hydroxyl ring of catecholamine at pHs higher than 7 [17], has no effect on HHMA instability. However, $CaCl_2$ and $NaHCO_3$ were the components which caused HHMA concentration to reduce. In case of $NaHCO_3$, the reduction of HHMA concentration was expected due to its ability in increasing the pH of solutions. However, the observed rate for concentration reduction of HHMA, was slower than the observed rate for HHMA in perfusion medium. In addition to $NaHCO_3$, $CaCl_2$ could cause reduction in concentration of HHMA in aqueous solution. When the concentration of $CaCl_2$ increased from 0.3 to 150 g/L, the AUC of HHMA peak reduced faster. Moreover, increasing the shaking time from 5 to 60 seconds reduced the AUC of HHMA peak, significantly.

The HPTLC analysis of HHMA aqueous solution in the presence of $CaCl_2$ showed that a new spot appeared in the chromatogram after adding $CaCl_2$ (150 g/L) with the Rf = 0.25. This spot did not exist in the chromatograms of HHMA or $CaCl_2$ aqueous solutions alone. Mass spectroscopic analysis of this spot on a triple quadruple mass detector revealed that its molecular weight is different from that of HHMA. Moreover, the UV spectrum of this spot was different from the UV spectrum of HHMA aqueous solution (Figures 5 and 6). The same results were obtained in all replication. These results indicated that HHMA has changed to other

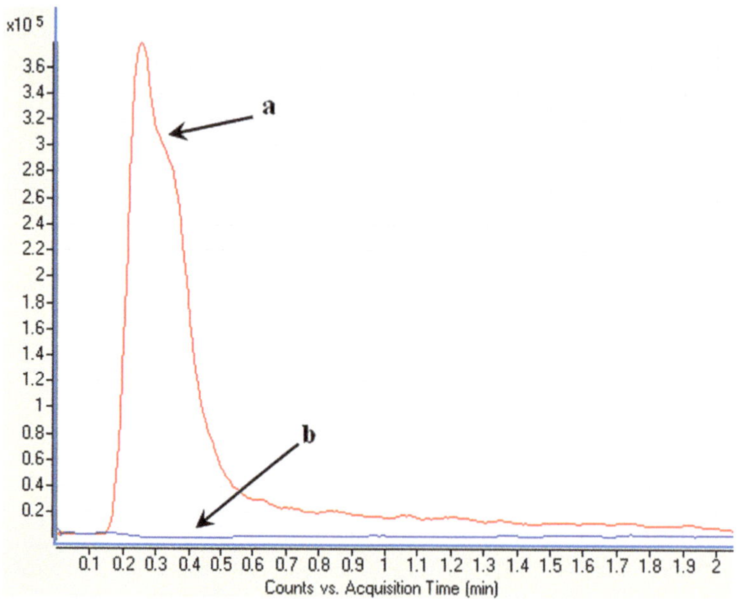

Figure 6 Extracted ion chromatogram at (*m/z* 182) of HHMA (1 µg/mL) in the absence (a) and in the presence (b) of $CaCl_2$ (150 g/L).

compounds in the presence of $CaCl_2$. There are no reports in the literature about a direct role of $CaCl_2$ in oxidation of catecolamines. It seems that Cl^- has no impact on stability of HHMA, because adding NaCl could not reduce the AUC of HHMA peak over 2 hours. It could be speculated that calcium cation (Ca^{2+}), due to free d-orbital in its electronic configuration, can act as a catalyst or something like that in this phenomenon, but magnesium cation (Mg^{2+}), due to the lack of this free d-orbital, cannot play such role.

It has been reported that HHMA can be oxidized to related ortho quinone compounds that react with nucleophilic groups of macromolecules or form neurotoxins [8,18]. Moreover, HHMA can change to carbene intermediate and covalently bind to heme iron of CYP2D6 in the biological systems [18,19]. Beside HHMA, dopamine, which is structurally the most similar compound to HHMA, is oxidized in the presence of MnO_2 and $NaIO_4$ to the reactive ortho quinone compounds which covalently bind to cysteinyl group of proteins and impair their functions. Moreover, reactive ortho quinone compounds are responsible for neurodegenerative process of dopaminergic system. When the oxidizing agents were added to the aqueous solutions of dopamine, the absorption intensity at λ = 280 nm decreased and two new peaks appeared at λ = 300 and 475 nm in the UV spectrum, which were associated with AC structure [10,11]. The similar pattern changes were reported in the UV spectrum of HHMA when oxidized electrochemicaly [8]. In our study, such a phenomenon was observed when the $CaCl_2$ was added to aqueous solution of dopamine. In the UV spectrum when $CaCl_2$ (150 g/L) was added to 1 μg/mL dopamine aqueous solution, the intensity of the absorption at λ = 276 nm decreased, and after 10 min a new peak at λ = 294 and a small peak at about 455 nm appeared.

In light of the above observations, it could be speculated that HHMA, in the presence of $CaCl_2$, is oxidized to its corresponding aminochrome like structures. Therefore, in study of MDMA effect on isolated organs, the perfusion medium should not contain $CaCl_2$ or Ca^{2+}. However, calcium cation has a crucial role in cell biological activity, vesicle movement and exocytosis [20]. The total vesicular concentration of Ca^{2+} is about 1.6 g/L and the main internal source of this cation is endoplasmic reticulum. In addition to, CYP450 isoenzymes are located and activated in endoplasmic reticulum. Therefore, the role of this cation in generating reactive ortho quinonic compounds and neurotoxicity associated with MDMA could be speculated.

Conclusion

Serotonin neuron damage which is related to the MDMA metabolites is one of crucial aspect of MDMA side effects. Different reports have been published about this effect, some of them suggesting HHMA as the neurotoxic metabolite of MDMA, while other reports suggest MDA as the neurotoxin. One of the possible reasons for this controversy can be due to failure in HHMA determination as a free form in these studies.

The results of our study indicated that Ca^{2+} besides sodium bicarbonate can be responsible components in HHMA concentration reduction in perfusion medium. In order to obtain reliable results in these cases, the perfusion medium should not contain Ca^{2+} and the pH of medium is better to be adjusted at acidic range. Moreover, Ca^{2+}can play a role in dopamine conversion to AC, which has a distinctive role in neurodegenerative process of dopaminergic system. In summary, it would be possible that Ca^{2+} accelerates HHMA degradation or plays a role in producing neurodegenerative diseases associated with dopamine or MDMA neurotoxicity.

Competing interests

The authors declare that they have no competing interests.

Authors' contributions

M-RR, YHA and BJ conceived the study. AF synthesized the required chemicals which were not available from chemical companies, BJ, YHA, SA, VHZA and FK performed the experimental work. All authors were involved in data analysis and interpretation. BJ, M-RR and FK drafted the manuscript. All authors read and approved the final version.

Acknowledgments

This work was part of a PhD thesis supported by Tehran University of Medical Sciences and was supported by a grant from Iran National Science Foundation (INSF).

Author details

[1]Department of Pharmaceutics, Biopharmaceutics and Pharmacokinetics Division, Faculty of Pharmacy, Tehran University of Medical Sciences, Tehran, Iran. [2]Drug design and Development Research Center, Tehran University of Medical Sciences, Tehran, Iran. [3]Department of Medicinal Chemistry, School of Pharmacy, Shahid Beheshti University of Medical Sciences, Tehran, Iran. [4]Central Research Laboratories, Shahid Beheshti University of Medical Sciences, Tehran, Iran.

References

1. Kreth K, Kovar K, Schwab M, Zanger UM: **Identification of the human cytochromes P450 involved in the oxidative metabolism of "ecstasy"-related designer drugs.** *Biochem Pharmacol* 2000, **59:**1563–1571.
2. De la Torre R, Farre M, Roset PN, Pizarro N, Abanades S, Segura M, Segura J, Cami J: **Human pharmacology of MDMA: pharmacokinetics, metabolism, and disposition.** *Ther Drug Monit* 2004, **26:**137–144.
3. National Institute on Drug Abuse (NIDA); 2011. http://www.drugabuse.gov/DrugPages/MDMA.html accessed in 1 September.
4. Sadeghi R, Agin K, Taherkhani M, Najm-Afshar L, Nelson LS, Abdollahi M, Shadnia S: **Report of methamphetamine use and cardiomyopathy in three patients.** *DARU Journal of Pharmaceutical Sciences* 2012, **20:**20–24.
5. Mehrpour O: **Methamphetamin abuse a new concern in Iran.** *DARU Journal of Pharmaceutical Sciences* 2012, **20:**73.
6. Mueller M, Yuan J, Felim A, Neudorffer A, Peters FT, Maurer HH, McCann UD, Largeron M, Ricaurte GA: **Further studies on the role of metabolites in (±)-3,4-methylenedioxymethamphetamine-induced serotonergic neurotoxicity.** *Drug Metab Dispos* 2009, **37:**2079–2086.
7. Segura M, Ortuno J, Farre M, McLure JA, Pujadas M, Pizarro N, Llebaria A, Joglar J, Roset PN, Segura J, De la Torre R: **3,4-**

Dihydroxymethamphetamine (HHMA). a major in vivo 3,4-methylenedioxymethamphetamine (MDMA) metabolite in humans. *Chem Res Toxicol* 2001, **14**:1203–1208.

8. Felim A, Neudörffer A, Monnet FP, Largeron M: **Environmentally friendly expeditious one-pot electrochemical synthesis of bis-catechol-thioether metabolites of ecstasy: in vitro neurotoxic effects in the rat hippocampus.** *Int J Electrochem Sci* 2008, **3**:266–281.
9. Ghanayem NS, Yee L, Nelson T, Wong S, Gordon JB, Marcdante K, Rice TB: **Stability of dopamine and epinephrine solutions up to 84 hours.** *Pediatr Crit Care Med* 2001, **2**:315–317.
10. Bisaglia M, Mammi S, Bubacco L: **Kinetic and structural analysis of the early oxidation products of dopamine analysis of the interaction with α-synuclein.** *J Biol Chem* 2007, **282**:15597–15605.
11. Barreto WJ, Ponzoni S, Sassi P: **A Raman and UV–vis study of catecholamines oxidized with Mn (III).** *Spectrochim Acta A* 1999, **55**:65–72.
12. Dostalek M, Pistovcakova J, Minarikova V, Jurica J, Tomandl J, Hadasova E: **Effect of acute and repeated administration of methamphetamine on the activity of CYP2D in isolated perfused rat liver.** *Acta Vet Brno* 2005, **74**:339–345.
13. Kłys M, Rojek S, Wozniak K, Rzepecka-Wozniak E: **Fatality due to the use of a designer drug MDMA (ecstasy).** *Leg Med* 2007, **9**:185–191.
14. Gouarne C, Foury A, Duclos M: **Critical study of common conditions of storage of glucocorticoids and catecholamines in 24-h urine collected during resting and exercising conditions.** *Clinica Chimica Acta* 2004, **348**:207–214.
15. Alegria AE, Sanchez-Cruz P, Rivas L: **Alkaline-earth cations enhance Ortho-quinone-catalyzed ascorbate oxidation.** *Free Radic Biol Med* 2004, **37**:1631–1639.
16. Mannisto PT, Kaakkola S: **Catechol-O-methyltransferase (COMT): biochemistry, molecular biology, pharmacology and clinical efficacy of the new selective COMT inhibitors.** *Pharmacol Rev* 1999, **51**:593–628.
17. Granot J: **Nuclear magnetic resonance studies of catecholamines, ternary complexes with adenosine 5′-triphosphate and divalent metal ions in aqueous solution.** *J Am Chem Soc* 1978, **100**:2886–2891.
18. Heydari A, Yeo KR, Lennard MS, Ellis SW, Tucker GT, Rostami-Hodjegan A: **Mechanism-based inactivation of CYP2D6 by methylenedioxymethamphetamine.** *Drug Metab Dispos* 2004, **32**:1213–1217.
19. Bertelsen KM, Venkatakrishnan K, Von Moltke LL, Obach RS, Greenblatt DJ: **Apparent mechanism-based inhibition of human CYP2D6 in vitro by Paroxetine: comparison with fluoxetine and quinidine.** *Drug Metab Dispos* 2003, **31**:289–293.
20. Borges R, Domínguez N, Estévez-Herrera J, Pereda D, Machado JD: **Vesicular Ca^{2+} mediates granule motion and exocytosis.** *Cell Calcium* 2012, **51**:338–341.

The efficacy of magnesium sulfate loading on microalbuminuria following SIRS: One step forward in dosing

Bahador Mirrahimi[1], Hadi Hamishehkar[2], Arezo Ahmadi[3], Mohamad Reza Mirjalili[4], Mostafa Aghamohamadi[5], Atabak Najafi[6], Mohammad Abdollahi[6] and Mojtaba Mojtahedzahed[1*]

Abstract

Backgrounds: Magnesium has been known for its antioxidative and antiinflammatory properties in many studies. In this study two dosing regimens of magnesium were compared with a placebo control group in order to investigate safety and efficacy of high doses of intravenous magnesium sulfate infusion on critically ill trauma patients. Inflammatory and oxidative factors were measured in this trial.

Methods: 45 trauma patients with systemic inflammatory response syndromes (SIRS) were randomly assigned into 2 treatment and one placebo groups. The high dose group received 15 g $MgSO_4$, low dose group received 7.5 g of $MgSO_4$ over 4 hour infusion, and placebo group received saline alone. The initial and post magnesium sulfate injections levels of tumor necrosis factor alpha (TNF-α), total antioxidant power and lipid peroxidation were measured after 6, 18 and 36 hours. The pre-infusion along with 6 and 36 hour level of microalbuminuria were also determined.

Results: Repeated measurements illustrated that there was no significant difference in TNF-α, total antioxidant power and lipid peroxidation levels among groups during the period of analysis. The microalbuminuria at 36 hour post infusion of high dose group was lower than that of control group ($p = 0.024$). Patient's mortality (28 day) was similar among all treatment groups. Both magnesium infusion groups tolerated the drug without experiencing any complications.

Conclusion: No evidence for antioxidative and antiinflammatory effects of magnesium in traumatic SIRS positive patients was found. Magnesium in high doses may be recommended for traumatic patients with SIRS status to prevent microalbuminuria.

Keyword: Magnesium, Microalbumin, TNF-α, Oxidative stress, Trauma, Critical care

Background

Magnesium is one of the four most common electrolytes in human body which is an essential co-factor in more than 300 enzymatic reactions. It is involved in many vital processes, such as cardiac excitability [1], transmembrane ion flux, and neurotransmitter release and gating of calcium ion channels [2]. In many respects magnesium serves as a physiological antagonist of calcium [3] and this is a very important theoretical role for magnesium in critical care medicine [4]. Calcium has a defined effect in inflammatory responses, cytokine release and programmed cell death [5]. Magnesium deficiency is common among hospitalized patients (7-11%) and it has been found in 20-60% of intensive care unit (ICU) admitted patients [6]. In near half of electrolyte abnormalities, hypomagnesaemia is found to be a co-morbid factor [7] which indicates its important role in ICU patients [4]. Microalbuminuria is defined as excretion of albumin in small amounts (between 30 and 300 mg/day) that indexed for reliability as microalbumin to creatinine ratio (MACR) [8]. In the past few years, microalbuminuria is utilized for determining severity of

* Correspondence: mojtahed@sina.tums.ac.ir
[1]Department of Clinical Pharmacy, Faculty of Pharmacy, Tehran University of Medical Sciences, Tehran 1417614411, Iran
Full list of author information is available at the end of the article

inflammatory cascade in ICU patients [9]. It is hypothesized that increasing pro-inflammatory and inflammatory factors will lead to increase in permeability of endothelium and consequent increase of albumin excretion through kidneys.

The relationships between oxidative stress, inflammation, proteinuria and hypomagnesaemia have been evaluated in previous animal and human studies [3,10-12] and cultured human cells [13]. However, we have not came across any study which was conducted in normomagnesemic patients, therefore the effectiveness of magnesium as a therapeutic agent in critical care medicine has not been validated [12,14]. It is hypothesized that high doses of magnesium infusion would be effective and safe for the management of oxidative stress and inflammation following SIRS/trauma.

Methods

Study design and setting

This randomized clinical trial study was conducted during 14 months at a University teaching hospital ICU. Block randomization method used to randomize the patient and both patient and researcher were blinded and a third party decides the treatment group designated to patients based on a randomization table.

Patient population

The study procedure was approved by the University ethics committee with code number (87-03-33-7752) according to the declaration of Helsinki. Patients or their relatives were informed of the study and a written consent was obtained from each individual. Severely ill patients who were admitted for multiple trauma with an Acute Physiology And Chronic Health Evaluation (APACHE II) score of more than 18 accompanied by SIRS criteria [15]. A normal ionized serum magnesium (isMg) level ($0.75 < isMg < 0.95$ mmol/l) [4] and albumin concentration (40–60 g/l) were the other criteria for acceptance of patients into clinical study pool.

The patient exclusion criteria were conditions that may cause pathological microalbuminuria (creatinine >1.5 mg/dl, metabolic syndrome and diabetes mellitus [16]). Patients with such conditions either before admitting or during stay at ICU were excluded from the study. Patients who had taken drugs which are known as endothelial active drugs (like angiotesin-converting-enzyme, C reactive proteins, corticosteroids and statins) [17], previous magnesium intake, hematologic diseases, neuromuscular disease, pregnancy, severe sepsis and septic shock also were also excluded.

Patients' ionized serum magnesium concentration was based for determination of magnesium status [18] and all of the patients considered not having serum hyper or hypomagnesaemia at the time of study enrollment. The ionized serum magnesium concentration was measured with ion selective electrodes by Stat Profile Critical Care Xpress analyzer (NOVA biomedical, Waltham, Massachusetts, USA).

Before enrollment a 5 ml blood sample was taken from a central catheter with a heparinized acid washed syringe. This sample was centrifuged in an acid washed test tube and serum derived from blood was used to assess isMg in sample. Before starting infusion and after 6, 18 and 36 hour blood samples were taken in order to measure TNF-α, total antioxidant power and lipid peroxidation.

Total antioxidant power was measured by ferric reducing ability of plasma (FRAP) and the extent of lipid peroxidation was determined with thiobarbituric acid (TBA) method called TBA reactive substances (TBARS) as both were described in our previous paper [1]. TNF-α was assessed with Enzyme-Linked ImmunoSorbaent Assay (ELISA) kit obtained from (BenderMed Systems, Austria) according to manufacturer manual. Creatinine in urine samples were measured with an immunoassay method utilizing BT3500 analyzer (Biotecnica instruments, Italy) by using Jaffe method [19] according to the manufacturer's brochure. Detection range was >3 mg/L. MACR was determined by ratio between urinary albumin and creatinine concentration. All the samples were tested twice in order to achieve a higher grade of precision. The average of both results were recorded and utilized in analysis.

Patient's demographic characteristics were recorded at the admission to ICU. The APACHE II scores for definition of severity of illness, and Sequential Organ Failure Assessment (SOFA) score for organ failure were calculated in the first day of admission. Therapeutic intervention scoring system (TISS) score was used to evaluate equal medical treatment among study groups. Deep tendon reflexes were checked hourly during infusion and routinely in the first three days of study. All the patients had urinary catheters and were under mechanical ventilation.

Patients were randomized in this study. High and moderate dose group received 70 or 35 ml of 20% $MgSO_4$ solutions, respectively. This amount is equivalent to 15 or 7.5 g of magnesium sulfate for high or moderate group which was diluted into 1000 ml of NaCl (0.9% v/v) and infused in 4 hours.

Three 5 ml midstream urine samples were obtained during the first two days of study. The samples were taken at the time of enrollment (0 hour), 2, 6 and 36 hours post infusion. The study period proceeded for 28 days.

Statistical analysis

Data are presented as mean with standard errors. Univariate comparisons of baseline characteristics were performed by the independent Student's t-test. Pearson's $\chi2$ was used to test differences in survival among groups. Two-way analysis of variance was applied for comparing the repeated measurements of microalbumin levels among groups with multiple comparisons (Scheffe's test) for each time period. A p value of less than 0.05 has been considered statistically significant. Values for microalbumin were log transformed to obtain proportionally constant variation and normally distributed data.

Results

Population Characteristics

53 trauma patients enrolled in this study and 8 were excluded. Four of these patients (2 moderate doses, 1 high dose and 1 control) dropped out due to their progression to acute renal injury, 1 patient died during study and 3 patients had developed severe sepsis manifestations. The patients (n = 45) were randomly divided into three groups. The two experimental groups consisted of high and medium level doses of magnesium. The remaining 15 patients were included in a placebo control group. Patient's demographic characteristics and clinical manifestation are summarized in Table 1. Subjects had no statistical differences in their age, sex, TNF-α, FRAP, TBARS, MACR, APACHE II and SOFA scores at the time of enrollment into the study.

It is important to note that patients ionized serum magnesium concentration was based for determination of magnesium status [18]. This method is considered to be the most accurate (Table 1). All the patients' baseline serum ionized magnesium concentration was in normal range at the start point of the study.

Effect of magnesium on oxidative & inflammatory factors

The TNF alpha levels remained steady for the control group at all time points. There was only a slight (statistically insignificant) decrease in TNF-α at 36-hour time point for both experimental groups (Table 2), suggesting that the blood retained its reductive characteristics. The level of FRAP remained steady for all the groups. However, TBARS level for the high dose group demonstrated a considerable drop in readings at 36 hour (3.0 ± 1.0) when it was compared to the 18 hour readings (3.6 ± 1.2) for the high dose group. The reduction in TBARS level is an indication of the positive effect of high dose of magnesium on traumatic patients who were positive for systemic inflammatory response syndromes (SIRS) normomagnesemic status (Table 2).

There were no significant difference in levels of TNF- α and TBARS. Another noticeable change was microalbuminuria, at 36 hours post magnesium infusion in high dose group which was determined to be statistically lower than the control group (p = 0.024)(Figure 1). The trends of other mentioned anti inflammatory and oxidative factors proved our hypothesis on existence of lower levels of MACR over time between high dose infusion and placebo groups.

Outcome

A trend toward mortality reduction was found in high dose magnesium recipients although this difference was not statistically significant. Patients tolerated $MgSO_4$ infusion very well with no significant difference between treatment and placebo groups (p = 0.61) and no serious adverse reaction were reported, except for 2 cases of hypermagnesaemia in the high dose group which did not have any clinical consequences.

Discussion

This study demonstrate that high doses of magnesium reduce microalbuminuria in traumatic critically ill patients at 36 hour post infusion. Although no significant difference observed among trends, there was a positive trend toward better outcomes in treatment groups in total antioxidant power, lipid peroxidation and TNF-α between treatment and placebo groups.

Microvascular changes induced by nitric oxide (NO) and other proinflammatory factors and their interaction

Table 1 Demographic data, Scoring systems and MACR at the beginning of the study

		Control	moderate dose	High dose	Sig.
Age(years)		49.33333 ± 5.30	39.86667 ± 5.51	48.33333 ± 5.29	NS
sex	Male	13 (86%)	13 (86%)	13 (86%)	NS
	Female	2 (14%)	2 (14%)	2 (14%)	NS
Mortality rate		6 (40%)	7 (46.7%)	5 (33.3%)	NS
APACHE II(0 h)		21.06 ± 0.69	21.20 ± 0.56	21.26 ± 0.58	NS
SOFA(0 h)		8.33 ± 0.30	8.53 ± 0.44	8.20 ± 0.29	NS
TNFα (pg/ml)(0 h)		36.37 ± 11.77	34.16 ± 9.99	32.71 ± 11.42	NS
TBARS (μM)(0 h)		3.89 ± 0.65	4.27 ± 1.44	3.76 ± 1.32	NS
FRAP (μM)		402.44 ± 65.33	399.61 ± 71.83	448.87 ± 85.03	NS
MACR(0 h)*		30.21 ± 5.69	27.59 ± 5.35	29.53 ± 5.35	NS

APACHE = Acute Physiology and Chronic Health Evaluation, SOFA = Sequential Organ Failure Assessment, MACR = microalbumin to creatinine ratio. * mg/mmol.

Table 2 Inflammatory and oxidative factors

		Control group	Medium dose group	High dose group
TNF-α pg/ml ± SD	0 h	36.0 ± 12.1	37.0 ± 12.2	38.1 ± 10.7
	6 h	37.4 ± 13.2	34.5 ± 8.1	35.6 ± 15.4
	18 h	35.6 ± 11.6	36.38 ± 10.8	30.1 ± 7.0
	36 h	36.3 ± 10.9	28.6 ± 6.5	26.9 ± 7.9
FRAP μM ± SD	0 h	421. ± 54.5	412.3 ± 69.9	424.7 ± 71.4
	6 h	397.1 ± 69.0	398.7 ± 73.0	427.5 ± 74.6
	18 h	407.7 ± 82.2	401.8 ± 90.7	452.7 ± 90.8
	36 h	383.4 ± 51.4	385.5 ± 53.8	490.5 ± 92.5
TBARS μM ± SD	0 h	4.1 ± 0.7	4.3 ± 1.7	4.4 ± 1.0
	6 h	3.7 ± 0.5	4.4 ± 1.0	3.9 ± 1.5
	18 h	3.9 ± 0.7	4.2 ± 1.1	3.6 ± 1.2
	36 h	3.7 ± 0.4	4.1 ± 1.4	3.0 ± 1.0

with leukocytes amplify inflammatory response in SIRS patients. Endothelial cells could be injured through inflammatory response and cause an increase in capillary permeability particularly in glomerular vessels [8] which induces kidneys to undergo transient proteinuria. The deleterious scale of these changes can be measured by increased levels of microalbuminuria [8]. The population enrolled in this study was homogenous and consisted of neurotraumatic critically ill only. The purpose of this study is to evaluate the efficacy and rational of magnesium infusion on neurotraumatic patients. In traumatic condition, an energy depletion dilemma emerges in cellular level. The consequence of this depletion is reduction in activity of transmembrane calcium ion transport channels which leads to distorted ion balance and permeability changes. Membrane permeability changes cause calcium influx in cells, which results in many deleterious reactions such as alternation of adenosine triphosphate (ATP) production in mitochondria, overproduction of reactive oxygen species (ROS), NO generation and release of proinflammatory factors [1,2]. Magnesium could serve as antagonist of calcium to inhibit these harmful effects [3] in traumatic patients.

In previous animal studies it was demonstrated that hypomagnesaemia can cause systemic inflammatory syndrome [12]. Magnesium deficiency opens N-methyl-D-aspartate (NMDA) calcium channels and activates nuclear factor-kappa B (NF-kB) as primary mechanism of inflammation [11]. However, in this study after magnesium infusion, the levels of TNF-α, total antioxidant power and lipid peroxidation did not demonstrate any significant change at various periods of analysis. Therefore, administration of magnesium salt did not display any anti-inflammatory activities in critically ill patients with normal levels of this ion. Effect of body magnesium levels (plasma, erythrocyte and urine) and its association with microalbuminuria has been previously studied on type 1 diabetic patients [20]. A negative relation between erythrocyte magnesium level and microalbuminuria was observed suggesting hypomagnesaemia as a risk factor

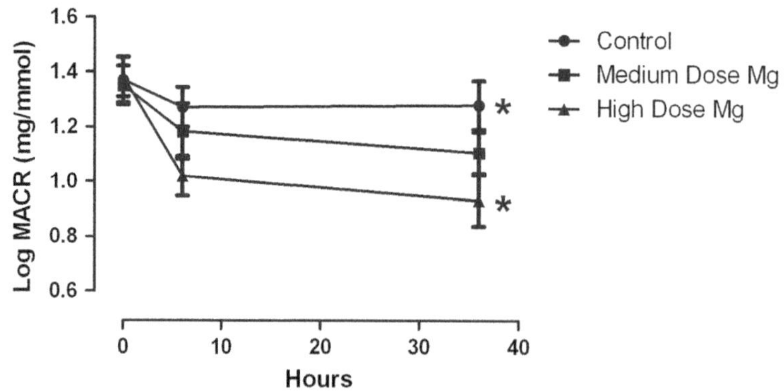

Figure 1 Changes in microalbumin/creatine in urine samples of control group vs. moderate dose and high dose magnesium group by hours. * $p < 0.05$ vs high dose magnesium group.

for proteinuria in diabetic patients. In another study, it was suggested that hypomagnesaemia is an independent risk factor for microalbuminuria in type two diabetic patients [20]. In the present study there has been a lag about 48–72 hour between hospital and ICU admission that might be the time that most critical changes in level of TNF-α and oxidative marker occurred and thus less significant changes were observed subsequently. As we mentioned in previous study with cytokines determination of cutoff point for cytokine measurement in ethnic populations remained unclear and problematic [21]. Our previous study verified that N-acetylcysteine performs as a free radical scavenger and an anti-inflammatory agent and improves microalbuminuria in acute respiratory distress syndrome patients [22]. It has been illustrated that severity of microalbuminuria has a direct relationship with mortality and morbidity rates [9,16]. Although, no significant change in TNF-α and oxidative factors showed up in the study time window, the change in microalbumin suggests that inflammation has been reduced in the high dose treatment subjects. In order to omit the bias of hypomagnesaemia effect on proteinuria [20], patients with normal levels of serum magnesium were allowed to be enrolled in this clinical study. Magnesium total serum concentration is the most studied laboratory parameter and considered poorly related to cellular status of magnesium in the patient's body. Magnesium loading test or ionized serum magnesium concentration is used for evaluation of magnesium sufficiency in the body [23]. Magnesium loading test was not utilized for evaluation of magnesium status in this study because patients received a large dose of magnesium before enrollment in the study and the result would be compromised and unreliable. Therefore, ionized serum magnesium test was utilized in order to establish magnesium status. Ionized serum magnesium test has been applied to establish magnesium status instead of magnesium loading test due to limitation of previous magnesium intake. In this study, the serum albumin concentration was assessed prior to the evaluation of magnesium status. High levels of albumin may interfere with ionized serum magnesium test [23] and may negatively impact the accurate evaluation for microalbuminuria.

Although, management of patients in ICU is somehow complicated and dependent of the status of each patient [24], it was decided to use an established protocol as a base amount for moderate dose of magnesium that was safe over the years in ICU [25]. Two fold of that dose has been assumed as high dose of magnesium for this study. The positive effect of magnesium dosing in critically ill patients is under debate and the results are controversial. Determination of a specific dose was difficult because compensation for magnesium depletion was not the aim of this study. The normomagnesemic populations have never been studied before to the extent of our knowledge. Therefore, clinically significant results would be due to the theoretical role of magnesium. There were no significant difference among groups during time, but after 36 hours, the MACR in high dose magnesium group was significantly lower than control group (Figure 1).

Mild bradycardia and hypotension were the only side effects observed in patients who received magnesium. Therefore we suggest that magnesium doses as high as the ones used in this study are relatively safe for infusion of critically ill patients. However magnesium therapy should be considered in special populations. Magnesium is generally cleared by kidneys and magnesium therapy in higher doses should be administered with more caution in patients with any risk of renal failure.

Administration of magnesium as a therapeutic agent is not a common approach, but it is routinely employed to correct the hypomagnesemic state. In this study magnesium sulfate infusion was administered as an anti-inflammatory therapeutic agent and some optimistic results were obtained. In order to obtain a more definitive conclusion, another more elaborated clinical trial is recommended.

There was a beneficial trend toward high magnesium load where we left the study (Figure 1). The number of subjects and the duration of study were limited in this trial. The results could not be generalized to the population in this condition, but it is recommended to conduct more studies with longer duration and greater sample size. It is also recommended to infuse magnesium in longer duration and more divided intervals.

Conclusion

We did not find conclusive evidence for antioxidative and antiinflammatory effects of magnesium in traumatic SIRS positive patients. However, high dose magnesium might be recommended as a safe option for preventing microalbuminuria in traumatic patients with SIRS criteria.

Abbreviations

ICU: Intensive care unit; SIRS: Systemic inflammatory response syndromes; TNF-α: Tumor necrosis factor alpha; MACR: Microalbumin to creatinine ratio; APACHE: II: Acute Physiology And Chronic Health Evaluation; isMg: Ionized serum magnesium; FRAP: Ferric reducing ability of plasma; TPTZ: 2,4,6 Tripyridyl-s-Triazine; HCl: Hydrochloric acid; TBARS: Thiobarbituric acid reactive substances; TCA: Trichloroacetic acid; ELISA: Enzyme-Linked ImmunoSorbaent Assay; SOFA: Sequential Organ Failure Assessment score; TISS: Therapeutic intervention scoring system; ROS: Reactive oxygen species; NO: Nitric oxide; NMDA: N-methyl-D-aspartate; NF-kB: Nuclear factor-kappa B; MLT: Magnesium loading test.

Competing interests

There are no conflicts of interest related to this publication.

Authors' contributions

BM and HH were responsible for drafting of the article, and gathering and analysis of data. AA, AN and MRM were responsible for patient inclusion, study design, implementation of study and gathering the data. MAM was responsible for analyzing the samples and laboratory data. MA shared in the idea and edited the paper. MM was responsible for conception of study, critical revision and drafting the article. All authors read and approved the final manuscript.

Acknowledgement

This research has been supported by Tehran University of Medical Sciences. Hereby we express our gratitude toward Sina hospital ICU and trauma center staff because this couldn't be accomplished without their dedication. Also we thank pharmaceutical science research center members and staff for their contributions to this study. We express our appreciation toward laboratory of Children's Medical Center hospital for measuring the isMg for us.

Author details

[1]Department of Clinical Pharmacy, Faculty of Pharmacy, Tehran University of Medical Sciences, Tehran 1417614411, Iran. [2]Department of Clinical Pharmacy, Faculty of Pharmacy, Tabriz University of Medical Science, Tabriz 1476651664, Iran. [3]Department of anesthesia and intensive care, Sina hospital, Tehran University of Medical Science, Tehran 1136746911, Iran. [4]Department of anesthesia and intensive care, Faculty of Medicine, Shahid Sadoghi University of Medical Science, Yazd 8915173143, Iran. [5]Sina hospital, Tehran University of Medical Science, Tehran 1136746911, Iran. [6]Department of Toxicology and Pharmacology, Faculty of Pharmacy, and Pharmaceutical Sciences Research Center, Tehran University of Medical Sciences, Tehran 1417614411, Iran.

References

1. Shafiee H, Mohammadi H, Rezayat SM, Hosseini A, Baeeri M, Hassani S, Mohammadirad A, Bayrami Z, Abdollahi M: **Prevention of malathion-induced depletion of cardiac cells mitochondrial energy and free radical damage by a magnetic magnesium-carrying nanoparticle.** *Toxicol Mech Methods* 2010, **20**:538–543.
2. Wolf FI, Trapani V: **Cell (patho)physiology of magnesium.** *Clin Sci (Lond)* 2008, **114**:27–35.
3. Romani AM: **Cellular magnesium homeostasis.** *Arch Biochem Biophys* 2011, **512**:1–23.
4. Noronha JL, Matuschak GM: **Magnesium in critical illness: metabolism, assessment, and treatment.** *Intensive Care Med* 2002, **28**:667–679.
5. Weglicki WB, Phillips TM, Freedman AM, Cassidy MM, Dickens BF: **Magnesium-deficiency elevates circulating levels of inflammatory cytokines and endothelin.** *Mol Cell Biochem* 1992, **110**:169–173.
6. Ryzen E, Wagers PW, Singer FR, Rude RK: **Magnesium deficiency in a medical ICU population.** *Crit Care Med* 1985, **13**:19–21.
7. Buckley MS, Leblanc JM, Cawley MJ: **Electrolyte disturbances associated with commonly prescribed medications in the intensive care unit.** *Crit Care Med* 2010, **38**:S253–S264.
8. Gosling P, Czyz J, Nightingale P, Manji M: **Microalbuminuria in the intensive care unit: Clinical correlates and association with outcomes in 431 patients.** *Crit Care Med* 2006, **34**:2158–2166.
9. Thorevska N, Sabahi R, Upadya A, Manthous C, Amoateng-Adjepong Y: **Microalbuminuria in critically ill medical patients: prevalence, predictors, and prognostic significance.** *Crit Care Med* 2003, **31**:1075–1081.
10. Mak IT, Komarov AM, Wagner TL, Stafford RE, Dickens BF, Weglicki WB: **Enhanced NO production during Mg deficiency and its role in mediating red blood cell glutathione loss.** *Am J Physiol* 1996, **271**:C385–C390.
11. Mazur A, Maier JA, Rock E, Gueux E, Nowacki W, Rayssiguier Y: **Magnesium and the inflammatory response: potential physiopathological implications.** *Arch Biochem Biophys* 2007, **458**:48–56.
12. Rayssiguier Y, Mazur A: **[Magnesium and inflammation: lessons from animal models].** *Clin Calcium* 2005, **15**:245–248.
13. Rochelson B, Dowling O, Schwartz N, Metz CN: **Magnesium sulfate suppresses inflammatory responses by human umbilical vein endothelial cells (HuVECs) through the NFkappaB pathway.** *J Reprod Immunol* 2007, **73**:101–107.
14. Malpuech-Brugere C, Nowacki W, Daveau M, Gueux E, Linard C, Rock E, Lebreton J, Mazur A, Rayssiguier Y: **Inflammatory response following acute magnesium deficiency in the rat.** *Biochim Biophys Acta* 2000, **1501**:91–98.
15. Bone RC, Balk RA, Cerra FB, Dellinger RP, Fein AM, Knaus WA, Schein RM, Sibbald WJ: **Definitions for sepsis and organ failure and guidelines for the use of innovative therapies in sepsis. The ACCP/SCCM Consensus Conference Committee. American College of Chest Physicians/Society of Critical Care Medicine.** *Chest* 1992, **101**:1644–1655.
16. Dubaybo BA: **Microalbuminuria: simple, inexpensive, and dynamic marker of critical illness.** *Chest* 2001, **120**:1769–1771.
17. Ruilope LM, Redon J, Schmieder R: **Cardiovascular risk reduction by reversing endothelial dysfunction: ARBs, ACE inhibitors, or both? Expectations from the ONTARGET Trial Programme.** *Vasc Health Risk Manag* 2007, **3**:1–9.
18. Huijgen HJ, Soesan M, Sanders R, Mairuhu WM, Kesecioglu J, Sanders GT: **Magnesium Levels in Critically Ill Patients: What Should We Measure?** *Am J Clin Pathol* 2000, **114**:688–695.
19. Vasiliades J: **Reaction of alkaline sodium picrate with creatinine: I.** *Kinetics and mechanism of formation of the mono-creatinine picric acid complex. Clin Chem* 1976, **22**:1664–1671.
20. Corica F, Corsonello A, Ientile R, Cucinotta D, Di Benedetto A, Perticone F, Dominguez LJ, Barbagallo M: **Serum ionized magnesium levels in relation to metabolic syndrome in type 2 diabetic patients.** *J Am Coll Nutr* 2006, **25**:210–215.
21. Hamishehkar H, Beigmohammadi MT, Abdollahi M, Ahmadi A, Mahmoodpour A, Mirjalili MR, Abrishami R, Khoshayand MR, Eslami K, Kanani M, *et al*: **Identification of enhanced cytokine generation following sepsis. Dream of magic bullet for mortality prediction and therapeutic evaluation.** *Daru* 2010, **18**:155–162.
22. Najafi A, Mojtahedzadeh M, Mahmoodpoor A, Aghamohammadi M, Ahmadi A, Nahreini S, Pazuki M, Khajavi MR, Abdollahi M: **Effect of N-acetylcysteine on microalbuminuria in patients with acute respiratory distress syndrome.** *Arch Med Sci* 2009, **5**:408–414.
23. Saris NE, Mervaala E, Karppanen H, Khawaja JA, Lewenstam A: **Magnesium. An update on physiological, clinical and analytical aspects.** *Clin Chim Acta* 2000, **294**:1–26.
24. Honarmand H, Abdollahi M, Ahmadi A, Javadi MR, Khoshaiand MR, Tabeefar H, *et al*: **Randomized trial of the effect of intravenous paracetamol on inflammatory biomarkers and outcome in febrile critically ill adults.** *DARU* 2012, **20**:12.
25. Hebert P, Mehta N, Wang J, Hindmarsh T, Jones G, Cardinal P: **Functional magnesium deficiency in critically ill patients identified using a magnesium-loading test.** *Crit Care Med* 1997, **25**:749–755.

Changes in gram negative microorganisms' resistance pattern during 4 years period in a referral teaching hospital; a surveillance study

Hossein Khalili[1*], Simin Dashti-Khavidaki[1], Mohammad-Reza Shahidi[1], Alireza Abdollahi[2], Sirous Jafari[3], Zahra Jahangard-Rafsanjani[1] and Azita-Hajhosssein Talasaz[1]

Abstract

Background and purpose: Surveillance studies evaluating antimicrobial susceptibilities are of great value in preventing the spread of resistant pathogens by elucidating the trend of resistance in commonly used antibiotics and as a consequence providing information for prescribing the most appropriate agent. This study is a longitudinal antimicrobial resistance surveillance study designed to evaluate the trend in antimicrobial resistance to gram negative microorganisms from 2007 to 2010.

Method: During a four-year period (2007–2010) isolates derived from all patients admitted to infectious diseases ward of Imam Khomeini Hospital, the major referral center for infectious disease in Iran with the highest admission rates, were evaluated. Based on disk diffusion method and zone of inhibition size, the microorganism was regarded as to be sensitive, resistant or has intermediate susceptibility to the antimicrobial agents.

Results: The widest spread Gram-negative microorganism in all of isolates taken together in our study was *E.coli* (30%) followed by *Stenotrophomonas maltophilia* in 28.6% and *Enterobacter spp.* in 11.9%, respectively. The susceptibility to amikacin, imipenem, piperacillin/tazobactam, and nitrofurantoin was equal or above 50% for all microorganisms over four years. However, the susceptibility to ampicillin, ampicillin/sulbactam, cefotaxim, and ceftriaxone was less than 50% in derived isolates during the study period.

Conclusion: In conclusion, the finding of the present study revealed that resistance rate to common antimicrobial agents in Iran is growing and isolates were susceptible mostly to broad-spectrum antibiotics including imipenem and piperacillin/tazobactam.

Keywords: Gram negative microorganism, Resistance pattern

Introduction

Antibiotic resistance is a critical challenge for infective diseases management around the word [1-3]. Infection with a resistant strain has been associated to higher rate of morbidity and mortality as well as prolonged length of hospital and intensive care unit stay and increased expenses for the healthcare systems [3,4].

Surveillance studies evaluating antimicrobial susceptibilities are of great value in providing information for prescribing the most appropriate agent [5]. These studies could be used as a guide in antimicrobial usage policies in order to halt the expansion of microorganism resistance [6-10].

Although there are few reports on the antibiotic resistance in Iran, many of them are simple point-in-time prevalence studies or evaluated pathogens involved in a specific infectious disease [11-14]. Present evaluation is a longitudinal antimicrobial resistance surveillance study designed to evaluate the trend in antimicrobial resistance to nosocomial origin gram negative microorganisms, from 2007 to 2010.

Methods

During a four-year period (2007–2010) isolates biological samples from all patients admitted to Infectious

* Correspondence: khalilih@tums.ac.ir
[1]Department of Clinical Pharmacy, Faculty of Pharmacy, Tehran University of Medical Sciences, Tehran, Iran
Full list of author information is available at the end of the article

Diseases Ward of Imam Khomeini Hospital Complex, the major referral center for infectious disease in Iran with the highest admission rates, were evaluated. The Institutional Review Board (IRB) and the Medical Ethics Committee of the hospital approved the study.

Isolates were sent to a central laboratory of the hospital for identification and antimicrobial susceptibility testing by Kirby – Bauer disc diffusion method. Based on zone of inhibition size the microorganism was regarded as to be sensitive, resistant or intermediate susceptibility to the antimicrobial agent. Microorganisms' susceptibilities were investigated against those antimicrobials of clinical utility for the treatment of infections caused by susceptible Gram- negative bacteria available in the hospital. β-lactams such as ampicillin and piperacillin from penicillin class; cephalosporins including cefixime, cefotaxim, ceftazidim, ceftriaxone, cefepime; and the carbapenems such as imipenem were among evaluated antimicrobials. Combinations of penicillins with β-lactamase inhibitors including piperacillin-tazobactam and ampicillin-sulbactam, fluroquinolones such as ciprofloxacin, aminoglycosides including amikacin and gentamicin, nitrofurantoin and cotrimoxazole were those studied for antimicrobial resistance pattern in this surveillance. The trend in this pattern over four years was reviewed and reported.

Results

In a four-year period from 2007 to 2010, 1745 isolates were sent to the central library of the hospital, from those 983 (56.3%) were confirmed to be Gram-negative pathogens. The most frequent specimen sources were blood (46.2%) followed by the urine (27%), and wound (13.7. The most wide spread Gram-negative microorganism in all of isolates taken together in our study was *E. coli* (30%) followed by *Stenotrophomonas maltophilia* in 28.6% and *Enterobacter spp.* in 11.9%, respectively. The frequency of microorganisms in terms of the derived isolates is shown in Table 1.

Table 1 Frequency of Gram-negative microorganisms according to the origins of specimen resource

Microorganism	Blood	Urine	Wound	Other	Total
E.Coli	14	201	40	30	285
Stenotrophomonas sp.	278	0	1	2	281
Enterobacter	64	42	5	6	117
Pseudomona	21	25	25	13	84
Acinetobacter	29	22	10	13	74
Kelebsiela	18	32	6	8	64
Proteus	2	9	20	11	42
Citrobacter	3	22	6	5	36
Total	429	353	113	88	983

The overall susceptibility of the specimens to antimicrobial agents did not remain the same over four years. For some of antimicrobial agents, the percentage of susceptible microorganisms was increased including ciprofloxacin (44.2 to 68.4%), piperacillin(33.3 to 66.7%) and piperacillin/tazobactam (77.8 to 89.5%). In contrast the susceptibility of nosocomial pathogens was reduced against nitrofurantoin (75.9 to 56%) in a four-year period. The susceptibility of microorganisms against all other antimicrobial agents showed non-steady pattern. The susceptibility to amikacin, imipenem, piperacillin/tazobactam, and nitrofurantoin was equal or above 50% for microorganisms all over four years. However, the susceptibility to ampicillin, ampicillin/sulbactam, cefotaxim, and ceftriaxone was less than 50% in derived isolates during the study period. The resistance rate of microorganism to Cefepime was increased in 2007–2008 while the susceptibilities were enhanced in 2009–2010. Comparison of the trend of resistance pattern of isolated bacteria of nosocomial originas well as the rate of frequency of each pathogen was illustrated in Table 2. Regarding the microorganisms, the most frequent resistances were seen in *Acientobacter* followed by *Citrobacter* with 50–73.7% and 58.3-65.8% resistant isolates, respectively. In contrast, *Enterobcter* was the most susceptible microorganism with resistance rate of 25.6-29.5% in the study period. The switches in the percent of resistant microorganism were not the same for all of the pathogens (Table 3). Proteus resistance was decreased in four-year period from 43.9% to 6.7% against all of the antibiotics taken together. *Acinetobacter* resistance to ciprofloxacin was increased whereas *Enterobacter* resistance rate to Gentamicin and Ciprofloxacin and *E.coli* resistance to Ceftazidim was decreased in four-year period. The number of resistant *Entrobacter i*solates to Cefixim was increased. From 2008 to 2010 the susceptibility rate of *Acinetobacter* against Ampicillin/sulbactam was reduced.

Discussion

Antimicrobial resistance is a widespread problem that health care providers are encountered with all over the world. Determining the specific pattern of antibiotic resistance especially in infectious diseases wards of main hospitals in every country is of great value for controlling the rate of increasing resistance as well as helping in empirical treatment. Since Imam Khomeini hospital Complex is the main center for infectious diseases in Iran with the highest admission rates, we can say that a serious problem of antimicrobial resistance to commonly used antibiotics exists among different isolates in Iran.

The most frequent isolated pathogen from all specimens taken together was *E. coli* followed by *S. maltophilia* and *Enterobacter sp.* with *E. coli* being the major

Table 2 Comparison of resistance pattern of isolated bacteria of nosocomial origin in four-year period

Antimicrobial agent/ microorganism	Susceptibility											
	Sensitive; n (%)				Intermediate; n (%)				Resistant; n (%)			
	2007	2008	2009	2010	2007	2008	2009	2010	2007	2008	2009	2010
Amikacin												
Acinetobacter	8	13	7	1	1	0	0	1	9	6	9	8
Citrobacter	4	5	11	N/A	1	0	0	N/	7	7	20	N/
E.Coli	62	85	53	26	2	0	0	A	10	8	16	A
Enterobacter	20	34	25	13	0	0	1	0	1	1	3	4
Kelebsiella	13	10	12	4	2	0	0	0	7	1	6	1
Proteus spp.	8	4	13	5	0	0	0	1	3	0	1	1
Pseudomonas sp.	9	18	12	11	0	0	0	0	2	3	11	6
Stenotrophomonas sp.	9	40	83	25	2	1	0	0	11	31	29	24
Total	133 (69.6%)	209 (78.3%)	216 (69.2%)	85 (64.4%)	8 (4.2%)	1 (0.3%)	1 (0.3%)	1 3 (2.3%)	50 (26.2%)	57 (21.3%)	95 (30.4%)	44 (33.3%)
Ampicillin/sulbactam												
Acinetobacter	1	5	11	3	0	0	0	0	3	3	10	5
E.Coli	3	6	15	7	0	0	2	1	2	12	49	15
Enterobacter	5	3	9	4	0	0	1	0	0	5	15	1
Kelebsiella	0	1	5	1	0	0	0	0	3	1	11	4
Proteus spp.	1	2	11	5	0	0	0	0	0	0	4	0
Pseudomonas sp.	0	0	3	0	0	0	0	0	2	4	20	14
Stenotrophomonas sp.	1	1	1	1	1	0	0	1	9	19	5	2
Total	11 (35.5%)	18 (29%)	55 (32%)	21 (32.8%)	1 (3.2%)	0 (0)	3 (1.7%)	2 (3.1%)	19 (61.3%)	44 (71%)	114 (66.3%)	41 (64.1%)
Ampicillin												
E.Coli	0	0	1	1	0	0	0	0	2	22	25	0
Enterobacter	0	0	2	0	0	0	0	0	1	5	4	2
Total	0 (0)	0 (0)	3 (9.4%)	1 (33.3%)	0 (0)	0 (0)	0 (0)	0 (0)	3 (100%)	27 (100%)	29 (90.6%)	2 (66.7%)
Cotrimoxazole												
Acinetobacter	7	6	5	1	0	0	0	0	14	10	13	8
Citrobacter	1	2	3	1	0	0	0	0	6	6	13	1
E.Coli	21	19	24	8	0	0	1	0	49	59	47	20
Enterobacter	12	24	21	8	0	0	0	0	11	13	7	4
Kelebsiella	6	5	7	2	0	0	0	0	17	3	12	4
Proteus spp.	4	2	4	3	0	1	0	0	7	3	9	1
Pseudomonas sp.	0	7	4	2	0	0	0	0	13	11	20	14
Stenotrophomonas sp.	22	78	107	35	0	0	0	0	1	2	2	10

Table 2 Comparison of resistance pattern of isolated bacteria of nosocomial origin in four-year period *(Continued)*

Total	73 (38.2%)	143 (57%)	173 (58.2%)	60 (49.2%)	0 (0)	1 (0.4%)	1 (0.4%)	0 (0)	118 (61.8%)	107 (42.6%)	123 (41.4%)	62 (51.8%)
Cefepim												
E.Coli	3	4	7	2	0	0	0	0	3	3	5	1
Enterobacter	0	4	5	1	0	0	0	0	1	6	2	1
Proteus spp.	1	0	4	1	0	1	0	0	1	2	0	0
Pseudomonas sp.	0	0	2	1	0	0	0	0	1	8	4	3
Total	4 (40%)	8 (28.6%)	18 (62.1%)	5 (50%)	0 (0)	1 (3.6%)	0 (0)	0 (0)	6 (60%)	19 (67.9%)	11 (37.9%)	5 (50%)
Cefixime												
Acinetobacter	0	0	1	0	0	0	0	0	4	7	3	1
E.Coli	3	2	2	0	0	0	0	0	11	10	0	1
Enterobacter	3	6	1	0	1	2	0	1	3	11	2	4
Proteus spp.	1	0	4	1	0	1	0	0	1	2	0	0
Pseudomonas sp.	0	0	2	1	0	0	0	0	1	8	4	3
Total	7 (25%)	8 (40%)	10 (52.6%)	2 (16.7%)	1 (3.6%)	3 (15%)	0 (0)	1 (8.3%)	20 (71.4%)	9 (45%)	9 (47.4%)	9 (75%)
Cefotaxim												
Acinetobacter	1	1	0	1	0	0	0	0	4	3	5	1
Citrobacter	0	1	0	1	0	0	0	0	5	1	2	1
Pseudomonas sp.	0	1	0	1	0	0	0	0	4	1	4	1
Stenotrophomonas sp.	1	0	0	0	2	0	0	0	5	8	3	1
Total	2 (10%)	3 (18.7%)	0 (0)	3 (42.8%)	0 (0)	0 (0)	0 (0)	0 (0)	18 (90%)	13 (91.3%)	14 (100%)	4 (57.2%)
Ceftazidim												
Acinetobacter	0	0	2	2	0	0	0	0	4	8	5	2
E.Coli	3	3	7	15	0	0	1	0	4	16	43	6
Enterobacter	5	1	12	7	0	0	1	0	0	9	8	4
Kelebsiella	2	1	6	0	0	1	0	0	0	4	7	2
Proteus spp.	2	0	8	4	0	1	0	0	2	3	1	0
Pseudomonas sp.	2	0	4	3	0	0	0	0	1	12	12	4
Stenotrophomonas sp.	0	5	1	2	0	1	0	0	9	31	1	6
Total	14 (41.2%)	10 (10.4%)	40 (33.6%)	33 (57.9%)	0 (0)	3 (3.1%)	2 (1.7%)	0 (0)	20 (58.8%)	83 (86.4%)	77 (64.7%)	24 (42.1%)
Ciprofloxacin												
Acinetobacter	9	4	7	1	0	1	0	0	8	8	13	6
E.Coli	19	26	24	13	0	0	0	0	44	51	49	18
Enterobacter	12	18	24	8	0	0	0	0	8	7	8	2
Kelebsiella	6	4	10	4	2	0	0	0	20	7	20	7
Proteus spp.	4	2	8	6	0	0	0	0	5	3	7	0

Table 2 Comparison of resistance pattern of isolated bacteria of nosocomial origin in four-year period *(Continued)*

Pseudomonas sp.	8	6	10	12	0	1	1	0	2	9	14	3
Stenotrophomonas sp.	15	39	109	45	0	0	0	0	3	0	0	1
Total	73 (44.2%)	99 (53.2%)	192 (63.2%)	80 (68.4%)	2 (1.2%)	2 (1.1%)	1 (0.3%)	0 (0)	90 (54.5%)	85 (45.7%)	111 (36.5%)	37 (31.6%)
Gentamicin												
Acinetobacter	5	9	4	1	1	0	0	0	9	2	6	5
E.Coli	18	49	24	12	1	1	2	0	32	35	36	8
Enterobacter	9	23	21	5	0	0	1	0	4	6	5	1
Kelebsiella	7	4	10	3	0	0	0	0	11	5	5	3
Proteus spp.	2	5	8	1	1	0	0	0	4	0	0	1
Pseudomonas sp.	5	12	1	4	0	0	0	0	3	7	10	2
Stenotrophomonas sp.	8	31	3	2	1	2	0	0	4	9	3	0
Total	54 (43%)	133 (66.5%)	71 (51.1%)	28 (58.3%)	4 (3%)	3 (1.5%)	3 (2.2%)	0 (0%)	67 (54%)	64 (32%)	65 (46.8%)	20 (51.7%)
Imipenem												
Acinetobacter	8	15	20	7	0	3	0	1	4	0	1	3
E.Coli	25	47	77	29	0	0	0	0	0	0	0	2
Enterobacter	12	30	31	13	0	0	0	0	0	0	0	1
Kelebsiella	10	8	19	8	0	0	0	0	0	0	0	0
Proteus spp.	7	6	17	6	0	0	0	0	0	0	0	0
Pseudomonas sp.	9	22	26	15	0	0	0	0	1	0	1	1
Stenotrophomona s sp.	2	10	2	2	0	1	1	0	20	49	7	9
Total	73 (74.5%)	132 (71.3%)	192 (95%)	80 (82.5%)	0 (0)	4 (2.2%)	1 (0.5%)	1 (1%)	25 (25.5%)	49 (26.5%)	9 (4.5%)	16 (16.5%)
Nitrofurantoin												
Acinetobacter	2	2	1	0	0	0	0	0	5	3	0	2
E.Coli	31	68	39	10	1	1	0	0	2	11	11	1
Enterobacter	4	8	8	1	1	1	0	0	1	8	3	0
Kelebsiella	5	2	5	3	0	0	1	0	1	3	3	2
Proteus spp.	1	1	0	0	0	0	0	0	2	0	1	1
Pseudomonas sp.	1	0	0	0	0	0	1	0	1	8	3	5
Total	44 (75.9%)	81 (69.8%)	53 (69.7%)	14 (56%)	2 (3.5%)	2 (1.7%)	2 (2.6%)	0 (0)	12 (20.7%)	33 (28.5%)	21 (27.6%)	11 (44%)
Piperacillin												
Acinetobacter	2	4	N/A	0	1	0	N/A	0	5	3	N/A	3
E.Coli	2	0	N/A	1	0	0	N/A	0	18	4	N/A	0
Enterobacter	9	14	N/A	6	0	0	N/A	0	2	4	N/A	1
Kelebsiella	3	2	N/A	1	0	0	N/A	0	6	4	N/A	0
Total	16 (33.3%)	20 (57.1%)	N/A	8 (66.7%)	1 (2.1%)	0 (0)	N/A	0 (0)	31 (64.6%)	15 (42.9%)	N/A	4 (33.3%)

Table 2 Comparison of resistance pattern of isolated bacteria of nosocomial origin in four-year period *(Continued)*

Ceftriaxone												
Acinetobacter	1	6	4	0	0	0	0	0	15	13	10	9
E.Coli	17	40	16	13	0	1	1	0	51	50	55	17
Enterobacter	9	19	19	10	0	0	1	0	9	12	8	5
Kelebsiella	3	3	5	2	1	0	0	0	16	6	13	4
Proteus spp.	5	3	14	6	0	0	0	0	5	0	2	0
Pseudomonas sp.	2	2	4	5	0	4	1	0	7	13	19	8
Stenotrophomonas sp.	1	5	3	2	0	0	1	0	16	65	91	49
Total	39 (24.5%)	78 (32.2%)	65 (24.3%)	38 (29.2%)	1 (0.6%)	5 (2.1%)	4 (1.5%)	0 (0)	119 (74.8%)	159 (65.7%)	198 (74.2%)	92 (70.8%)
Piperacillin/tazobactam												
Acinetobacter	2	1	12	3	0	0	0	0	1	1	5	0
E.Coli	1	3	22	18	0	0	0	0	0	1	0	0
Proteus spp.	1	1	12	5	0	0	0	0	0	0	0	3
Pseudomonas sp.	1	3	13	6	0	0	0	1	1	0	4	0
Stenotrophomonas sp.	2	3	5	2	0	0	0	0	0	1	1	0
Total	7 (77.8%)	11 (78.6%)	64 (86.5%)	34 (89.5%)	0 (0)	0 (0)	0 (0)	1 (2.6%)	2 (22.2%)	3 (21.4%)	10 (13.5%)	3 (7.9%)

Table 3 Comparison of resistance pattern of isolated bacteria against different antimicrobial agents in four-year period

Microorganism / Antimicrobial agent	Susceptibility											
	Sensitive; n (%)				Intermediate; n (%)				Resistant; n (%)			
	2007	2008	2009	2010	2007	2008	2009	2010	2007	2008	2009	2010
Acinetobacter												
Amikacin	8	13	7	1	1	0	0	1	9	6	9	8
Ampicillin/sulbactam	1	5	11	3	0	0	0	0	4	8	21	8
Cotrimoxazole	7	6	5	1	0	0	0	0	14	10	13	8
Cefixime	0	0	1	0	0	0	0	0	4	7	3	1
Cefotaxime	1	1	0	1	0	0	0	0	4	3	5	1
Ceftazidim	0	2	2	0	0	0	0	0	4	10	7	2
Ciprofloxacin	9	4	7	1	0	1	0	0	8	8	13	6
Gentamicin	5	9	4	1	1	0	0	0	9	2	6	5
Imipenem	8	15	20	7	0	3	0	1	4	0	1	3
Nitrofurantoine	2	2	1	0	0	0	0	0	5	3	0	2
Piperacillin	2	4	N/A	0	1	0	N/A	0	5	3	N/A	3
Ceftriaxone	1	6	4	0	0	0	0	0	15	13	10	9
Piperacillin/ tazobactam	2	1	12	3	0	0	0	0	1	1	5	0
Total	46 (34.1%)	68 (45.9%)	74 (44.3%)	18 (23.7%)	3 (2.2%)	4 (2.7%)	0 (0)	2 (2.6%)	86 (63.7%)	74 (50%)	93 (55.7%)	56 (73.7%)
Citrobacter												
Amikacin	4	5	11	N/A	1	0	0	N/A	2	2	9	N/A
Cotrimoxazole	1	2	3	N/A	0	0	0		6	6	13	N/A
Cefixime	0	1	0	N/A	0	0	0	N/A	1	1	1	N/A
Ciprofloxacin	2	3	3	N/A	0	0	0		6	4	21	N/A
Gentamicin	1	5	4	N/A	0	0	0	N/A	5	1	11	N/A
Imipenem	4	3	20	N/A	0	0	0	N/A	0	0	0	N/A
Ceftriaxone	0	1	3	N/A	0	0	1	N/A	5	14	16	N/A
Total	12 (31.6%)	20 (41.7%)	44 (37.9%)	N/A	1 (2.6%)	0 (0)	1 (0.9%)	N/A	25 (65.8%)	28 (58.3%)	71 (61.2%)	N/A
E. coli												
Amikacin	62	85	53	26	2	0	0	0	10	8	16	4
Ampicillin/sulbactam	3	6	15	7	0	0	2	1	2	12	49	15
Ampicillin	0	0	1	1	0	0	0	0	2	22	26	1
Cotrimoxazole	21	19	24	8	0	0	1	0	49	59	47	20
Cefepime	3	4	7	2	0	0	0	0	3	23	5	1
Cefixime	3	2	2	0	0	0	0	0	11	10	0	1
Ceftazidim	3	3	7	15	0	0	1	0	4	16	43	6
Ciprofloxacin	19	26	24	13	0	0	0	0	44	51	49	18

Table 3 Comparison of resistance pattern of isolated bacteria against different antimicrobial agents in four-year period *(Continued)*

Gentamicin	18	49	24	12	1	1	2	0	32	35	26	8
Imipenem	25	47	77	29	0	0	0	0	0	0	0	2
Nitrofurantoine	31	68	39	10	1	1	0	0	2	11	11	1
Ceftriaxone	17	40	16	13	0	1	1	0	51	50	55	17
Piperacillin/ tazobactam	1	3	22	18	0	1	1	0	0	1	0	0
Total	206 (49.1%)	352 (53.8%)	311 (48.1%)	154 (61.8%)	4 (0.9%)	4 (0.6%)	8 (1.2%)	1 (0.4%)	210 (50%)	298 (45.6%)	327 (50.6%)	94 (37.7%)
Enterobacter	20	34	25	13	0	0	1	0	1	1	3	1
Amikacin	5	3	9	4	0	0	1	0	0	5	15	1
Ampicillin/sulbactam	0	0	2	0	0	0	0	0	1	5	4	2
Ampicillin	12	24	21	8	0	0	0	0	11	13	7	4
Cotrimoxazole	0	4	5	1	0	0	0	0	1	6	2	1
Cefepime	3	6	1	0	1	2	0	1	3	11	2	4
Cefixime	5	11	12	7	0	0	1	0	0	9	8	4
Ceftazidim	12	18	24	8	0	0	0	0	8	7	8	2
Ciprofloxacin	9	23	21	5	0	0	1	0	4	6	5	1
Gentamicin	12	30	31	13	0	0	0	0	0	0	0	1
Imipenem	4	8	8	1	1	1	0	0	1	8	3	0
Nitrofurantoine	9	19	19	10	0	0	1	0	9	12	8	5
Ceftriaxone												
Total	91 (68.9%)	180 (67.7%)	178 (72.3%)	70 (72.2%)	2 (1.5%)	3 (1.1%)	5 (20.3%)	1 (0.1%)	39 (29.5%)	83 (31.2%)	63 (25.6%)	26 (26.8%)
Kelebsiella												
Amikacin	13	10	12	4	2	0	0	1	7	1	6	1
Ampicillin/sulbactam	0	1	5	1	0	0	0	0	3	1	11	4
Cotrimoxazole	6	5	7	2	0	0	0	0	17	3	12	4
Cefixime	1	3	1	0	0	0	0	0	9	3	0	1
Ceftazidim	2	1	6	0	0	1	0	0	0	4	7	2
Ciprofloxacin	6	4	10	4	2	0	0	0	12	3	10	3
Gentamicin	7	4	10	3	0	0	0	0	11	5	5	3
Imipenem	10	8	19	8	0	0	0	0	0	0	0	0
Nitrofurantoine	5	2	5	3	0	0	1	0	1	3	3	2
Ceftriaxone	3	3	5	2	1	0	0	0	16	6	13	4
Total	53 (39.5%)	41 (57.7%)	70 (50.7%)	27 (51.9%)	5 (3.7%)	1 (1.4%)	1 (0.7%)	1 (1.9%)	76 (56.7%)	29 (40.8%)	67 (48.5%)	24 (46.1%)
Proteus												
Amikacin	8	4	13	5	0	0	0	0	3	0	1	0
Ampicillin/sulbactam	1	2	11	5	0	0	0	0	0	0	4	0
Cotrimoxazole	4	2	4	3	0	1	0	0	7	3	9	1

Table 3 Comparison of resistance pattern of isolated bacteria against different antimicrobial agents in four-year period *(Continued)*

Cefepime	1	0	4	1	0	1	0	0	1	2	0	0
Ceftazidim	2	0	8	4	0	1	0	0	2	3	1	0
Ciprofloxacin	4	2	8	6	0	0	0	0	5	3	7	0
Gentamicin	2	5	8	1	1	0	0	0	4	0	0	1
Imipenem	7	6	17	6	0	0	0	0	0	0	0	0
Nitrofurantoine	1	1	0	0	0	0	0	0	2	0	1	1
Ceftriaxone	5	3	14	6	0	0	0	0	5	0	2	0
Piperacillin/ tazobactam	1	1	12	5	0	0	0	0	0	0	0	0
Total	36 (54.5%)	26 (65%)	99 (79.8%)	42 (93.3%)	1 (1.5%)	3 (7.5%)	0 (0)	0 (0)	29 (43.9%)	11 (27.5%)	25 (20.2%)	3 (6.7%)
Pseudomona												
Amikacin	9	18	12	11	0	0	0	0	2	3	11	6
Ampicillin/sulbactam	0	0	3	0	0	0	0	0	2	4	20	14
Cotrimoxazole	0	7	4	2	0	0	0	0	13	11	20	14
Cefepime	0	0	2	1	0	0	0	0	1	8	4	3
Ceftazidim	2	0	4	3	0	0	0	0	1	12	12	4
Ciprofloxacin	8	6	10	12	0	1	1	0	2	9	14	3
Gentamicin	5	12	1	4	0	0	0	0	3	7	10	2
Imipenem	9	22	26	15	0	0	0	0	1	0	1	1
Nitrofurantoine	1	0	0	0	0	0	1	0	1	8	3	5
Ceftriaxone	2	2	4	5	0	4	1	0	7	13	19	8
Piperacillin/ tazobactam	1	3	13	6	0	0	0	1	1	0	4	3
Total	37 (52.1%)	70 (46.7%)	79 (39.9%)	59 (48%)	0 (0)	5 (3.3%)	3 (1.6%)	1 (0.8%)	34 (47.9%)	75 (50%)	118 (62.1%)	63 (51.2%)
Stenotrophomonas sp.												
Amikacin	9	40	83	25	2	1	0	1	11	31	29	24
Ampicillin/sulbactam	1	1	1	1	1	0	0	1	9	19	5	2
Cotrimoxazole	22	78	107	35	0	0	0	0	1	2	2	10
Cefixime	0	0	0	0	0	0	0	0	12	44	2	9
Cefotaxime	1	0	0	0	2	0	0	0	5	8	3	1
Ceftazidim	0	5	1	2	0	1	0	0	9	31	1	6
Ciprofloxacin	15	39	109	45	0	0	0	0	3	0	0	1
Gentamicin	8	31	3	2	1	2	0	0	4	9	3	0
Imipenem	2	10	2	2	1	1	0	0	20	49	7	9
Ceftriaxone	1	5	3	2	0	0	1	0	16	65	91	49
Piperacillin/ tazobactam	2	3	5	2	0	0	0	0	0	1	1	0
Total	61 (38.6%)	212 (44.5%)	314 (68.4%)	116 (50.6%)	7 (4.4%)	5 (1%)	1 (0.2%)	2 (0.9%)	90 (57%)	259 (54.5%)	144 (31.4%)	111 (48.5%)

derived pathogen from urine and *S. maltophilia* from bloodstream samples. In a similar Korean study, E. coli had the first rank in terms of the most prevalent organism isolated, *Pseudomona sp.,* and *Klebseilla sp.* had the next ranks among isolated gram-negative pathogens [15]. During 2000 to 2002, more than 220,000 isolated were collected from intensive care units of five countries including France, Germany, Italy, Canada and United States, in which the most common gram-negative pathogen was *E. coli* followed by *Pseudomona sp.* [16]. *S. maltophilia* which was the most common pathogen for bloodstream samples in the present study, were less common in western countries, however it was also seen frequently in Saudi isolates [17].

Antibiotic resistance among *Acinetobacter spp.*, and *Citrobacter spp.* were more frequent in comparison with other isolated pathogens, and our susceptibility rates were similar to rates reported from other regions of the world [18,19]. However, the susceptibility rate of *Acinetobacter spp.* in our study was less than similar surveillance five-year study in Children Medical Center in Iran [20] and was more consistent with reports of antimicrobial resistance from other parts of the world [19,21]. Since that Iranian report dated back to approximately a decade ago, this may demonstrate the increase in the rate of *Acinetobacter* resistance in Iran like other countries over the world. Moreover, the resistance frequency rate of *Acinetobacter* to Ampicillin/sulbactam had an increasing trend after 2007. This was because the availability of generic Iranian formulation of this specific antibiotic in 2007 as well as the administration of oral dosage forms which was used widespread in that year.

The most commonly administered antibiotics in different countries all over the world are β-lactams, and decreased susceptibility of nosocomial pathogens to this therapeutic class of antibiotics has resulted in a major clinical disaster [22]. Iran is not an exception for this statement, and cephalosporines are commonly used in the country because of their availability as well as low rate of adverse events [12]. With respect to antibiotics, the most frequent resistance to antibiotics was observed in ampicillin (66.7-100%) and third generation cephalosporines consisting of cefotaxime (57.2-100%), ceftazidim (42.1-86.4%), cefixime (45-75%) and ceftriaxone (65.7-74.8%). To elucidate the importance of increasing resistance, it is worth mentioning that even the resistant rate of *Enterobacter* as the most susceptible microorganism to cefixime was increased in a four-year period. In contrast, the lowest resistant rates were seen with imipenem (4.5-26.5%),piperacillin/tazobactam (7.9-22.2%), and amikacin (21.3-33.3%). Resistance to third generation cephalosporines in this study was higher than similar studies evaluating the susceptibility rates of gram-negative pathogens [23-25]. This higher resistance can be attributed to the frequent use of third generation cephalosporines in the empirical management of infectious in Iran as the resistance rate of *E.coli* to ceftazidim was reduced after its administration was reduced and it was omitted from local protocols of empiric treatment for a period of time. Resistance of microorganisms to Cefepime, as a fourth generation cephalosporine, had an increasing trend in 2007–2008 but with restrictions in its usage the susceptibility rates were improved in 2009–2010.In contrast to previous studies that reported an increase in the resistance rate to fluoroquinolones [26,27], we found an improving susceptibility to ciprofloxacin in our study in a four-year period with *Acinetobacter* as an exception. This can be partly explained by the fact that fluoroquinolones are not routinely used as an empirical antibiotic for infectious diseases in Imam Hospital. In the present study, resistance to ciprofloxacin was 31.6-54.5% that was less than similar previous evaluation in Argentina with resistance rate of more than 80% [28]. On the other hand, the majority of the nosocomial pathogens from various specimen resources in the present study were susceptible to imipenem and this was consistent through the assessment period. As there was a correlation between previous use of fluoroquinolones and imipenem resistance [29,30], the low administration rate of ciprofloxacin and as a consequence improved sensitivity of organisms to this agent can be the reason behind the susceptibility of most of the organisms to imipenem. The low resistance rate of isolates to imipenem was also reported in previous Belgian and Polish studies with 13% and 8% resistant isolated, respectively [23,25]. In contrast, in Turkish patients resistance to imipenem was slightly more prevalent than that of our study [31]. Amikacin was among the most active antimicrobial agents against isolates with the low resistant rate of 21.3-33.3%. Studies performed over a long time period revealed that the increase in resistance to aminoglycosides is milder than for any other antimicrobial agent even with continued administration [32,33].

In conclusion, the finding of the present study revealed that resistance rate to common antimicrobial agents in Iran is growing and isolates were susceptible mostly to broad-spectrum antibiotics including imipenem and piperacillin/tazobactam. As the antibiotic resources of developing countries including Iran are limited, periodic surveillances of antimicrobial resistance patterns play a vital role in controlling the spread of resistant strains as well as implementing protocols for halting the process. Moreover, it is rational to establish a committee for appropriate antibiotic administration to control the use of antimicrobial agents at the same time of performing surveillance studies for the aim of effective infection management. Such surveillance studies could help in limiting the rate of antimicrobial resistance all over the world.

Competing interests

The authors have not any conflict of interest about this work and have not any financial support.

Authors' contributions

MRS collected the culture and anti-biogram results of the patients from the microbiology laboratory. HK is main supervisor of the study and organized the data, SJ was responsible for clinical interpretation of the results, AA was responsible for the laboratory data analysis, Statistical analysis was done by ZJR and SDK and AH-T prepared the manuscript. All authors read and approved the final manuscript.

Acknowledgement

We must appreciate the staffs of Valiasr Laboratory Department for their supports.

Author details

[1]Department of Clinical Pharmacy, Faculty of Pharmacy, Tehran University of Medical Sciences, Tehran, Iran. [2]Department of Pathology, Faculty of Medicine, Tehran University of Medical Sciences, Tehran, Iran. [3]Department of Infectious Diseases, Faculty of Medicine, Tehran University of Medical Sciences, Tehran, Iran.

References

1. Masterton RG: **Surveillance studies: how can they help in the management of infection?** *J Antimicrob Chemother* 2000, **46**:53–58.
2. Masterton R, Drusano G, Paterson DL, Park G: **Appropriate antimicrobial treatment in nosocomial infections—the clinical challenges.** *J Hosp Infect* 2003, **55**:1–12.
3. Kollef MH, Fraser VJ: **Antibiotic resistance in the intensive care unit.** *Ann Intern Med* 2001, **134**:298–314.
4. Kollef M: **Appropriate empirical antibacterial therapy for nosocomial infections: getting it right the first time.** *Drug* 2003, **63**:2157–2168.
5. Turner PJ: **Trends in antimicrobial susceptibilities among bacterial pathogens isolated from patients hospitalized in European medical centers: 6-year report of the MYSTIC Surveillance Study (1997–2002).** *Diagn Microbiol Infect Dis* 2005, **51**:281–289.
6. Morris AK, Masterton RG: **Antibiotic resistance surveillance: action for international studies.** *J Antimicrob Chemother* 2002, **49**:7–10.
7. Lewis D: **Antimicrobial resistance surveillance: methods will depend on objectives.** *J Antimicrob Chemother* 2002, **49**:3–5.
8. Fontana R, Lo CG, Giacobone E, Romero E, Cipriani P, Sessa R, Franchino L: **Resistance surveillance in Italy: four-year results from the MYSTIC Program.** *J Chemother* 2002, **14**:323–331.
9. Garcia-Rodriguez JA, Jones RN, The MYSTIC Programme Study Group: **Antimicrobial resistance in Gram-negative isolates from European intensive care units: data from the Meropenem Yearly Susceptibility Test Information Collection (MYSTIC) Programme.** *J Chemother* 2002, **14**:25–32.
10. Masterton RG, Kuti JL, Turner PJ, Nicolau DP: **The OPTAMA Programme: utilizing MYSTIC (2002) to predict critical pharmacody- namic target attainment against nosocomial pathogens in Europe.** *J Antimicrob Chemother* 2005, **55**:71–77.
11. Aslani MM, Alikhani MY, Zavari A, Yousefi R, Zamani AR: **Characterization of enteroaggregative Escherichia coli (EAEC) clinical isolates and their antibiotic resistance pattern.** *Int J Infect Dis* 2011, **15**:e136–e139.
12. Hadadi A, Rasoulinejad M, Maleki Z, Yonesian M, Shirani A, Kourorian Z: **Antimicrobial resistance pattern of Gram-negative bacilli of nosocomial origin at 2 university hospitals in Iran.** *Diagn Microbiol Infec Dis* 2008, **60**:301–305.
13. Vessal G, Afhami S, Gholami K, Shafaghi B, Yazdi SH: **Evaluation of antimicrobial resistance among gram-negative isolates collected from intensive care units and reliability of routine disc susceptibility tests at a teaching hospital in tehran.** *Iranian Journal of Pharmaceutical Research* 2006, **2**:89–100.
14. Bush K: **Bench-to-bedside review: The role of β-lactamases in antibiotic-resistant Gram-negative infections.** *Crit Care* 2010, **14**:224.
15. Lee K, Lee MA, Lee CH, Lee J, Roh KH, Kim S, Kim JJ, Koh E, Yong D, Chong Y: **KONSAR Group. Increase of ceftazidime- and fluoroquinolone-resistant Klebsiellapneumoniae and imipenem-resistant Acinetobacter spp. in Korea: analysis of KONSAR study data from 2005 and 2007.** *Yonsei Med J* 2010, **51**:901–911.
16. Jones ME, Darghi DC, Thornsberry C, Karlowsky JA, Sahm DF, Wenzel RB: **Emerging resistance among bacterial pathogens in the intensive care unit: A European and North American Surveillance study 2000–2002.** *Ann Clin Microbiol Antimicrob* 2004, **3**:14.
17. Al-Johani SM, Akhter J, Balkhy H, El-Saed A, Younan M, Memish Z: **Prevalence of antimicrobial resistance among gram-negative isolates in an adult intensive care unit at a tertiary care center in Saudi Arabia.** *Ann Saudi Med* 2010, **30**:364–369.
18. Winokur PL, Canton R, Casellas JM, Legakis N: **Variations in the prevalence of strains expressing an extended spectrum β-lactamase phenotype and characterization of isolates from Europe, the Americas, and the Western Pacific region.** *Clin Infect Dis* 2001, **32**:S94–S103.
19. Gales AC, Jones RN, Forward KR, Linares J, Sader HS, Verhoef J: **Emerging importance of multi-drug resistant *Acinetobacter* species and *Stenotrophomonas maltophilia*as pathogens in seriously ill patients: geographic patterns, epidemiological features, and trends in the SENTRY Antimicrobial Surveillance Program (1997–1999).** *Clin Infect Dis* 2001, **32**:S104–S113.
20. Mamishi S, Pourakbari B, Ashtiani MH, Hashemi FB: **Frequency of isolation and antimicrobial susceptibility of bacteria isolated from bloodstream infections at Children's Medical Center, Tehran, Iran, 1996–2000.** *Int J Antimicrob Agents* 2005, **26**:373–379.
21. Fluit AC, Jones ME, Schmitz FJ, Acar J, Gupta R, Verhoef J: **Antimicrobial susceptibility and frequency of occurrence of clinical blood isolates in Europe from the SENTRY antimicrobial surveillance pro- gram, 1997 and 1998.** *Clin Infect Dis* 2000, **30**:454–460.
22. Jean SS, Teng LJ, Hsueh PR, Ho SW, Luh KT: **Antimicrobial susceptibilities among clinical isolates of extended-spectrum cephalosporin-resistant Gram-negative bacteria in a Taiwanese University Hospital.** *J Antimicrobiol Chemother* 2002, **49**:69–76.
23. Glupczynski Y, Delmee M, Goossens H, Struelens M: **Belgian Multicenter ICU Study Group. Distribution and prevalence of antimicrobial resistance among gram-negative isolates in intensive care units (ICU) in Belgian hospitals between 1996 and 1999.** *Acta Clin Belg* 2001, **56**:297–306.
24. Ishii Y, Alba J, Kimura S, Yamaguchi K: **Evaluation of antimicrobialactivity of betalactam antibiotics by E-test against clinical isolates from100 medical centers in Japan.** *Diagn Microbiol Infect Dis* 2006, **55**:143–148.
25. Patzer J, Dzierzanowska D, Turner P: **Susceptibility patterns of Gram-negative bacteria from a Polish intensive care unit, 1997–2000.** *Int J Antimicrob Agents* 2002, **9**:431–434.
26. Ko WC, Hsueh PR: **Increasing extended-spectrum b-lactamase production and quinolone resistance among Gram-negative bacilli causing intra-abdominal infections in the Asia/Pacific region: Data from the Smart Study 2002–2006.** *J Infect* 2009, **59**:95–103.
27. Karlowsky JA, Jones ME, Draghi DC, Thornsberry C, Sahm DF, Volturo GA: **Prevalence and antimicrobial susceptibilities of bacteria isolated from blood cultures of hospitalized patients in the United States in 2002.** *Ann Clin Microbiol Antimicrob* 2004, **3**:7–14.
28. Rodriguez CH, Juarez J, de Mier C, Pugliese L, Blanco G, Vay C: **Bacterial resistance to antibiotics in gram-negative rods isolated from intensive care units. Comparative analysis between two periods (1998 and 2001).** *Medicina* 2003, **63**:21–27.
29. Lautenbach E, Weiner MG, Nachamkin I, Bilker WB, Sheridan A, Fishman NO: **Imipenem resistance among Pseudomonas aerugi- nosa isolates: risk factors for infection and impact of resis- tance on clinical and economic outcomes.** *Infect Control Hosp Epidemiol* 2006, **27**:893–900.
30. Tanimoto K, Tomita H, Fujimoto S, Okuzumi K, Ike Y: **Fluoroquinolone enhances the mutation frequency for meropenem-selected carbapenem resistance in Pseudomonas aeruginosa, but use of the high-potency drug doripenem inhibits mutant formation.** *Antimicrob Agents Chemother* 2008, **52**:3795–3800.
31. Kucukates E: **Antimicrobial resistance among Gram-negative bacteria isolated from intensive care units in a Cardiology Institute in Istanbul Turkey.** *Jpn J Infect Dis* 2005, **58**:228–231.

32. Gerding DN, Larson TA, Hughes RA, *et al*: **Aminoglycoside resistance and aminoglycoside usage: ten years of experience in one hospital.** *Antimicrob Agents Chemother* 1991, **35**:1284–1290.
33. Hsueh PR, Chen WH, Luh KT: **Relationships between antimicrobial use and antimicrobial resistance in Gram-negative bacteria causing nosocomial infections from 1991–2003 at a university hospital in Taiwan.** *Int J Antimicrob Agents* 2005, **26**:463–472.

Tribulus terrestris for treatment of sexual dysfunction in women: randomized double-blind placebo - controlled study

Elham Akhtari[1], Firoozeh Raisi[2*], Mansoor Keshavarz[1], Hamed Hosseini[3,4], Farnaz Sohrabvand[5], Soodabeh Bioos[1], Mohammad Kamalinejad[6] and Ali Ghobadi[7]

Abstract

Background: Tribulus terrestris as a herbal remedy has shown beneficial aphrodisiac effects in a number of animal and human experiments. This study was designed as a randomized double-blind placebo-controlled trial to assess the safety and efficacy of Tribulus terrestris in women with hypoactive sexual desire disorder during their fertile years. Sixty seven women with hypoactive sexual desire disorder were randomly assigned to Tribulus terrestris extract (7.5 mg/day) or placebo for 4 weeks. Desire, arousal, lubrication, orgasm, satisfaction, and pain were measured at baseline and after 4 weeks after the end of the treatment by using the Female Sexual Function Index (FSFI). Two groups were compared by repeated measurement ANOVA test.

Results: Thirty women in placebo group and thirty women in drug group completed the study. At the end of the fourth week, patients in the Tribulus terrestris group had experienced significant improvement in their total FSFI ($p < 0.001$), desire ($p < 0.001$), arousal ($p = 0.037$), lubrication ($p < 0.001$), satisfaction ($p < 0.001$) and pain ($p = 0.041$) domains of FSFI. Frequency of side effects was similar between the two groups.

Conclusions: Tribulus terrestris may safely and effectively improve desire in women with hypoactive sexual desire disorder. Further investigation of Tribulus terrestris in women is warranted.

Keywords: Tribulus terrestris, Sexual dysfunction, Women, Traditional medicine

Background

Hypoactive sexual desire disorder (HSDD) is a multi factorial and multifaceted disorder which has been entangled with biologic and psychological considerations and interpersonal relations. HSDD is a common sexual complaint affecting approximately 1 in 10 adult women in the USA [1,2], and its prevalence appears to be similar in Europe (7%-16%) [3] and Australia (16%) [4]. According to some scientific reports the prevalence in Iran is 30% [5].

Currently there are two therapeutic modalities for women who suffer from the lack of libido: psychotherapy and pharmacotherapy. Several drugs have been suggested for treating women's loss of libido including estrogen, methyl testosterone [4], phenethylamin [5], bupropion [6] and saffron [7]. However, there is no Food and Drug Administration (FDA) approved drug for treating women's HSDD [8,9].

Avicenna's *The Canon of Medicine* (1025 AD) provides a full chapter to the description of libido, its disorders and treatments. Twentieth chapter of the book discusses the libido under rubric of "*Bah*", its disorders and causes that may boost and reduce the sex drive as well as treatments for each cause [10]. According to *the Canon of Medicine* and Aghili Khorasani's *Makhzan al-Advia* (The treasury of Spices) (18th AD), Bindii or *Tribulus terrestris* influences libido [11] and is able to boost sex drive in human beings. According to the Iranian Traditional Medicine (ITM) deregulation and disorders of libido in both sexes is considerably common. It is worthy to mention that, ITM is based on principles of Humorist school and

* Correspondence: Fraisi@gmail.com
[2]Psychiatry, Fellow of the European Committee of Sexual Medicine (FECSM), Roozbeh Psychiatric Hospital, Psychiatric and Clinical Psychology, Research Center, Tehran University of Medical Sciences, South Kargar Street, Tehran 13337, Iran
Full list of author information is available at the end of the article

four humors (black bile, yellow bile, phlegm and blood), but the mentioned herbal medicine, Tribulus terrestris, has been classified as an experimental remedy because it affects all four humors and boosts the libido.

Recent scientific studies on medicinal herbs have referred to Tribulus terrestris as an effective drug of women's sex drive [12]. A study on mice hypothesized that the drug may affect follicle-stimulating hormone (FSH) and luteinizing hormone (LH); injecting 10 mg of Tribulus extract into female mice resulted in significant increase in both growth rate and size of follicles in comparison to the control mice [13].

The aim of our clinical trial was to analyze the effect of Tribulus on women with HSDD in childbearing age.

Methods

Trial design

This was a randomized, double-blind, placebo-controlled clinical trial study, performed in two medical centers in Tehran Province, Rostamabad Neighborhood Health Center, part of the 1st district of the greater Tehran Municipality, and Sajjad Hospital in city of Shahryar. This study was approved by the ethics committee of School of Medicine, Tehran University of Medical Sciences (TUMS), and it was registered in the clinical trial center under reg. no. of IRCT201211111111425N1

Participants

Participants of the study were selected after responding to this specific question *"Do you suffer from loss of libido?"* in a direct and face to face encounter, and the study was conducted from June 2012 to July 2013. Then a phone interview was scheduled for all 96 women who were selected; and subsequently they were invited for a screening visit after verification of their disorder. The inclusion criteria of the study were: being married and actively living with a partner at least 15 days per month, being in childbearing age, lack and or loss of libido which causes distress, having normal pelvic exam, negative pap smear test conducted at least within past six months, and having normal breast exam. The exclusion criteria were: lack of steady sexual partner, suffering from a serious medical condition (any disease which may force the participant to use drugs during the study), any history of genital tract or breast cancers, suffering from major depression disorder or other psychiatric disorders, menopause, pregnancy, husband's sexual problems and active plans for divorce. Participants with the mentioned inclusion criteria were allowed to start the next stage which was a face to face interview based on Diagnostic and Statistical Manual of Mental Disorders (DSM-IV-TR) codes for HSDD [14]. Finally patients were asked to sign the informed consent forms.

Preparations of tribulus terrestris

Tribulus is widely scattered across the planet a herbal plant [15]. Tribulus belongs to Zygophyllaceae family. Alpha amyrin constitutes over 60% of active ingredient (AI) of the herb [16]. Dried leaves of Tribulus were obtained from a licensed distributer of herbs and natural remedies in Tehran. They were approved and registered by the SHUM herbarium (voucher number: SHUM 8051).

Preparations of syrup and placebo

Traditional Medicine Department, School of Medicine, TUMS used the whole vaporized ethanolic extract of Tribulus terrestris for preparing the syrup. There was 3.5 grams of ethanolic extract in every 5 ml of the syrup. The placebo was prepared via the same method without Tribulus terrestris extract as a sucrose syrup.

Treatment and assessment

Each participant was initially asked to fill the Female Sexual Function Index (FSFI) (21) a self-reported questionnaire under supervision of an Iranian traditional medicine intern who was already trained by a gynecologist and a psychiatrist for conducting the trial, and then she was provided with a drug bottle with specific cod*ing*. Drug Product Information Form (DPIF) was inscribed on a label attached to the bottle. The specific code was recorded on both questionnaire and participant's data sheet. The DPIF instructions included this information: 7.5 ml of the drug should be used two times a day for four full weeks since the day after the completion of menstruation period. Two days after submitting the drug, the patient was checked by a physician through a phone call in order to make sure that the drug was used correctly. Again, after a week a second phone call was made to make sure of continuity of the mentioned order. Patients, who forgot to use more than three doses of their drugs, were excluded. Another interview according to the DSM-IV-TR criteria for HSDD was made four weeks after completion of the drug therapy, side effects (if any) were checked and FSFI questionnaire was refilled. The participants were allowed to call their therapist during the treatment period.

Outcomes

The participants filled the FSFI questionnaire [1,17] two times: 1) at the beginning of the study, 2) four weeks after finishing their drug. The questionnaire have 19 questions with six domains included desire, arousal, lubrication, orgasm, satisfaction and pain, and a general score in which higher scores reflected better sexual activity. Questions 1 and 2 were related to the sexual desire and its score varied between 1.2 and 6. Questions 3, 4, 5 and 6 analyzed arousal of the patient. Another domain of the questionnaire was lubrication which covered questions 7, 8, 9, and 10. The orgasm domain included questions 11, 12 and 13. Questions

14, 15 and 16 all were related to the sexual satisfaction and finally questions 17, 18 and 19 analyzed pain.

The initial outcome was the assessment of desire and total score of our samples with FSFI before and after intervention. Likewise, different subscales including arousal, lubrication, orgasm, satisfaction and pain were compared as the secondary targets using the questionnaire before and after treatment. The FSFI question contained 19 questions which analyzed five domains of women's sexual function. Side effects were recorded systematically within the trial period through visits made within 1, 2 and 4 weeks and after the end of pharmacotherapy.

Sample size

The statistical power was set at 80% in order to achieve a minimum score of 3, to improve the "sexual desire" score in the intervention (experimental) group in comparison with the control group. The standard deviation (SD) was 3.5 (resulted from our pilot study). In regards to possibility of loss measuring 20% during the study period, we achieved significance level of 95% and a bilateral t-test.

Randomization, allocation concealment, and blinding

The randomized sequence was produced by a methodology using randomization permuted block technique with blocks size of 4 which was submitted to therapists with ratio 1:1 divided in two groups. The randomized sequence for allocating the main or placebo treatment was concealed through producing unknown codes; hence, pre-provided drugs and placebo were submitted through similar packs but different codes, as neither therapists nor patients were aware of the active ingredient of the drug packs.

Statistical analysis

Descriptive baseline characteristics for two groups comparisons were tabulated as means and SD or as percentages. All analyses comparing the efficacy of our primary and secondary outcomes were by intention-to-treat principles. Using General Linear Model (GLM) score of desire, arousal, lubrication, orgasm, satisfaction, and pain between two groups were compared by repeated measurement ANOVA test. Compound symmetry assumption was tested using Mauchley's Sphericity test. The time groups cross-product (interaction term) was considered as group differences in their response over time with the baseline values as a covariate in this model. Significance level of 5% (alpha = 0.05) was used for all statistical tests.

Results

A total of 96 women were enrolled for the study (Figure 1), and 67 women were identified as qualified (out which two women decided not to participate after acquiring DSM IV codes and upon issuing the informed consent, three other women stopped participating at the second phone call time point despite receiving drug and answering the first phone call. According to the code recorded on the questionnaire, (before taking drug) it was turned out that two women were from the placebo group and another one was from the drug group. Their reasons for stopping participating at the studying included very sweet taste of the drug (one woman) and anxiety due to using an investigational drug (two women). Another two women were not available after getting off the study; they signed the consent form, but there was no drug available at that time when they were in the center, and they never came back to receive their ration. Between June 2012 and July 2013, participants took part in an interview and then they filled the FSFI questionnaire; then they were assigned randomly in drug and placebo groups. There was a second visit a week after starting pharmacotherapy and third visit was made four weeks after termination of the treatment which was accompanied with the filling of the questionnaire for the second time. Hence patients in average were followed up for two consecutive months (Figure 1).

60 women out of 67 participants completed their treatment process and the results were analyzed according to what was recorded in their questionnaires. The mean ages of drug and control groups were 36 ± 6.24 years and 36.13 ± 5.88 years, respectively. 70% and 66.6% of participants in drug and control groups had bachelor or higher educational degrees (Table 1). 30 members of Tribulus and 30 members of the placebo group completed their treatment process.

Patients' desire was the main measured outcome of the study in both groups (Table 2) which was measured after four weeks of pharmacotherapy process by using the Female Sexual Function Index (FSFI) questionnaire and the following scores were gained: score of placebo group, before and after intervention, respectively: 2.66 ± 0.75 and 2.86 ± 0.79; scores of Tribulus group, before and after intervention, respectively: 3.06 ± 0.69 and 3.90 ± 0.71. After matching the effect of the possible effective variables (age, pregnancy rate, method of delivery, method of contraception), the difference became significant statistically ($p < 0.001$).

Another variable analyzed in this study was arousal which was measured four weeks after completion of the treatment process through the FSFI questionnaire. Scores of placebo group before and after pharmacotherapy were 3.16 ± 0.95 and 3.17 ± 0.75; Scores of intervention group before and after using Tribulus terrestris were 3.61 ± 0.92 and 4.21 ± 0.67. After matching the effect of the possible effective variables (age, pregnancy rate, method of delivery, method of contraception), the difference became significant statistically ($p = 0.037$).

According to the FSFI another secondary variable was lubrication. Similar to two previous variables lubrication

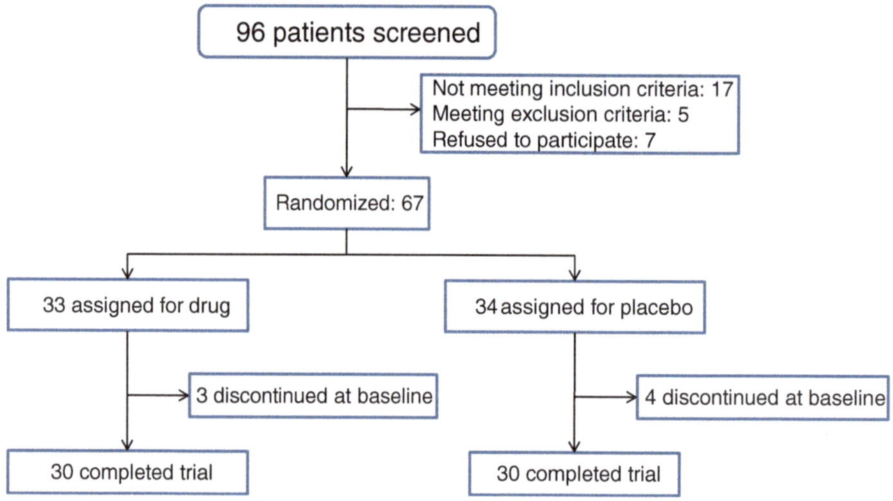

Figure 1 Flow chart indicating subject enrolment, group allocation and analysis according to CONSORT guidelines.

was analyzed four weeks after completion of the treatment. Scores of this domain gained by placebo group before and after usage were 4.15 ± 1.15 and 4.18 ± 0.79 while scores won by intervention group were 4.15 ± 1.13 and 4.66 ± 0.87. After matching the effect of the possible effective variables (age, pregnancy rate, method of delivery, method of contraception), the difference became significant statistically ($p < 0.001$).

Orgasm was analyzed using the FSFI questionnaire after four weeks of completion of treatment with Tribulus terrestris. Scores of this domain gained by placebo group before and after usage were 3.31 ± 0.97 and 3.59 ± 0.85 while scores won by intervention group were 3.21 ± 0.98 and 4.20 ± 0.72. After matching the effect of the possible effective variables (age, pregnancy rate, method of delivery, method of contraception), the difference became significant statistically ($p < 0.001$).

Satisfaction was measured four weeks after completion of treatment process through the FSFI questionnaire. Scores of this domain gained by placebo group before and after pharmacotherapy were 3.43 ± 1.13 and 3.75 ± 1.12; scores won by intervention group before and after

Table 1 Demographic and baseline characteristics of patients

		Tribulus (n = 30)	Placebo (n = 30)
Age (years), mean ± SD		36 ± 6.24	36.13 ± 5.88
Partner age, mean ± SD		39.87 ± 7.13	40.43 ± 7.74
BMI kg/m^2		26.25 ± 3.75	24.67 ± 2.92
Education	Diploma	9	10
	Bachelor	21	17
	MA	0	3
Delivery (mean ± SD)			
Type of delivery	No	10%	6.7%
	NVD	60%	40%
	C/S	30%	53.3%
Contraception	Natural	33.3%	43.3%
	OCP	10%	6.7%
	Candom	23.3%	13.3%
	IUD	16.7%	13.3%
	None	10%	3.3%
	Tubectomy	6.7%	20%
Marriage years mean ± SD		14 ± 5.97	12.73 ± 6.22

Table 2 Summary results for each study group

			Mean differences (CI 95%)	Placebo N = 30	Tribulus terrestris N = 30
	Control Mean ± SD	Baseline Mean ± SD	Control mean ± SD	Baseline mean ± SD	
Desire	3.66 ± 0.69	3.90 ± 0.71	2.66 ± 0.75	2.86 ± 0.79	0.71 (0.41 – 1.01) p < 0.001
Arousal	3.61 ± 0.92	4.21 ± 0.67	3.16 ± 0.95	3.17 ± 0.75	0.75 (0.47 – 1.46) p = 0.037
Lubrication	4.15 ± 1.13	4.66 ± 0.87	4.15 ± 1.15	4.18 ± 0.79	0.50 (0.32 – 0.68) p < 0.001
Orgasm	3.21 ± 0.98	4.20 ± 0.72	3.31 ± 0.97	3.59 ± 0.85	0.85 (0.56 – 1.14) p < 0.001
Satisfaction	3.44 ± 1.15	4.61 ± 0.93	3.43 ± 1.13	3.75 ± 1.12	1.10 (0.73– 1.48) p < 0.001
Pain	4.19 ± 1.56	5.07 ± 1.01	4.19 ± 1.51	4.87 ± 1.42	0.37 (0.16 – 0.73) p < 0.001
General score	22.41 ± 2.87	26.80 ± 3.03	20.39 ± 4.64	21.25 ± 4.72	4.32 (3.33 – 5.31) p = 0.040

using Tribulus terrestris were 3.44 ± 1.15 and 4.61 ± 0.93. After matching the effect of the possible effective variables (age, pregnancy rate, method of delivery, method of contraception), the difference became significant statistically ($p < 0.001$).

Pain was measured four weeks after completion of treatment process through the FSFI questionnaire. Scores of this domain gained by placebo group before and after pharmacotherapy were 4.19 ± 1.51 and 4.87 ± 1.42; scores won by intervention group before and after using Tribulus terrestris were 4.19 ± 1.56 and 5.07 ± 1.01. After matching the effect of the possible effective variables (age, pregnancy rate, method of delivery, method of contraception), the difference became significant statistically ($p = 0.041$).

Finally general scores of both drug and placebo groups were analyzed and compared based on FSFI questionnaire four weeks after completion of intervention. The general scores in placebo and intervention groups before using Tribulus terrestris were 20.89 ± 6.46 and 21.25 ± 4.72, respectively; and four weeks after its completion were 22.41 ± 2.87 and 26.80 ± 3.03, respectively (p = 0.040). These results confirmed by the interviews using DSM-IV-TR (Table 2).

Safety assessment

Possible side effects including abdominal pain, cramping, nausea, vomiting, diarrhea or constipation were recorded using Common Terminology Criteria for Adverse Events (CTCAE) Version 4.02 during the scheduled visits. Only one patient reported grade 1 abdominal cramp.

Discussion

Our findings showed that Tribulus terrestris was effective in improving women's sex drive based on the questions of FSFI questionnaire. Since the basic findings of two groups were similar, the improved score of the Tribulus group can be attributed to libido boosting effects of the plant. Our findings confirmed what has already been described in the Iranian Traditional Medical textbooks about libido boosting effects of Tribulus. There is also more recent evidence that Tribulus can be used as a libido booster plant in women [12]. There may be a possible synergy between Tribulus and FSH-LH mechanism. For instance, one animal experiment showed that mice, injected with 10 mg Tribulus extract, developed thicker theca internal layer and more follicles in comparison with control mice in the same period of time [13].

Prescribing Tribulus extract for women can increase desire score in women who suffer from loss of sex desire. However, according to our knowledge there has not been any similar research on the impact of Tribulus extract in improving women's sex desire in childbearing age. The effect of testosterone in improving desire in menopausal women has been confirmed by studies that have looked at women's sex drive and how to boost it [18,19]. The role of conjugated testosterone in treating lack of sex drive has been emphasized [20]. Currently testosterone is the only approved drug for treatment of HSDD in menopausal women, particularly for those have surgically-induced menopause [21]. In one study on women with SSRI induced desire disorder, it was shown that Saffron was an effective herbal remedy which could improve desire [7]. Another study showed that Bupropion was effective in improving women's desire [6]. However, Tribulus is the only drug which not only improves the sexual desire in women but also it does not have any unexpected side effects in patients.

Our study showed very clearly through acquired scores of the FSFI questionnaire that patients had significant increase in their scores related to questions about desire, arousal and satisfaction. Our results indicated a considerable improvement in scores of desire. Thus, Tribulus had apparent boosting effects on desire, and it was able to improve sexual satisfaction and sexual behavior.

Although our study showed the effect of Tribulus on improving the desire, it must be noticed that Iranian women are generally modest and shy because of their cultural beliefs about sexual concepts, and our sample size was small. In order to produce consistent results and more reliable evidence, more studies with a large sample size must be carried out.

Conclusion

Tribulus terrestris may safely and effectively improve desire in women with HSDD. Further investigation of Tribulus terrestris in women is warranted.

Competing interests

The authors do not have any financial/commercial competing interest in the study presented here. This study was supported with Tehran University of Medical Sciences, School of Traditional Medicine.

Authors' contribution

EA was responsible for recruiting, visiting and evaluating patients; she was also involved in designing the study, analyzing the data and writing the manuscript. FR (the corresponding author) supervised the trial and was involved in all aspects of the study including designing and coordinating the study as well as analyzing the data and drafting the manuscript. MK gave his valuable comments throughout the study and was involved in the original design of the proposal, and also the final revision of the manuscript. HH performed all statistical analysis of the data and interpreted the results of the study. FS was the consultant gynecologist who recommended and supervised the gynecological evaluations of the patients. SB was consulted for a list of medications or herbal products that could interfere with the results of this study. MK participated in the identification of the plants, plant extraction and supervised preparing the placebo and Tribulus terrestris extract. AG prepared the placebo and Tribulus terrestris extract under supervision of MK. All authors read and approved the final manuscript.

Acknowledgements

This study was part of Dr. Elham Akhtari's postgraduate dissertation. The authors like to thank Dr. Roshanak Mokaberinejad at Shahid Behehshti University of Medical Sciences and Dr. Padideh Ghaeli at Tehran University of Medical Sciences for their valuable help throughout the study.

Author details

[1]Department of Traditional Medicine, School of Medicine, Tehran University of Medical Sciences, Tehran, Iran. [2]Psychiatry, Fellow of the European Committee of Sexual Medicine (FECSM), Roozbeh Psychiatric Hospital, Psychiatric and Clinical Psychology, Research Center, Tehran University of Medical Sciences, South Kargar Street, Tehran 13337, Iran. [3]School of Public Health, Tehran University of Medical Sciences, Tehran, Iran. [4]Clinical Trial Center, Tehran University of Medical Sciences, Tehran, Iran. [5]Department of Gynecology and Infertility, Imam Khomeini Hospital, Tehran University of Medical Sciences, Tehran, Iran. [6]Department of Pharmacognosy, School of Pharmacy, Shaheed Beheshti University of Medical Sciences, Tehran, Iran. [7]Department of Traditional Medicine, School of Traditional Pharmacology, Tehran University of Medical Sciences, Tehran, Iran.

References

1. Shifren JL, Monz BU, Russo PA, Segreti A, Johannes CB: **Sexual problems and distress in United States women: prevalence and correlates.** *Obstet Gynecol* 2008, **112**(5):970–978.
2. Leiblum SR, KKoochaki PE, Rodenberg CA, Barton IP, Rosen RC: **Hypoactive Sexual desire disorder in postmenopausal women: US results from the Women's International Study of Health and Sexuality (WISHeS).** *Menopause* 2006, **13**(1):46–56.
3. Dennerstein L, Koochaki P, Barton I, Graziottin A: **Hypoactive sexual desire disorder in menopausal women: a survey of western European women.** *J Sex Med* 2006, **3**(2):212–22.
4. Hayes RD, Dennerstein L, Bennett CM, Fairley CK: **What is the "true" prevalence of female sexual dysfunctions and does the way we assess these conditions have an impact?** *J Sex Med* 2008, **5**(4):777–778.
5. Safarinejad MR: **Female sexual dysfunction in population based study in Iran: prevalence and associated risk factors.** *Int J Impot Res* 2006, **18**(4):382–395.
6. Davis SR, van der Mooren MJ, van Lunsen RH, Lopes P, Ribot J, Rees, Moufarege A, Rodenberg C, Buch A, Purdie DW: **Efficacy and safety of a testosterone patch for the treatment of hypoactive sexual desire disorder in surgically menopausal women: a randomized, placebo-controlled trial.** *Menopause* 2006, **13**(3):387–396.
7. Berman JR, Berman LA, Werbin TJ, Goldstein I: **Female sexual dysfunction: anatomy, physiology, evaluation and treatment options.** *Curr Opin Urol* 1999, **9**(6):563–568.
8. Segraves RT, Clayton A, Croft H, Wolf A, Wamock J: **Bupropion sustained release for the treatment of hypoactive sexual desire disorder in premenopausal women.** *J Clin Psychopharmacol* 2004, **24**(3):339–342.
9. Kashani L, Raisi F, Saroukhani S, Sohrabi H, Modabbernia A, Nasehi AA, Jamshidi A, Ashrafi M, Mansouri P, Ghaeli P, Akhondzadeh S: **Saffron for treatment of fluoxetine-induced sexual dysfunction in women: randomized double-blind placebo-controlled study.** *Hum Psychopharmacol* 2013, **28**(1):54–60.
10. Simon JA: **Opportunities for intervention in HSDD.** *J Fam Pract* 2009, **58**(7 Suppl Hypoactive):S26–30.
11. Basson R, Leiblum S, Brotto L, Derogatis L, Fourcroy J, Fugl-Meyer K, Graziottin A, Heiman JR, Laan E, Meston C, Schover L, van Lankveld J, Schultz WW: **Definitions of women's sexual dysfunction reconsidered: advocating expansion and revision.** *J Psychosom Obstet Gynaecol* 2003, **24**(4):221–229.
12. Clayton AH: **The pathophysiology of hypoactive sexual desire disorder in women.** *International J of Gynecol Obstet* 2010, **110**(1):7–11.
13. Ibn-e-sina (Avicenna Husain): *Al-Qanun fit-tib [The Canon of Medicine]*, (Research of Ebrahim Shamsedine). Beirut, Lebanon: Alaalami Beirut library Press; 2005.
14. Aghili Khorasani MH: *Makhzan al Advieh.* Tehran, Iran: Bavardaran Press. Research Institute for Islamic and Complementary Medicine, Iran University of Medical Sciences; 2001.
15. Mazaro-Costa R, Andersen ML, Hachul H, Tufik S: **Medicinal plants as alternative treatments for female sexual dysfunction: Utopian vision or possible treatment in climacteric women?** *J Sex Med* 2010, **7**(11):3695–3714.
16. Esfandiari A, Dehghan A, Sharifi S, Vesali E: **Effect of Tribulus Terresteris extract on ovarian activity in immature wistar rat: a histological evaluation.** *J Anim Vet Adv* 2011, **7**(10):883–886.
17. Brotto LA: **The DSM4 diagnostic criteria for hypoactiove sexual desire disorder in women.** *Arch Sex Behav* 2010, **39**(2):221–239.
18. Zargari A: *Medicinal plants, Vol 1; Tehran.* Iran: Tehran University of Medical Sciences Press; 1989.
19. Abirami P, Rajendran A: **GC-MS analysis of Tribulus terrestris. 1.** *Asian J Plant Sci Res* 2011, **1**(4):13–16.
20. Wiegel M, Meston C, Rosen R: **The female sexual function index (FSFI): cross validation and development of clinical cutoff scores.** *J Sex Marital Ther* 2005, **31**(1):1–20.
21. Rosen R, Brown C, Heiman J, Meston C, Shabsigh R, Ferguson D, Agostino R Jr: **The female sexualfunction index (FSFI): a multidimensional self-report instrument of female sexual function.** *J Sex Marital Thera* 2000, **26**(2):191–208.

A study on quantitative structure–activity relationship and molecular docking of metalloproteinase inhibitors based on L-tyrosine scaffold

Maryam Abbasi[1,2], Fatemeh Ramezani[1], Maryam Elyasi[3], Hojjat Sadeghi-Aliabadi[2] and Massoud Amanlou[1*]

Abstract

Background: MMP-2 enzyme is a kind of matrix metalloproteinases that digests the denatured collagens and gelatins. It is highly involved in the process of tumor invasion and has been considered as a promising target for cancer therapy. The structural requirements of an MMP-2 inhibitor are: (1) a functional group that binds the zinc ion, and (2) a functional group which interacts with the enzyme backbone and the side chains which undergo effective interactions with the enzyme subsites.

Methods: In the present study, a QSAR model was generated to screen new inhibitors of MMP-2 based on L–hydroxy tyrosine scaffold. Descriptors generation were done by Hyperchem 8, DRAGON and Gaussian98W programs. SPSS and MATLAB programs have been used for multiple linear regression (MLR) and genetic algorithm partial least squares (GA-PLS) analyses and for theoretical validation. Applicability domain of the model was performed to screen new compounds. The binding site potential of all inhibitors was verified by structure-based docking according to their binding energy and then the best inhibitors were selected.

Results: The best QSAR models in MLR and GA-PLS were reported, with the square correlation coefficient for leave-one-out cross-validation (Q^2_{LOO}) larger than 0.921 and 0.900 respectively. The created MLR and GA-PLS models indicated the importance of molecular size, degree of branching, flexibility, shape, three-dimensional coordination of different atoms in a molecule in inhibitory activities against MMP-2.

The docking study indicated that lipophilic and hydrogen bonding interactions among the inhibitors and the receptor are involved in a ligand-receptor interaction. The oxygen of carbonyl and sulfonyl groups is important for hydrogen bonds of ligand with Leu82 and Ala83. R_2 and R_3 substituents play a main role in hydrogen bonding interactions. R_1 is sited in the hydrophobic pocket. Methylene group can help a ligand to be fitted in the lipophilic pocket, so two methylene groups are better than one. The Phenyl group can create a π-π interaction with Phe86.

Conclusions: The QSAR and docking analyses demonstrated to be helpful tools in the prediction of anti-cancer activities and a guide to the synthesis of new metalloproteinase inhibitors based on L-tyrosine scaffold.

Keywords: GA-PLS, Metalloproteinase inhibitors, MLR, Molecular docking, QSAR

* Correspondence: amanlou@tums.ac.ir
[1]Department of Medicinal Chemistry, Faculty of Pharmacy, Pharmaceutical Science Research Center, Tehran University of Medical Science, Tehran, Iran
Full list of author information is available at the end of the article

Introduction

The matrix metalloproteinases (MMPs) function predominantly as enzymes that degrade structural components of the extracellular matrix (ECM) [1-4]. MMPs play a substantial role in tumor progression and invasion of inflammatory cells. Among MMPs, MMP-2 easily digests the denatured collagens and gelatins [5,6]. It is highly involved in the process of tumor invasion and has been considered as a promising target for cancer therapy [3,7,8]. MMP-2 has a catalytic center) zinc (II) ion (and two hydrophobic domains (S1′ pocket and S1 pocket). S1′ pocket, the key domain of MMP-2, is deeper and narrower than other MMP subtypes and S1 pocket is a solvent exposure domain [3,9,10].

The structural requirements of an MMP-2 inhibitor are: (1) a functional group that binds the zinc ion (zinc-binding group; ZBG), capable of chelating the active site zinc ion; (2) a functional group which interacts with the backbone of enzyme; (3) side chains that undergo effective interactions with the enzyme subsites, such as S1′ pocket and S1 pocket [3,11,12].

Cheng et al. studied the L–hydroxy proline scaffold-based MMP-2 inhibitors in 2008 [13], and, in order to identify more potent MMP-2 inhibitors, replaced L-hydroxy proline with the L-tyrosine scaffold to form a new integrated structural pattern. They reported that the alteration in substitution pattern at R_1, R_2 and R_3 positions alter MMP-2 inhibitory activity [1].

In 2012, 30 L–hydroxy tyrosine scaffold-based MMP-2 inhibitors were identified. It seems that finding a relationship between the structure of these compounds and their inhibitory activities in order to design structures with better activities and to predict their activity would be essential.

Quantitative structure activity relationships (QSARs), one of the most extensively used methods in chemometrics, and molecular docking are two of the helpful methods for drug design and prediction of drug activity [14-16]. QSAR models are mathematical equations which generate a communication between chemical structures and their biological activities, while molecular docking is done to specify the structural features that are important for interaction with a receptor.

In this report, we have performed a QSAR study and a molecular docking examination on 30 compounds of L-tyrosine derivatives which had been synthesized and evaluated as metalloproteinase (MMP-2) inhibitors [1].

Materials and methods

QSAR

All calculations were implemented using an Intel Core i5 2.4 GHz processor, with the windows 7 operating system. Geometry optimization was done by Hyperchem 8.0 software. Descriptor generation was performed by Hyperchem 8.0, DRAGON package and Gaussian 98 W programs. SPSS software (version 11.5) and MATLAB software (version 7.12.0) were used for model creation and validation methods.

Activity data and descriptors generation

In this study, the biological data employed is MMP-2 inhibitory activity of 30 compounds. The synthesis and determination of biological activity of these inhibitors have been reported by Cheng et al. [1]. The structure of these compounds and their biological activity are shown in Table 1. The two-dimensional structures of molecules were drawn using Hyperchem 8.0 software. At the beginning, pre-optimization was conducted using the MM + molecular mechanic force field and then a more accurate optimization was performed with the semi-empirical PM3 method. The optimization was performed using the Polak–Ribiere algorithm until the root mean square gradient reached 0.01 kcal/ (Å mol). Hyperchem 8.0 program was also used to calculate chemical descriptors including: surface area, molecular volume, hydration energy, octanol/water partition coefficient (logP), molar refractivity, molar polarisability and molar mass.

The output files of Hyperchem 8.0 software (.hin files) were transferred to DRAGON package to calculate four classes of descriptors (0D, 1D, 2D and 3D) including 28 constitutional descriptors, 10 functional groups, 18 atom-centered fragments, 216 topological descriptors, 15 molecular walk counts, 64 BCUT descriptors, 24 Galvestopol.charge indices, 96 2D autocorrelations, 14 charge descriptors, 41 Randic molecular profiles, 27 geometrical descriptors, 150 radial distribution function descriptors (RDF), 160 3D-MoRSE descriptors, 99 WHIM descriptors and 196 GETAWAY descriptors.

The z-matrix files of compounds were also provided by Hyperchem 8.0 program (.zmt files) and then were transferred as input files to the Gaussian98W program [17]. Semi-empirical molecular orbital calculation by PM3 method was performed using Gaussian98W program. Different quantum chemical descriptors were obtained by this method including highest occupied molecular orbital energy (E_{HOMO}), lowest unoccupied molecular orbital energy (E_{LUMO}), and molecular dipole moment. Local charge was obtained by PM3 method in Gaussian98W. Hardness ($\eta = 0.5\ (E_{HOMO} + E_{LUMO})$), softness ($S = 1/\eta$), electronegativity ($\chi = 0.5\ (E_{HOMO} - E_{LUMO})$) and electrophilicity ($\omega = \chi^2/2\eta$) were calculated according to the method proposed by Thanikaivelan et al. [18].

Data processing and models building

All calculated descriptors were collected in a data matrix, D, the number on rows was representative of molecule numbers and the numbers on columns accounted for

Table 1 Chemical structures of L-tyrosine derivatives and their experimental and predicted activity by MLR and GA-PLS models

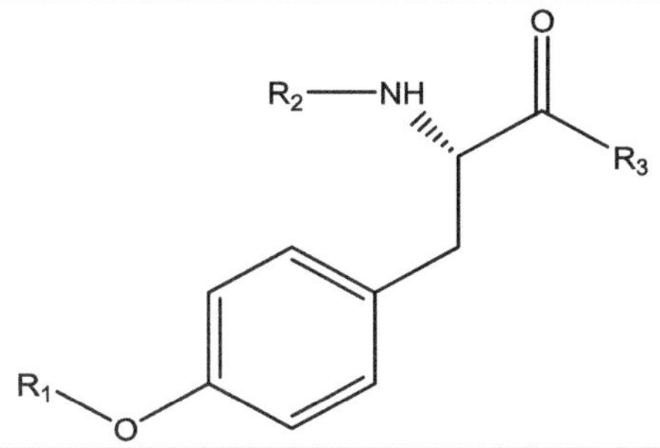

Comp.	R_1	R_2	R_3	Experimental pIC_{50}	Predicted pIC_{50}	
					MLR	GA-PLS
4a	$C_6H_5CH_2$	C_6H_5CO	OCH_3	4.17	4.01	3.90
4b	$C_6H_5CH_2$	p-$CH_3C_6H_4CO$	OCH_3	4.08	3.82	3.92
4c	$C_6H_5CH_2$	CH_3CO	OCH_3	4.56	4.42	4.61
4d	$C_6H_5CH_2$	CH_3SO_2	OCH_3	4.75	4.74	4.74
4e	$C_6H_5CH_2$	p-$CH_3C_6H_4SO_2$	OCH_3	4.97	4.75	4.86
4f	$C_6H_5CH_2CH_2$	C_6H_5CO	OCH_3	4.13	4.16	3.79
4 g	$C_6H_5CH_2CH_2$	p-$CH_3C_6H_4CO$	OCH_3	4.07	3.94	4.42
4 h	$C_6H_5CH_2CH_2$	CH_3CO	OCH_3	4.90	4.98	4.97
4i	$C_6H_5CH_2CH_2$	CH_3SO_2	OCH_3	5.62	5.82	5.98
4j	$C_6H_5CH_2CH_2$	p-$CH_3C_6H_4SO_2$	OCH_3	5.20	5.24	5.44
5a	$C_6H_5CH_2$	C_6H_5CO	OH	5.01	4.39	4.78
5b	$C_6H_5CH_2$	p-$CH_3C_6H_4CO$	OH	5.09	4.77	4.3
5c	$C_6H_5CH_2$	CH_3CO	OH	5.52	5.68	5.66
5d	$C_6H_5CH_2$	CH_3SO_2	OH	5.85	6.03	6.06
5e	$C_6H_5CH_2$	p-$CH_3C_6H_4SO_2$	OH	5.60	5.99	5.91
5f	$C_6H_5CH_2CH_2$	C_6H_5CO	OH	5.12	5.57	5.33
5 g	$C_6H_5CH_2CH_2$	p-$CH_3C_6H_4CO$	OH	5.35	5.90	5.82
5 h	$C_6H_5CH_2CH_2$	CH_3CO	OH	6.12	6.67	6.08
5i	$C_6H_5CH_2CH_2$	CH_3SO_2	OH	6.92	6.69	6.48
5j	$C_6H_5CH_2CH_2$	p-$CH_3C_6H_4SO_2$	OH	6.57	6.49	6.52
6a	$C_6H_5CH_2$	C_6H_5CO	NHOH	5.77	6.04	5.84
6b	$C_6H_5CH_2$	p-$CH_3C_6H_4CO$	NHOH	6.34	6.42	6.82
6c	$C_6H_5CH_2$	CH_3CO	NHOH	7.43	7.32	6.84
6d	$C_6H_5CH_2$	CH_3SO_2	NHOH	7.17	7.44	7.39
6e	$C_6H_5CH_2$	p-$CH_3C_6H_4SO_2$	NHOH	7.60	7.19	7.14
6f	$C_6H_5CH_2CH_2$	C_6H_5CO	NHOH	6.05	6.05	6.86
6 g	$C_6H_5CH_2CH_2$	p-$CH_3C_6H_4CO$	NHOH	5.41	5.57	5.95
6 h	$C_6H_5CH_2CH_2$	CH_3CO	NHOH	7.89	7.55	7.53
6i	$C_6H_5CH_2CH_2$	CH_3SO_2	NHOH	7.54	7.91	7.94
6j	$C_6H_5CH_2CH_2$	p-$CH_3C_6H_4SO_2$	NHOH	7.77	7.49	7.73

descriptors (30 × 1168). At the beginning, the columns which had constant and near constant values were removed from the original data matrix. Since collinear variables disrupt the models in MLR analysis, collinear descriptors needed to be detected and removed. The correlation of descriptors with one another and with activity data was then investigated. In the pairs with collinearity higher than 0.9, one which had the highest correlation versus the activity was retained and the rest were omitted. The number of total descriptors for each molecule reached 291.

The data set (30 compounds) was split into a calibration set and validation set. Validation subset was made of 20% of the total data (here, 6 biological activity data). An MLR analysis was performed by the stepwise regression SPSS (version 12.0) software and the model was built.

Since the data splitting has a considerable influence on the final selected model, a combined data splitting-feature selection (CDFS) strategy was employed [19]. In the CDFS methodology, several subdivisions of calibration and validation set were made (10 times). In each case, the best model was chosen with a correlation coefficient higher than 0.95. The created models were validated by leave-one out (LOO) cross-validation method and Y-randomization test to investigate their predictability.

Molecular docking

Molecular docking has become an increasingly main tool for drug discovery. Docking is a method which predicts the preferred orientation of one ligand when bound in an active site to form a stable complex. In this study, molecular docking of L-tyrosine derivatives with MMP-2 was studied by AutoDock 4.2 program [20] to find their binding site and the best direction based on the binding energy. Pdb file of MMP-2 was obtained from www.pdb.org (PDB: 3AYU) [21]. All water molecules were deleted, polar hydrogens were added and the Kollman charge [22] was computed. A 120 x 120 x 120 Å size was chosen for the grid box, which covers the whole protein. In all of the ligands, the same as protein, polar hydrogens were added and the Gasteiger charge was computed [23]. After preparation of ligand and protein files, the map files were created. Docking process with 50 runs and maximum number of evaluations 2500000 were performed. The final .dlg files were analyzed and the interaction between ligands and the active site of protein were studied. The ligand-protein interactions were analyzed and visualized by Discovery studio Ver. 3.

Result and discussion

Multiple linear regression analysis (MLR)

This study made use of an MLR analysis, as a simple regression method. The stepwise regression (using SPSS software) was also utilized to choose the most relevant set of descriptors for each type of the split data. The model coefficients were calculated using calibration data and then were used to predict the biological activity of validation samples. Several models were constructed by running a typical stepwise regression which is ranked based on calibration correlation coefficient (R^2c). A model with calibration correlation coefficient higher than 0.9 was selected. The created model needed to be validated. The theoretical validation is generally classified into two groups: internal and external validation. Two of the internal validation methods include Leave-one out cross validation (LOO) and Y-randomization [24]. The offered model was evaluated for both over-fitting and avoidance of chance correlations by the leave-one-out cross-validation (LOO) method and Y-randomization test respectively.

MLR method was repeated several times by different splitting data. In each case, one model was proposed. Leave-one-out cross-validation was performed and lastly, the best ten models were obtained with R^2 and Q^2_{LOO} higher than 0.9 in as reported in Table 2. The statistical qualities of models were acceptable and all of them had Q^2_{LOO} larger than 0.92; hence, the predicted models can make over 92% of variances in the inhibitory activity. In addition, results were acceptable in the prediction sets. The values of prediction correlation coefficient (R^2_p) are listed in Table 2 for the ten final models. All of the

Table 2 The best ten models were selected for future analysis in MLR

NO.	Descriptor used	R^2_c [a]	S.E [b]	R^2_p [c]	Q^2_{LOO} [d]	RMS_{CV} [e]
1	IC1, RDF135e, Mor24m, RDF035u, E3u, RDF120m, Mor15e	0.985	0.177	0.988	0.956	0.250
2	IC1, Mor24m, Mor15e, R7e0, G3p	0.989	0.154	0.90	0.967	0.218
3	IC1, Mor24m, Mor15e, dipx, GATS8p, RDF065m	0.986	0.170	0.952	0.962	0.230
4	IC1, SP20, RDF115m, RDF115e, Mor28e	0.988	0.148	0.972	0.972	0.199
5	IC1, Mor24m, Mor15e, Mor09e, G2u, Mor27u	0.976	0.228	0.951	0.940	0.300
6	IC1, Mor24m, Mor15e, Mor09e, G2u, Mor27u	0.969	0.243	0.962	0.932	0.309
7	IC1, Mor28e, HATS3p, RDF120m, RDF115m	0.987	0.152	0.974	0.969	0.203
8	IC1, Mor28e, HATS3p, RDF115m, RDF120m, G3m	0.978	0.194	0.972	0.952	0.245
9	IC1, Mor24m, RDF135e, RDF035v, RDF135m, Mor26m	0.977	0.223	0.979	0.918	0.354
10	IC1, Mor26m, G3p, GATS8p, HATS7e	0.976	0.214	0.953	0.942	0.284

[a] R^2_c = Correlation Coefficient of calibration set.
[b] S.E = Standard error of regression.
[c] R^2_p = Correlation Coefficient of prediction set.
[d] Q^2_{LOO} = Leave-one-out cross-validation correlation coefficient.
[e] $RMSE_{CV}$ = Root mean square error of cross validation.

squared correlation coefficients were higher than 0.90, so the resultant linear models can predict 90% of variances in the inhibitory activity in the ten prediction sets.

The total number of descriptors, which existed in all the ten models, was 22. These descriptors are briefly described in Table 3. Among these, 3 descriptors were common. Some of the descriptors such as E3u, HATS7e, RDF065m, SP20, RDF115e, G3m and dipx were observed only in one model. The repeated descriptors were IC1, Mor24m and Mor15e. IC1 descriptor existed in all the ten models. IC1 is topological descriptor and Mor24m and Mor15e are 3D-MoRSE ones.

The repetition of IC1 in all the ten models indicated that this descriptor has a main effect on L-tyrosine scaffold-based MMP-2 inhibitors. 3D-MoRSE descriptors also have significant effects. The quantum descriptors such as (dipx) that were seen only in one model have lower effects on MMP-2 inhibitors. The observation of the models, as listed in Table 2, revealed that there is a high degree of resemblance between the subset of descriptors (without considering the difference between the chosen descriptors in different models).

To create a general model, all of the 22 descriptors were used and an MLR analysis was applied with the stepwise variable selections. Finally, one model with balance between the highest R^2, Q^2_{LOO} and the lowest number of descriptors was opted for further analysis, as reported in MLR Equation 1:

$$\begin{aligned} pIC_{50} = & -13.428\ (\pm 1.720) + 5.965\ (\pm 0.488)\ IC1 \\ & + 1.464\ (\pm 0.618)\ Mor24m - 0.187\ (\pm 0.044) \\ & RDF115m + 0.307\ (\pm 0.067)\ SP20 \\ & + 1.284\ (\pm 0.514)\ Mor15e \end{aligned} \quad (1)$$

$$N = 24,\ R^2_c = 0.958,\ S.E = 0.285,\ Q^2_{LOO} = 0.921,\ RMS_{CV} = 0.346$$

In this equation, N represents the number of molecules in the calibration set. R^2_c and Q^2_{LOO} are respectively the squared correlation coefficients for calibration and cross-validation. In addition, S.E is the standard error of calibration and RMS_{CV} is the root mean square error of cross-validation. This equation has three common descriptors (IC1, Mor24m and Mor15e), with high calibration statistics and prediction ability.

Topological descriptors, such as IC1, explain the size, degree of branching, flexibility and overall shape. 3D-MoRSE descriptors explain three-dimensional coordination of the different atoms in a molecule. IC1, Mor24m and Mor15e have positive signs which indicate that pIC_{50} is directly related to these descriptors. The radial distribution function (RDF) descriptors are based on the distance distribution in the molecule. RDF115m has a negative sign which indicates that pIC_{50} is inversely related to this descriptor.

For the MMP-2 inhibition activity, a higher value of molecular size, degree of branching, flexibility, shape, three-dimensional coordination of the different atoms in a molecule (IC1) and a lower value of radial distribution function, RDF115m, are beneficial to the activity.

The general model has a Q^2_{LOO} equal to 0.921; hence, the predicted model can make over 92% of variances in the inhibitory activity. The predicted values of pIC_{50} were obtained for all the molecules by MLR equation which was listed in Table 1 and were plotted against the experimental values (Figure 1A).

Table 3 Brief description of the descriptors in ten models

NO.	Name	Description
1	IC1	Information content index (neighborhood symmetry of 1-order)
2	RDF135e	Radial Distribution Function −3.5/ weighted by atomic Sanderson electronegativities
3	Mor24m	3D-MoRSE – signal 24/ weighted by atomic masses
4	RDF035u	Radial Distribution Function −3.5/ unweighted
5	E3u	3rd component accessibility directional WHIM index/ unweighted
6	RDF120m	Radial Distribution Function −12.0/ weighted by atomic masses
7	Mor15e	3D-MoRSE – signal 15/ weighted by atomic Sanderson electronegativities
8	G3p	3st component symmetry directional WHIM index/weighted by atomic polarizabilities
9	R7e0	R maximal autocorrelation of lag 7/weighted by atomic Sanderson electronegativities
10	dipx	Molecular dipole moment at X-direction
11	GATS8p	Geary autocorrelation -lag 8/ weighted by atomic polarizabilities
12	RDF065m	Radial Distribution Function −6.5/ weighted by atomic masses
13	SP20	Shape profile no. 20
14	Mor28e	3D-MoRSE – signal 28/ weighted by atomic Sanderson electronegativities
15	Mor09e	3D-MoRSE – signal 09/ weighted by atomic Sanderson electronegativities
16	G2u	2st component symmetry directional WHIM index/ unweighted
17	Mor27u	3D-MoRSE – signal 27/unweighted
18	RDF115m	Radial Distribution Function −11.5/ weighted by atomic masses
19	RDF115e	Radial Distribution Function −11.5 / weighted by atomic Sanderson electronegativities
20	HATS3p	Leverage- weighted autocorrelation of lag 3/ weighted by atomic polarizabilities
21	G3m	3st component symmetry directional WHIM index/ weighted by atomic masses
22	Mor26m	3D-MoRSE – signal 26/ weighted by atomic masses

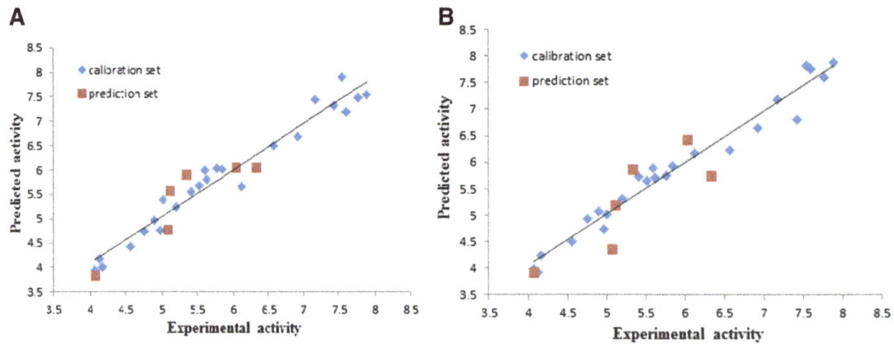

Figure 1 Plot of predicted pIC_{50} versus the experimental values for MLR model **(A)**, and GA-PLS model **(B)**.

The Y-randomization test was performed to evaluate the robustness of the general model. In the Y-randomization test, the activity data were randomly permuted in the original model and 10 models were generated. All of the models were expected to have lower R^2 and Q^2_{LOO} values than the original MLR model. If the reverse occurs, a suitable MLR model cannot be generated. The lower R^2 and Q^2_{LOO} values are shown in Table 4.

Genetic algorithm partial least squares (GA-PLS)

Since the variable selection method, that is the stepwise regression, may not be a suitable selection, variable selection methods such as the genetic algorithm, which demonstrate much better outcomes in comparison with the stepwise regression, are more favorable [25,26].

In genetic algorithm, if its corresponding descriptor is contained, a gene receives a value of 1 in the subset; otherwise, it takes a value of zero. The number of genes at each chromosome is equivalent to the number of descriptors. The population size varied between 80 and 125 for different GA runs. The number of genes with the values of 1 was relatively lower than the number of genes with the values of 0. The genes with the values of 1 were maintained. The chromosomes with the smallest numbers of chosen descriptors (total number of descriptors for each molecule reached 105) and the highest fitness were selected as the intended model. The predicted model was tested by leave-n-out cross-validation [27]. A leave-one-out cross-validation was triggered and the value of Q^2_{LOO} was obtained 0.850.

In GA-PLS, the resulted model with higher cross-validation statistics is reported in Equation 2 and the predicted values of pIC_{50} are shown in Table 1 and plotted against the experimental values in Figure 1B.

$$pIC_{50} = -12.589\ (\pm 1.208) + 6.363\ (\pm 0.394)\ IC1 + 2.119\ (\pm 0.485)\ Mor24m - 0.665\ (\pm 0.189)$$

$$Mor15e - 0.784\ (\pm 0.370)\ Mor32e \quad (2)$$

$$N = 24 \quad R^2_c = 0.932 \quad S.E = 0.328 \quad Q^2_{LOO} = 0.900 \quad RMSCV = 0.391$$

This equation has three MLR descriptors (IC1, Mor24m and Mor15e) with high calibration statistics and prediction ability. IC1 and Mor24m have a display positive effect and Mor15e and Mor32e have a display negative effect on inhibitory activity in GA-PLS. Unlike MLR, The radial distribution function (RDF) descriptors have no effect on inhibitory activity in GA-PLS.

As observed from Equation 2, the variables used in this equation can explain 93.2% of the variances in the inhibitory activity of the MMP-2 inhibitors used in this study.

The Y-randomization test was performed to evaluate the robustness of the created model in GA-PLS and 10 models were generated. All of the models were expected to have lower R^2 and Q^2_{LOO} values than the original GA-PLS model, as shown in Table 4.

Applicability domain of the model

A QSAR model is exploited to screen new compounds when its domain of application has been defined [28]. The prediction may be assumed reliable for only those

Table 4 R^2 and Q^2_{LOO} values after ten Y-randomization tests

Iteration	MLR		GA-PLS	
	R^2	Q^2_{LOO}	R^2	Q^2_{LOO}
1	0.204	0.001	0.319	0.102
2	0.048	0.265	0.048	0.244
3	0.314	0.068	0.206	0.016
4	0.075	0.260	0.040	0.235
5	0.118	0.022	0.097	0.028
6	0.106	0.069	0.132	0.020
7	0.256	0.010	0.394	0.194
8	0.096	0.099	0.038	0.296
9	0.068	0.175	0.062	0.175
10	0.191	0.007	0.177	0.002

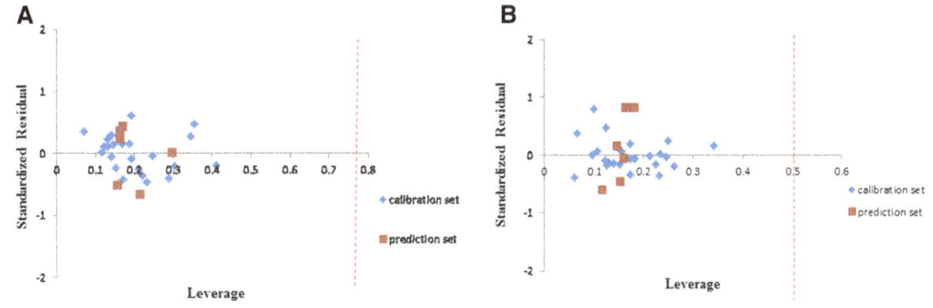

Figure 2 William's plot of generated MLR model **(A)**, and GA-PLS model **(B)**.

compounds which fall into this domain [29]. Standardized residuals of the activity were computed and were plotted versus leverage values (h). The value of leverage was calculated for every compound. Values are always between 0 and 1. A value of 0 is indicative of perfect prediction and usually is not accessible, and a value of 1 indicates very poor prediction. The lower the value, the higher confidence in the prediction. Warning leverage (h*) is another standard for explanation of the results and is, generally, fixed at 3 (k + 1)/ n, where k is the number of model parameters and n is the number of calibration set [29]. Calculated leverage for calibration set is useful for determining the compounds which affect the model and, in terms of validation set, useful for assigning the applicability domain of the model. The William's plot for the developed models in MLR and GA-PLS are shown in Figure 2.

Response outliers are compounds that have standard residual points higher than ± 2.0 standard deviation units and a leverage value higher than the warning leverage, which is 0.75 and 0.5 for MLR and GA-PLS respectively. As can be seen in Figure 2, all studied molecules in calibration and validation set lie with high degree of confidence in application domain of the developed models in both methods.

Molecular docking studies

To explore the ligand binding modes, and to find amino acids, which are essential in ligand binding to MMP-2, molecular docking was performed on a ligand-binding pocket. The way the compound was bound with the lowest free energy was studied. Interactions between MMP-2 and ligand N-4-[(1-hydroxycarbamoyl-2-methyl-propyl)-(2-morpholin-4-yl-ethyl)-sulfamoyl]-4- pentyl-benzamide (SC-74020) were obtained by Feng et al. and were reported. According to their results, the catalytic zinc is chelated by His120, His124, His130 and ligand, and the structural zinc is coordinated by His70, Asp72, His85 and His98. In addition, hydrogen bond was bound by Leu82 and Ala83 to a sulfoneoxygen atom of the inhibitor [30].

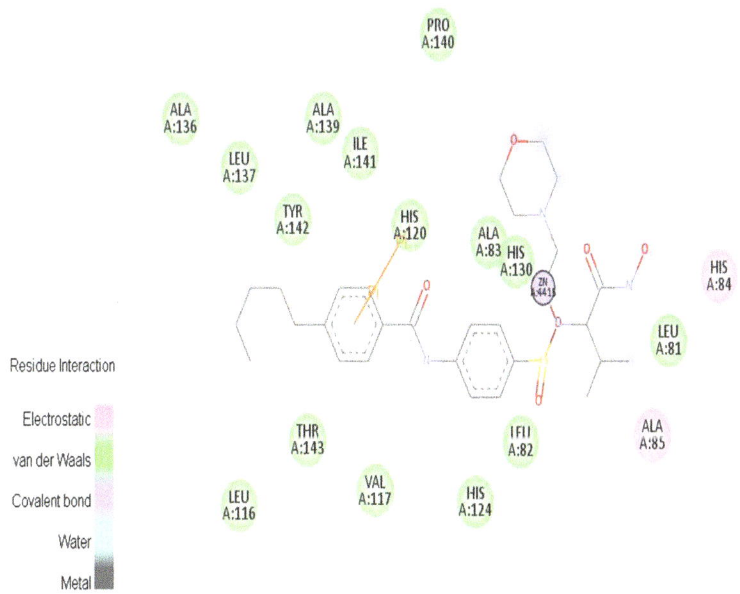

Figure 3 Interactions between ligand and MMP-2.

Table 5 The obtained binding energy by AutoDock

Compound	Binding energy (kcal/mol)	Compound	Binding energy (kcal/mol)
4a	−5.90	5f	−6.13
4b	−5.57	5 g	−6.34
4c	−5.96	5 h	−5.93
4d	−5.39	5i	−5.92
4e	−6.88	5j	−6.79
4f	−5.88	6a	−7.08
4 g	−5.67	6b	−7.07
4 h	−6.23	6c	−7.01
4i	−6.21	6d	−7.27
4j	−5.98	6e	−7.29
5a	−6.68	6f	−7.16
5b	−6.76	6 g	−6.92
5c	−6.85	6 h	−7.35
5d	−6.47	6i	−7.30
5e	−6.67	6j	−7.29

Initially, to assure binding mode of ligand and protein, ligand docking with MMP-2 protein has been validated by Feng. All of the interactions between the ligand and catalytic zinc with the protein from our results are shown in Figure 3. Root mean square deviation (RSMD) was lower than 1. Both of the prior cases proposed high reliability of docking program. Therefore, the AutoDock 4.2 could be used to find the binding mode of other inhibitors of MMP-2.

All of the 30 compounds were docked into the binding site of protein by AutoDock 4.2 and were studied. The binding energy of all the compounds is reported in Table 5. The obtained energies were compared with the experimental IC_{50}, and the 6a-6j compounds have the lowest binding energy. This means that based on the binding energy of the active site, these compounds, especially compound (6 h), are the best L-tyrosine scaffold based inhibitors. The binding orientation of compound (6 h) and hydrogen bond of the ligand with Leu82 and Ala83 are depicted in Figure 4. This compound was fitted into the active site of MMP-2. In all of the compounds, the oxygen of carbonyl and sulfonyl groups are important for hydrogen bond of the ligand with Leu82 and Ala83. R_2 and R_3 substituents have the main role for hydrogen bonding interactions. In 4a-4j compounds, IC_{50} is higher than 5a-5j and 6a-6j compounds. When R_3 is OH and NHOH groups, hydrogen bond can be created better than when R_3 is $-OCH_3$. Moreover, when R_2 is sulfonyl, because of two oxygen groups, a stronger hydrogen bond can be created than that of carbonyl.

R_1 is sited in hydrophobic pocket. Methylene group can help the ligand to be fitted in lipophilic pocket, so two Methylene groups are better than one. Phenyl group can create a π- π interaction with Phe86. Therefore, phenethyl ($C_6H_5CH_2CH_2$) is better than benzyl ($C_6H_5CH_2$).

To design L-tyrosine based inhibitors and prediction of their activity against MMP-2 based on AutoDock 4.2 and QSAR studies, addition to a higher value of molecular size, degree of branching, flexibility, shape and three-dimensional coordination of the different atoms in a molecule, hydrophobicity and hydrophilicity of R_1, R_2 and R_3 are highly important. When R_1 is more hydrophobic, and R_2, is more hydrophilic, there is a stronger inhibition against MMP-2.

Conclusion

In this study, quantitative relationships between molecular structure and inhibitory effect of L-tyrosine scaffold based

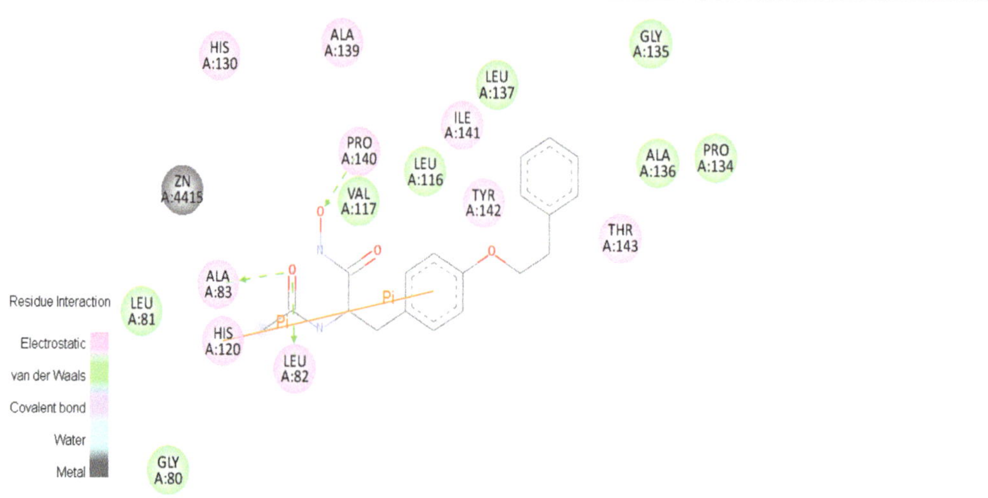

Figure 4 The best orientation of 6 h ligand.

MMP-2 inhibitors were investigated by MLR and GA-PLS. In MLR, A combined data splitting-feature selection method (CDFS) was offered to develop a quantitative structure–activity relationship model. It was found that topological parameter (IC1) has a main effect on the inhibitory activity of the compounds, among the different QSAR models. By this simple procedure, a multilinear 5-parametric model was created out of 22 descriptors. This method yielded acceptable results for the prediction set which was measured by cross-validation and Y-randomization. The findings indicate that the linear model produced by CDFS methodology could reproduce more than 92% of variances in the inhibitory activity. In addition to MLR, genetic algorithms, which demonstrated much better outcomes in comparison with stepwise regression, were used. By GA-PLS, the model with higher cross-validation statistics was created and the results indicated that IC1, Mor24m, Mor15e and Mor32e are main descriptors. It can be concluded from the two methods that higher values of molecular size, degree of branching, flexibility, shape and three-dimensional coordination of the different atoms in a molecule are particularly important

The docking study revealed that two hydrogen bonds between all of the inhibitors and the active site of MMP-2 (Leu82 and Ala83) are formed, as well as a π-π interaction between phenyl group and Phe86.

The information above could be used to design new inhibitors, and to show higher inhibitory activities and chemical synthesis of new inhibitors.

Abbreviations

MMP: Matrix metalloproteinase; QSAR: Quantitative structure activity relationship; MLR: Multiple linear regression; ECM: Extracellular matrix; CDFS: Combined data splitting-feature selection; Q^2_{LOO}: Square correlation coefficient for leave-one-out cross-validation; R^2_c: Calibration correlation coefficient; R^2_p: Prediction correlation coefficient; RSMD: Root-mean-square deviation; SE: standard error of calibration; RMS_{CV}: root mean square error of cross-validation; RDF: radial distribution function descriptors; GA-PLS: Genetic algorithm partial least squares.

Competing interests

The authors declare that they have no competing interests.

Authors' contributions

MA: Participated in the design of the study, carried out the QSAR study, performed molecular docking and drafted the manuscript. FR: Carried out the QSAR study and drafted the manuscript. ME: Helped the QSAR analysis. HAS: Participated in the design of the study drafted the manuscript. MA: Was responsible for the study registration, financial and administrative support, and also gave final approval of the version to be published. All authors read and approved the final manuscript.

Author details

[1]Department of Medicinal Chemistry, Faculty of Pharmacy, Pharmaceutical Science Research Center, Tehran University of Medical Science, Tehran, Iran. [2]Department of Medicinal Chemistry, Faculty of Pharmacy, Isfahan University of Medical Sciences, 81746-73461 Isfahan, Iran. [3]Medicinal & Natural Product Chemistry Research Center, Shiraz University of Medical Sciences, Shiraz, Iran.

References

1. Cheng X-C, Wang R-L, Dong Z-K, Li J, Li Y-Y, Li R-R. Design, synthesis and evaluation of novel metalloproteinase inhibitors based on L-tyrosine scaffold. Bioorg Med Chem. 2012;20:5738–44.
2. Lerchenberger M, Uhl B, Stark K, Zuchtriegel G, Eckart A, Miller M, et al. Matrix metalloproteinases modulate ameboid-like migration of neutrophils through inflamed interstitial tissue. Blood. 2013;122:770–80.
3. Page-McCaw A, Ewald AJ, Werb Z. Matrix metalloproteinases and the regulation of tissue remodelling. Nat Rev Mol Cell Bio. 2007;8:221–33.
4. Sapna G, Gokul S, Bagri-Manjrekar K. Matrix metalloproteinases and periodontal diseases. Oral Dis. 2013;20:538–50.
5. Bouloumié A, Sengenès C, Portolan G, Galitzky J, Lafontan M. Adipocyte produces matrix metalloproteinases 2 and 9 involvement in adipose differentiation. Diabetes. 2001;50:2080–6.
6. Visse R, Nagase H. Matrix metalloproteinases and tissue inhibitors of metalloproteinases structure, function, and biochemistry. Circ Res. 2003;92:827–39.
7. Hu Q, Yu L, Liao Q. Methylation of matrix metalloproteinases-2 promoter in endometrial cancer invasion. Beijing Da Xue Xue Bao. 2012;44:911–5.
8. Wang Y, Hu C, Dong R, Huang X, Qiu H. Platelet-derived growth factor-D promotes ovarian cancer invasion by regulating matrix metalloproteinases 2 and 9. Asian Pac J Cancer Prev. 2011;12:3367–70.
9. Maskos K. Crystal structures of MMPs in complex with physiological and pharmacological inhibitors. Biochimie. 2005;87:249–63.
10. Zucker S, Cao J. Selective matrix metalloproteinase (MMP) inhibitors in cancer therapy. Cancer Biol Ther. 2009;8:2371–3.
11. Di Pizio A, Laghezza A, Tortorella P, Agamennone M. Probing the S1′ Site for the Identification of Non-Zinc-Binding MMP-2 Inhibitors. Chem Med Chem. 2013;8:1475–82.
12. Wojtowicz-Praga SM, Dickson RB, Hawkins MJ. Matrix metalloproteinase inhibitors. Invest New Drugs. 1997;15:61–75.
13. Cheng X-C, Wang Q, Fang H, Tang W, Xu W-F. Design, synthesis and evaluation of novel sulfonyl pyrrolidine derivatives as matrix metalloproteinase inhibitors. Bioorg Med Chem. 2008;16:5398–404.
14. Hansch C, Hoekman D, Gao H. Comparative QSAR: toward a deeper understanding of chemicobiological interactions. Chem Rev. 1996;96:1045–76.
15. Hansch C, Kurup A, Garg R, Gao H. Chem-bioinformatics and QSAR: a review of QSAR lacking positive hydrophobic terms. Chem Rev. 2001;101:619–72.
16. Sabet R, Mohammadpour M, Sadeghi A, Fassihi A. QSAR study of isatin analogues as in vitro anti-cancer agents. Eur J Med Che. 2010;45:1113–8.
17. Frisch M, Trucks G, Schlegel H, Scuseria G, Robb M, Cheeseman J, et al. Gaussian 98, revision A. 7. Pittsburgh, Pa: Gaussian, Inc; 1998. p. 12.
18. Thanikaivelan P, Subramanian V, Raghava Rao J, Unni Nair B. Application of quantum chemical descriptor in quantitative structure activity and structure property relationship. Chem Phys Lett. 2000;323:59–70.
19. Hemmateenejad B, Shamsipur M, Miri R, Elyasi M, Foroughinia F, Sharghi H. Linear and nonlinear quantitative structure–property relationship models for solubility of some anthraquinone, anthrone and xanthone derivatives in supercritical carbon dioxide. Anal Chim Acta. 2008;610:25–34.
20. Morris GM, Huey R, Lindstrom W, Sanner MF, Belew RK, Goodsell DS, et al. AutoDock4 and AutoDockTools4: Automated docking with selective receptor flexibility. J Comput Chem. 2009;30:2785–91.
21. Hashimoto H, Takeuchi T, Komatsu K, Miyazaki K, Sato M, Higashi S. Structural basis for matrix metalloproteinase-2 (MMP-2)-selective inhibitory action of β-amyloid precursor protein-derived inhibitor. J Biol Chem. 2011;286:33236–43.
22. Singh UC, Kollman PA. An approach to computing electrostatic charges for molecules. J Comput Chem. 1984;5:129–45.
23. Azizian H, Bahrami H, Pasalar P, Amanlou M. Molecular modeling of Helicobacter pylori arginase and the inhibitor coordination interactions. J Mol Graph Model. 2010;28:626–35.
24. Shahlaei M, Madadkar-Sobhani A, Saghaie L, Fassihi A. Application of an expert system based on Genetic Algorithm–Adaptive Neuro-Fuzzy Inference System (GA–ANFIS) in QSAR of cathepsin K inhibitors. Expert Syst Appl. 2012;39:6182–91.
25. Barros A, Rutledge D. Genetic algorithm applied to the selection of principal components. Chemometr Intell Lab Syst. 1998;40:65–81.
26. Liu S-S, Liu H-L, Yin C-S, Wang L-S. VSMP: a novel variable selection and modeling method based on the prediction. J Chem Inform Comput Sci. 2003;43:964–9.
27. Fernández M, Caballero J. Modeling of activity of cyclic urea HIV-1 protease inhibitors using regularized-artificial neural networks. Bioor Med Chem. 2006;14:280–94.

28. Tropsha A, Gramatica P, Gombar VK. The importance of being earnest: validation is the absolute essential for successful application and interpretation of QSPR models. QSAR Comb Sci. 2003;22:69–77.
29. Mansourian M, Fassihi A, Saghaie L, Madadkar-Sobhani A, Mahnam K, Abbasi M. QSAR and docking analysis of A_{2B} adenosine receptor antagonists based on non-xanthine scaffold. Med Chem Res. 2015;24:394–407.
30. Feng Y, Likos JJ, Zhu L, Woodward H, Munie G, McDonald JJ, et al. Solution structure and backbone dynamics of the catalytic domain of matrix metalloproteinase-2 complexed with a hydroxamic acid inhibitor. BBA Proteins Proteom. 2002;1598:10–23.

Can donepezil facilitate weaning from mechanical ventilation in difficult to wean patients? An interventional pilot study

Saeed Abbasi[1], Shadi Farsaei[2*], Kamran Fazel[3], Samad EJ Golzari[4] and Ata Mahmoodpoor[5]

Abstract

Background: Management of difficult to wean patients is a dilemma for health care system. Recently published studies demonstrated efficacy of donepezil to counteract respiratory depression in sleep apnea. However, to the best of our knowledge, pharmaceutical interventions with donepezil to facilitate weaning have not been tested so far. Therefore in the present study, we evaluated the efficacy of using donepezil on weaning course in difficult to wean patients.

Methods: In this non-randomized interventional clinical study, difficult to wean patients with prior inappropriately depressed respiratory responses were included from two referral intensive care units (ICU) in Iran. Patients with another potentially reasons of weaning failure were excluded from the study. Donepezil was started for eligible patients at dose of 10 mg daily for 2–4 weeks. For the primary outcomes, arterial blood gas (ABG) parameters were also measured before and after intervention to evaluate the possible effects of donepezil on them. In addition, weaning outcomes of patients were reported as final outcome in response to this intervention.

Results: Twelve out of 16 studied patients experienced successful results to facilitate weaning with donepezil intervention. The mean duration of donepezil treatment until outcome measurement was 12 days. There were not any significant differences in ABG parameters among patients with successful and failed weaning trial on day of donepezil initiation. However after donepezil intervention, mean of PCO2 and HCO3 decreased in patients with successful weaning trial and mean of PCO2 increased in those with weaning failure.

Conclusions: Reduced central respiratory drive was infrequently reason of failed weaning attempts but it must be considered especially in patients with hypercapnia secondary to inefficient gas exchange and slow breathing. Our results in the clinical setting suggest that, the use of donepezil can expedite weaning presumably by stimulation of respiratory center and obviate the need to re-intubation in cases of respiratory drive problem in difficult to wean patients. We suggest decrease PCO2 and HCO3 during donepezil steady could be valuable predictors for positive response to donepezil intervention.

Background

Difficult weaning is a common problem of patients in whom weaning trials were attempted [1]. Since, 26% of medical and surgical patients were considered difficult-to-wean in a prospective cohort study [2]. Similarly, another prospective cohort study found that the incidence of difficult weaning was 39% among patients who needed mechanical ventilaion for more than 12 hours [3].

* Correspondence: farsaei@pharm.mui.ac.ir
[2]Department of Clinical Pharmacy and Pharmacy Practice, Isfahan University of Medical Sciences, Isfahan, Iran
Full list of author information is available at the end of the article

Both prolonged weaning and duration of mechanical ventilation are associated with increased risk of mortality. Therefore, difficult weaning is an important challenge for critically ill patients with mechanical ventilation support [4]. Management of patients who are difficult-to-wean is based on identification and correction of potential causes related to ventilator dependency [5].

Although impaired respiratory drive is an uncommon cause of weaning failure, but its important role should be highlighted if any definite reason is not found for weaning failure [1]. Therefore, treatment targeting the respiratory drive can be helpful in facilitating weaning of difficult-to-wean patients [6]. Respiratory stimulants such as caffeine, aminophylline and doxapram have been used effectively to increase central respiratory drive and subsequently weaning from mechanical ventilation and avoiding post-extubation apnea in preterm infants [7-9]. In addition, some studies showed beneficial effects of cholinergic drugs like donepezil to stimulate respiratory drive [10,7].

Some advances in understanding the role of central cholinergic modulation in the process of respiration provide a pharmacological basis for explaining beneficial effects of cholinergic drugs as therapeutic agents for disorders related to neural control of breathing [10]. Donepezil is cholinergic drug which reversibly and noncompetitively inhibits centrally-active acetyl cholinesterase [11]. It was first introduced for Alzheimer treatment but many studies showed efficacy and safety of donepezil for different clinical problems such as cognitive impairment resulting from severe traumatic brain injury [12-14]. Nausea, diarrhea, insomnia and infection were reported the most prevalent adverse reactions of donepezil with prevalence of less than 20% in high doses of donepezil [15].

Moreover, findings of conducted animal studies indicated the beneficial effect of systemically administered donepezil to counteract respiratory depression in anesthetized rabbits [16,17]. Recently published clinical studies showed donepezil may improve sleep apnea [18,19]. As a result, it seems donepezil is safe and may be effective medication to stimulate respiratory drive. To the best of our knowledge, pharmaceutical interventions with donepezil in difficult-to-wean patients have not been tested so far. Therefore, in the present study we hypothesized that using donepezil could facilitate weaning course in difficult-to-wean patients.

Methods

This is an interventional non-randomized clinical study approved by medical ethics committee of Isfahan University of Medical Sciences (Code Number: 292232) and conducted in the intensive care units (ICUs) of two referral hospitals in Iran (Alzahra and Imam reza hospitals).

Intubated patients who failed the first spontaneous breathing trial (SBT) on weaning trial and required up to three SBTs or 7 days to pass a SBT were defined as difficult-to-wean. Difficult-to-wean patients with prior inappropriately depressed respiratory responses when removed from the ventilator were considered eligible to enter in this study.

According to clinical judgment of intensivist, when other possible reasons of weaning failure such as electrolytes and acid–base disorders were ruled out, depressed respiratory response could be considered the cause of this failure.

Since electrolytes and acid–base imbalances (in particular metabolic alkalosis from volume depletion which promoted hypoventilation) could interfere in weaning process, we did our best to control and maintain normal ranges of serum electrolytes and nutritional support in this study and preserve the pH less than 7.45 during the time of active weaning [20].

Patients with unconsciousness and need for sedation or hypothyroidism were excluded from this study.

A continuous electrocardiograms (ECG), heart rate, mean arterial blood pressure, and oxygen saturation were also monitored during SBT. Therefore, patients with weaning-related myocardial ischemia or hemodynamic instability were excluded from the study to omit the potentially negative effects of these confounding factors on weaning failure [21]. Treatment with other potentially respiratory stimulants such as doxapram and medroxyprogesterone was additional criterion to exclude patients from this study.

Donepezil was started for eligible patients according to inclusion and exclusion criteria at dose of 10 mg daily. Because time to steady state for donepezil was expected 15 days [22], donepezil administration was continued at least for 2 weeks and patients were followed up daily during this period and evaluated for readiness of weaning and other endpoints of the study. If weaning was failed during first two weeks, patients would be assessed again for another potential barrier to extubation. In cases with strong clinical suspicion of central respiratory drive problem during weaning, donepezil was continued for another two weeks until 4-week duration of donepezil treatment [23].

For the primary outcomes of the study, oxygenation variables such as partial pressures of oxygen (PO2) and carbon dioxide (PCO2), pH and hemoglobin oxygen saturation (SO2) were measured on day of donepezil initiation and on day of outcome evaluation. Moreover, weaning outcomes of patients were reported as final outcome in response to this intervention. Thereafter for statistical analysis patients were categorized in two groups: patients with successful or failure weaning and then oxygenation variables mentioned above were compared between two groups.

Statistical analysis: Descriptive and statistical analyses were performed. The distribution of continuous variables was assessed by the Kolmogrov-Smirnov test, and continuous data were expressed as mean ± SD. The Mann–Whitney U test and independent sample t-tests were used to assess differences in quantitative data of patients' characteristics for nonparametric and parametric variables, respectively. For categorical data expressed as percentage, chi-squared test was applied.

Results

Eighteen difficult-to-wean patients with suspicion of depressed respiratory response (62 ± 18 years old) were included in this study and finally 16 patients completed the study for outcome measurement. Two patients of enrolled subjects died before any evaluations, therefore data were not applicable to evaluate weaning outcome of them (Figure 1). Characteristics of the patients were summarized in Table 1.

The study patients had been on mechanical ventilation for 32 ± 21 days prior to study enrollment. In addition, more than 80% of patients had been failed weaning trial more than 2 times before enter to study. Among 16 studied patients, 13 patients had pneumonia, whereas; 30% of them experienced concomitant acute exacerbation of COPD. Pulmonary edema was also reported in 3 patients (Table 1).

The results showed 12 out of 16 patients experienced successful weaning during donepezil intervention. However, in one of the successful weaning trial, re-intubation was occurred during 24 hours and therefore considered as final unsuccessful weaning outcome.

Therefore, 11 patients were categorized as successful weaning and remained patients were classified in unsuccessful weaning group. In comparison of these two groups of patients (successful or failure weaning), there were not any significant differences in age, duration of mechanical ventilation and number of failed weaning trial before donepezil initiation (p-value > 0.05) (Table 2).

The effects of donepezil on arterial blood gas (ABG) were also evaluated on day of donepezil initiation and on day of outcome measurement. Variations in arterial PH, PO2, PCO2, HCO3 and oxygen saturation were demonstrated in part A, B, C, D and E of Figure 2 respectively. Results showed patients had no evidence of primary metabolic alkalosis at weaning time.

According to independent sample t-test, there were not any significant differences in ABG parameters between successful and unsuccessful weaning patients on day of donepezil initiation (p-value > 0.05). In patients with successful weaning trial, paired sample analyses revealed mean of PCO2 and HCO3 decreased, whereas mean of PO2 and PO2 saturation increased after donepezil intervention. Although, in those with failed weaning, mean of PCO2 increased after donepezil intervention. However none of these statistical analyses were significant (Table 3).

Discussion

This present study was performed in difficult-to-wean patients with potential respiratory drive problems which caused repeatedly failing spontaneous breathing attempts. Donepezil administration in our study enabled successful SBT and weaning in nearly 70% of patients. Our patients manifested hypercapnia and hypopnea when removed from the ventilator in prior weaning trials which promoted the probability of reduced ventilator central drive before donepezil initiation. Since, we initially could find neither reversible causes for repeated failure to prior weaning trials, nor any contraindication for the use of donepezil, we empirically used donepezil to facilitate weaning in these patients.

According to recent systematic review and meta-analysis, 10 mg donepezil was well tolerated without any life threatening effect [24]. In addition, regarding to the long half-life of donepezil (70 hours) it is unlikely that adverse reactions of donepezil occurs in first days of its initiation [25]. Therefore, deaths of two patients in the initial days of donepezil intervention might be related to poor clinical condition of them not donepezil adverse reactions. Also it should be mentioned that no related adverse reaction of donepezil was reported during follow up of our study.

Etiologies of failures upon removal from the ventilator in spite of donepezil treatment in our study were not readily clear. Although it seems patients apparently had a depressed ventilatory drive initially, but possible inadequate resolution of the illness that had caused mechanical ventilation and/or progress of new problem could incorporate to weaning failure in few patients.

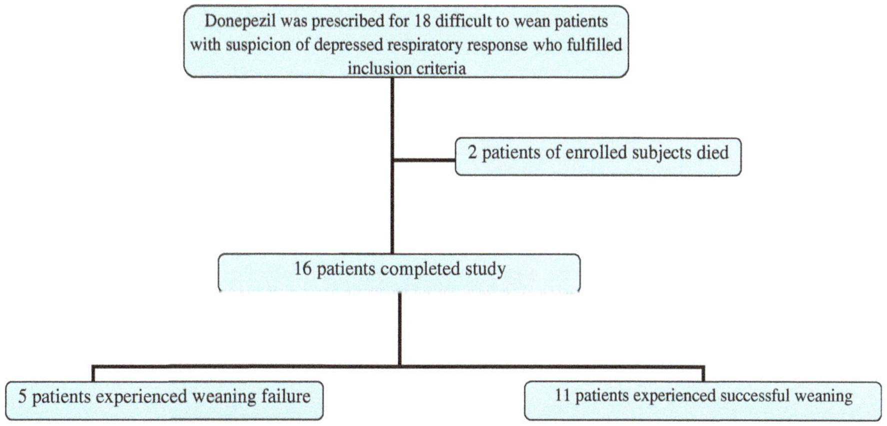

Figure 1 Flow diagram of the patients received donepezil during study follow up. Eleven out of 16 difficult to wean patients who completed the study experienced successful weaning in our study.

Table 1 Demographic and clinical characteristics of the patients with donepezil intervention to facilitate weaning

Patient	Age	Sex	Diagnosis	Number of failed weaning trial[α]	Duration of MV[α]	Days of donepezil treatment*	Outcome of weaning	ICU outcome
1	73	M	COPD exacerbation, pneumonia, pulmonary edema	2	10	28	S but re-intubated	D
2	26	M	Opioid intoxiction, seizure	2	30#	6	S	A
3	55	M	COPD exacerbation, PTE, pneumonia	2	5	4	S	A
4	73	M	COPD exacerbation, Pneumonia	2	5	8	S	D
5	72	M	Brain tumor, PTE, pneumonia	2	10	15	F'	D
6	64	F	Abdominoplasty, PTE	2	19	9	S	A
7	80	F	PTE, dyspnea, pneumonia, pulmonary edema	1	18	8	S	A
8	68	M	Arrest, pneumonia	3	60#	6	S	A
9	41	F	Arnoldikiary, pneumonia	2	25#	13	S	A
10	81	F	cholecystectomy	2	32#	10	S	A
11	78	M	COPD exacerbation, pneumonia	3	33#	17	F'	A
12	68	M	CVA, pneumonia	3	65#	27	S	A
13	67	M	PTE, dyspnea, pneumonia	3	60#	4	S	A
14	81	M	Massive pleural effusion, pneumonia, pulmonary edema	3	57#	15	F'	A
15	24	M	Multiple trauma, pneumonia	1	57#	21	S	A
16	46	M	Cerebral tumor, pneumonia, PTE	1	33#	15	F'	A

[α]Before donepezil initiation.
*From initial donepezil treatment until outcome measurement.
#Tracheostomy tube used for mechanical ventilation.
A, alive; COPD, chronic obstructive pulmonary disease; CVA, cerebrovascular accident; D, died; F, female; F', failure; MV, mechanical ventilation; M, male; NA, not applicable and excluded; PTE, pulmonary thromboembolism; S, success.

Muscle fatigue is one of the frequent causes of weaning failure manifested ultimately by rising in PCO2 [26]. Weaning failure in our study might be contributed to muscle fatigue during donepezil intervention. Because as mentioned in results, mean PCO2 rose in patients with unsuccessful weaning in this period. If fatigue developed during donepezil treatment, further stimulation of the respiratory muscles with donepezil would have inevitably made the fatigue worse and patients would have weaning failure or required re-intubation.

In addition, in a patient with cervical tumor, phrenic nerve was involved and patient had also peripheral neuropathy. Since, diaphragm muscle is primarily innervated by the phrenic nerve, partial damage of that in surgical removal of cervical tumor could be a reason for failed response to donepezil intervention. Moreover, metabolic alkalosis may be another causative factor for re-intubation of the first patient in our study because compensatory hypoventilatory response to metabolic alkalosis disposed patient to weaning failure or re-intubation [27]. Some studies maintained pH less than 7.4 during the time of active weaning [28].

Most of patients had history of pneumonia in our study which justified extubation failure and predisposition of them in difficult-to-wean condition. Pneumonia at the initiation of ventilation was one of the best predictors of extubation failure for patients following a successful SBT [29].

Cholinergic stimulation to develop respiratory coordination [30], increasing neuromuscular transmission and improving the effectiveness of upper airways muscles are some reasons which donepezil can accelerate weaning [31].

Table 2 Comparison of clinical parameters in patients with successful and unsuccessful weaning trial

Parameters	Successful weaning (N = 11)	Unsuccessful weaning (N = 5)	p-value *
Age (Mean ± SD)	58.8 ± 20.1	70.0 ± 14.0	0.22
duration of mechanical ventilation (Mean ± SD)	34.2 ± 22.6	28.6 ± 19.6	0.83
duration of donepezil treatment (Mean ± SD)	10.6 ± 7.3	18.0 ± 5.7	0.03

*Mann–Whitney U test was performed.

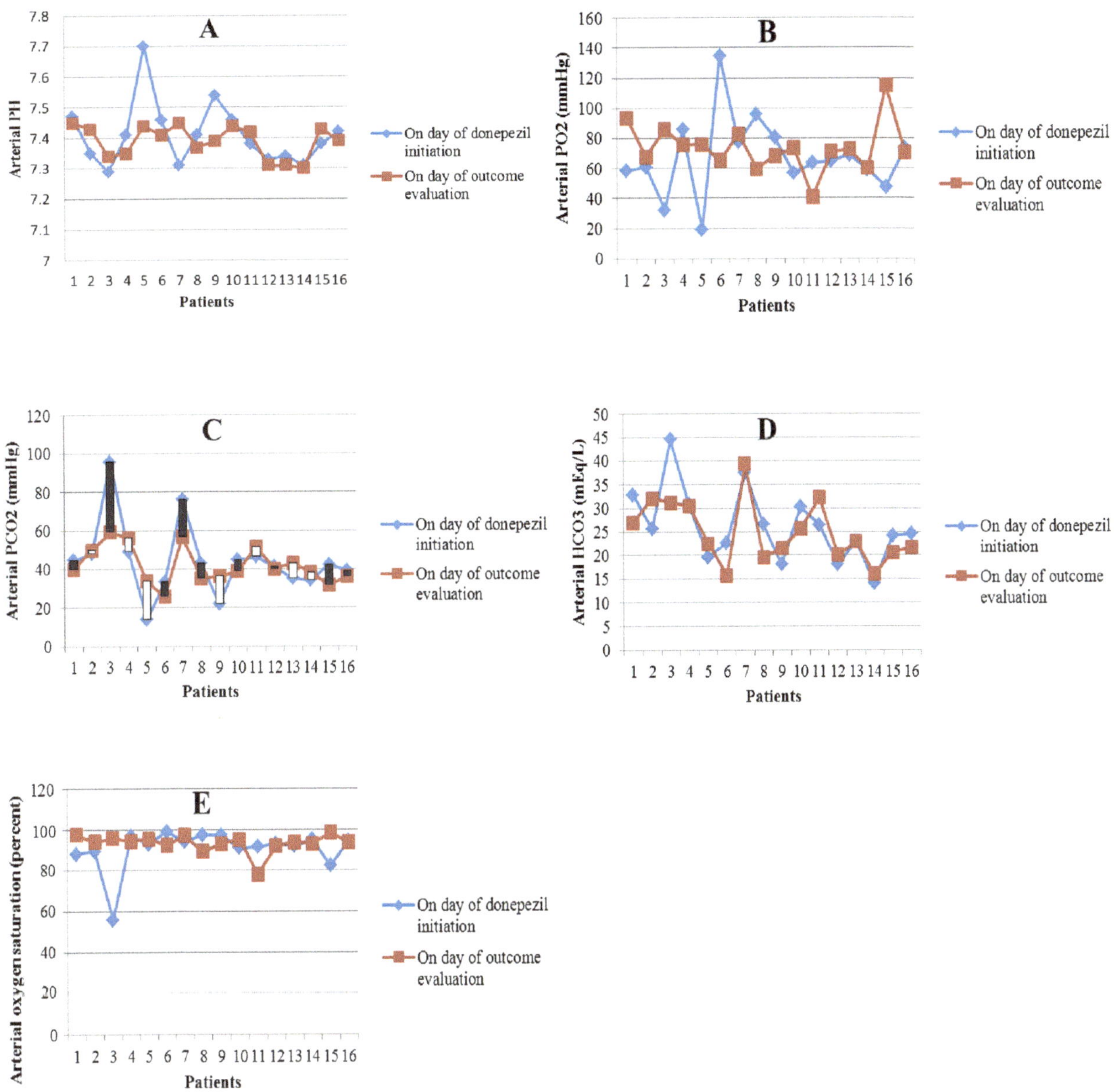

Figure 2 Variation of Arterial blood gas during donepezil treatment. Variations in arterial PH, PO2, PCO2, HCO3 and oxygen saturation were demonstrated in part **A**, **B**, **C**, **D** and **E** respectively. For each patient the first reported parameter was related to donepezil initiation day and the last one demonstrated that parameter on weaning day or until donepezil treatment was continued in cases of weaning failure. Patients with number 5, 11, 14 and 16 had unsuccessful attempts for weaning.

Not only cholinergic drugs can increase chemoreflex response to hypoxia by acting upon carotid body and stimulate respiratory center, but also play an important role in the neural control of respiration [31-33]. In addition, beneficial effects of cholinergic drugs to increase saliva secretion can reduce collapsibility of upper airways and contribute in this result [34]. Although different mechanisms can explain the beneficial effect of donepezil to expedite weaning but the exact mechanism is not clear.

By considering these mechanisms, donepezil facilitated the weaning of most patients in our study. We conclude that ABG parameters can be valuable factors to predict patient response to donepezil intervention. As our results also showed, decrease of PCO2 and HCO3 during donepezil steady state would give us good news about positive response of donepezil and possibly successful weaning trial in near future. Conversely, increase or unchanged PCO2 during steady state of donepezil could promote clinicians to seek for other reasons of weaning failure such as muscle fatigue. However, because of small sample size analyzed in this study differences in ABG parameters between two groups

Table 3 Arterial blood gas parameters before and after donepezil intervention

	ABG parameters	Group	Mean ± SD	p-value
Successful weaning (N = 11)	PH	Before	7.39 ± .076	0.96
		After	7.38 ± .047	
	PO2	Before	73.2 ± 27.1	0.84
		After	75.5 ± 15.3	
	PCO2	Before	48.2 ± 20.6	0.23
		After	42.8 ± 11.3	
	HCO3	Before	27.4 ± 8.0	0.19
		After	25.1 ± 7.4	
	PO2 saturation	Before	89.9 ± 12.1	0.29
		After	94.49 ± 2.4	
Unsuccessful weaning or re-intubation (N = 5)	PH	Before	7.46 ± 0.15	0.19
		After	7.40 ± 0.06	
	PO2	Before	54.7 ± 20.9	0.67
		After	68.2 ± 19.6	
	PCO2	Before	35.5 ± 13.0	0.192
		After	39.8 ± 7.0	
	HCO3	Before	23.5 ± 7.1	0.132
		After	23.9 ± 6.1	
	PO2 saturation	Before	92.4 ± 2.7	0.99
		After	91.7 ± 7.8	

PCO2: carbon dioxide, PO2: Partial pressures of oxygen, SO2: hemoglobin oxygen saturation and SD: standard deviation.

(successful and failure weaning) were not statistically significant.

Various pharmacokinetic parameters in population study and contribution of different factors in weaning process might be the reasons of diverse time needed for donepezil treatment to achieve its response goal during the study. As expected, mean duration of donepezil until successful weaning was 12 days which was parallel to the time required for donepezil to receive its steady state [20]. However, clinical benefit of donepezil may occur before or after steady state of donepezil. Therefore we suggest if weaning is not facilitated during 2 weeks of donepezil initiation and clinician do not find any other factor for this failure, patient may benefit from 4 weeks therapy. This study protocol justify the significant higher duration of donepezil treatment in patients who failed weaning trial compared to those with successful weaning outcomes.

Finally, potential limitations of the present study should be mentioned. First, however patients ruled out for other potential barriers of weaning in our study but other reasons of weaning failure might not be completely resolved or some new barriers evolved during the study. So, outcome of weaning failure in our population is not necessarily or primarily related to respiratory drive problem which is discussed in patients with unsuccessful weaning trial. Another limitation which should be pointed out is that relatively small number of studied patients. Despite more than 1 year study duration and inclusion of consecutive patients in two centers; only limited number of patients entered the study according to inclusion and exclusion criteria. A non-randomized design of this study without control group is the third limitation. Therefore, these results require further confirmation with larger controlled clinical trials to clarify and establish donepezil role in the management of difficult-to-wean patients. Additional studies should be conducted to compare the efficacy of donepezil with other respiratory center stimulants such as doxapram or cholinergic drugs to facilitate weaning in difficult-to-wean patients with respiratory drive problem. Moreover, the effect of donepezil on weaning of patients with different diagnoses can be evaluated in future studies.

Conclusion

According to safety consideration and previous study in obstructive sleep apnea (OSA) we evaluated 10 mg of donepezil during 2–4 weeks in our study [19]. In accordance with our findings, donepezil also supported breathing regulation in OSA patients [19]. To the best of our knowledge, this is the first study in which donepezil was given as respiratory drive stimulant in difficult-to-wean patients in order to expedite the weaning.

However ventilator drive failure uncommonly exists on the list of reversible causes of weaning problem, but it may prolong mechanical ventilation and lead impaired weaning. We think this condition may be overlooked by the other factors which contribute to weaning failure and may remain unrecognized. Our results showed donepezil could be considered as useful treatment option in this condition.

Competing interests
The authors declare that they have no competing interests.

Authors' contributions
SA carried out patient assessment for inclusion and exclusion criteria, donepezil prescription and patient follow up to evaluate outcome of donepezil intervention in Alzahra hospital. He is also participated in design of study and revising the manuscript. SF conceived of the study, and participated in its design and coordination and participated in sequence alignment and drafted the manuscript. She also helped acquisition and interpretation of data and statistical analysis. KF carried out patient assessment for inclusion and exclusion criteria, donepezil prescription and patient follow up to evaluate outcome of donepezil intervention in Alzahra hospital and helped acquisition of data. SEJG and AM carried out patient assessment for inclusion and exclusion criteria, donepezil prescription and patient follow up to evaluate outcome of donepezil intervention in Imam reza hospital. SEJG also helped acquisition of data. All authors read and approved the final manuscript.

Acknowledgements
This work was financially supported by anesthesiology and critical care research center of Isfahan University of Medical Sciences, Iran.

Author details
[1]Anesthesiology and Critical Care Research Center, Isfahan University of Medical Sciences, Isfahan, Iran. [2]Department of Clinical Pharmacy and Pharmacy Practice, Isfahan University of Medical Sciences, Isfahan, Iran. [3]Department of Anesthesia and Critical Care Medicine, Bagiatalla University of Medical Sciences, Tehran, Iran. [4]Medical Education Research Center, Tabriz University of Medical Sciences, Tabriz, Iran. [5]Cardiovascular Research Center, Tabriz University of Medical Sciences, Tabriz, Iran.

References
1. Heunks LM, van der Hoeven JG. Clinical review: the ABC of weaning failure–a structured approach. Crit Care. 2010;14:245.
2. Funk GC, Anders S, Breyer MK, Burghuber OC, Edelmann G, Heindl W, et al. Incidence and outcome of weaning from mechanical ventilation according to new categories. Eur Respir J. 2010;35:88–94.
3. Penuelas O, Frutos-Vivar F, Fernandez C, Anzueto A, Epstein SK, Apezteguia C, et al. Characteristics and outcomes of ventilated patients according to time to liberation from mechanical ventilation. Am J Respir Crit Care Med. 2011;184:430–7.
4. Thille AW, Cortes-Puch I, Esteban A. Weaning from the ventilator and extubation in ICU. Curr Opin Crit Care. 2013;19:57–64.
5. Grasso S, Pisani L. Weaning and the heart: from art to science*. Crit Care Med. 2014;42:1954–5.
6. Durbin Jr CG, Blanch L, Fan E, Hess DR. Respiratory care year in review 2013: airway management, noninvasive monitoring, and invasive mechanical ventilation. Respir Care. 2014;59:595–606.
7. Bancalari E, Claure N. Strategies to accelerate weaning from respiratory support. Early Hum Dev. 2013;89 Suppl 1:S4–6.
8. Parnell H, Quirke G, Farmer S, Adeyemo S, Varney V. The successful treatment of hypercapnic respiratory failure with oral modafinil. Int J Chron Obstruct Pulmon Dis. 2014;9:413–9.
9. Kim DW, Joo JD, In JH, Jeon YS, Jung HS, Jeon KB, et al. Comparison of the recovery and respiratory effects of aminophylline and doxapram following total intravenous anesthesia with propofol and remifentanil. J Clin Anesth. 2013;25:173–6.
10. Shao XM, Feldman JL. Central cholinergic regulation of respiration: nicotinic receptors. Acta Pharmacol Sin. 2009;30:761–70.
11. Seltzer B. Donepezil: a review. Expert Opin Drug Metab Toxicol. 2005;1:527–36.
12. Hansen RA, Gartlehner G, Webb AP, Morgan LC, Moore CG, Jonas DE. Efficacy and safety of donepezil, galantamine, and rivastigmine for the treatment of Alzheimer's disease: a systematic review and meta-analysis. Clin Interv Aging. 2008;3:211–25.
13. Ballesteros J, Guemes I, Ibarra N, Quemada JI. The effectiveness of donepezil for cognitive rehabilitation after traumatic brain injury: a systematic review. J Head Trauma Rehabil. 2008;23:171–80.
14. Foster M, Spiegel DR. Use of donepezil in the treatment of cognitive impairments of moderate traumatic brain injury. J Neuropsychiatry Clin Neurosci. 2008;20:106.
15. Donepezil. In: Lexi-Comp Online™, Lexi-Drugs Online™. Hudson (OH): Lexi-Comp, Inc.; Accessed via UpToDate 2014 Dec 9.
16. Sakuraba S, Tsujita M, Arisaka H, Takeda J, Yoshida K, Kuwana S. Donepezil reverses buprenorphine-induced central respiratory depression in anesthetized rabbits. Biol Res. 2009;42:469–75.
17. Tsujita M, Sakuraba S, Kuribayashi J, Hosokawa Y, Hatori E, Okada Y, et al. Antagonism of morphine-induced central respiratory depression by donepezil in the anesthetized rabbit. Biol Res. 2007;40:339–46.
18. Moraes W, Poyares D, Sukys-Claudino L, Guilleminault C, Tufik S. Donepezil improves obstructive sleep apnea in Alzheimer disease: a double-blind, placebo-controlled study. Chest. 2008;133:677–83.
19. Sukys-Claudino L, Moraes W, Guilleminault C, Tufik S, Poyares D. Beneficial effect of donepezil on obstructive sleep apnea: a double-blind, placebo-controlled clinical trial. Sleep Med. 2012;13:290–6.
20. Gruber PC, Gomersall CD, Leung P, Joynt GM, Ng SK, Ho KM, et al. Randomized controlled trial comparing adaptive-support ventilation with pressure-regulated volume-controlled ventilation with automode in weaning patients after cardiac surgery. Anesthesiology. 2008;109:81–7.
21. Routsi C, Stanopoulos I, Zakynthinos E, Politis P, Papas V, Zervakis D, et al. Nitroglycerin can facilitate weaning of difficult-to-wean chronic obstructive pulmonary disease patients: a prospective interventional non-randomized study. Crit Care. 2010;14:15.
22. Liptzin B, Laki A, Garb JL, Fingeroth R, Krushell R. Donepezil in the prevention and treatment of post-surgical delirium. Am J Geriatr Psychiatry. 2005;13:1100–6.
23. Rogers SL, Cooper NM, Sukovaty R, Pederson JE, Lee JN, Friedhoff LT. Pharmacokinetic and pharmacodynamic profile of donepezil HCl following multiple oral doses. Br J Clin Pharmacol. 1998;46 Suppl 1:7–12.
24. Tan CC, Yu JT, Wang HF, Tan MS, Meng XF, Wang C, et al. Efficacy and safety of donepezil, galantamine, rivastigmine, and memantine for the treatment of Alzheimer's disease: a systematic review and meta-analysis. J Alzheimers Dis. 2014;41:615–31.
25. Prvulovic D, Schneider B. Pharmacokinetic and pharmacodynamic evaluation of donepezil for the treatment of Alzheimer's disease. Expert Opin Drug Metab Toxicol. 2014;10:1039–50.
26. Laghi F, D'Alfonso N, Tobin MJ. A paper on the pace of recovery from diaphragmatic fatigue and its unexpected dividends. Intensive Care Med. 2014;40:1220–6.
27. Lian JX. Using ABGs to optimize mechanical ventilation: three case studies illustrate how arterial blood gas analyses can guide appropriate ventilator strategy. Dimens Crit Care Nurs. 2013;32:204–9.
28. Haake RE, Saxon LA, Bander SJ, Haake RJ. Depressed central respiratory drive causing weaning failure. Its reversal with doxapram. Chest. 1989;95:695–7.
29. Frutos-Vivar F, Ferguson ND, Esteban A, Epstein SK, Arabi Y, Apezteguia C, et al. Risk factors for extubation failure in patients following a successful spontaneous breathing trial. Chest. 2006;130:1664–71.
30. Haxhiu MA, Cherniack NS, Mitra J, van Lunteren E, Strohl KP. Nonvagal modulation of hypoglossal neural activity. Respiration. 1992;59:65–71.
31. Hedner J, Kraiczi H, Peker Y, Murphy P. Reduction of sleep-disordered breathing after physostigmine. Am J Respir Crit Care Med. 2003;168:1246–51.

32. Bellingham MC, Ireland MF. Contribution of cholinergic systems to state-dependent modulation of respiratory control. Respir Physiol Neurobiol. 2002;131:135–44.
33. Gilman S, Chervin RD, Koeppe RA, Consens FB, Little R, An H, et al. Obstructive sleep apnea is related to a thalamic cholinergic deficit in MSA. Neurology. 2003;61:35–9.
34. Proctor GB, Carpenter GH. Salivary secretion: mechanism and neural regulation. Monogr Oral Sci. 2014;24:14–29.

Effect of myrtle fruit syrup on abnormal uterine bleeding: a randomized double-blind, placebo-controlled pilot study

Marzieh Qaraaty[1], Seyed Hamid Kamali[2*], Fataneh Hashem Dabaghian[3], Nafiseh Zafarghandi[4*], Roshanak Mokaberinejad[5], Masumeh Mobli[6], Gholamreza Amin[6], Mohsen Naseri[1], Mohammad Kamalinejad[7], Mohsen Amin[8], Azizeh Ghaseminejad[9], Seyedeh jihan HosseiniKhabiri[10] and Daryush Talei[11]

Abstract

Background: Myrtle (*Myrtus communis* L.) has been used in the Iranian Traditional Medicine as a treatment for abnormal uterine bleeding-menometrorrhagia. The main aim of this study is to evaluate the effect of myrtle fruit syrup on abnormal uterine bleeding-menometrorrhagia.

Methods: A randomized, double-blind, placebo-controlled pilot study was conducted on 30 women suffering from abnormal uterine bleeding-menometrorrhagia. Treatment comprised of giving 15 ml oral myrtle syrup daily (5 ml three times a day) for 7 days starting from the onset of bleeding. The myrtle syrup along with placebo was repeated for 3 consecutive menstrual periods. Menstrual duration and number of used pads were recorded by the Pictorial Blood loss Assessment Chart at the end of each menstrual period. The quality of life was also evaluated using the menorrhagia questionnaire.

Results: The mean number of bleeding days significantly declined from 10.6 ± 2.7 days to 8.2 ± 1.9 days after 3 months treatment with the syrup ($p = 0.01$) and consequently the participants in the intervention group used fewer pads after 3 months (16.4 ± 10.7) compared with the number of pads used at the beginning of the treatment (22.7 ± 12.0, $p = 0.01$). Bleeding days and number of pads used by the participants in the placebo group did not change significantly. Also significant changes of quality of life scores were observed in the intervention group after 3 months compared to the baseline.

Conclusion: Myrtle syrup is introduced as a potential remedy for abnormal uterine bleeding-menometrorrhagia.

Keywords: Abnormal uterine bleeding-menometrorrhagia, Effrat-e-tams, Iranian traditional medicine, *Myrtus communis* L, Myrtle, Myrtaceae

Introduction

Abnormal uterine bleeding (AUB) is one of the main reasons of visiting gynecologists [1]. AUB affects up to one-third of sexually active women [2] and the overall prevalence of this abnormality is 11%-13%, reaching 24% at the age of 36–40 [3]. AUB has a considerable high morbidity rate among women of childbearing age and imposes major medical, social and financial burdens on women, their families and health services [4]. Different types of AUB include a range of dysfunctional conditions affecting regularity, frequency, duration or volume of menstrual flow [5,6]. Menorrhagia or hypermenorrhea is defined as menstrual blood loss of more than 80 ml per cycle or longer than 7 days or both of them [7], while polymenorrhea is defined as having menstruations about every 21 days and occasionally at even shorter intervals causing irregular ovulation. Metrorrhagia is uterine bleeding at irregular intervals, particularly between the expected menstrual periods [8]. Abnormal uterine bleeding-Menometrorrhagia (AUB-MM) is defined as prolonged and excessive uterine bleeding in irregular intervals [9]. The most common

* Correspondence: kamaliseyyedhamid@yahoo.com; nafis_zafar@ymail.com
[2]Department of Traditional Medicine, Faculty of Traditional Medicine, Shahid Beheshti University of Medical Sciences, Tehran, Iran
[4]Department of Gynecology and Obstetrics, Faculty of Medical Sciences, Shahed University, Tehran, Iran
Full list of author information is available at the end of the article

causes of AUB may be pregnancy, genital tract diseases, certain medical conditions such as thyroid dysfunctions and hypothalamic suppressions including stress, weight loss, excessive exercise, and even coagulopathies [1,10]. AUB treatment includes administration of non-steroidal anti-inflammatory drugs (NSAIDs), antifibrinolytics such as tranexamic acid, cyclic oral progestins, oral contraceptives and levonorgestrel-releasing intra-uterine system [1,5,11]. Hormone therapies have many side effects [12] and the common complication of tranexamic acid is gastrointestinal disturbances [13]. AUB involves two-thirds of all hysterectomies leading to several complications [14,15].

Iranian Traditional Medicine (ITM) practitioners such as Ibn Sina (Avicenna, 980–1037 A.D) believed that the normal menstruation is a good sign of healthy status of a woman which results in chastity and modesty [16-18]. In ITM literature, AUB is described under the title of "Effrat-e-Tams" or "Kasrat-e-Tams" [7,18]. Menometrorrhagia is more compatible with Effrat-e-Tams in ITM [17-20].

Based on ITM literature, particularly Avicenna's book (Al-Qanun fit-teb or Canon of medicine, 1025 A.D), myrtle is known as "*mourd*" or "aass" (مورد یا آس) and its fruit that called *Habbol- aass*, is one of the effective medicinal herbs for decreasing the menstrual bleeding [18]. Myrtle is a fragrant evergreen shrub belonging to *myrtaceae* family, growing wild in Iran [21,22] and the Mediterranean area. The fruits have sweet-spicy tastes that are very astringent [23]. Myrtle has been used as antiviral, antifungal, antiseptic and antioxidant agent [24,25]. Myrtle berries extract has ulcer-protective properties [26] and anti-inflammatory effects [27]. The essential oils obtained from leaves, flowers and fruits have been used in flavor and fragrance industries [28]. Its biological effect in menstrual disturbances has been described in ITM which may be novel in modern medicine [18].

There is a lack of detailed trials on the effects of myrtle syrup on menstruation. The main objective of the present study was to investigate the effects of myrtle syrup on reducing AUB-MM in a pilot placebo-controlled clinical trial.

Materials and methods

Study design and target group

In this randomized, double-blinded, placebo-controlled pilot study, 30 patients were randomly assigned into two groups of placebo (n = 15) and myrtle treatment (n = 15). Participants were treated with either 15 ml of myrtle fruit syrup or placebo, 3 times a day for seven days starting from the onset of bleeding. The treatment was performed for 3 consecutive menstrual periods. Randomization of equal number of subjects to placebo or treated group was achieved using a simple random allocation strategy, using block randomization method. The participants were selected according to the defined inclusion criteria: 20 to 55 years old, married women, not disposed toward hormone therapy, not pregnant, not lactating, normal gynecological observations, normal pap smear, endometrial thickness less than 12 mm, menstrual period more than 7 days in duration and/or less than 21 days from the start of one period until the start of the next menstrual period and/or clot excretion, use of more than 10 sanitary product items in a cycle. Sexually active women were required to use a suitable non-hormonal birth control. Initially, 92 patients were interviewed from which, 35 patients were recruited and randomized in two groups of placebo and extract treatment. 30 participants completed the study, 15 in each group (Figure 1). Two participants in the placebo group discontinued their therapy because of increasing bleeding during first cycle. One subject in the intervention group did not use the syrup completely and two persons discontinued the study because of personal reasons.

Women were excluded from the study if they had a history of significant medical problems (coagulopathies, diabetes mellitus, chronic inflammatory disease, thyroid dysfunctions); had a history of endometrial abnormalities (such as hyperplasia), cervical carcinoma, uterine or ovary malignancy; sub-mucosal or intramural fibroids more than 5 cm; needed surgery and emergency procedure because of increasing bleeding during the study. All of the subjects were free to withdraw at any time during the course of study.

Participants were not permitted to use mefenamic acid, tranexamic acid, any hormonal therapy, herbal medicine and medicinal herb during the study. Use of acetaminophen, oral iron therapy and analgesic opioids was permitted throughout the study.

All participants signed a written informed consent before recruiting in the study. The Ethics Committee of Shahed University approved the protocol (approval number: 41/138342). In addition, the trial was registered in the Iranian Registry of Clinical Trials under the number IRCT 201109077511 N1.

Plant material

Myrtle dried berries were collected from Manjil on road to Gilan (North of Iran) in 2011 and its identity was authenticated by Professor Gholamreza Amin. A voucher specimen of the plant has been deposited in Herbarium Tehran University of Medical Sciences, Faculty of Pharmacy under the voucher No 6632-TEH.

Preparation of syrup and placebo

Traditional decoction was prepared as described in "Qarabadin" (Ghayeni, Qarabadin-e-Salehi, 1765 AD; Aghili, Qarabadin-e-Kabir, 1781 AD) [29,30] texts belonging to ITM pharmaceutical discipline. 63 g of the

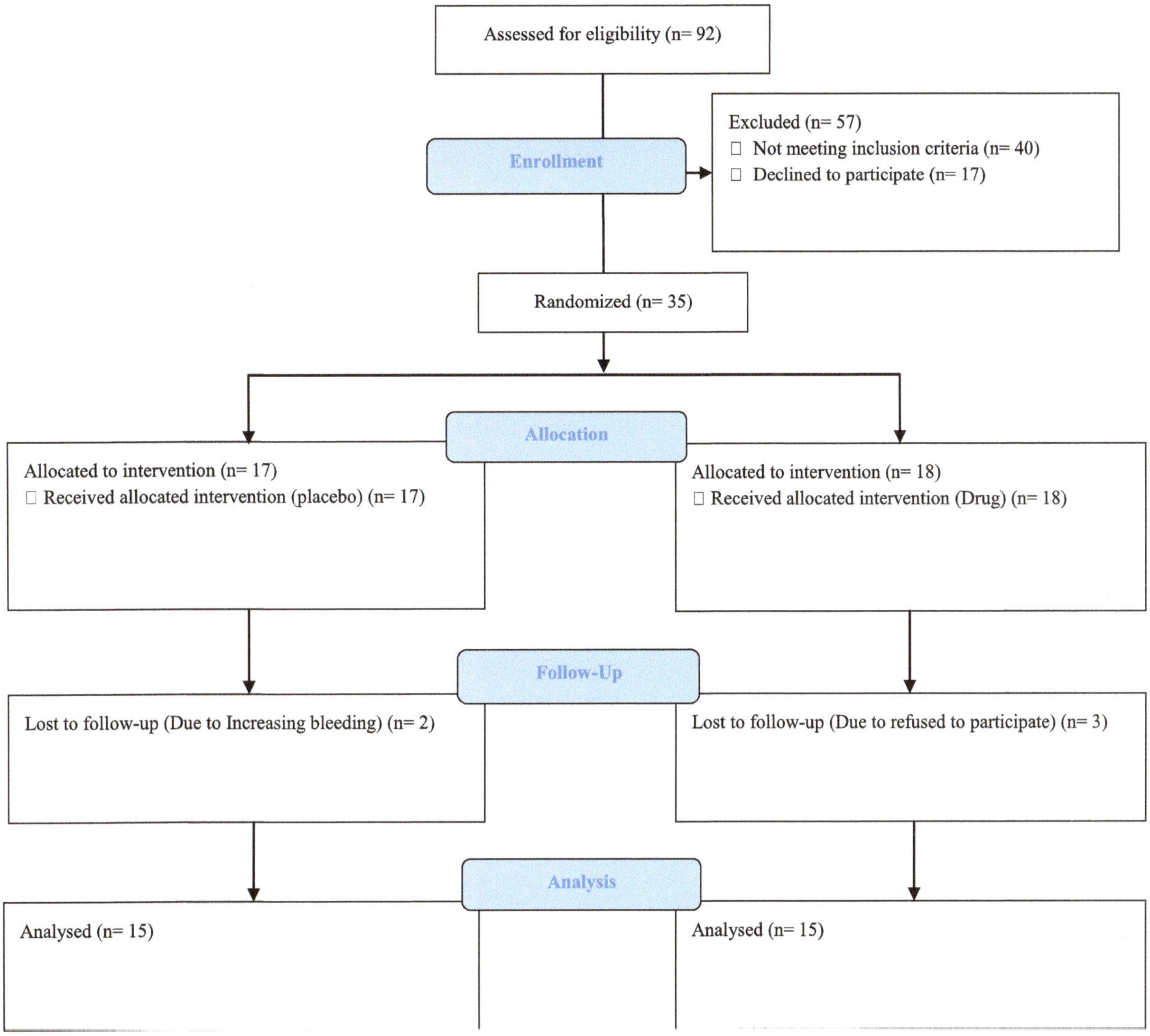

Figure 1 Study flow chart.

pulverized samples of myrtle fruits were macerated for 24 hours with 200 ml of distilled water, filtered and boiled for 15 min. 108 g sucrose was added to the extract in order to prepare the syrup. The medication was supplied in bottles of 120 ml, containing either drug or placebo.

Placebo was prepared based on pharmacopoeia simple syrup formula including approved color additives and looked the same as the myrtle syrup.

Myrtle syrup is standardized based on total phenols (Folin-Ciocalteau method) and gallic acid (Rhodanine assay) content. Each 5 ml of syrup contains 0.05 ± 0.03 g dry residue and 41 mg total phenols as gallic acid equivalents.

The participants were given either 5 ml of prepared syrup or placebo three times a day, 30 minute after each meal for seven days starting from the onset of bleeding. This treatment was repeated for three consecutive menstruation cycle.

The myrtle syrup and placebo were identical in the same physical form, packaging and labeling and divided to groups 1 and 2. Physician prescribed syrups to the patients according to the label numbers. Physician and presenter of the myrtle syrup or placebo were blind for the contents. The pharmacist was the only person who was aware of the numbers assigned to the myrtle syrup or placebo.

Bleeding measurements

All the participants were evaluated based on a complete medical history and gynecological examination. Menstrual blood loss was assessed with Pictorial Blood loss Assessment Chart (PBAC). The quality of life was evaluated with menorrhagia questionnaire (MQ-Iranian Version) [31,32] before treatment and at the end of the study. Certain blood test including complete blood count (CBC), prothrombin time (PT), partial thromboplastin time (PTT), follicle-stimulating hormone (FSH), luteinizing hormone (LH) and thyroid stimulating hormone (TSH) were done before the study. PT and PTT were done to exclude bleeding disorders. TSH, FSH and LH were done to exclude thyroid dysfunction and hypothalamic pituitary dysfunction, respectively. CBC was performed to determine hemoglobin (Hb) and hematocrit (Hct). Trans-vaginal ultra sonography was also performed to find out if the subject had any pelvic pathological disorders and to determine the endometrial thickness. Cervical cytology (Pap smear) was done to rule out other abnormalities.

Menstrual blood loss and menstrual duration were measured using PBAC chart during three consecutive treatment cycles and was compared with the ones at the beginning of the treatment (baseline). The participants were requested to report the details of their menstrual cycle i.e., the start date, duration of menstruation, the number of sanitary pads used (considered as the intensity of bleeding) and any adverse effects. The information was recorded at the beginning of the treatment and at the end of each menstrual cycle. The PBAC chart had a sensitivity of 80% and specificity of 88% in diagnosing menorrhagia (as defined in the alkaline hematin method) [33].

Statistical analysis

The primary outcome measures included the duration of menstrual period, number of pads used during menstruation. The MQ score and the side effects were the secondary outcome measures.

Normal probability plot was used to test for normality of data in GraphPad Prism version 5. The data points appeared linear on the plot and the data were considered as normal distribution. Repeated-measures ANOVA function in the program GraphPad Prism version 5 was used to test for differences of primary outcomes within the groups. Repeated-measures ANOVA compares the means of more than two matched groups in a longitudinal study in which change over time is assessed. Student's *t*-test was used to compare the MQ scores before and after the treatment.

Results

Baseline characteristics

The baseline characteristics of the subjects are described on Table 1. There were no statistically significant differences in baseline characteristics between the groups. Hence, the groups were homogenous with respect to age, level of education and investigations. Age of the patients ranged from 20 to 55 years with the mean age 41.2 ± 6.9 years.

Table 1 Baseline characteristics of study subjects

Parameter	Intervention group	Placebo group	P value
Age	41.33 ± 7.228	41.13 ± 6.978	0.5
BMI	28.86 ± 4.68	31.99 ± 6.29	0.2
MQ score	47.8 ± 15.7	41.2 ± 15.3	0.2
Duration of abnormality (month)	53.93 ± 61.46	72.33 ± 69.92	0.3

Effects of myrtle fruit syrup on duration and intensity of bleeding

The average number of bleeding days and number of pads used during the study are summarized on Table 2. There was not statistically significant difference between the groups in terms of bleeding days and number of pads at the beginning of the study.

The number of bleeding days and consequently number of pads used by the participants significantly decreased in the intervention group after 3 months (P = 0.01), while changes of these variables were not significant in the placebo group.

Significant changes of MQ score was observed in the intervention group after 3 months compared to the baseline (P = 0.02).

Discussion

To the best of our knowledge, the present study is the first randomized placebo-controlled trial on the effects of myrtle fruit in women with AUB-MM. The results of this study showed that myrtle syrup had notable advantages over placebo in women with AUB-MM. Also, the quality of life was significantly improved in the intervention group with minor side effects.

During luteal phase in menstrual cycle, some inflammatory processes lead to tissue edema in endometrium and continue with excessive menstrual bleeding (EMB). Unusual secretion of local pro-inflammatory cytokines responsible in the vascular tone has been observed [2,4]. In these women, endometrium synthesizes much more prostaglandin E_2 (PGE_2) than it does with vasoconstrictor $PGF_{2\alpha}$. A noticeable increased $PGE_2/PGF_{2\alpha}$ ratio happens during luteal phase in women with menstrual blood loss (>90 ml). Endometrial synthesis of PGs and signaling in women with profuse menstruation is greater than women with normal menstrual bleeding [4]. These inflammatory molecules can be targeted to treat the disturbances in women suffering from AUB.

Myrtle berries aqueous extract contains phenolic-like tannins (galllic acid derivatives), anthocyanins and flavonoids [34]. Tannin-containing medications have been used traditionally as styptics [35]. Anti-inflammatory activities of anthocyanins have been proven in some studies [36]. Some studies have demonstrated that flavonoids can

Table 2 The effect of myrtle fruit syrup in bleeding at baseline and post treatment

Variable	Group	Title	Mean(±SD)	Mean difference (±SE) compared with baseline	95% CI*	P values**
Menstrual duration (day)	Intervention (n = 15)	Baseline	10.6(2.7)			
		After 1st cycle	8.8(2.3)	1.7(0.6)	−0.3– 3.8	0.08
		After 2nd cycle	8.9(3.8)	1.6(0.9)	−1.3– 4.7	0.08
		After 3rd cycle	8.2(1.9)	2.3(0.6)	0.3– 4.3	0.01
	Placebo (n = 15)	Baseline	9.8(3.5)			
		After 1st cycle	8.8(3.2)	1(0.5)	−0.7– 2.7	0.6
		After 2nd cycle	8.7(2.6)	1.1(0.6)	−0.8– 3.1	0.5
		After 3rd cycle	8.6(3.2)	1.2(0.4)	−0.08– 2.6	0.5
Number of pads used	Intervention (n = 15)	Baseline	22.7(12)			
		After 1st cycle	20(14)	2.6(1.6)	−2.4-−7.7	0.5
		After 2nd cycle	21.4(17.9)	1.3(2.7)	−7.1– 9.7	0.8
		After 3rd cycle	16.4(10.7)	6.3(1.5)	1.6– 11	0.01
	Placebo (n = 15)	Baseline	15.4(9.8)			
		After 1st cycle	13.9(7.2)	1.5(1.7)	−3.7– 6.8	0.6
		After 2nd cycle	11.6(7.8)	3.8(1.5)	−0.7– 8.4	01
		After 3rd cycle	15(8.7)	0.4(2)	−5.9– 6.7	0.9
MQ score	Intervention (n = 15)	Baseline	47.8(15.7)			
		After 3 months	39.4(16.7)	8.4(3.7)	0.4-16.4	0.02
	Placebo (n = 15)	Baseline	41.2(15.3)			
		After 3 months	39.2(14.5)	2(2.03)	−2.3- 6.4	0.7

*One-way analysis of variance (ANOVA) was used to compare the groups before and after each treatment with either placebo or extract. There was statistically significant difference between groups before and after three rounds of treatment with myrtle syrup, while the difference between groups before and after placebo treatment was not statistically significant.
**P values <0.05 are significant.

inhibit inflammatory mediators [37]. According to a preliminary study, micronized flavonoids suppressed endometrial prostaglandins and were safe and effective in AUB [38]. Another phytochemical compound in myrtle that suppresses prostaglandin E_2 formation efficiently is myrtucommulon [39]. Therefore, the presence of the effective anti-inflammatory components in the myrtle extract can render the myrtle syrup a potential source to reduce prostaglandin secretion and to cure AUB subsequently. Further mechanistic studies are suggested to prove the anti-inflammatory effects of the components in the myrtle extract.

This study had some potential limitations which are usually part of the nature of human studies. Firstly, ITM has two groups of principal variables: one is part of human nature, *mezaj* (temperament), racial/ethnic, sex, age, season, zone, profession [40], and the second factor is the composition of the herbal preparations which may vary based on the geographical habitat of the plant, the climate, and the time of reaping [41]. These factors have not been considered in our study.

In the present study, the subjects received syrup only for three cycles; therefore we cannot comment on any long-term efficacy of myrtle syrup. Also, the subjects were not followed up after finishing the study and the long-lasting effects are not clear to us.

Conclusion

The outcomes of this study showed that myrtle syrup is an effective drug as a short-term treatment of AUB-MM. Women in the test group experienced significant reductions of bleeding duration, as well as a significant decline of the intensity of bleeding while placebo did not affect the variables significantly. The quality of life improved among the subjects in the syrup-treated group. Based on the current novel results, a therapeutic role of myrtle syrup is suggested for women with AUB-MM, which is accessible and cost-effective therapy. Larger and longer randomized trials are being planned in our research group to confirm the long-term effects of myrtle on bleeding reduction in AUB-MM.

Abbreviations

AUB-MM: Abnormal uterine bleeding-menometrorrhagia; CBC: Complete blood count; EMB: Excessive menstrual bleeding; FSH: Follicle- stimulating hormone; Hb: Hemoglobin; Hct: Hematocrit; HMB: Heavy menstrual bleeding; ITM: Iranian traditional medicine; LH: Luteinizing hormone; MQ: Menorrhagia questionnaire; PG: Prostaglandin; PT: Prothrombin time; PTT: Partial thomboplastin time; TSH: Thyroid stimulating hormone.

Competing interests

The authors do not have any financial/ commercial competing interest in the study presented here.

Authors' contributions

MQ has made substantial contribution in designing, acquisition of data, and drafting the manuscript and has given the final approval of the version to be published. SHK participated involved in design, and revising, have given the final approval of the version to be published. FHD analyzed and interpreted the data. NZ the supervisor of conduction of the study, participated involved in design, and revising, have given the final approval of the version to be published. RM participated involved in revising. MM participated involved in revising. GHA participated in the identification of the plants, plant extraction and made substantial contributions in the study. MN co- study designer. MK participated involved in revising. MA participated involved in revising and analyzing the data of the manuscript. AGH participated involved in recruitment. SJHK participated involved in randomization procedure. DT participated involved in revising. All authors read and approved the final manuscript.

Acknowledgements

The authors thank all the study participants for their participation. The authors gratefully acknowledge the help of the following individuals: Dr Jale aliasl Mamaghani for editing the data and revising; Dr Zahra Ghorbanifar for editing and Dr. Maliheh Tabarrai for revising. This was supported by a research grant provided by Shahed University.

Author details

[1]Traditional Medicine Clinical Trial Research Center, Shahed University, Tehran, Iran. [2]Department of Traditional Medicine, Faculty of Traditional Medicine, Shahid Beheshti University of Medical Sciences, Tehran, Iran. [3]Research Institute for Islamic and Complementary Medicine, Iran University of Medical Sciences, Tehran, Iran. [4]Department of Gynecology and Obstetrics, Faculty of Medical Sciences, Shahed University, Tehran, Iran. [5]Department of Traditional Medicine, School of Traditional Medicine, Shahid Beheshti University of Medical Sciences, Tehran, Iran. [6]Department of Traditional Pharmacy, Faculty of Traditional Medicine, Tehran University of Medical Sciences, Tehran, Iran. [7]Department of Pharmacognosy, School of Pharmacy Shahid Beheshti University of Medical Sciences, Tehran, Iran. [8]Department of Drug and Food control, Faculty of Pharmacy, Tehran University of Medical Sciences, Tehran, Iran. [9]Department of Gynecology and Obstetrics, Tehran University of Medical Sciences, Tehran, Iran. [10]Khatam Hospital, Tehran, Iran. [11]Medicinal Plant Research Centre, Shahed University, Tehran, Iran.

References

1. Gibbs R, Karlan B, Haney A, Nygaard I: *Danforth's obstetrics and gynecology.* 10th edition. Philadelphia: Lippincott Williams & Wilkins; 2008:664–671.
2. Livingstone M, Fraser IS: **Mechanisms of abnormal uterine bleeding.** *Hum Reprod Update* 2002, **8**(1):60–67.
3. Marret H, Fauconnier A, Chabbert-Buffet N, Cravello L, Golfier F, Gondry J, Agostini A, Bazot M, Brailly-Tabard S, Brun JL: **Clinical practice guidelines on menorrhagia: management of abnormal uterine bleeding before menopause.** *Eur J Obstet Gynecol Reprod Biol* 2010, **152**(2):133–137.
4. Critchley HO, Maybin JA: **Molecular and cellular causes of abnormal uterine bleeding of endometrial origin.** *Semin Reprod Med; Thieme Med Pub* 2011, **29**(5):400–409. doi: 10.1055/s-0031-1287664.
5. Shobeiri S, Sharei S, Heidari A, Kianbakht S: **Portulaca oleracea L. in the treatment of patients with abnormal uterine bleeding: a pilot clinical trial.** *Phytother Res* 2009, **23**(10):1411–1414.
6. Telner DE, Jakubovicz D: **Approach to diagnosis and management of abnormal uterine bleeding.** *Can Fam Physician* 2007, **53**(1):58–64.
7. Fathima A, Sultana A: **Clinical efficacy of a Unani formulation 'Safoof Habis' in menorrhagia:A randomized controlled trial.** *Eur J Integr Med* 2012, **4**(3):e315–e322.
8. Speroff I, Glass R, Kase N: *Clinical gynecology endocrinology and infertility.* 8th edition. Philadelphia, USA: lippincott williams and wilkins; 2011:592–617.
9. Bereak SJ: *Break and Novaks Gynecology.* 15th edition. Philadelphia, USA: lippincott williams and wilkins; 2012:403–409.
10. JANET RA, Sharon K, Robert M: **Abnormal uterine bleeding.** *Am Fam Physician* 2004, **69**(8):1915–1926.
11. Leminen H, Hurskainen R: **Tranexamic acid for the treatment of heavy menstrual bleeding: efficacy and safety.** *Int J Womens Health* 2012, **4**:413–421.
12. Canonico M, Oger E, Plu-Bureau G, Conard J, Meyer G, Lévesque H, Trillot N, Barrellier MT, Wahl D, Emmerich J, the ESTHER study: **Hormone therapy and venous thromboembolism among postmenopausal women impact of the route of estrogen administration and progestogens.** *Circulation* 2007, **115**(7):840–845.
13. Muoukhah S, Mazari Z, Ghoshtasbi A, Moayed Mohseni S: **The effect of tranexamic acid on the quality of life and blood loss of woman with menorrhagia: A clinical trial.** *Arak Med Uni J* 2012, **15**(3):75–84.
14. Zafarghandi N, Torkestani F, Hadavand S, Zaeri F, Jalilinejad H: **Evaluation of libido in post hystrectomy patients.** *Tehran Uni Med J* 2006, **64**(11):77–80.
15. Jensen JT, Parke S, Mellinger U, Machlitt A, Fraser IS: **Effective treatment of heavy menstrual bleeding with estradiol valerate and dienogest: a randomized controlled trial.** *Obstet Gynecol* 2011, **117**(4):777–787.
16. Jorjani SE: *Al- Aghraz al- Tibbia val Mabohess al- Alaiia.* Iran, Tehran: Tehran university press; 2005:761–764.
17. Zafarghandi N, Jafari F, Moradi F, Alizade F, Karimi M, Alizade M: **A study on the frequency of signs and symptoms of dystemperament in hypermenorrhea from viewpoint of Traditional Iranian Medicine.** *IJOGI* 2012, **15**(24):8–16.
18. Ibn-e-sina AH: *Al-Qanun fit-tib [The Canon of Medicine].* Beirut, Lebanon: Alaalami Beirut library Press (research of shamsedine); 2005:442–443.
19. Aqili khorasani SMHIMH: *Moalejate Aqili (medicine).* Iran, Qom: Jalaleddin; 2008:771–773.
20. Arzani MA: *Tebbe Akbari 2.* 1st edition. Iran, Qom: Jalaleddin; 2008:961–964.
21. Mozaffarian V: *Trees and Shrubs of Iran.* 1st edition. Tehran: Farhang Moaser Publishers; 2005:357.
22. Amin G: *Popular Medicinal plants of Iran.* 2nd edition. Tehran: Vice-chancellorship of Research, Tehran University of Medical sciences; 2005:254.
23. Fleming T: *PDR for herbal medicine.* 4th edition. Montvale: THomson; 2007:596–597.
24. Zanetti S, Cannas S, Molicotti P, Bua A, Cubeddu M, Porcedda S, Marongiu B, Sechi LA: **Evaluation of the Antimicrobial Properties of the Essential Oil of Myrtus communis L. against Clinical Strains of Mycobacterium spp.** *Interdiscip Perspect Infect Dis* 2010. doi: 10.1155/2010/931530.
25. Jorsaraei SG, Moghadamnia AA, Firoozjahi AR, Miri SM, Omranirad A, Saghebi R, Hashemi SF: **A comparison on histopathological effects on Myrtle extract and silver sulfadiazine 1% on healing of second degree burn wound in rats.** *J Qazvin Univ Med Sci* 2006, **10**(1):6–15.
26. Sumbul S, Ahmad MA, Asif M, Saud I, Akhtar M: **Evaluation of Myrtus communis Linn. berries (common myrtle) in experimental ulcer models in rats.** *Hum Exp Toxicol* 2010, **29**(11):935–944.
27. Zaidi SF, Muhammad JS, Shahryar S, Usmanghani K, Gilani A, Jafri W, Sugiyama T: **Anti-inflammatory and cytoprotective effects of selected Pakistani medicinal plants in Helicobacter pylori-infected gastric epithelial cells.** *J Ethnopharmacol* 2012, **141**(1):403–410.
28. Serce S, Ercisli S, Sengul M, Gunduz K, Orhan E: **Antioxidant activities and fatty acid composition of wild grown myrtle (Myrtus communis L.) fruits.** *Pharmacogn Mag* 2010, **6**(21):9.
29. Ghayeni M: *Salehi Garabadin.* Tehran: Islamic medicine and complementary medicine institute press; 2004:156.
30. Aghili M: *Kabir Garabadin.* Tehran: Islamic medicine and complementary medicine institute press; 2004:571–576.
31. Mazari Z, Ghoshtasbi A, Muoukhah S, Saki F: **Translation of Iranian version of Menorrhagia questionaire.** *Payesh* 2011, **11**(1):83–88.
32. Ruta D, Garratt A, Chadha Y, Flett G, Hall M, Russell I: **Assessment of patients with menorrhagia: how valid is a structured clinical history as a measure of health status?** *Qual Life Res* 1995, **4**(1):33–40.
33. Wyatt KM, Dimmock PW, Walker TJ, O'Brien P: **Determination of total menstrual blood loss.** *Fertil Steril* 2001, **76**(1):125–131.
34. Tuberoso CIG, Rosa A, Bifulco E, Melis MP, Atzeri A, Pirisi FM, Dessì MA: **Chemical composition and antioxidant activities of Myrtus communis L. berries extracts.** *Food Chem* 2010, **123**(4):1242–1251.
35. Evans WC: *Trease and evans pharmacognosy.* United Kingdom: Saunders; 2009:228.
36. Wang H, Nair MG, Strasburg GM, Chang Y-C, Booren AM, Gray JI, DeWitt DL: **Antioxidant and antiinflammatory activities of anthocyanins and their aglycon, cyanidin, from tart cherries.** *J Nat Prod* 1999, **62**(2):294–296.

37. Gonzalez-Gallego J, Sánchez-Campos S, Tunon M: **Anti-inflammatory properties of dietary flavonoids.** *Nutr Hosp* 2007, **22**(3):287–293.
38. Mukherjeea GG, Gajarajb AJ, Mathiasc J, Marya D: **Treatment of abnormal uterine bleeding with micronized flavonoids.** *Int J Gynecol Obstet* 2005, **89**(2):156–157.
39. Koeberle A, Pollastro F, Northoff H, Werz O: **Myrtucommulone, a natural acylphloroglucinol, inhibits microsomal prostaglandin E2 synthase 1.** *Br J Pharmacol* 2009, **156**(6):952–961.
40. Mokaberinejad R, Zafarghandi N, Bioos S, Dabaghian FH, Naseri M, Kamalinejad M, Amin G, Ghobadi A, Tansaz M, Akhbari A: **Mentha longifolia syrup in secondary amenorrhea: a double-blind, placebo-controlled, randomized trials.** *DARU J Pharm Sci* 2012, **20**(1):1–8.
41. Kamali SH, Khalaj AR, Hasani-Ranjbar S, Esfehani MM, Kamalinejad M, Omidmalayeri S, Kamali SA: **Efficacy of 'Itrifal Saghir', a combination of three medicinal plants in the treatment of obesity; A randomized controlled trial.** *DARU J Pharm Sci* 2012, **20**:33.

Molecular docking and inhibition studies on the interactions of *Bacopa monnieri's* potent phytochemicals against pathogenic *Staphylococcus aureus*

Talha Bin Emran[1,2*], Md Atiar Rahman[2], Mir Muhammad Nasir Uddin[3], Raju Dash[1], Md Firoz Hossen[1], Mohammad Mohiuddin[1] and Md Rashadul Alam[1]

Abstract

Background: *Bacopa monnieri* Linn. (Plantaginaceae), a well-known medicinal plant, is widely used in traditional medicine system. It has long been used in gastrointestinal discomfort, skin diseases, epilepsy and analgesia. This research investigated the *in vitro* antimicrobial activity of *Bacopa monnieri* leaf extract against *Staphylococcus aureus* and the interaction of possible compounds involved in this antimicrobial action.

Methods: Non-edible plant parts were extracted with ethanol and evaporated *in vacuo* to obtain the crude extract. A zone of inhibition studies and the minimum inhibitory concentration (MIC) of plant extracts were evaluated against clinical isolates by the microbroth dilution method. Docking study was performed to analyze and identify the interactions of possible antimicrobial compounds of *Bacopa monnieri* in the active site of penicillin binding protein and DNA gyrase through GOLD 4.12 software.

Results: A zone of inhibition studies showed significant ($p < 0.05$) inhibition capacity of different concentrations of *Bacopa monnieri's* extract against *Staphylococcus aureus*. The extract also displayed very remarkable minimum inhibitory concentrations (≥16 μg/ml) which was significant compared to that (≥75 μg/ml) of the reference antibiotic against the experimental strain *Staphylococcus aureus*. Docking studies recommended that luteolin, an existing phytochemical of *Bacopa monnieri*, has the highest fitness score and more specificity towards the DNA gyrase binding site rather than penicillin binding protein.

Conclusions: *Bacopa monnieri* extract and its compound luteolin have a significant antimicrobial activity against *Staphylococcus aureus*. Molecular binding interaction of an *in silico* data demonstrated that luteolin has more specificity towards the DNA gyrase binding site and could be a potent antimicrobial compound.

Keywords: *Bacopa monnieri* L, *Staphylococcus aureus*, Antibacterial activity, MIC, Molecular docking, GOLD, *in silico* drug discovery

* Correspondence: talhabmb@gmail.com
[1]Department of Pharmacy, BGC Trust University Bangladesh, Chittagong 4000, Bangladesh
[2]Department of Biochemistry and Molecular Biology, University of Chittagong, Chittagong 4331, Bangladesh
Full list of author information is available at the end of the article

Background

Effective therapeutic options to combat *Staphylococcus aureus* infection are still limited. And this makes a major burden to control *Staphylococcus aureus* [1]. *S. aureus* is a commensal Gram-positive bacterium, which colonizes in human nasal mucosa either permanently or transiently [2], causing severe infections eventually [3,4]. But the clinical symptoms are not visualized until the immune system is affected [5]. However, the major problem in controlling the *S. aureus* infection is the occurrence of multi-drug resistance produced mainly due to the misuse of antibiotics. This is also caused by the treatment of non-bacterial infections with antibiotics or inadequate compliance with the regulations for drug ingestion. Therefore, new therapeutic molecule is an urgence to be introduced as antibiotic in the treatment of multi-drug resistant *S. aureus.* Several studies have proposed that phytocompounds are the best alternative to develop therapies for multidrug resistant bacterial infections [6-8].

Bacopa monnieri (L.) Wellst. (Family: Plantaginaceae) is known as *Herpestis monniera.* It is a water hyssop or "Brahmi" and is reputed as Ayurvedic medicine. It is used for gastrointestinal discomfort, rejuvenation, promoting memory and intellect, skin disorders, epilepsy, pyrexia and analgesia [9]. Number of biologically active compounds has been isolated from this plant. GC-MS analysis of the leaf extract of this plant showed the presence of tetracyclic triterpenoids, saponin, bacosides A and B phytosterols, hersaponin, D-mannitol, flavonoids viz., luteolin-7-glucoside, apigenin-7-glucocronide, alkaloids such as nicotine and herpestine, betulic acid, β-sitosterol, stigma-sterol and its esters, aspartic acid, glutamic acid and serine [10]. Despite enormous possibilities of this plant, no compound-activity relationship study has been conducted yet to investigate the phytochemicals responsible for its antimicrobial action. This research evaluates the *in vitro* antimicrobial activity of *B. monnieri* against *S. aureus* establishing the interaction of existing phytocompounds involved in this antimicrobial activity through *an in silico* molecular docking analysis [11,12].

Methods

Media and chemicals

Mueller-Hinton broth and agar media (Hi media, India; final pH 7.3 ± 0.2 at 25°C), was used for the determination of MIC and antibacterial activity. Tetracycline (50 μg/disk) and ampicillin disks (50 μg/disk) were procured from Oxoid, England.

Collection and identification of plant materials

The plant *B. monnieri* was selected by Talha Bin Emran, Lecturer, Department of Pharmacy, BGC Trust University Bangladesh. Fresh leaves of *B. monnieri* were collected from the Chittagong University hilly forest on December 2013. The plant was identified by Dr. Shaikh Bokhtear Uddin, Taxonomist and Associate Professor, Department of Botany, University of Chittagong-4331, Bangladesh. A voucher specimen (Accession Number: 36285) containing the identification characteristics of the plant has been preserved in the Bangladesh National Herbarium for future reference.

Preparation of crude ethanol extract

The fresh leaves of *B. monnieri* were washed immediately after collection and chopped into small pieces, air dried and ground (Moulinex Blender AK-241, Moulinex, France) into powder (40-80 mesh, 500 g). The resulting powder was soaked in an Erlenmeyer flask of absolute ethanol (2.0 L, at room temperature) and left for seven days allowing occasional stirring of the flask. Filtrate obtained through cheesecloth and Whatman filter paper No. 1 was concentrated under reduced pressure at the temperature below 50°C using a rotatory evaporator (RE 200, Bibby Sterling Ltd., UK). The extracts (yield 4.4 - 5.6% w/w) were all placed in glass Petri dishes (90 × 15 mm, Pyrex, Germany) to allow an air-dry for complete evaporation of solvent.

Study of antibacterial activity

Bacterial strain

Gram-positive *Staphylococcus aureus* (ATCC6538) was used for screening the antibacterial effect of the plant extract. Bacterial strain was collected from the Microbiology Division of Bangladesh Council of Scientific and Industrial Research (BCSIR), Chittagong-4220, Bangladesh.

Preparation of sample solutions

Small amount (1, 2 and 3 mg) of solid sample was dissolved in a definite volume (1 ml) of DMSO to make a solution of 1 mg/ml. DMSO was chosen as solvent because it does not have any inhibitory effect on bacterial cultures and it has extraordinary capacity to dissolve solid sample completely.

Media preparation

The bacterial strain was grown and maintained on Standard Nutrient Agar (DIFCO) media (Hi media, India) at 37°C and pH 7.3 ± 0.2. The bacterium was sub-cultured overnight in nutrient agar broth which was further adjusted to obtain turbidity comparable to McFarland (0.5) standard when required. Test tube slants of nutrient agar medium were prepared for the maintenance of culture. Then a small amount of the collected microorganism was transferred to the test tubes with the help of sterilized needles. A number of test tubes were freshly cleaned for bacterial pathogen. The inoculated slants were inoculated at temperature below laboratory condition.

Antibacterial screening through disk diffusion technique

The antibacterial activity of the extract was determined by disk diffusion technique (National Committee for Clinical Laboratory Standards, NCCLS, 2002). The test microbes were taken from the broth culture with inoculating loop and transferred to test tubes containing 5.0 ml sterile distilled water. The inoculums were added until the turbidity was equal to 0.5 McFarland standards. Cotton swab was then used to inoculate the test tube suspension onto the surface of the Muller Hinton agar plate and the uniformly swabbed plates were then allowed to dry. On the dry inoculated surfaces prepared paper disks were placed as follows. Sterilized Whatman paper disks (6 mm in diameter) were prepared previously by punching the filter paper with the help of a punch machine. After that the disks were placed upon 0.5 ml of the desired solution (1, 2 and 3 mg/disk) of the extract. After each application the disks were allowed to the temperature 40°C (one minute) for drying purposes. The disks containing plant extract were placed with blunt-nosed thumb forceps on the inoculated plates at equidistance in a circle. These plates were kept for 4-6 h at a low temperature (<8°C) to allow for diffusion of the extract from the disk into the medium. The same was done for negative control (ethanol). The plates were incubated at 37°C for 24 h. The experiment was conducted in triplicates. Antimicrobial activity was determined by a measurement of the inhibition zone diameter (mm) around each test organism.

Minimum inhibitory concentration (MIC) determination

Minimum inhibitory concentration was determined by the microdilution method using serially diluted (2 folds) plant extract according to the National Committee for Clinical Laboratory Standards (NCCLS) (National Committee for Clinical Laboratory Standards, 2000). The MIC of the extract was determined by the dilution of *B. monnieri* extract with the concentrations of 0.0-25, 0.0-50, 0.0-75, 0.0-100, 0.0-125, and 0.0-150 μg/ml. Equal volume of each extract and nutrient broth was mixed in a test tube. Specifically 0.1 ml of standardized inoculum ($1\text{-}2 \times 10^7$ cfu/ml) was added in each tube. The tubes were incubated aerobically at 37°C for 18-24 h. Two control tubes were maintained for each test batch. These included antibiotic control (a tube containing extract and growth media without inoculum) and organism control (a tube containing the growth medium, saline and the inoculum). The lowest concentration (highest dilution) of the extract that produced no visible bacterial growth (no turbidity) was considered as MIC.

Statistical analysis

All data are presented as mean ± standard deviation (SD). The data were analyzed by a statistical software statistical package for social science (SPSS, version 18.0, IBM Corporation, NY, USA) using Tukey's multiple range *post hoc* tests. The values were considered significantly different at $p < 0.05$.

Docking approach

To have a better understanding about the inhibitory mechanism as well as the mode of interactions of the phytochemical compounds of the crude extract, docking analysis was accomplished using the GOLD 4.12 package. Two primary drug-target-pathways, i.e., penicillin-binding protein [13] and DNA gyrase [14] of *S. aureus* were subject to forecast the mechanism of plant derived compounds. Protein X-ray structure pdb ID: 3vsl and 3g7b was retrieved from protein data bank [15] and compared with standard inhibitor orientation in crystal structure. From the literature review, all compounds represented in Figure 1 were drawn in Symyx Draw 4.0 and to prepare for docking using the Sybyl 7.3 Molecular Modeling Suite of Tripos, Inc. Three dimensional (3D) conformations generated by using Concord 4.0 [16]; hydrogen atoms were added and charges were loaded using the Gasteiger and Marsili charge calculation method [17]. Basic amines were protonated and acidic carboxyl groups were de-protonated prior to charge calculation. The ligands were minimized with the Tripos Force Field prior to docking using the Powell method with an initial Simplex [18] optimization and 1000 interactions or gradient termination at 0.01 kcal/(mol*A). The input ligand file format was mol2 for all docking programs investigated. Three dimensional structure of standard drugs i.e., penicillin G and ciprofloxacin was occupied from zinc databases. The docking tool "GOLD" utilizes genetic algorithm to explore the rotational flexibility of receptor hydrogen's and ligand conformational flexibility [19]. Such GOLD docking was carried out using the wizard with default parameters population size (100); selection pressure (1.1); number of operations (10,0 00); number of islands (1); niche size (2); and operator weights for migrate (0), mutate (100), and crossover (100). The active site with a 10 Å radius sphere was defined by selecting an active site residue of protein. Default genetic algorithm settings were used for all calculations and a set of 10 solutions was saved for each ligand. GOLD was used by a GoldScore fitness function. GoldScore is a molecular mechanism like function and has been optimized for the calculation of binding positions of ligand. It takes into account for four terms:

$$\mathbf{Fitness} = \mathbf{S}_{(hb\_ext)} + \mathbf{1.3750} * \mathbf{S}_{(vdw\_ext)} + \mathbf{S}_{(hb\_int)} + \mathbf{1.0000} * \mathbf{S}_{(int)}$$

$$\mathbf{S}_{(int)} = \mathbf{S}_{(vdw\_int)} + \mathbf{S}_{(tors)}$$

Where, S_{hb_ext} is the protein-ligand hydrogen bonding

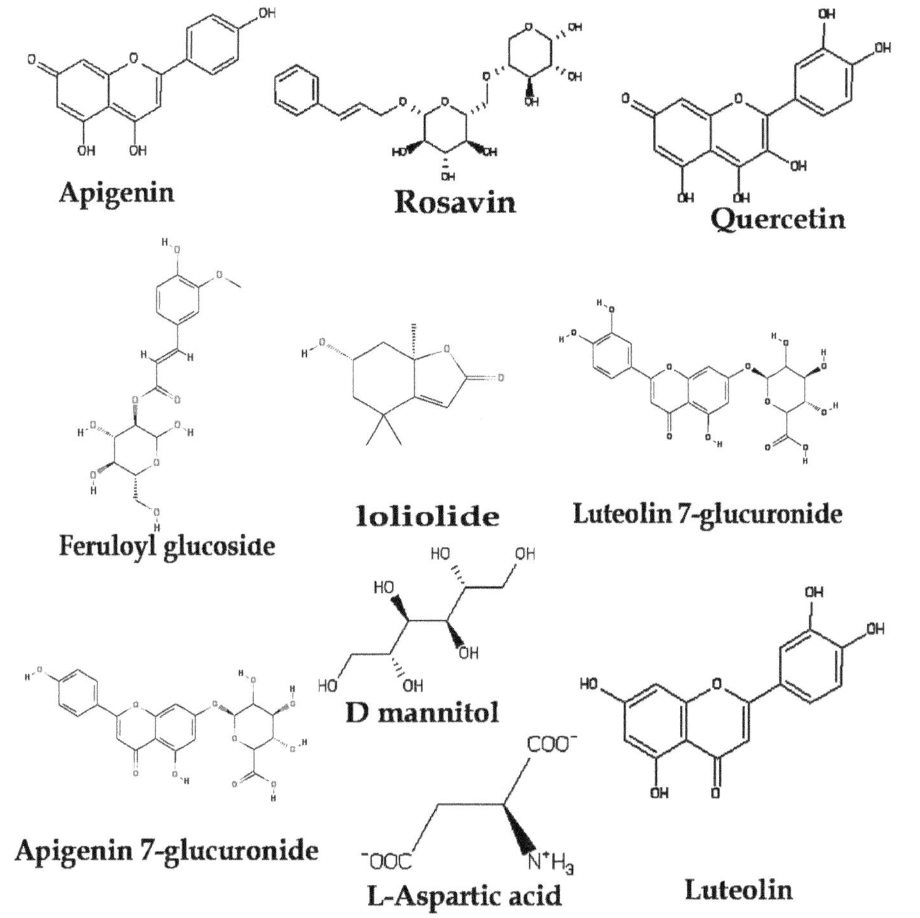

Figure 1 2D structure of all compounds of *B. monnieri.*

and s $_{vdw\_ext}$ are the Vanderwaals interactions between protein and ligand. S $_{hb\_int}$ are the intramolecular hydrophobic interactions whereas S $_{vdw\_int}$ is the contribution due to intramolecular strain in the ligand.

Results

In vitro antimicrobial assay

Results for the antibacterial activity of *B. monnieri* extract showed that the mean zone of inhibition (13.0-15.0 mm) produced by the extract was close to those produced by the reference antibiotics, i.e., tetracycline and ampicillin which had the zone of inhibitions between 16 to 20 mm. The extract of three different concentrations (1, 2 and 3 mg/disk) produced significant ($p < 0.05$) zone of inhibition against *S. aureus* and the values were 13.33 ± 2.08, 13.33 ± 2.08 and 15.33 ± 1.52 for 1, 2 and 3 mg/disk, respectively. The result of antibacterial activity of *B. monnieri* ethanol extract is shown in Table 1.

Minimum inhibitory concentration

The minimum inhibitory concentrations of *B. monnieri* leaf extract for different bacterial strains were ranged from 25 to 100 μl/ml (Table 2). The arbitrary MIC against the Gram-positive bacteria *S. aureus* was greater than or equal to 75 for the extract and 16 for the reference antibiotic tetracycline.

Docking experiments

Considering the results obtained in *in vitro* study, it was thought worthy to perform molecular docking studies which correlate both *in silico* and *in vitro* results. Docking studies are used at different stages of drug discovery such as to predict a ligand-receptor interaction and also to rank the compounds based on the binding energies or fitness score [20]. In our present study, docking of tested compounds with the primary drug pathway for *S. aureus* was performed, and the corresponding fitness score was also determined as shown in Table 3. The interacting energies followed the order of the best fitness core. Highest fitness scored compound was further subjected to compare its binding pattern and molecular interaction with the standard drug penicillin G and ciprofloxacin.

In the docking studies of DNA gyrase binding site, luteolin among the other tested compounds has the

Table 1 *in vitro* antibacterial activity of *B. monnieri* ethanol extract

Bacterial type	Test organism	Source ID (ATCC)	Diameter of zone of inhibition (mm)				
			Bacopa monnieri			Standard antibiotics	
Gram + ve			1 mg/disk	2 mg/disk	3 mg/disk	Tetracycline (50 μg/disk)	Ampicillin (50 μg/disk)
	Staphylococcus aureus	6538	13.33 ± 2.08^{a}	13.33 ± 2.08^{b}	15.33 ± 1.52^{c}	16.00 ± 3.54^{d}	20.00 ± 1.60^{e}

Data are shown as mean ± SD for triplicate of concentration. Different superscript letters (a-e) shown in the data indicate that the values are significantly different (Tukey's multiple range, *post hoc* test, $p < 0.05$) from each other.

highest fitness score 53.77 compared with the highest fitness score 46.48 of ciprofloxacin. Molecular binding pattern of ciprofloxacin revealed that it has two hydrogen bonds with ARG144 and GLY85 consisting of hydrogen bonding distances 2.634 Å and 2.476 Å shown in Figure 2. These two hydrogen bonding residues in luteolin are found to be similar with different hydrogen bonds viz. 2.641 Å for ARG144 and 2.520 Å for GLY85. Additionally, it also formed two other hydrogen bonds with ARG84 and ASP81 having a bonding distance of 2.932 Å and 2.956 Å.

For the most potent inhibitor of penicillin binding protein, luteolin showed the highest fitness score among the other tested compounds viz., 45.35 fitness score compared to its reference standard drug penicillin G 46.48. In context of different binding patterns, luteolin has formed the three hydrogen bonds SER429, THR621 and THR619 where bonding distances were 3.020, 2.798 and 2.331. On the other hand, reference drug penicillin G formed hydrogen bonds with ASN450, SER778, THR621 and GLN524 with corresponding hydrogen bonds 2.956 Å, 2.968 Å, 2.556 Å and 3.031 Å, respectively. Binding mode and related interactions are summarized in Figure 3.

The emergence of bacterial resistance to current clinical drugs has brought intention to develop novel antimicrobial agents for selectively inhibiting the constantly evolved bacterial targets which have been also continually promoted with challenges. Presently known target of *Staphyloccus* sp. includes PBP (penicillin binding protein) of peptidoglycan biosynthesis pathway where beta-lactam antibiotics were known to be effective against it [21]. A different prescribing drug i.e. Fluroquinolone, DNA Gyrase A enzyme which is essential for the replication and super-coiling of DNA, is the main target at this case. But according to Stephen *et al.*, a highly significant association between Levofloxacin and Ciprofloxacin treatment and consequent isolation of MRSA is reported [22]. However, in this research, molecular docking analysis suggested that luteolin has the more specificity towards the DNA gyrase binding site than penicillin binding protein. Regarding the obtained results, luteolin could serve as an appropriate starting point for designing new chemical entities as potent *S. aureus* inhibitor.

Table 2 Minimum inhibitory concentrations (MIC) of *B. monnieri* and tetracycline against *Staphylococcus aureus*

Test organism	MIC of *Bacopa monnieri* extract (μg/ml)	MIC of tetracycline (μg/ml)
Staphylococcus aureus	≥75	≥16

Discussion

Plants have long been a very important source of drug and many plants have been screened whether they contain compounds with therapeutic activity. Therefore, it is vital to evaluate the antimicrobial activity of *B. monnieri*. The bacterial strain was chosen to be studied as it is an important pathogen and rapidly develop antibiotic resistance with its increased uses. In disk diffusion technique, the mean zone of inhibition produced by the commercial antibiotic, tetracycline and ampicillin, was larger than that produced by ethanol extract. It may be attributed to the fact that the plant extract being in crude form contains a smaller concentration of bioactive compounds. In classifying the antimicrobial activity it would be generally expected that a greater number would be active against Gram-positive than Gram-negative bacteria. Apart from this, the higher MIC value is an indication that either the plant extracts are less effective on bacteria or the organism has the potential to develop antibiotic resistance. On the contrary, the low MIC value for bacteria is an indication of the higher efficacy of the plant extracts.

Most of the pathogenic bacteria have developed resistance to currently available antibiotics due to their misuse or overuse. This situation has led to an urgent need to explore different sources of efficient, less toxic and cost-effective antimicrobial agents [23,24]. Medicinal plants play a major role and constitute the backbone of traditional medicine. According to the World Health Organization (WHO) estimate, 80% of populations in developing countries rely exclusively on traditional medicine for their healthcare need. Moreover, 20% of the available allopathic drugs have an active principal obtained from higher plants [25]. Recognizing the significance of indigenous medicinal plants WHO states in its 1997 guideline that locally available effective plants may

Table 3 Gold fitness score of *B. monnieri's* all compounds against DNA gyrase and penicillin binding protein

DNA gyrase						Penicillin binding protein				
Compound name	Fitness score	S(hb_ext)	S(vdw_ext)	S(hb_int)	S(int)	Fitness Score	S(hb_ext)	S(vdw_ext)	S(hb_int)	S(int)
Apigenin	46.59	5.57	36.00	0.00	-8.48	41.73	7.29	30.70	0.00	-7.77
Rosavin	51.58	5.44	42.31	0.00	-12.03	41.96	8.88	31.27	0.00	-9.92
Quercetin	45.71	6.04	37.32	0.00	-11.64	40.14	9.37	30.55	0.00	-11.23
Feruloyl glucoside	49.23	8.14	42.78	0.00	-17.74	32.42	4.76	35.88	0.00	-21.68
Loliolide	29.61	0.10	23.41	0.00	-2.68	31.02	3.34	22.10	0.00	-2.71
Luteolin-7-glucoside	47.87	10.04	42.46	0.00	-20.56	43.85	2.46	42.08	0.00	-16.48
Apigenin-7- glucocronide	45.63	8.34	39.19	0.00	-16.59	43.35	8.74	37.80	0.00	-17.36
D-mannitol	32.55	9.88	23.13	0.00	-9.13	30.21	8.15	20.48	0.00	-6.11
L-asperatic acid	33.35	17.74	17.07	0.00	-7.86	28.29	14.01	16.69	0.00	-8.66
Luteolin	53.77	11.23	37.44	0.00	-8.94	45.35	7.81	41.67	0.00	-19.77
Penicillin G	-------	-------	-------	-------	-------	46.48	2.62	35.14	0.00	-4.46
Ciprofloxacine	46.48	0.21	42.47	0.00	-8.94	--------	-------	-------	------	-------

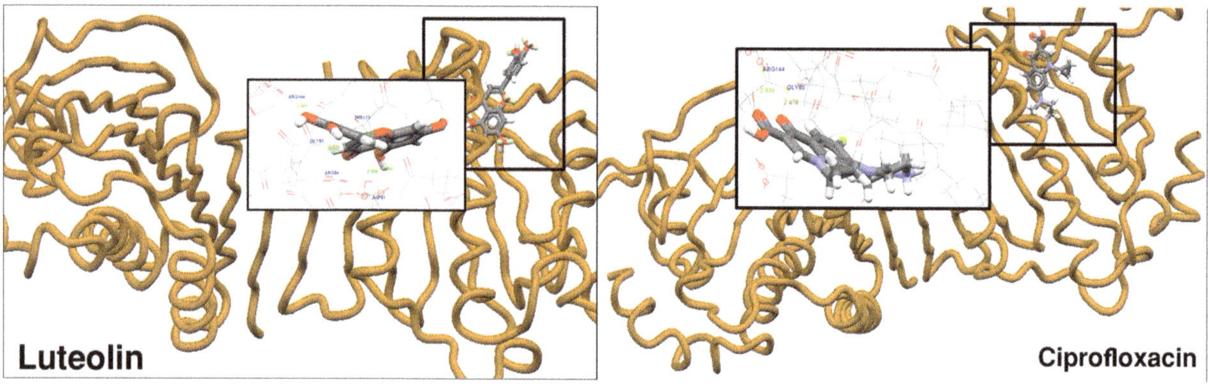

Figure 2 Interaction and superimposed structure of compound of luteolin and ciprofloxacin with DNA gyrase.

be used as substitutes for drugs. Research work on medicinal plants and exchange of obtained information will go a long way in scientific exploration of medicinal plants for the benefit of mankind. This will ultimately decrease our dependence on synthetic drugs [26]. Plant synthesizes natural products as its chemical weapon that arrests the growth of environmental microbes [27] and some plants inhibit the growth of potential human pathogens too. In the current study, *in vitro* MIC of *B. monnieri* leaf parts, prescribed in indigenous system of medicine, that are available in the local market or growing in Bangladesh and India were evaluated against local clinical bacterial isolate of *S. aureus*. Determination of MIC of this plant is important to find out the best plant that eradicates infectious agents (Table 2). Clinicians also select the antibiotic on the basis of their MIC value to treat infectious diseases. Plant extracts having MIC below 8000 μg/ml have been reported as therapeutically effective [28]. Our results for *B. monnieri* implicated a significant MIC value (below or equal to 75 μg/ml) in this study. This significance suggests that we have identified antimicrobial activity of plant that is effective for arresting the growth of *S. aureus* causing hospital-,-acquired- and opportunistic-infections.

Conclusions

B. monnieri extract and its compound luteolin have a significant antimicrobial activity against *S. aureus*. Molecular binding interaction of *in silico* data demonstrated that luteolin has more specificity towards the DNA gyrase binding site and could be a potent antimicrobial compound. However several scientific reports manifested that lead-drug discovery projects on the basis of binding efficiency indices would afford bioactive compounds with better pharmacokinetic outcomes. Hence, isolated bioactive compounds should be employed for establishing more rational structure activity relationships in the era of antimicrobial drug development.

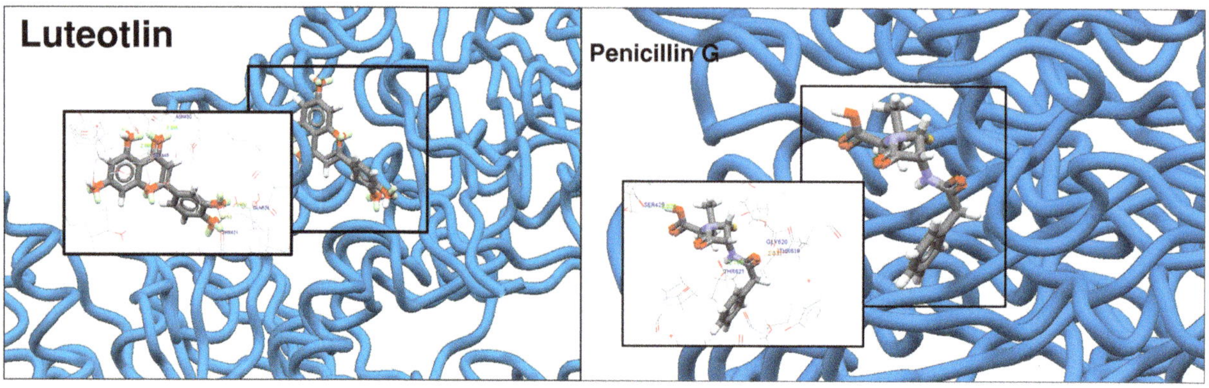

Figure 3 Interaction and superimposed structure of compound of luteolin and penicillin G with penicillin binding protein.

Competing interests

The authors declare that they have no competing interests.

Authors' contributions

TBE has designed the study, performed data analysis and interpretation and written the manuscript. MAR has revised the whole manuscript and also helped in the grammatical corrections. MMNU has modified the *in silico* sections. RD has performed data analysis and written the *in silico* sections. MFH and MM have participated in experiments, data collection and literature search. MRA has provided assistance in taxonomical identification and collections of voucher specimen's number of the plant. All authors read and approved the final version of the manuscript.

Acknowledgements

Authors are thankful to Dr. Shaikh Bokhtear Uddin, Taxonomist and Associate Professor, Department of Botany, University of Chittagong, Chittagong-4331, Bangladesh for identifying the plant sample. We are also grateful to Bangladesh Council of Scientific and Industrial Research (BCSIR), Chittagong-4220, Bangladesh for supplying the microbial strains.

Author details

[1]Department of Pharmacy, BGC Trust University Bangladesh, Chittagong 4000, Bangladesh. [2]Department of Biochemistry and Molecular Biology, University of Chittagong, Chittagong 4331, Bangladesh. [3]Department of Pharmacy, University of Chittagong, Chittagong 4331, Bangladesh.

References

1. Boucher HW, Talbot GH, Bradley JS, Edwards JE, Gilbert D, Rice LB, et al. Bad bugs, no drugs: no ESKAPE! An update from the Infectious Diseases Society of America. Clin Infect Dis. 2009;48(1):1–12.
2. Kluytmans J, van Belkum A, Verbrugh H. Nasal carriage of Staphylococcus aureus: epidemiology, underlying mechanisms, and associated risks. Clin Microbiol Rev. 1997;10(3):505–20.
3. Kuehnert MJ, Hill HA, Kupronis BA, Tokars JI, Solomon SL, Jernigan DB. Methicillin-resistant-*Staphylococcus aureus* hospitalizations, United States. Emerg Infect Dis. 2005;11(6):868–72.
4. Klevens RM, Morrison MA, Nadle J, Petit S, Gershman K, Ray S, et al. Invasive methicillin-resistant *Staphylococcus aureus* infections in the United States. Jama. 2007;298(15):1763–71.
5. Diefenbeck M, Mennenga U, Guckel P, Tiemann AH, Muckley T, Hofmann GO. Vacuum-assisted closure therapy for the treatment of acute postoperative osteomyelitis. Z Orthop Unfall. 2011;149:336–41.
6. Garo E, Eldridge GR, Goering MG, DeLancey PE, Hamilton MA, Costerton JW, et al. Asiatic acid and corosolic acid enhance the susceptibility of *Pseudomonas aeruginosa* biofilms to tobramycin. Antimicrob Agents Chemother. 2007;51(5):1813–7.
7. Coutinho HD, Costa JG, Lima EO, Falcao-Silva VS, Siqueira-Junior JP. Enhancement of the antibiotic activity against a multiresistant *Escherichia coli* by *Mentha arvensis* L. and chlorpromazine. Chemotherapy. 2008;4:328–30.
8. Coutinho HD, Costa JG, Lima EO, Falcao-Silva VS, Siqueira Jr JP. Herbal therapy associated with antibiotic therapy: potentiation of the antibiotic activity against methicillin–resistant Staphylococcus aureus by *Turnera ulmifolia* L. BMC Complement Altern Med. 2009;9(13):1472–6882.
9. Aguiar S, Borowski T. Neuropharmacological review of the nootropic herb *Bacopa monnieri*. Rejuvenation Res. 2013;16(4):313–26.
10. Chopra RNNL, Chopra IC. Glossary of Indian Medicinal Plants. New Delhi: Council of Scientific and Industrial Research; 1956. p. 32.
11. Ghosh S, Nie A, An J, Huang Z. Structure-based virtual screening of chemical libraries for drug discovery. Curr Opin Chem Biol. 2006;10(3):194–202.
12. Dash R, Emran TB, Uddin MM, Islam A, Junaid M. Molecular docking of fisetin with AD associated AChE, ABAD and BACE1 proteins. Bioinformation. 2014;10(9):562–8.
13. Yoshida H, Kawai F, Obayashi E, Akashi S, Roper DI, Tame JR, et al. Crystal structures of penicillin-binding protein 3 (PBP3) from methicillin-resistant *Staphylococcus aureus* in the apo and cefotaxime-bound forms. J Mol Biol. 2012;423(3):351–64.
14. Ronkin SM, Badia M, Bellon S, Grillot AL, Gross CH, Grossman TH, et al. Discovery of pyrazolthiazoles as novel and potent inhibitors of bacterial gyrase. Bioorg Med Chem Lett. 2010;20(9):2828–31.
15. Berman HM, Westbrook J, Feng Z, Gilliland G, Bhat TN, Weissig H, et al. The Protein Data Bank. Nucleic Acids Res. 2000;28(1):235–42.
16. Hevener KE, Zhao W, Ball DM, Babaoglu K, Qi J, White SW, et al. Validation of molecular docking programs for virtual screening against dihydropteroate synthase. J Chem Inf Model. 2009;49(2):444–60.
17. Hristozov DP, Oprea TI, Gasteiger J. Virtual screening applications: a study of ligand-based methods and different structure representations in four different scenarios. J Comput Aided Mol Des. 2007;21(10–11):617–40.
18. Osolodkin DI, Palyulin VA, Zefirov NS. Structure-based virtual screening of glycogen synthase kinase 3-beta inhibitors: analysis of scoring functions applied to large true actives and decoy sets. Chem Biol Drug Des. 2011;78(3):378–90.
19. Jones G, Willett P, Glen RC, Leach AR, Taylor R. Development and validation of a genetic algorithm for flexible docking. J Mol Biol. 1997;267(3):727–48.
20. Kitchen DB, Decornez H, Furr JR, Bajorath J. Docking and scoring in virtual screening for drug discovery: methods and applications. Nat Rev Drug Discov. 2004;3(11):935–49.
21. Hao H, Cheng G, Dai M, Wu Q, Yuan Z. Inhibitors targeting on cell wall biosynthesis pathway of MRSA. Mol Biosyst. 2012;8(11):2828–38.
22. Weber SG, Gold HS, Hooper DC, Karchmer AW, Carmeli Y. Fluoroquinolones and the risk for methicillin-resistant *Staphylococcus aureus* in hospitalized patients. Emerg Infect Dis. 2003;9(11):1415–22.
23. Russell AD. Bacterial resistance to disinfectants: present knowledge and future problems. J Hosp Infec. 1999;43(0):S57–68. Supplement 1.
24. Sheldon Jr AT. Antibiotic resistance: a survival strategy. Clin Lab Sci. 2005;18(3):170–80.
25. Gurib-Fakim A. Medicinal plants: traditions of yesterday and drugs of tomorrow. Mol Aspects Med. 2006;27(1):1–93.
26. Veerappan A, Miyazaki S, Kadarkaraisamy M, Ranganathan D. Acute and subacute toxicity studies of *Aegle marmelos* Corr., an Indian medicinal plant. Phytomedicine. 2007;14(2-3):209–15.
27. Gibbons S. Anti-staphylococcal plant natural products. Nat Prod Rep. 2004;21(2):263–77.
28. Fabry W, Okemo PO, Ansorg R. Antibacterial activity of East African medicinal plants. J Ethnopharmacol. 1998;60(1):79–84.

Anti-cancer effect of *Cordyceps militaris* in human colorectal carcinoma RKO cells via cell cycle arrest and mitochondrial apoptosis

Hwan Hee Lee[1,2], Seulki Lee[1,2], Kanghyo Lee[3], Yu Su Shin[4], Hyojeung Kang[5*] and Hyosun Cho[1,2*]

Abstract

Background: *Cordyceps militaris* has been used as a traditional medicine in Asian countries for a long time. Different types of Cordyceps extract were reported to have various pharmacological activities including an anti-cancer effect. We investigated the inhibitory effect of *Cordyceps militaris* ethanol extract on a human colorectal cancer-derived cell line, RKO.

Methods: RKO cells were treated with various concentrations of nucleosides-enriched ethanol extract of *Cordyceps militaris* for 48 h and cytotoxicity was measured using a CCK-8 assay. Then, xenograft Balb/c nude mice were injected with RKO cells and subsequently orally administered with ethanol extract of *Cordyceps militaris* every day for 3 weeks to examine the inhibitory effect on tumor growth. Lastly, the effect of *Cordyceps militaris* on cell cycle as well as apoptosis was measured using flow cytometry. Also, the expression of p53, caspase 9, cleaved caspase-3, cleaved PARP, Bim, Bax, Bak, and Bad were detected using western blot assay.

Results: RKO cells were highly susceptible to the ethanol extract of *Cordyceps militaris* (CME) and the growth of RKO cells-derived tumor was significantly delayed by the treatment of *Cordyceps militaris*. *Cordyceps militaris* induced cell cycle arrest in G2/M phase (untreated; 20.5 %, CME 100 μg/ml; 61.67 %, CME 300 μg/ml; 66.33 %) and increased early apoptosis (untreated; 1.01 %, CME 100 μg/ml; 8.48 %, CME 300 μg/ml; 18.07 %). The expression of p53, cleaved caspase 9, cleaved caspase-3, cleaved PARP, Bim, Bak, and Bad were upregulated by the treatment of *Cordyceps militaris*.

Conclusion: Ethanol extract of *Cordyceps militaris* was highly cytotoxic to human colorectal carcinoma RKO cells and inhibited the growth of tumor in xenograft model. The anti-tumor effect of *Cordyceps militaris* was associated with an induction of cell cycle arrest and mitochondrial-mediated apoptosis.

Keywords: *Cordyceps militaris*, Human colorectal carcinoma, p53, Mitochondrial-mediated apoptosis

Background

A large number of edible mushrooms have been shown to possess various biological activities [1–5]. Edible mushrooms from Pleurotus species showed the antioxidative, antimicrobial and anrifungal properties when they were cultivated on banana agrowastes [1, 2]. Antimetastatic activity of *Hericium erinaceus* edible mushroom extracts was reported using murine colon carcinoma cells [3]. Antioxidant and cytotoxic activities of ethanolic extracts of *Phellinus Quél* were recently reported [4]. An extract of *Agaricus blazei Murill* was shown to stimulate immunocytes and regulate immune response in leukemia mice [5]. *Cordyceps* mushrooms also have received extensive attention owing to their potent pharmacological activities. *Cordyceps sinensis* and *Cordyceps militaris* are representative species for their medicinal uses in China and Korea. Both of them are fungi on the larvae of caterpillars of moths and traditional medicine involves both mushroom fruitbody and parasitized larvae. A couple of well-known active ingredients in these mushrooms include cordycepin, cordycepic acid, sterols (ergosterol), nucleosides, and polysaccharides [6, 7]. *Cordyceps militaris* is a traditional Chinese

* Correspondence: hkang72@gmail.com; hyosun1102@gmail.com
[5]College of Pharmacy, Research Institute of Pharmaceutical Sciences and Institute for Microorganisms, Kyungpook National University, Daegu 702-701, Republic of Korea
[1]College of Pharmacy, Duksung Women's University, Seoul 132-714, Republic of Korea
Full list of author information is available at the end of the article

medicine, which has been cultured successfully and has been shown to have a higher content of cordycepin and cordycepic acid than *Cordyceps sinensis* [8]. Diffferent types of extracts of *Cordyceps militaris* have been reported to exert immunomodulatory, anti-inflammatory, antimicrobial and antitumor effects although the primary pharmacological activity is a little bit different depending on the main ingredients of extract [7–10]. Recently, we found that ethanol extract of *Cordyceps militaris*, which has a couple of nucleoside analogs as the main components, had an anti-influenza effect in a DBA2 mouse model [11].

Beside the routine methods of surgery, radiotherapy and chemotherapy, traditional herb medicine is one of the major complementary and alternative medicines for treating various malignant diseases, including colorectal cancer [12–14].

Colorectal cancer is a serious health problem that has progressively increased to be one of the most common cancers in Asian countries [15]. *Cordyceps* extract has been reported to have a potent cytotoxic effect on various human cancer cells, including human lung carcinoma cells [16, 17]. However, the anti-tumor effect of *Cordyceps* extract on human colorectal cancer cells was not precisely examined *in vivo* model. Xenograft mouse model is immunocompromised animal, which could be implanted with the human tumor cells either under the skin or into any organ and does not reject the tumor. Therefore, it has been an indispensable model system for the preclinical screen and the development of novel anti-cancer agents.

p53 is known to play a critical role in the induction of cell apoptosis in response to DNA damage [18]. A typical pro-apoptotic molecule activated by p53 is Bax, a member of the Bcl-2 family [19]. The Bcl-2 family of proteins includes both pro-apoptotic members (Bak, Bax, and Bad) as well as anti-apoptotic members (Bcl-2, Bcl-xL, and Bcl-w). Mitochondria-dependent cell apoptosis is regulated mainly by the ratio of expression of Bcl-2 family proteins [20]. The activation of Bax results in the release of cytochrome c into the cytosol, which leads to the activation of caspases 9 and 3, effector caspases, in the mitochondrial pathway of cell apoptosis [21, 22].

In the present study, we investigated the cytotoxic effect of *Cordyceps militaris* ethanol extract on human colorectal carcinoma RKO cells and evaluated the anti-cancer effect of *Cordyceps militaris* in mice bearing RKO cell-derived tumors. Subsequently, the underlying mechanisms, which mediate the anti-cancer effect of *Cordyceps militaris* on human colorectal cancer, were precisely examined. We found that the anti-cancer effect of nucleosides-enriched ethanol extract of *Cordyceps militaris* was highly associated with the increased expression of p53, Bax, Bim, Bak, Bad, cleaved-caspases 9 and 3, and PARP.

Material and methods

Specimen preparation

The fungus strain *Cordyceps militaris* was from Dong-Chong-Xia-Cao Culture Collection (Mushtech, Hoengseong, Kangwondo, Reupblic of Korea). Fresh fruiting bodies or mycelia of *Cordyceps militaris* were extracted with 50 % ethanol at room temperature for 3 days. The extracts were filtered, concentrated, sterilized and dried as previously described [23]. The major compounds of extract are cordycepin, adenosine, urasil and guanosine, which structurally belong to nucleoside family (provided by Dong-a Pharm. Co., LTD, Yongin, Republic of Korea). Extracts of specimens were diluted with distilled water for RKO cell treatment as well as for oral administration in the mouse experiment.

Cell culture and treatment

Human colorectal carcinoma (RKO) cells were obtained from ATCC and cultured in Dulbecco's Modified Eagle's medium (DMEM, Gibco, USA) supplemented with 10 % heat-inactivated fetal bovine serum (FBS, Hyclone, USA), 100 U/ml penicillin and streptomycin (Gibco, USA) at 37 °C in a humidified atmosphere with 5 % CO_2.

Cell cytotoxicity

Cytotoxicity of ethanol extract of *Cordyceps militaris* on human colorectal carcinoma (RKO) cells was assessed with the Cell Counting Kit-8 (CCK-8, Dojindo, Japan) as previously described [24]. Briefly, cells were seeded in 96-well plates at a density of 3 × 103 cells/well and treated with different concentrations of ethanol extract of *Cordyceps militaris* (0, 25, 50, 100, 250, 500, and 1000 μg/ml) for 24 h or 48 h. CCK-8 solution was added to each well and incubated for another 3 h. The absorbance was measured using a microplate reader (BMG Labtech, Germany) at 450 nm.

Cell morphology

Cells were seeded at a density of 4 × 104 cells/well in 6-well plates. After incubation for 24 h, the cells were treated with different concentrations of ethanol extract of *Cordyceps militaris* (0, 100, and 300 μg/ml) and incubated for 24 h. The cells were observed by light microscopy (×200) (Nikon eclipse TS100, Japan).

Cell cycle analysis

Cells were seeded at a density of 1 × 106 cells/well in 6-well plates, and treated with different concentrations of ethanol extract of *Cordyceps militaris* (0, 100, and 300 μg/ml) for 24 h. Cells were harvested by trypsinization and fixed with 70 % ethanol at 4 °C overnight. The next day, cells were resuspended in PBS buffer containing 0.2 mg/ml RNase A (Qiagen, USA) and incubated for 1 h at 37 °C. Cells were then stained with propidium iodide for 30 min in the dark. Stained cells were analyzed using a flow cytometer (EasyCyte guava, Merck Millipore).

Annexin V-FITC and propidium iodide assay

Cell apoptosis was analyzed using the Annexin V-FITC Apoptosis Detection Kit (Roche, USA) as previously described [24]. Briefly, RKO cells were plated in 6-well plates at a density of 1 × 106 cells/well and incubated for 24 h. Cells were treated with different concentrations (0, 100, and 300 μg/ml) of ethanol extract of *Cordyceps militaris* for 24 h or 48 h and then Annexin V and PI solution were added. Cells were analyzed by flow cytometry (EasyCyte guava, Merck Millipore).

Western blot analysis

Western blot assays were performed as previously described with modification [24]. Briefly, RKO cells were treated with ethanol extract of *Cordyceps militaris* (100 and 300 μg/ml) for 48 h. Protein from cell lysates was measured using the Bradford assay, separated by electrophoresis, and transferred onto nitrocellulose membranes. Membranes were subsequently incubated with 1st and 2nd antibody, and the blots were visualized by enhanced chemiluminescent (ECL) detection solutions (GE Healthcare, USA).

Xenograft mouse model experiments

All animal experiments were conducted in accordance with recommendations in the National Research Council's Guide (IACUC, Republic of Korea) for the Care and Use of Laboratory Animals. The experimental protocol was approved by the Animal Experiments Committee of Duksung Women's University (permit number: 2014-015-007). Balb/c nude mice (female, 5 weeks old; Joong-ang Animal Experiment Company, Republic of Korea) were used as our xenograft animal model. Mice were housed individually on a 12-h day/12-h night cycle at 23 ~ 27 °C and had access to food and water. Mice were randomly divided into two groups (n = 10/group): (1) a drinking water group (n = 10): animals received oral administration of drinking water; (2) a CME group (n = 10): animals received oral administration of *Cordyceps militaris* ethanol extract (100 mg/kg). To produce tumors, each mouse was implanted with RKO cells (1×10^6 cells per animal), subcutaneously in the back next to the right hind leg. Next, *Cordyceps militaris* ethanol extract (100 mg/kg) or drinking water was administered orally every day for 3 weeks. Fourteen days later, the tumors were identified and then measured every 2 days with a Standard Caliper. Tumor volume was calculated as follows: tumor volume (mm^3) = [tumor length (mm) × tumor width $(mm)^2$]/2. Once tumor volume reached up to 2000 mm^3, animals were euthanized.

Statistical analysis

Data were processed using Microexcel software and were expressed as mean ± SD. Comparisons of several means were performed using one-way or two-way analysis of variance followed by the Fisher's exact test to identify significant differences between groups. P values of less than 0.05 were considered significant.

Results

Cytotoxicity of *Cordyceps* extract in RKO cells

To investigate the cytotoxic effect of ethanol extract of *Cordyceps militaris* on human colorectal carcinoma RKO cells, cells were treated with serially diluted extract of *Cordyceps militaris* (0, 25, 50, 75, 100, 250, 500, and 1000 μg/ml) for 48 h and cytotoxicity was determined by CCK-8. Figure 1a shows that ethanol extract of *Cordyceps militaris* starts to inhibit cell viability at a concentration of 75 μg/ml compared to untreated cells ($P < 0.0001$). In Fig. 1b, cell morphological changes by two different concentrations of ethanol extract of *Cordyceps militaris* (100 and 300 μg/ml) were observed. There were fewer cells in the extract-treated conditions.

In vivo evaluation of anti-cancer effect of *Cordyceps militaris* ethanol extract in a xenograft mouse model

To evaluate the anti-cancer effect of ethanol extract of *Cordyceps militaris in vivo*, mice were injected subcutaneously with human colorectal cancer RKO cells (1×10^6 cells per mouse) and then ethanol extract of *Cordyceps militaris* (100 mg/kg) or drinking water was orally administrated every day for 3 weeks. Tumor growth was detected from all 20 mice and tumor volume was measured every two days until it reached 2000 mm^3. Figure 2a displays the overall study design for animal experiment. Figure 2b shows representative photographs of xenograft mice bearing RKO cell-derived human colorectal cancer. The pictures of the extract fed and water fed groups were taken at 13 days since the tumor volume was measured. The size of tumors from the extract fed mice was smaller than that from water fed mice. In Fig. 2c, we confirmed that continuous feeding of ethanol extract of *Cordyceps militaris* (100 mg/kg) significantly inhibited the growth of RKO cell-derived tumors. We further determined whether inhibition of tumor growth directly correlates with survival rate in the xenograft animals. As expected, we observed a reduced mortality in mice administered 100 mg/kg of ethanol extract of *Cordyceps militaris* in Fig. 2d.

Evaluation of cell cycle arrest in RKO cells treated with *Cordyceps militaris* ethanol extract

To clarify the molecular mechanism of *Cordyceps militaris*, we analyzed the effect on cell cycle regulation in RKO cells using flow cytometry. Interestingly, ethanol extract of *Cordyceps militaris* (100 or 300 μg/ml) induced

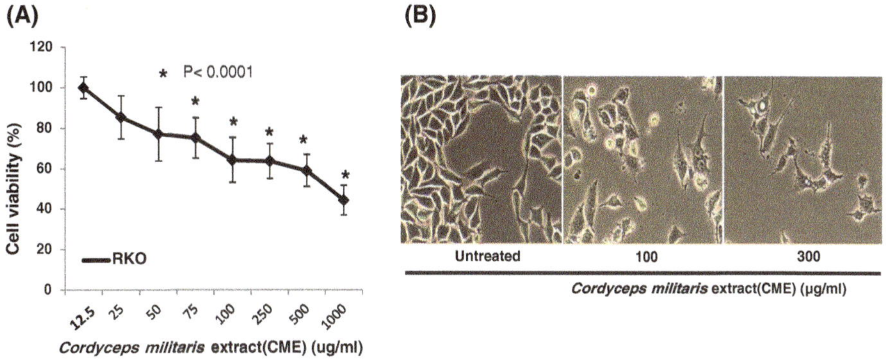

Fig. 1 Cell cytotoxicity of *Cordyceps militaris* in human colorectal carcinoma RKO cells. **a** RKO cells were treated with various concentrations (0–1000 μg/mL) of ethanol extract of *Cordyceps militaris* (CME) for 48 h, and cell viability was determined by CCK-8 assay. The results are presented as mean ± standard deviation (SD) for five independent experiments. **b** Cells were treated with or without ethanol extract of *Cordyceps militaris* (CME) for 24 h or 48 h. Cell morphology was observed by light microscopy (×200)

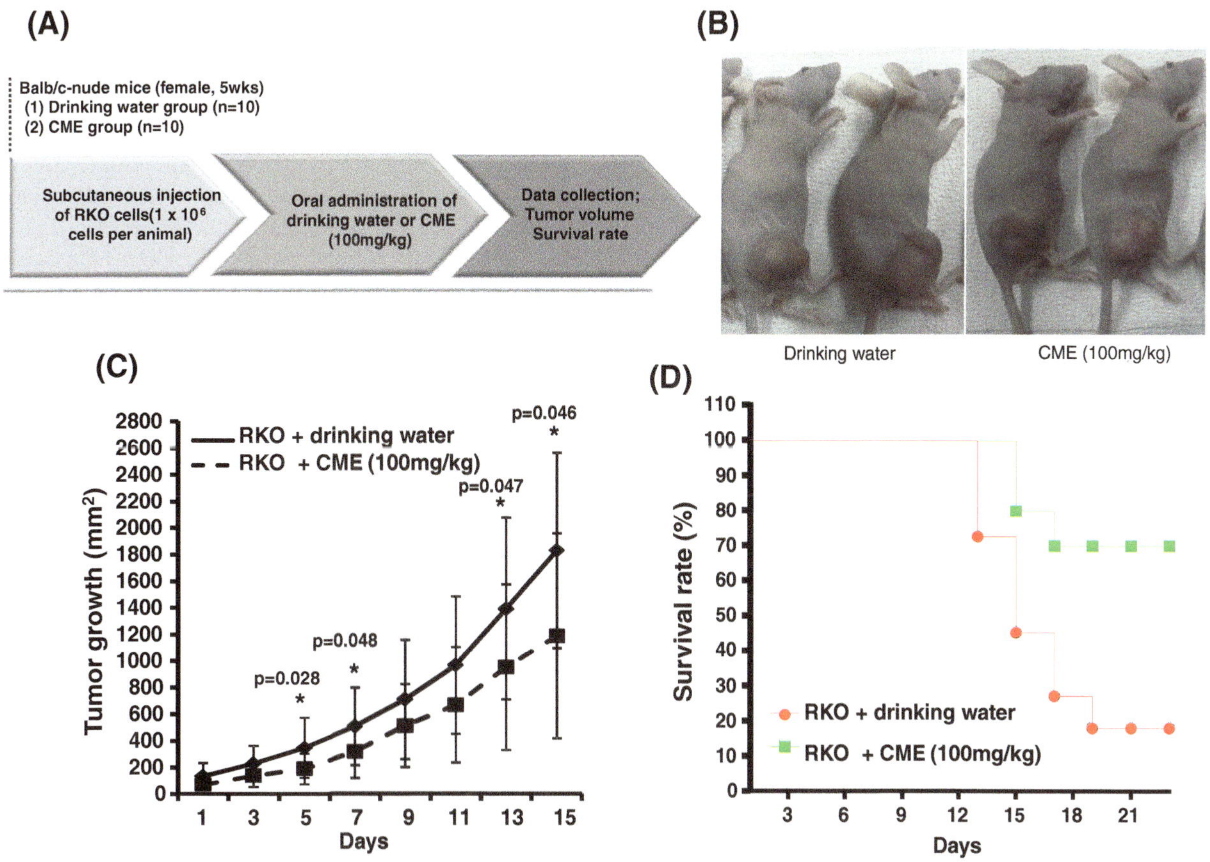

Fig. 2 Anti-cancer effect of *Cordyceps militaris* in a xenograft mouse bearing RKO cell-derived human colorectal cancer. Mice were injected with human colorectal carcinoma RKO cells (1×10^6 cells per mouse) subcutaneously into the back next to the right hind leg. Mice were sorted into 2 groups ($n = 10$/group) and orally administered ethanol extract of *Cordyceps militaris* (CME) (100 mg/kg) or drinking water. 14 days later, tumors were identified and measured every two days until the experimental endpoint. **a** Study design for animal experiment. **b** Photograph of xenograft mice bearing RKO cell-derived human colorectal cancer in right hind leg. The pictures of untreated and treated groups were taken at 13 days since the tumor volume was measured. **c** Inhibitory effect of *Cordyceps militaris* (CME) on RKO cell-derived tumor growth. Compared between drinking water group and CME group *$P < 0.05$. **d** Correlation of survival rate of xenograft mice bearing human colorectal cancer

an increase in the G2/M phase distribution of cells (100 μg/ml; 61.67 %, 300 μg/ml; 66.33 %) as compared to untreated cells (20.5 %) (Fig. 3a). and the quantitative analysis gave a statistically significant difference (Fig. 3b).

Evaluation of cell apoptosis in RKO cells treated with *Cordyceps militaris* ethanol extract

We further examined its effect on cell apoptosis using Annexin V-FITC and propidium iodide (PI) staining. As shown in Fig. 4a, 100 or 300 μg/ml of ethanol extract of *Cordyceps militaris* induced 8.37 % or 22.5 %, respectively, early apoptosis in RKO cells. Five times of independent experiments showed that ethanol extract of *Cordyceps militaris* significantly increased early apoptosis compared to untreated cells(untreated; 1.01 %, 100 μg/ml; 8.48 %, 300 μg/ml; 18.07 %) (Fig. 4b).

Evaluation of apoptotic-related protein expression in RKO cells treated with *Cordyceps militaris* ethanol extract

To identify the responsible apoptotic-related molecules, we examined the expression of p53, Bcl-2 family proteins, caspases, and poly (ADP-ribose) polymerase (PARP) using western blot analysis. Mitochondria-mediated apoptosis involves a variety of signaling molecules including p53, caspase activators, the proapoptotic and antiapoptotic Bcl-2 family proteins [18–20]. We found increased expression of p53 and proapoptotic Bcl-2 family proteins (Bim, Bax, Bak, and Bad) in RKO cells treated with ethanol extract of *Cordyceps militaris*.

In addition, the release of cytochrome *c* is known to activate caspase-9 and caspase-3. Activation of caspase 3 triggers the cleavage of PARP (89 and 24 kDa), which functions to prevent DNA damage [25]. As shown in Fig. 5b, the extract of *Cordyceps militaris* increased the cleaved forms of caspases 9 and 3, which are final effector molecules in mitochondrial apoptosis.

Discussion

In this study, we investigated the anti-cancer effect of ethanol extract of *Cordyceps militaris* in human colorectal carcinoma RKO cells. *Cordyceps militaris* showed potent cell cytotoxicity to RKO cells (Fig. 1), which is consistent with previous studies conducted in other human cancer cell lines [26, 27]. Our *in vitro* cell cytotoxicity was correlated with inhibition of tumor growth of human colorectal cancer observed in a xenograft mouse model (Fig. 2c). A few research groups have studied the anti-cancer effect of *Cordyceps militaris* in a xenografted animal model before. Park *et al.* reported an anti-tumor effect with a water extract of *Cordyceps militaris* in lung cancer cell-derived tumors [28]. The amount of *Cordyceps militaris* extract used in that study was either 150 mg/kg or 300 mg/kg, which is slightly higher than the amount (100 mg/kg) we used in this study. Therefore, we speculate that ethanol extract of *Cordyceps militaris* is more potent than water extract [28].

We also found that the anti-cancer effect of *Cordyceps militaris* in RKO cells was directly associated with induction of cell cycle arrest and apoptosis (Figs. 3 and 4). In fact, Yang *et al.* previously reported that *Cordyceps militaris* arrested human glioblastoma cells in the G0/G1 phase of the cell cycle. Further, Mollah *et al.* reported that *Cordyceps militaris* arrested human colon cancer HT-29 cells in the G2/M phase of the cell cycle, which agrees with our results [26, 29]. Therefore, there may be a differential regulation in cell cycle progression between human glioblastoma cells and human colon-related carcinoma HT-29 or RKO cells. In terms of apoptosis, *Lee et al.* reported that cordycepin, the major ingredient of *Cordyceps militaris*, induced cell apoptosis in HT-29 cells, which is consist with our present study in RKO cells treated with ethanol extract of *Cordyceps militaris* [30]. Also, cordycepin was reported to stimulate

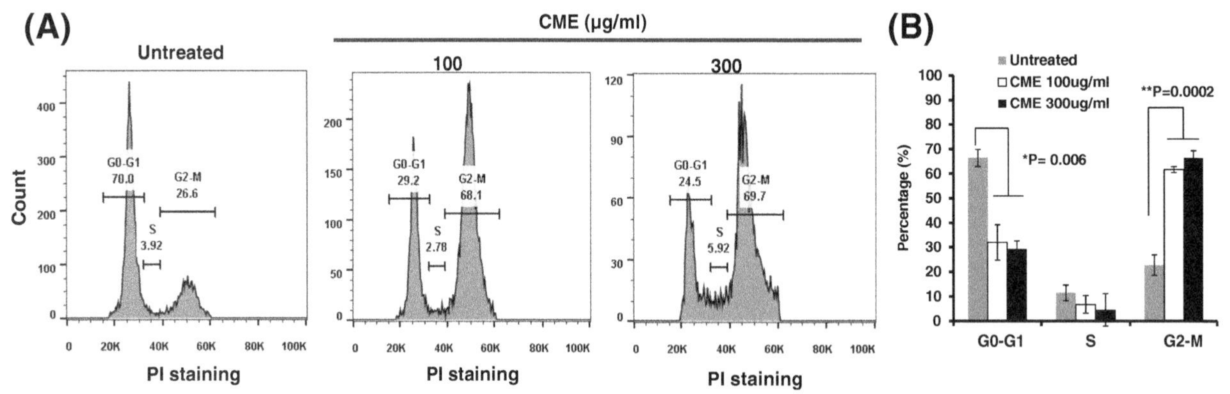

Fig. 3 Induction of cell cycle arrest by *Cordyceps militaris* in RKO cells. Cells were treated with or without ethanol extract of *Cordyceps militaris* (CME) (100 and 300 μg/ml) for 24 h. Then, cells were harvested for PI staining, which was measured by flow cytometry. **a** Representative PI staining for cell cycle progress in RKO cells. **b** The percentage of cell cycle distribution is presented as mean ± standard deviation (SD) for five independent experiments. Compared with other groups *P =0.006, **p = 0.0002

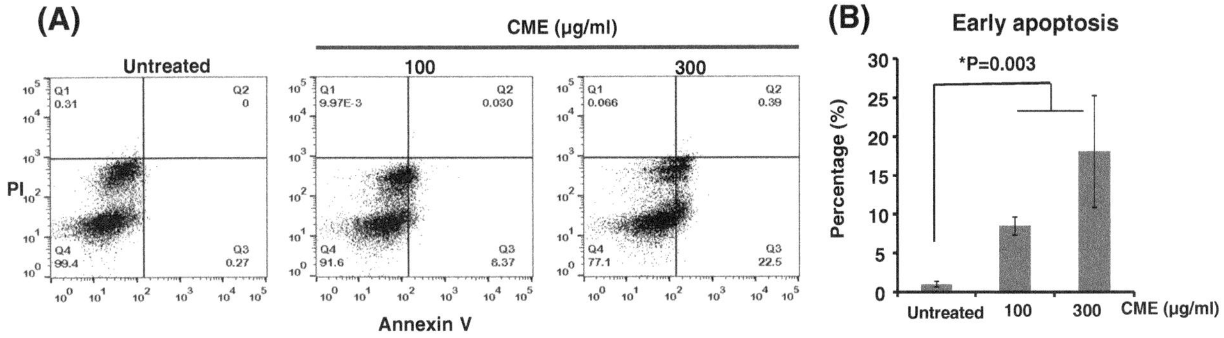

Fig. 4 Induction of cell apoptosis by *Cordyceps militaris* in RKO cells. Cells were treated with or without ethanol extract of *Cordyceps militaris* (CME) (100 and 300 µg/mL) for 48 h and then stained with Annexin V and propidium iodide (PI). Apoptosis of RKO cells was analyzed by flow cytometry. **a** Representative Annexin V and PI staining for cell apoptosis in RKO cells. **b** The percentage of early apoptosis is presented as mean ± standard deviation (SD) for five independent experiments. Compared with other groups *$P = 0.003$

Hep3B human hepatocellular carcinoma cells to TRAIL-mediated apoptosis [31]. In addition, Cordycepol C, one of sesquiterpene compounds from Cordyceps extract, showed to cause poly(ADP-ribose)polymerase-1 (PARP-1) cleavage and triggered the loss of mitochondrial membrane potential ($\Delta\Psi_m$) in HepG2 cells in a time- and dose-dependent manner [32].

Finally, we identified that the responsible molecules for cell apoptosis by *Cordyceps militaris* are caspases 3 and 9, Bim, Bax, Bak, and Bad, which are critical components in the mitochondrial pathway of cell apoptosis. This result is consistent with a recent study by Zhang *et al.* [33]. Interestingly, we also found increased expression of cleaved PARP (89 kDa) in RKO cells treated with

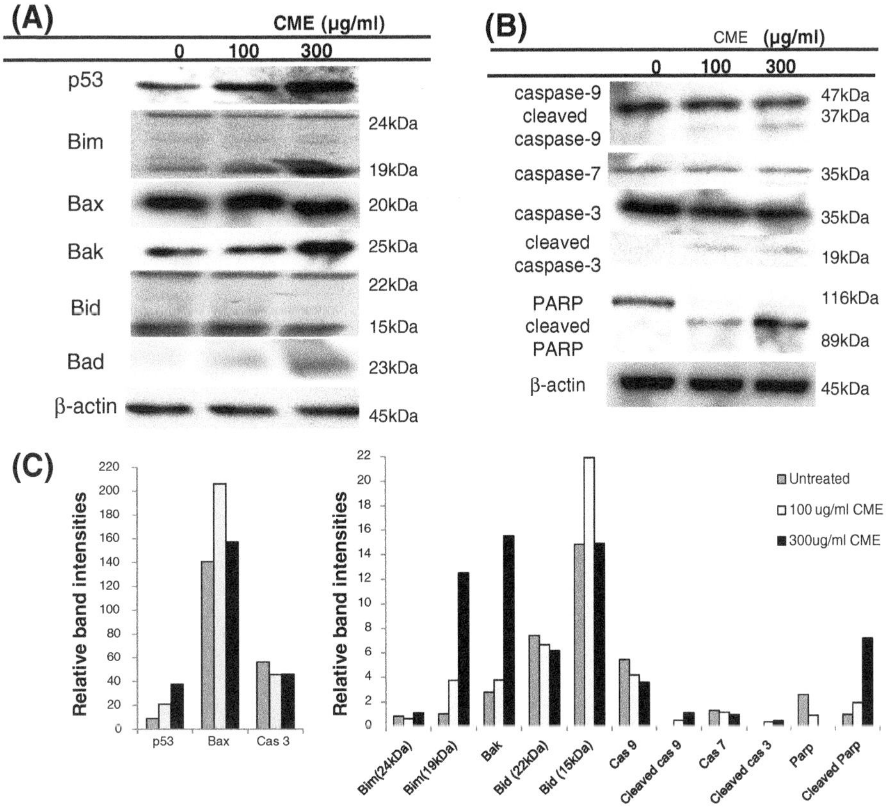

Fig. 5 Induction of mitochondrial-mediated apoptosis by *Cordyceps militaris* in a p53-dependent manner. Cells were treated with or without ethanol extract of *Cordyceps militaris* (CME) (0, 100, and 300 µg/ml) for 48 h and then western blot analysis for various apoptotic related molecules were performed. β-actin served as the loading control. **a** Expression of p53 and Bcl-2 family proteins. **b** Expression of caspases 9, 7, and 3, and PARP proteins. **c** The relative intensity of each band compared to the loading control

ethanol extract of *Cordyceps militaris* (Fig. 5b). As mentioned earlier, the activation of caspase-3 is known to trigger the cleavage of PARP, which indicates the halt of PARP function [25]. Therefore, *Cordyceps militaris* induces mitochondria-dependent apoptosis in RKO cells, which involves an increase of pro-apoptotic Bcl-2 family proteins, activation of caspases 9 and 3 and cleavage of PARP.

As mentioned early, traditional herbal medicines have become one of the most important alternative treatments for cancer therapy. These days, publics are also aware of the significance of prophylactic medications to complement or prevent various cancers. Therefore, we consider our ethanol extract of *Cordyceps militaris* could be a good nutritional supplement for cancer therapy. We will further characterize the active compounds from our extract for anti-cancer effect and investigate the responsible molecular mechanisms in detail.

Conclusions

Ethanol extract of *Cordyceps militaris* inhibited the growth of human colorectal carcinoma RKO cells as well as the *in vivo* growth of tumor in xenograft mice. The inhibitory effect on human colorectal carcinoma cells was highly connected with cell cycle arrest and p53-dependent, mitochondrial mediated apoptosis.

Abbreviations

CME: Extract of *Cordyceps militaris*; ATCC: American type culture collection; ECL: Enhanced chemiluminescene; FITC: Fluorescein isothiocyanate.

Competing interests

The authors declare that they have no competing interests.

Authors' contributions

HHL, HK and HC conceived and designed the study. HHL, SL, HK and HC carried out the study and the data analysis. HHL and HC wrote the manuscript. KL, YS, and HK revised the manuscript. All authors read and approved the final version of the manuscript.

Acknowledgements

This work was carried out with the support of "Cooperative Research Program for Agriculture Science & Technology Development (Project No. PJ0092412015)" Rural Development Administration, Republic of Korea.

Author details

[1]College of Pharmacy, Duksung Women's University, Seoul 132-714, Republic of Korea. [2]Innovative Drug Center, Duksung Women's University, Seoul 132-714, Republic of Korea. [3]Mushroom Research Division, National Institute of Horticultural and Herbal Science, Rural Development Administration, Eumseong 369-873, Republic of Korea. [4]Department of Medicinal Crop Research, National Institute of Horticultural and Herbal Science, Rural Development Administration, Eumseong 369-873, Republic of Korea. [5]College of Pharmacy, Research Institute of Pharmaceutical Sciences and Institute for Microorganisms, Kyungpook National University, Daegu 702-701, Republic of Korea.

References

1. Kunjadia PD, Nagee A, Pandya PY, Mukhopadhyaya PN, Sanghvi GV, Dave GS. Medicinal and antimicrobial role of the oyster culinary-medicinal mushroom Pleurotus ostreatus (higher Basidiomycetes) cultivated on banana agrowastes in India. Int J Med Mushrooms. 2014;16:227–38.
2. Phan CW, Lee GS, Macreadie IG, Malek SN, Pamela D. Lipid constituents of the edible mushroom, Pleurotus giganteus demonstrate anti-Candida activity. Nat Prod Commun. 2013;8:1763–5.
3. Kim SP, Nam SH, Friedman MJ. Hericium erinaceus (Lion's Mane) mushroom extracts inhibit metastasis of cancer cells to the lung in CT-26 colon cancer-tansplanted mice. Agric Food Chem. 2013;61:4898–904.
4. Yang Y, Hu J, Liu Y, Feng N, Chen H, Tang Q, et al. Antioxidant and cytotoxic activities of ethanolic extracts and isolated fractions of species of the genus Phellinus Quél. (Aphyllophoromycetideae). Int J Med Mushrooms. 2011;13:145–52.
5. Lin JG, Fan MJ, Tang NY, Yang JS, Hsia TC, Lin JJ, et al. An extract of Agaricus blazei Murill administered orally promotes immune responses in murine leukemia BALB/c mice in vivo. Integr Cancer Ther. 2012;11:29–36.
6. Tuli HS, Sharma AK, Sandhu SS, Kashyap D. Cordycepin: a bioactive metabolite with therapeutic potential. Life Sci. 2013;93:863–9.
7. Yue K, Ye M, Zhou Z, Sun W, Lin X. The genus Cordyceps: a chemical and pharmacological review. J Pharm Pharmacol. 2013;65:474–93.
8. Zhou X, Gong Z, Su Y, Lin J, Tang K. Cordyceps fungi: natural products, pharmacological functions and developmental products. J Pharm Pharmacol. 2009;61:279–91.
9. Park C, Hong SH, Lee JY. Growth inhibition of U937 leukemia cells by aqueous extract of *Cordyceps militaris* through induction of apoptosis. Oncol Rep. 2005;13:1211–6.
10. Lee H, Kim YJ, Kim HW, Lee DH, Sung MK, Park T. Induction of apoptosis by *Cordyceps militaris* through activation of caspase-3 in leukemiaHL-60 cells. Biol Pharm Bull. 2006;29:670–4.
11. Lee HH, Park H, Sung GH, Lee K, Lee T, Cho H. Anti-influenza effect of Cordyceps militaris through immunomodulation in a DBA/2 mouse model. J Microbiol. 2014;52:696–701.
12. Zhai XF, Chen ZB, Shen LF, Fan J, Zhou WP, Yang YK, et al. Traditional herbal medicine in preventing recurrence after resection of small hepatocellular carcinoma: a multicenter randomized controlled trial. J Integr Med. 2013;11:90–100.
13. Ling CQ, Yue XQ, Ling C. Three advantages of using traditional Chinese medicine to prevent and treat tumor. J Integr Med. 2014;12:331–5.
14. Li ZP, Zeng JQ, Hu AM. Clinical study on the qi and xue dual-supply therapy with chemotherapy to prevent the recurrence and metastasis from colorectal carcinoma. Shi Yong Ai Zheng Za Zhi. 2010;25:618–20.
15. John A, Kaabi SA, Dweik N, Yakoub R, Abdulla F. Emerging role for colorectal cancer screening in Asian countries. Trop Gastroenterol. 2014;35:21–4.
16. Lim HW, Kwon YM, Cho SM, Kim JH, Yoon GH. Antitumor activity of *Cordyceps militaris* on human cancer cell line. Korean J Pharmacogn. 2009;35:364–7.
17. Park SE, Yoo HS, Jin CY, Hong SH, Lee YW, Kim BM. Induction of apoptosis and inhibition of telomerase activity in human lung carcinoma cells by the water extract of *Cordyceps militaris*. Food Chem Toxicol. 2009;47:1667–75.
18. Lakin ND, Jackson SP. Regulation of p53 in response to DNA damage. Oncogene. 1999;18:7644–55.
19. Wu X, Deng Y. Bax and BH3-domain-only proteins in p53-mediated apoptosis. Front Biosci. 2002;7:151–6.
20. Murphy KM, Ranganathan V, Farnsworth M, Kavallaris LM, Lock RB. Bcl-2 inhibits Bax translocation from cytosol to mitochondria during drug-induced apoptosis of human tumor cells. Cell Death Differ. 2000;7:102–11.
21. Cain K, Brown DG, Langlais C, Cohen GM. Caspase activation involves the formation of the aposome, a large (approximately 700 kDa) caspase-activating complex. J Biol Chem. 1999;274:22686–92.
22. Adrain C, Slee EA, Harte MT, Martin SJ. Regulation of apoptotic protease activating factor-1 oligomerization and apoptosis by the WD-40 repeat region. J Biol Chem. 1999;274:20855–60.
23. Won SY, Park EH. Anti-inflammatory and related pharmacological activities of cultured mycelia and fruiting bodies of *Cordyceps militaris*. J Ethnopharmacol. 2005;96:555–61.
24. Son M, Lee M, Ryu E, Moon A, Jeong CS, Jung YW, et al. Genipin as a novel chemical activator of EBV lytic cycle. J Microbiol. 2015;53:155–65.
25. Boulares AH, Yakovlev AG, Ivanova V, Stoica BA, Wang G, Iyer S, et al. Role of poly(ADP-ribose) polymerase (PARP) cleavage in apoptosis; Caspase 3-resistant PARP mutant increases rates of apoptosis in transfected cells. J Biol Chem. 1999;274:22932–40.

26. Yang CH, Kao YH, Huang KS, Wang CY, Lin W. *Cordyceps militaris* and mycelial fermentation induced apoptosis and autophagy of human glioblastoma cells. Cell Death Dis. 2012;3, e431. doi:10.1038/cddis.
27. Park BT, Na KH, Jung EC, Par JW, Kim HH. Antifungal and anticancer activities of a protein from the mushroom cordyceps militaris. Korean J Physiol Pharmacol. 2009;1:49–54. doi:10.4196/kjpp.
28. Park SE, Kim JS, Lee YW, Yoo HS, Cho CK. Antitumor activity of water extracts from *Cordyceps Militaris* in NCI-H460 cell xenografted nude mice. J Acupunct Meridian Stud. 2009;2:294–300.
29. Mollah ML, Park DL, Park HJ. *Cordyceps militaris* grown on germinated soybean induces G2/M cell cycle arrest through down regulation of Cyclin B1 and Cdc25c in human colon cancer HT-29 Cells. Evid Based Complement Alternat Med. 2012;2012:249217.
30. Lee SY, Debnath T, Kim SK, Lim BO. Anti-cancer effect and apoptosis induction of cordycepin through DR3 pathway in the human colonic cancer cell HT-29. Food Chem Toxicol. 2013;60:439–47.
31. Lee HH, Jeong JW, Lee JH, Kim GY, Cheong J, Jeong YK, et al. Cordycepin increases sensitivity of hep3b human hepatocellular carcinoma cells to trail-mediated apoptosis by inactivating the jnk signaling pathway. Oncol Rep. 2013;30:1257–64.
32. Sun YS, Lv LX, Zhao Z, He X, You L, Liu JK, et al. Cordycepol c induces caspase-independent apoptosis in human hepatocellular carcinoma hepg2 cells. Biol Pharm Bull. 2014;37:608–17.
33. Zhang Y, Bao YL, Wu Y, Yu CL, Huang YX, Sun Y, et al. Alantolactone induces apoptosis in RKO cells through the generation of reactive oxygen species and the mitochondrial pathway. Mol Med Rep. 2013;4:967–72.

Hydroxylation index of omeprazole in relation to CYP2C19 polymorphism and sex in a healthy Iranian population

Maryam Payan[1], Mohammad Reza Rouini[1*], Nader Tajik[2], Mohammad Hossein Ghahremani[3] and Reza Tahvilian[4]

Abstract

Background: Polymorphism of *CYP2C19* gene is one of the important factors in pharmacokinetics of CYP2C19 substrates. Omeprazole is a proton pump inhibitor which is mainly metabolized by cytochrome P450 2C19 (*CYP2C19*). The aim of present study was to assess omeprazole hydroxylation index as a measure of CYP2C19 activity considering new variant allele (*CYP2C19*17*) in Iranian population and also to see if this activity is sex dependent.

Methods: One hundred and eighty healthy unrelated Iranian individuals attended in this study. Blood samples for genotyping and phenotyping were collected 3 hours after administration of 20 mg omeprazole orally. Genotyping of *2C19* variant alleles **2*, **3* and **17* was performed by using polymerase chain reaction-restriction fragment length polymorphism (PCR-RFLP) and semi-nested PCR methods. Plasma concentrations of omeprazole and hydroxyomeprazole were determined by high performance liquid chromatography (HPLC) technique and hydxroxylation index (HI) (omeprazole/ hydroxyomeprazole) was calculated.

Results: The *CYP2C19*17* was the most common variant allele in the studied population (21.6%). Genotype frequencies of *CYP2C19*17*17*, **1*17*, and **2*17* were 5.5%, 28.8% and 3.3% respectively. The lowest and the highest median omeprazole HI was observed in **17*17* and **2*2* genotypes respectively (0.36 vs. 13.09). The median HI of omeprazole in subjects homozygous for *CYP2C19*1* was 2.16-fold higher than individuals homozygous for *CYP2C19*17* ($P < 0.001$) and the median HI of *CYP2C19*1*17* genotype was 1.98-fold higher than *CYP2C19 *17*17* subjects ($P < 0.001$). However, subjects with *CYP2C19*2*17* (median HI: 1.74) and *CYP2C19*1*2* (median HI: 1.98) genotypes and also *CYP2C19*1*17* (median HI: 0.71) and *CYP2C19*1*1* (mean HI: 0.78) did not show any significantly different enzyme activity. In addition, no statistically significant difference was found between women and men in distribution of *CYP2C19* genotypes. Furthermore, the hydroxylation index of Omeprazole was not different between women and men in the studied population.

Conclusion: Our data point out the importance of *CYP2C19*2* and *CYP2C19*17* variant alleles in metabolism of omeprazole and therefore CYP2C19 activity. Regarding the high frequency of *CYP2C19*17* in Iranian population, the importance of this new variant allele in metabolism of CYP2C19 substrates shall be considered.

Keywords: CYP2C19, Enzyme activity, Genotype, Omeprazole, Phenotype

* Correspondence: rouini@tums.ac.ir
[1]Biopharmaceutics and Pharmacokinetics Division, Department of Pharmaceutics, School of Pharmacy, Tehran University of Medical sciences, Tehran, Iran
Full list of author information is available at the end of the article

Introduction

Cytochrome P450 includes a wide variety of phase I metabolizing enzymes which are involved in metabolism of drugs and endogenic substances [1,2]. CYP2C19 is one of the members of cytochrome iso enzyme superfamily which contributes in metabolism of important drugs such as proton pump inhibitors (PPI) [3] psychotic drugs like venlafaxine [4] and citalopram [5,6], voriconazol [7], and clopidogrel [8,9].

CYP2C19 is represented by a gene located on chromosome 10 [10]. Genetic polymorphism of CYP2C19 is one of the major reasons of inter-individual variability in response to CYP2C19 substrate [11-13]. The main CYP2C19 polymorphisms that are associated with difference in therapeutic response are attributed to *CYP2C19*2, CYP2C19*3* and *CYP2C19*17* [14,15].

A point mutation in exon 5 (*681 G > A*, designated **2*) causes a cryptic splice defect (*CYP2C19*2*) and a single nucleotide polymorphism (SNP) in exon 4 (*636 G > A* designated **3*) creates a stop codon. Both mutations predominantly result in decreased CYP2C19 activity [9,16]. A recently discovered SNP in 5′ –flanking region (*-806 C > T* and *-3402 C > T*) leads to increased CYP2C19 activity and therefore produces ultra rapid metabolizer phenotype [17,18].

The *CYP2C19*2*2* and **3*3* genotypes are more prevalent in oriental and Asian populations than in Caucasian (12-23% vs 3-5%). In contrast the *CYP2C19*17*17* is more frequent in Caucasian than in Asian populations (18-26% vs 0.4-1.4%) [19,20].

Omeprazole is a proton pump inhibitor that is administered in treatment of gastric acid related disease [21]. Polymorphism of CYP2C19 can affect pharmacokinetic and therefore efficacy of proton pump inhibitors [21,22]. Additionally non genetic factors like age, liver disease and combination therapy can result in resistance to *Helicobacter Pylori* eradication treatment [23,24].

Several studies have used hydroxylation index of omeprazole as an indicator of CYP2C19 activity however this enzyme activity, was mainly measured in relation to **2* and **3* variant alleles and not the new variant allele (**17*) [16,25-28]. Although Sim *et al.* studied the effect of *CYP2C19*17* variant allele on enzyme activity, they only reported this activity in extensive metabolizers (**17*17, *1*17* and **1*1*) and they did not determine CYP2C19 activity in *CYP2C19*2*17* carriers [17]. *CYP2C19*2* leads to decreased enzyme activity and *CYP2C19*17* causes increased enzyme activity [16,17] but the impact of combined alleles (*CYP2C19*2*17*) on CYP2C19 activity has not been reported comprehensively and it is unknown that the effect of which allele is more predominant in *CYP2C19*2*17* carriers.

Furthermore there are some controversies in publications about impact of sex on CYP2C19 activity [29,30]. To our best knowledge, currently there is no published data regarding CYP2C19 activity in relation to new variant allele in Iranian population. Thus, the objects of this study were to assess effect of *CYP2C19*17* on enzyme activity and also to see if there is any sex-dependent difference in CYP2C19 activity and finally to investigate genotype-phenotype relationship of CYP2C19 considering new variant allele (*CYP2C19*17*) in Iranian population.

Material and methods

Study subjects

The study protocol was approved by ethics committee of Tehran University of Medical Sciences (ethical no. 11208). Generally one hundred and eighty (60 women and 120 men) unrelated healthy Iranian volunteers with the mean age of between 20–55 years and average body weight of 45–89 kg took part in this study. All participants signed written informed consent of this project. The study was completed by contribution of faculties of pharmacy of Tehran, Yazd, Kermanshah and Kerman University of Medical Sciences. The participants were students or stuffs of pharmacy schools, with no history of any illness or medicine consumption. No smoking and consumption of medicine that would affect CYP2C19 activity was permitted for one week before and during the study.

CYP2C19 phenotyping

After an overnight fast for at least 8 hours, volunteers took 20 mg omeprazole capsule (Abidi pharmaceuticals) with 250 milliliter tap water. Ten ml venous blood sample was collected from each subject 3 hours after administration of omeprazole and transferred into tubes containing 10 μl of 10% EDTA. Five ml of blood samples were centrifuged for 5 min at 4000 rpm and the plasma was separated and transferred to Eppendorf tube and stored at −80°C up to the day of analysis. The other 5 ml blood samples were stored directly in −80°C for genotyping analysis.

Analytical procedure

Omeprazole powder was purchased from TMAD (Iran). 5-hydroxyomeprazole was a kind donation by AstraZeneca (Sweden). The concentration of omeprazole and 5-hydroxyomeprazole was analyzed by HPLC method as described by Rezk *et al.* with a few modifications [31]. Briefly 500 μl plasma was extracted by liquid-liquid extraction using 1500 μl ethyl acetate. After orbital mixing for 10 min and centrifuging at 4000 × g for 10 min, the upper organic layer was separated and transferred to glass tube and then evaporated to dryness under gentle stream of air. Finally the residue was dissolved in 250 μl mobile phase and 100 μl of this sample was injected to HPLC system. The mobile phase was a combination of dibasic sodium phosphate buffer (0.025 mol/lit, pH 6): acetonitrile: methanol (73: 18: 8 V/V/V). The HPLC apparatus consisted of a low pressure HPLC pump, UV detector ($\lambda = 302$ nm) all from Knauer (Berlin, Germany). The chromatographic separation was performed by using Chromolit™ Performance RP-18e 100 mm × 4.6 mm, 5 μm particle size. Flow rate was adjusted to 1 ml/min. The limits of quantification were about 15 μg/ml for both compounds. Intraday and between day precisions were < 5% for both omerpazole and 5-hydroxyomeprazole.

CYP2C19 genotyping

The DNA was extracted from blood leucocytes by standard salting out method as explained by Miller *et al.* [32]. The extracted DNA was dissolved in sterile distilled water and stored at 4 °C until the day of analysis. Amplification of *CYP2C19*2* and **3* allele was implemented using polymerase chain reaction-restriction fragment length polymorphism (PCR-RFLP) as described by De Morias [33]. The PCR product of each reaction was digested by specific endonuclease (all from New England Biolabs GmbH, Frankfurt, Germany); the 169 bp *CYP2C19*2* product was digested by SmaI to 40 and 129 bp fragments. The 329 bp PCR product of *CYP2C19*3* was digested by BamHI to 233 and 96 bp pieces. Genotyping of *CYP2C19*17 -3402 C > T* and *–806 C > T* polymorphisms was done by PCR-RFLP and nested-PCR assays as defined by Sim *et al.* [17]. For *CYP2C19*17 -3402 C > T* the PCR product (504 bp) was digested by MnlI and resulted in 224 and 280 bp fragments. But the PCR product of *CYP2C19*17 -806 C > T* (200 bp) was separated directly on 2.5% agarose gel without any digestion. In all PCR-RFLP assays mutation caused abolishment of restriction site and thus PCR product was not digested.

Statistical analysis

The allele frequencies differences between population were estimated using two-tailed Fisher's exact test. The 95% confidence intervals (CI) were calculated using Confidence Interval Analysis software. The relation of sex and genotype was assessed by two tailed Fisher's exact test. The observed and expected frequencies were calculated by using Hardy-Weinberg equation. The two-tailed Fisher's exact test was used to evaluate deviation of genotype frequencies in the studied population from Hardy-Weinberg equilibrium. The enzyme activity was compared by using omeprazole hydroxylation index. The hydroxylation index (HI) of omeprazole 3 hours after administration of omeprazole was calculated by dividing omeprazole to 5-hydroxyomeprazol plasma concentration. The mean HI in different genotypes were compared by Mann–Whitney two tailed test. The impact of sex on HI of omeprazole was also evaluated using Mann–Whitney two tailed test. The inter-individual variability in metabolism of omeprazole was represented by probit plot. For drawing probit plot, the log of HI was calculated, the antimode value was determined using Microsoft office excel 2010. The normality of HI distribution was analyzed by frequency distribution histogram and also by Kolmogorov-Smirnov test. All statistical analyses were performed by Sigma Plot version 12.0 and Graph Pad Prism version 5 softwares and $P < 0.05$ was considered as statistically significant difference.

Results

The genotype and allele frequencies of CYP2C19 are reported in Table 1. According to the data presented in Table 1, *CYP2C19 *17*17, *1*17* and **1*1* were detected in 10 (5.5%), 52 (28.9%) and 75 (41.7%) subjects respectively. The *CYP2C19 *2*17* and **1*2* were identified in 6 (3.3%) and 33 (18.3%) individuals and finally the *CYP2C19*2*2* was recognized in 4 (2.2%) of volunteers. *CYP2C19*17* was the most common variant allele in Iranian population.

The hydroxylation index of omeprazole as mean ± SD, median and 95% confidence interval is reported in Table 2. Subjects with *CYP2C19 *17*17* genotype had a very high metabolic capacity with median hydroxylation index of 0.36 and were classified as Ultra-Rapid Metabolizers (URM). The median hydroxylation index of omeprazole in subjects homozygous for *CYP2C19*1* was 2.17 fold higher than individual homozygous for *CYP2C19*17* ($P < 0.001$) and the median hydroxylation index of *CYP2C19*1*17* genotype was 1.97 fold higher than *CYP2C19*17*17* subjects ($P < 0.001$). There was not a significant difference between HI of omeprazole in *CYP2C19*1*17* and **1*1* carriers ($P > 0.05$) and these two groups were stratified as extensive metabolizers (EM).

The median HI of omeprazole was 1.74 in *CYP2C19*2*17* and 1.98 in *CYP2C19*1*2* carriers respectively. The difference in HI of omeprazole in *CYP2C19*1*2* carriers were statistically significant with other CYP2C19 genotypes ($P < 0.05$) except for *CYP2C19*2*17* genotype ($p > 0.05$). Individuals in these two groups had intermediate metabolic capacity and were designated as Intermediate-Metabolizers (IM). Homozygous carrier of *CYP2C19*2* had a very low metabolic capacity with the median hydroxylation index of 13.03 and they were classified as poor metabolizers (PM). There was a significant difference between HI index of homozygous carriers of *CYP2C19*2* with the other five genotypes ($p < 0.001$).

The plasma concentration of omeprazole and hydroxyomeprazole is illustrated in Figure 1. According to this figure there is a significant difference between omeprazole plasma concentration in individuals with *CYP2C19*17*17* genotype with all other groups ($P < 0.01$), but the omeprazole plasma concentration was neither different between *1*17* and *1*1*(EM) ($P > 0.5$) nor between *2*17* and *1*2* (IM)

Table 1 Genotype and allele frequencies of CYP2C19 in 180 healthy Iranian volunteers

CYP2C19 Genotype	Number of subjects		Frequency (%)	95% CI
	Men (120)	Women (60)		
*17*17	5	5	5.5	2.7 - 10.0
*1*17	37	15	28.8	22.4 - 36.1
*1*1	53	22	41.7	34.4 - 49.2
*1*2	20	13	18.3	13.0 - 24.7
*2*17	4	2	3.3	1.23 - 7.1
*2*2	1	3	2.2	0.6 - 5.5
CYP2C19 Alleles	**No. of alleles**		**Frequency (%)**	**95% CI**
CYP2C19*17	78		21.6	17.5 - 26.3
CYP2C19*1	235		65.3	60.1 - 70.2
CYP2C19*2	47		13.1	9.7 - 16.9
CYP2C19*3	0		0	0

*CI: Confidence Interval. (The 95% confidence intervals (CI) were calculated using Confidence Interval Analysis software).

genotypes. However, omeprazole plasma concentration was significantly different between EM (*1*17* and *1*1)* and IM *(2*17* and *1*2*). The plasma concentration of hydroxyomeprazole was significantly different between *2*2 and all other 5 genotypes while the plasma concentration of hydroxyomeprazole was not significantly different between other 5 genotypes *(17*17, 1*17, *1*1, 2*17, 1*2*).

Figure 2 indicates the hydroxylation index of omeprazole in 6 genotypes and also in predicted phenotype groups. As it is observed there is no significant difference between hydroxylation index of omeprazole in *1*17* and *1*1* groups or between *2*17* and *1*2* groups. While the difference between *17*17* or *2*2* with all other genotype groups were statistically significant.

The summary of omeprazole, hydroxyomeprazole plasma concentration and omeprazole HI in the total population, women and men is reported in Table 3. Omeprazole plasma concentration was significantly higher in *2*2* genotype than other genotype groups. Additionally there was a significant difference in omeprazole plasma concentration between different groups ($P < 0.001$) except for *CYP2C19*1*17* and **1*1* ($P > 0.05$), *CYP2C19*1*2* and *CYP2C19*2*17* ($P > 0.05$). Mean omeprazole plasma concentration was 19.0 fold higher in *CYP2C19*2*2* than *CYP2C19*17*17* and 11 fold higher than *CYP2C19*1*1* ($P < 0.001$), however hydroxyomeprazole concentration was not statistically different among genotype groups ($P > 0.05$) except for *CYP2C19*2*2.* Moreover, omeprazole and hydroxyomeprazole plasma concentrations as well as omeprazole HI were not statistically different among women and men in the studied population ($P > 0.05$).

The effect of sex on hydroxylation index of omeprazole is illustrated in Figure 3. According to this figure there is not any significant difference between median hydroxylation index in women (0.84) and men (0.86) ($p > 0.05$).

The frequency distribution histogram of omeprazole hydroxylation index in 180 healthy Iranian volunteers is indicated in Figure 4. The graph shows a bimodal distribution with the antimode of around 0.8. Kolmogorov-Smirnov test showed that the omeprazole hydroxylation index was not normally distributed in the studied population (K-S Dist. = 0.296 $p < 0.001$). The bimodal distribution was also confirmed by probit plot.

The correlation of CYP2C19 genotype and phenotype was tested using Spearman rank correlation, and the results showed a well correlation between CYP2C19 genotype and phenotype ($r_s = 0.64$, $P < 0.0001$).

Discussion

Inter-individual variability in drug response always has been one of the main concerns in drug discovery and development. The important factors resulting in such

Table 2 Hydroxylation index of omeprazole (omeprazole/hydroxyomeprazole) in relation to CYP2C19 genotype in 180 healthy Iranian subjects

	*17*17	*1*17	*1*1	*2*17	*1*2	*2*2
Mean (SD)	0.35(0.06)	0.75(0.28)	0.85(0.30)	2.02(0.84)	2.27(1.04)	13.59(3.13)
Median	0.36[a]	0.71	0.78	1.74[b]	1.98[b]	13.03[a]
95% CI	0.31 - 0.39	0.68 -0.83	0.79 – 0.92	1.33 – 2.72	1.92 – 2.63	10.51– 16.67

[a]Represent statistically significant difference with other 5 genotypes.
[b]Represent statistically significant difference with *17*17, *1*17, *1*1 and *2*2.
CI: Confidence Interval.

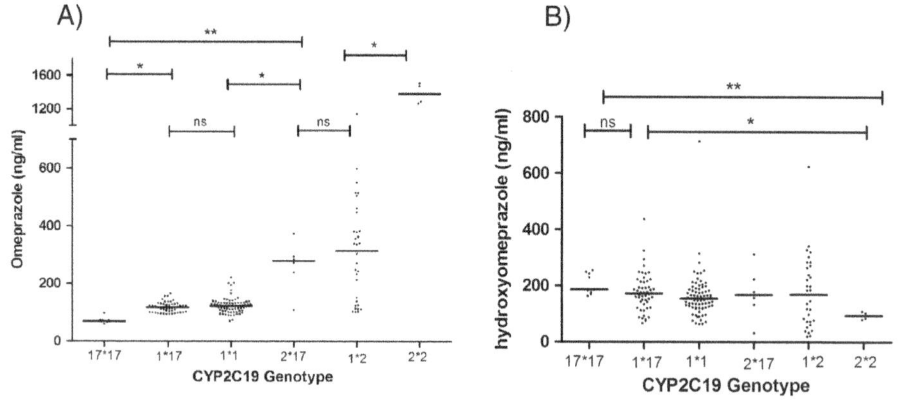

Figure 1 Plasma concentrations of Omeprazole (A) and hydroxyomerpazole (B) in different genotypes 3 hours after administration of Omeprazole orally. ns: not significant, * $p < 0.05$, ** $p < 0.001$.

variation include genetic, nongenetic and physiologic agents like change in protein structure, combination therapy, alcohol, smoking, sex, age and disease condition [34].

*CYP2C19*17* is a new variant allele which is associated with increased gene transcription and therefore higher enzyme activity [17]; which may lead to several clinical consequences including the lower susceptibility to breast cancer risk [35], higher risk of peptic ulcer disease [36], greater response to clopidogrel treatment and more risk of bleeding [37] in addition to a better treatment with tamoxifen [38].

In this study, omeprazole HI after 3 hours administration of omeprazole was used as indicator of CYP2C19 activity. The HI in *CYP2C19*17*17* was significantly different with *CYP2C19*1*17* and *CYP2C19*1*1* genotypes and people in this group had very high metabolic activity, which is in agreement with what was reported by Sim *et al.* They found that median HI of omeprazole in homozygous carriers of *CYP2C19*1* is 2 fold higher than homozygous carriers of *CYP2C19*17* and 1.2 fold higher than *CYP2C19*1*17* [17]. Ramsjö *et al.* has also reported that mean HI of omeprazole in *CYP2C19*1*1* was 3.2 fold higher than *CYP2C19*17*17* and 1.1 fold higher than *CYP2C19*1*17* [27].

*CYP2C19*2* allele is associated with decreased enzyme activity and *CYP2C19*17* variant allele is connected with increased enzyme activity. In Most of the genotype phenotype studies of *CYP2C19*17* variant allele, only HI of omeprazole in *CYP2C19*17*17, CYP2C19*1*17* and *CYP2C19*1*1* genotypes has been reported [17,27]. However, the capacity of CYP2C19 enzyme activity in people carrying both defective mutant alleles of *2 and *17 (CYP2C19*2*17)* was still unclear. Although Ragia *et al.* in the study for evaluation of distribution of *CYP2C19*17* genetic polymorphism in Greece people defined CYP2C19*2*17 carriers as EM and people with *CYP2C19*1*2* as IM, they only predicted phenotype based on genotype and CYP2C19 activity was not determined by using a probe drug [39]. Sugimito *et al.* did not see any difference between metabolic capacities of *CYP2C19*1*1, *1*17, 2*17* and *1*2* for metabolism of

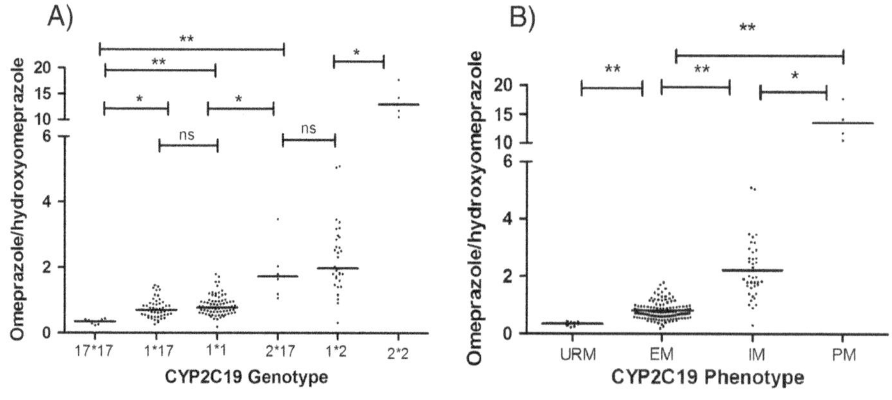

Figure 2 The hydroxylation index of Omeprazole in different genotypes (A) and in predicted phenotype groups (B) 3 hours after administration of Omeprazole orally. ns: not significant, * $p < 0.05$, ** $p < 0.001$.

Table 3 Plasma concentration of omeprazole (OMP) and hydroxyomeprazole (OH-OMP) and hydroxylation index (HI) of omeprazole in relation to genotype in 60 women and 120 men 3 hour after administration of single oral dose of 20 mg omeprazole

Genotype	No of subjects	Mean OMP concentration (ng/ml) ± SD	Mean OH-OMP concentration (ng/ml) ± SD	Mean HI ± SD
17*17	Total (10)	71.01 ± 10.28	203.31 ± 34.93	0.35 ± 0.06
	Women (5)	68.32 ± 5.73	204.92 ± 41.35	0.34 ± 0.08
	Men (5)	73.71 ± 13.67	201.69 ± 32.08	0.36 ± 0.04
1*17	Total (52)	118.28 ± 10.19	177.05 ± 37.53	0.75 ± 0.28
	Women (15)	120.22 ± 20.12	174.51 ± 28.01	0.72 ± 0.18
	Men (37)	117.49 ± 16.10	178.07 ± 44.57	0.77 ± 0.32
1*1	Total (75)	124.75 ± 27.18	163.74 ± 32.25	0.85 ± 0.30
	Women (22)	128.06 ± 39.90	194.40 ± 60.84	0.78 ± 0.27
	Men (53)	123.38 ± 20.83	151.01 ± 26.38	0.89 ± 0.30
2*17	Total (6)	289.01 ± 97.45	172.79 ± 63.58	2.02 ± 0.54
	Women (4)	324.25 ± 39.90	178.72 ± 33.59	1.97 ± 0.62
	Men (2)	271.39 ± 118.56	169.82 ± 84.95	2.05 ± 0.67
1*2	Total (33)	319.45 ± 150.34	177.79 ± 38.39	2.27 ± 1.04
	Women (13)	364.92 ± 265.16	194.66 ± 52.56	2.24 ± 0.79
	Men (20)	289.89 ± 167.55	165.53 ± 23.55	2.29 ± 1.19
2*2	Total (4)	1388.99 ± 123.41	104.67 ± 10.55	13.59 ± 3.13
	Women (3)	1359.84 ± 133.23	105.03 ± 13.80	13.37 ± 3.80
	Men (1)	1476.4	103.58	14.25

HI = (omerpazole concentration/hydroxyomeprazole concentration).

omeprazole and stratified these individuals as EM [20]. The omeprazole HI in subjects with *CYP2C19*2*17* genotype in this study was not significantly different from *CYP2C19*1*2* genotype (P = 0.33) so we designated them as IM. It seems that in heterozygous carriers of *CYP2C19*2* and **17* allele, the effect of **2* allele is more predominant than **17* allele and it can suppress induced enzyme activity by **17* allele. This observation is in agreement with classification of *CYP2C19*2*17* as IM by Gurbel *et al.* based on the study for genotype phenotype analysis of 2C19 in stented patient [40]. In contrast to these findings, in a study for evaluation of CYP2C19 enzyme activity in Turkish children using lansoprazole as a probe drug, individuals with *CYP2C19*2*17* had similar enzyme activity to *CYP2C19*1*17* and *CYP2C19*1*1*; and this activity was significantly different from *CYP2C19*1*2* [41]. Involvement of individual with different age groups could possibly explain such different observations. Our study was conducted in adult individuals with the average age of 32 years but Gumus implemented the study in children with mean age of 10.2 years. The lower frequency of *CYP2C19*2*17* in our studied subjects in comparison to Turkish individuals (6 vs 16) can be considered as another justification.

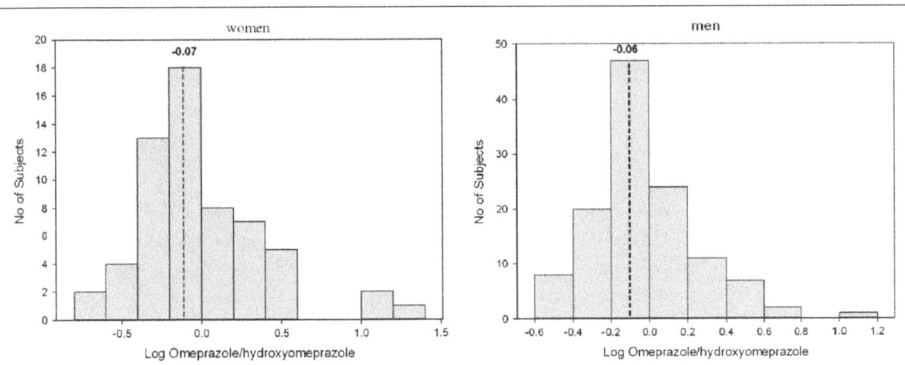

Figure 3 The effect of sex on hydroxylation index of omeprazole in 60 women and 120 men. The median hydroxylation index is indicated by dashed line.

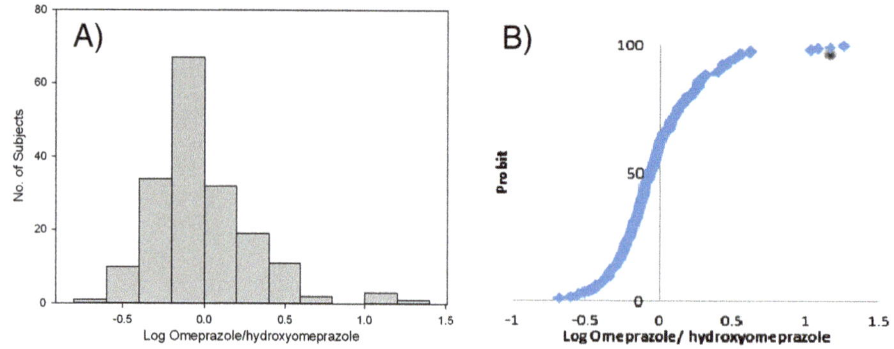

Figure 4 A) Frequency histogram distribution and B) Probit plot of log omeprazole hydroxylation index in 180 healthy Iranian volunteers. Subjects with log HI > 1.0 were phenotyped as poor metabolizers.

In the present study effect of CYP2C19 genetic polymorphism and sex on metabolic activity of CYP2C19 was also assessed. Sex is an important factor in activity of some cytochrome P450 enzymes. CYP3A4 is an example of cytochrome enzymes which has higher activity in women than men [2]. There were some controversies in the previous published reports for impact of sex on CYP2C19 activity. Ramsjö *et al.* indicated a sex difference in CYP2C19 activity between Korean subjects and not in Swedish volunteers using Omeprazole as a probe drug [27]. Tamminga *et al.* observed a sex related decreased CYP2C19 activity in women when used mephenytoin as a probe for evaluation of CYP2C19 activity, however the author declared this reduction was more obvious in those who used oral contraceptive [42]. In contrast, Hägg *et al.* did not see any sex differences in CYP2C19 activity after administration of mephenytoin in Norwegian population [43]. By considering these reports one may conclude that sex dependency of CYP2C19 activity is influenced by environmental and epigenetic factors like diet and ethnic differences. The other possibility can be attributed to some new genetic mutation in some populations which has not been studied well. The result of this study represents no effect of sex on CYP2C19 activity which is in line with what is reported in Swedish and Norwegian population.

The frequency of PM and URM in Iranian population in this study was about 2.2% and 5.5% which is close to the study by Zand *et al.* [44] and other Caucasian population. In previous report by Akhlaghi *et al.* in Iranian patients with coronary artery disease the genotype frequency of *CYP2C19*2*2* was reported 4.7% which is quite different from our results [45]. This can be due to difference in studied population (healthy volunteer's vs specific patients). The genotype frequency of *CYP2C19*17*17* (URM) was 4% in Swedish and 3% in Ethiopian [17], 5.1% in Danish [19], 3.18% in Greece [39], 7% in Saudi Arabian [46] 1.2% in Indian [16] and 0% in Japanese, Korean and Thai population [20,27,47]. Accordingly the genotype frequency of *CYP2C19*2*2* (PM) is 2.2% in Danish [19], 2.1% in Greece [39], 0.4% in Saudi Arabian [46], 18.4% in Indian [16] and 18% in Japanese people [20].

To the best of authors' knowledge, this is the first study evaluating CYP2C19 genotype and phenotype in Iranian population in relation to new variant allele (CYP2C19*17). In the previous report, Zendehdel *et al.* investigated impact of CYP2C19 on therapeutic efficacy of omeprazole in Iranian patients with erosive reflux esophagitis; patients were genotyped only for CYP2C19*2 and CYP2C19*3, Individuals with HetEM genotype had better response to treatment with omeprazole than EM (95% vs 43% successful treatment response respectively) [48]. The high frequency of CYP2C19*17 allele (21.6%) detected in this study maybe one justification for 50% resistance rate in the EM group in Iranian patients in previous report. However impact of this variant allele (CYP2C19*17) on the efficacy of PPIs like omeprazole shall be evaluated in controlled clinical trials.

In this study the antimode of 0.8 was calculated for Iranian population. Different antimodes for HI of omeprazole have been reported in different ethnics groups: 14.4 in Indian [16], 7.0 in Koreans [25] and Thai population [47], 0.63 in Colombians [26], and 3.98 in West Mexicans [49]. The calculated antimode for Iranian population is similar to Colombian population, indicating comparable CYP2C19 activity in Iranians and Colombians and faster enzyme activity than Asian people.

A complete genotype phenotype correlation was observed in this study. However it should be noted that enzyme activity and therefore metabolic ratio may vary during some disease condition which may result in discrepancy in genotype-phenotype relationship of specific enzyme. Kimura *et al.* [50] indicated discordance of genotype-phenotype relationship of omeprazole in 14.5% of EM patients who had peptic ulcer disease. However this discrepancy was not observed in healthy individuals. Reduced hepatic enzyme activity as a result of old age or liver disease was reported as an explanation for such finding. Long term treatment with omeprazole which has auto inhibition effect was the other possibility. Williams *et al.* [51] also did not see genotype-phenotype relationship of 2C19 using omeprazole in patients with advanced cancer. The authors concluded that increased level of some signaling molecules like interleukin (IL) and tumor necrosis factors (TNFα) may result in down-regulation of metabolizing enzymes [51,52]. So it should be considered that factors like age, disease state, and concomitant medication may have pronounced effect on enzyme activity. Although omeprazole hydroxylation index has been used as an indicator of CYP2C19 activity, it should be considered that hydroxyomeprazole which is formed by CYP2C19 is further metabolized by CYP3A4 to hydroxyomeprazole sulfone [53] which in turn may indirectly affect the hydroxylation index of omeprazole. Therefore the high concentration of CYP3A4 in liver microsomes of some human can explain the deviation from CYP2C19 genotype and also the sex dependent enzyme activity observed in some ethnic groups [54].

The prevalence of *CYP2C19*2*17* in this study was only 6% which is a limitation of this study. Future studies to investigate impact of *CYP2C19*2*17* genotype on CYP2C19 enzyme activity in larger groups specially by using drugs with narrow therapeutic window is suggested.

In conclusion, the result of this study shows that *CYP2C19*2*17* has an intermediate metabolic activity which maybe important for drug dose adjustment regimens for treatment, specially in those having narrow therapeutic indices like clopidogrel. Additionally no effect of sex on CYP2C19 activity was observed in this study. Regarding the high frequency of *CYP2C19*17* in Iranian population, the importance of this new variant allele in metabolism of CYP2C19 substrates shall be considered.

Abbreviations

CYP2C19: Cytochrome P450 2C19; PCR-RFLP: Polymerase chain reaction-restriction fragment length polymorphism; HPLC: High performance liquid chromatography; HI: Hydxroxylation index; SNP: Single nucleotide polymorphism; URM: Ultra-rapid metabolizers; EM: Extensive metabolizers; IM: Intermediate metabolizers; PM: Poor metabolizers; OMP: Omeprazole; OH-OMP: Hydroxyomepazole.

Competing interests

The authors declare that they have no competing interests.

Authors' contributions

M-RR, MP, NT, M-H GH and RT conceived the study. MP performed the experimental work. All authors were involved in data analysis and interpretation. MP prepared the manuscript. All authors read and approved the final version.

Acknowledgement

This project was supported by a grant from Tehran University of Medical Sciences. We thank Dr. Kjell Andersson, AstraZeneca, Sweden, for kind donation of pure powder of 5 -hydroxyomeprazole. We are grateful to Dr. Mehdi Ansari Dogaheh, Department of Pharmaceutics, Faculty of Pharmacy, Kerman Medical Sciences and Dr. Mohsen Nabimeybodi, Department of pharmaceutics, Faculty of Pharmacy, Yazd University of Medical Sciences, for kind assistance in collection of blood samples.

Author details

[1]Biopharmaceutics and Pharmacokinetics Division, Department of Pharmaceutics, School of Pharmacy, Tehran University of Medical sciences, Tehran, Iran. [2]Cellular and Molecular Research Center (CMRC), Iran University of Medical Sciences, Tehran, Iran. [3]Department of Pharmacology and Toxicology, School of Pharmacy, Tehran University of Medical sciences, Tehran, Iran. [4]Department of pharmaceutics, School of Pharmacy, Kermanshah University of Medical Sciences, Kermanshah, Iran.

References

1. Sim SC, Nordin L, Andersson TM-L, Virding S, Olsson M, Pedersen NL, Ingelman- Sundberg M: **Association Between CYP2C19 Polymorphism and Depressive Symptoms.** *Am J Med Genet* 2010, **153**(B):1160–1166.
2. Zanger UM, Schwab M: **Cytochrome P450 enzymes in drug metabolism: Regulation of gene expression, enzyme activities, and impact of genetic variation.** *J Pharmacol Ther* 2013, **138**:103–141.
3. Qiao H-L, Hu Y-R, Tian X, Jia L-J, Gao N, Zhang L-R, Guo Y-z: **Pharmacokinetics of three proton pump inhibitors in Chinese subjects in relation to the CYP2C19 genotype.** *Eur J Clin Pharmacol* 2006, **62**:107–112.
4. Weide JVD, Baalen-Benedek EHV, Kootstra-Ros JE: **Metabolic ratios of psychotropics as indication of cytochrome P450 2D6/2C19 genotype.** *Ther Drug Monit* 2005, **27**:478–483.
5. Yu B-N, Chen G-L, He N, Ouyang D-S, Chen X-P, Liu Z-Q, Zhou HH: **Pharmacokinetic of citalopram in relation to genetic polymorphism of CYP2C19.** *Drug Metabol Dispos* 2003, **31**(10):1255–1259.
6. Mrazek DA, Biernacka JM, O'Kane DJ, Black JL, Cunningham JM, Drews MS, Snyder KA, Stevens SR, Rush AJ, Weinshilboum RM: **CYP2C19 variation and citalopram response.** *Pharmacogenet Genomics* 2011, **21**:1–9.
7. Wang G, Lei HP, Li Z, Tan Z-R, Guo D, Fan L, Chen Y, Hu D-L, Wang D, Zhou H-H: **The CYP2C19 ultra rapid metabolizer genotype influences the pharmacokinetics of voriconazol in healthy male volunteers.** *Eur J Clin Pharmacol* 2009, **65**:281–285.
8. Sibbing S, Koch W, Gebhard D, Schuster T, Braun S, Stegherr J, Morath T, Scho¨mig A, Beckerath NV, Kastrati A: **Cytochrome *2C19*17* allelic variant, platelet aggregation, bleeding events, and stent thrombosis in clopidogrel-treated patients with coronary stent placement.** *Circulation* 2010, **121**:512–518.
9. Hulot JS, Collet JP, Silvain J, Pena A, Bellemain-Appaix A, Barthélémy O, Cayla G, Beygui F, Montalescot G: **Cardiovascular risk in clopidogrel-treated patients according to cytochrome P450 2C19*2 loss-of-function allele or proton pump inhibitor coadministration: a systematic meta-analysis.** *J Am Coll Cardiol* 2010, **56**(2):134–143.
10. Mathijssen RHJ, Schaik RHN: **Genotyping and phenotyping cytochrome P450: Perspectives for cancer treatment.** *Eur J Cancer* 2006, **42**:141–148.
11. Gabriella Scordo M, Caputi AP, D'Arrigo C, Fava G, Spina E: **Allele and genotype frequencies of CYP2C9, CYP2C19 and CYP2D6 in an Italian population.** *Pharmacol Res* 2004, **50**:195–200.
12. Ingelman-Sundberg M, Sim SC, Ingelman-Sundberg A, Rodriguez-Antona C: **Influence of cytochrome P450 polymorphism on drug therapies: Pharmacogenetic and clinical aspects.** *Pharmacol Ther* 2007, **116**:496–526.
13. Chaudhry AS, Kochhar R, Kohli KK: **Genetic polymorphism of CYP2C19 & therapeutic response to proton pump inhibitors.** *Indian J Med Res* 2008, **127**(6):521–530.
14. Lee S-J, Kim W-Y, Kim H, Shon J-H, Lee SS, Shin J-G: **Identification of new CYP2C19 variants exhibiting decreased enzyme activity in the metabolism of S-Mephenytoin and Omeprazole.** *Drug Metab Dispos* 2009, **37**(11):2262–2269.
15. Li-Wan-Po A, Girard T, Farndon P, Cooley C, Lithgow J: **Pharmacogenetics of CYP2C19: functional and clinical implications of a new variant *CYP2C19*17*.** *Br J Clin Pharmacol* 2010, **69**(3):222–230.
16. Rosemary J, Adithan C, Padmaja N, Shashindran CH, Gerard N, Krishnamoorthy R: **The effect of the CYP2C19 genotype on the hydroxylation index of Omeprazole in south Indians.** *Eur J Clin Pharmacol* 2005, **61**:19–23.
17. Sim SC, Risinger C, Dahl ML, Aklillu E, Christensen M, Bertilsson L, Ingelman-Sundberg M: **A common novel CYP2C19 gene variant causes ultrarapid drug metabolism relevant for the drug response to proton pump inhibitors and antidepressants.** *Clin Pharmacol Ther* 2006, **79**:103–113.

18. Anichavezhi D, Roa C, Shewade DG, Krishnamoorthy R, Adithan C: **Distribution of *CYP2C19*17* allele and genotype in an Indian population.** *J Clin Pharmacy Ther* 2012, **37**:313–318.
19. Pedersen RS, Brasch-Andersen C, Sim SC, Bergmann TK, Halling J, Petersen MS, Weihe P, Edvardsen H, Kristensen VN, Brøsen K, Ingelman-Sundberg M: **Linkage disequilibrium between the *CYP2C19*17* allele and wide type CYP2C8 and CYP2C9 alleles: identification of CYP2C haplotypes in healthy Nordic population.** *Eur J Clin Pharmacol* 2010, **66**:1199–1205.
20. Sugimito K, Uno T, Yamazaki H, Tateishi T: **Limited frequency of the *CYP2C19*17* allele and its minor role in a Japanese population.** *Br J Clin Pharmacol* 2008, **65**(3):437–439.
21. Sakai T, Aoyama N, Kita T, Sakaeda T, Nishiguchi K, Nishitora Y, Hohda T, Sirasaka D, Tamura T, Tanigawara Y, Kasuga M, Okumura K: **CYP2C19 genotype and pharmacokinetics of three proton pump inhibitors in healthy subjects.** *Pharm Res* 2001, **18**(6):72–77.
22. Cho H, Choi MK, Cho DY, Yeo CW, Jeong HE, Shon JH, Lee JY: **Effect of CYP2C19 genetic polymorphism on pharmacokinetics and pharmacodynamics of a new proton pump inhibitor, ilaprazole.** *J Clin Pharmacol* 2012, **52**(7):976–984.
23. Ammon S, Treiber G, Kees F, Klotz U: **Influence of age on the steady state disposition of drugs commonly used for the eradication of *Helicobacter pylori*.** *Aliment Pharmacol Ther* 2000, **14**(6):759–766.
24. Ishizawa Y, Yasui-Furukori N, Takahata T, Sasaki M, Tateishi T: **The effect of aging on the relationship between the cytochrome P450 2C19 genotype and Omeprazole pharmacokinetics.** *Clin pharmacokinetics* 2005, **44**:1179–1189.
25. Chong E, Ensom M: **Pharmacogenetics of the Proton Pump Inhibitors: A Systematic Review.** *Pharmacotherapy* 2003, **23**(4):460–471.
26. Isaza C, Henao J: **Isaza Martínez J H, Sepúlveda Arias J, Beltrán L: Phenotype-genotype analysis of CYP2C19 in Colombian mestizo individuals.** *BMC Clin Pharmacol* 2007, **7**(6):1–5.
27. Ramsjö M, Aklillu E, Bohman L, Ingelman-Sundberg M, Roh HK: **CYP2C19 activity comparison between Swedish and Koreans: effect of genotype, sex, oral contraceptive use and smoking.** *Eur J Clin Pharmacol* 2010, **66**:871–877.
28. Niioka T, Uno T, Sugimoto K, Sugawara K, Hayakari M, Tateishi T: **Estimation of CYP2C19 activity by the Omeprazole hydroxylation index at a single point in time after intravenous and oral administration.** *Eur J Clin Pharmacol* 2007, **63**(11):1031–1038.
29. Xie HG, Huang SL, Xu ZH, Xiao ZS, He N, Zhou HH: **Evidence for the effect of gender on activity of (S)-mephenytoin 4′-hydroxylase (CYP2C19) in a Chinese population.** *Pharmacogenetics* 1997, **7**(2):115–119.
30. Laine K, Tybring G, Bertilsson L: **No sex-related differences but significant inhibition by oral contraceptives of CYP2C19 activity as measured by the probe drugs mephenytoin and Omeprazole in healthy Swedish white subjects.** *Clin Pharmacol Ther* 2000, **68**(2):151–159.
31. Rezk NL, Brown KC, Kashuba ADM: **A simple and sensitive bioanalytical assay for simultaneous determination of Omeprazole and its three major metabolites in human blood plasma using RP-HPLC after a simple liquid–liquid extraction procedure.** *J Chromatogr B* 2006, **844**:314–321.
32. Miller SA, Dykes DD, Polesky HF: **A simple salting out procedure for extracting DNA from human nucleated cells.** *Nucleic Acids Res* 1988, **16**:1215.
33. De Morais SM, Wilkinson GR, Blaisdell J, Nakamura K, Meyer UA, Goldstein JA: **The major genetic defect responsible for the polymorphism of S-mephenytoin metabolism in humans.** *J Bio Chem* 1994, **269**(22):15419–15422.
34. Qiang M, Anthony YHL: **Pharmacogenetics, Pharmacogenomics, and Individualized Medicine.** *Pharmacol Rev* 2011, **63**:2437–2459.
35. Justenhoven C, Hamann U, Pierl CB, Baisch C, Harth V, Rabstein S, Spickenheuer A, Pesch B, Brüning T, Winter S, Ko YD, Brauch H: **CYP2C19*17 is associated with decreased breast cancer risk.** *Breast Cancer Res Treat* 2009, **115**(2):391–396.
36. Musumba CO, Jorgensen A, Sutton L, Eker DV, Zhang E, Hara NO, Carr DF, Pritchard DM, Pirmohamed M, Eker DV, Zhang E, Hara NO, Carr DF, Pritchard DM, Pirmohamed M: **CYP2C19*17 Gain-of-function polymorphism is associated with peptic ulcer disease.** *Clin Pharmacol Ther* 2013, **93**(2):195–203.
37. Li Y, Tang HL, Hu YF, Xie HG: **The gain-of-function variant CYP2C19*17: a double-edged sword between thrombosis and bleeding in clopidogrel-treated patients.** *J Thromb Haemost* 2012, **10**(2):199–206.
38. Schroth W, Antoniadou L, Fritz P, Schwab M, Muerdter T, Zanger UM, Simon W, Eichelbaum M, Brauch H: **Breast cancer treatment outcome with adjuvant tamoxifen relative to patient CYP2D6 and CYP2C19 genotypes.** *J Clin Oncol* 2007, **25**(33):5187–5193.
39. Ragia G, Arvanitidis KI, Tavridou A, Manolopoulos VG: **Need for reassessment of reported CYP2C19 allele frequencies in various populations in view of *CYP2C19*17* discovery: the case of Greece.** *Pharmacogenomics* 2009, **10**(1):43–49.
40. Gurbel PA, Shuldiner AR, Bliden KP, Ryan K, Pakyz RE, Tantry US: **The relation between CYP2C19 genotype and phenotype in stented patients on maintenance dual antiplatelet therapy.** *Am Heart J* 2011, **161**:598–604.
41. Gumus E, Karaca O, Babaoglu MO, Baysoy G, Balamtekin N, Demir H, Uslu N, Bozkurt A, Yuce A, Yasar U: **Evaluation of lansoprazole as a probe for assessing cytochrome P450 2C19 activity and genotype-phenotype correlation in childhood.** *Eur J Clin Pharmacol* 2012, **68**(5):629–636.
42. Tamminga WJ, Wemer J, Oosterhuis B, Weiling J, Wilffert B, de Leij LF, de Zeeuw RA, Jonkman JH: **CYP2D6 and CYP2C19 activity in a large population of Dutch healthy volunteers: indications for oral contraceptive-related gender differences.** *Eur J Clin Pharmacol* 1999, **55**(3):177–184.
43. Hägg S, Spigset O, Dahlqvist R: **Influence of gender and oral contraceptives on CYP2D6 and CYP2C19 activity in healthy volunteers.** *Br J Clin Pharmacol* 2001, **51**(2):169–173.
44. Zand N, Tajik N, Moghaddam AS, Milanian I: **Genetic polymorphisms of cytochrome P450 enzymes 2C9 and 2C19 in a healthy Iranian population.** *Clin Exp Pharmacol Physiol* 2007, **34**(1–2):102–105.
45. Akhlaghi A, Shirani S, Ziaie N, Pirhaji O, Yaran M, Shahverdi G, Sarrafzadegan N, Khosravi A, Khosravi E: **Cytochrome P450 2C19 Polymorphism in Iranian Patients with Coronary Artery Disease.** *ARYA Atheroscler* 2011, **7**(3):106–110.
46. Saeed LH, Mayet AY: **Genotype-Phenotype analysis of CYP2C19 in healthy Saudi individuals and its potential clinical implication in drug therapy.** *Int J Med Sci* 2013, **10**:1497–1502.
47. Tassaneeyakul W, Tawalee A, Tassaneeyakul W, Kukongaviriyapan V, Blaisdell J, Goldstein JA, Gaysornsiri D: **Analysis of the CYP2C19 polymorphism in a North-eastern Thai population.** *Pharmacogenetics* 2002, **12**:221–225.
48. Zendedel N, Biramijamal F, Hossein-Nezad A, Zendedel N, Sarie H, Doughaiemoghaddam M, Pourshams A: **Role of Cytochrome P450 2C19 genetic polymorphism in the therapeutic efficacy of omeprazole in Iranian patients with erosive reflux esophagitis.** *Arch Iran Med* 2010, **13**(5):406–412.
49. Gonzalez HM, Romero EM, Peregrina AA, de J Chavez T T, Escobar-Islas E, Lozano F, Hoyo-Vadillo C: **CYP2C19- and CYP3A4-dependent Omeprazole metabolism in West Mexicans.** *J Clin Pharmacol* 2003, **43**:1211–1215.
50. Kimura M, Ieiri I, Wada Y, Mamiya K, Urae A, Iimori E, Sakai T, Otsubo K, Higuchi S: **Reliability of the omeprazole hydroxylation index for CYP2C19 phenotyping: possible effect of age, liver disease and length of therapy.** *Br J Clin Pharmacol* 1999, **47**(1):115–119.
51. Williams ML, Bhargava P, Cherrouk I, Marshall JL, Flockhart DA, Wainer IW: **A discordance of the cytochrome P450 2C19 genotype and phenotype in patients with advanced cancer.** *Br J Clin Pharmacol* 2000, **49**(5):485–488.
52. Helsby NA, Lo WY, Sharples K, Riley G, Murray M, Spells K, Dzhelai M, Simpson A, Findlay M: **CYP2C19 pharmacogenetics in advanced cancer: compromised function independent of genotype.** *Br J Cancer* 2008, **99**(8):1251–1255.
53. Hagymási K, Müllner K, Herszényi L, Tulassay Z: **Update on the pharmacogenomics of proton pump inhibitors.** *Pharmacogenomics* 2011, **12**(6):873–888.
54. Yamazaki H, Inoue K, Shaw PM, Checovich WJ, Guengerich FP, Shimada T: **Different contributions of cytochrome P450 2C19 and 3A4 in the oxidation of omeprazole by human liver microsomes: effects of contents of these two forms in individual human samples.** *J Pharmacol Exp Ther* 1997, **283**(2):434–442.

Cost analysis of pharmaceutical care provided to HIV-infected patients: an ambispective controlled study

Renata Cavalcanti Carnevale[1], Caroline de Godoi Rezende Costa Molino[1], Marília Berlofa Visacri[1*], Priscila Gava Mazzola[1] and Patricia Moriel[1,2]

Abstract

Background: Studies have shown that pharmaceutical care can result in favorable clinical outcomes in human immunodeficiency virus (HIV)-infected patients, however, few studies have assessed the economic impact. The objective of this study was to evaluate the clinical and economic impact of pharmaceutical care of HIV-infected patients.

Methods: A controlled ambispective study was conducted in Brazil from January 2009 to June 2012. Patients were allocated to either intervention or control group. The control group was followed according to standard care while the intervention group was also followed by a pharmacist at each physician appointment for one year. Effectiveness outcomes included CD4+ count, viral load, absence of co-infections and optimal immune response, and economic outcomes included expenses of physician and pharmaceutical appointments, laboratory tests, procedures, and hospitalizations, at six months and one year.

Results: Intervention and control groups included 51 patients each. We observed significant decreases in total pharmacotherapy problems during the study. At six months, the intervention group contained higher percentages of patients without co-infections and of patients with CD4+ >500 cells/mm^3. None of the differences between intervention and control group considering clinical outcomes and costs were statistically significant. However, at one year, the intervention group showed higher percentage of better clinical outcomes and generated lower spending (not to procedures). An additional health care system daily investment of US$1.45, 1.09, 2.13, 4.35, 1.09, and 0.87 would be required for each additional outcome of viral load <50 copies/ml, absence of co-infection, CD4+ >200, 350, and 500 cells/mm^3, and optimal immune response, respectively.

Conclusion: This work demonstrated that pharmaceutical care of HIV-infected patients, for a one-year period, was able to decrease the number of pharmacotherapy problems. However, the clinical outcomes and the costs did not have statistical difference but showed higher percentage of better clinical outcomes and lower costs for some items.

Keywords: Pharmacoeconomics, Pharmaceutical care, HIV-infected patients

* Correspondence: mariberlofa@gmail.com
[1]Department of Clinical Pathology, Faculty of Medical Sciences (FCM), University of Campinas (UNICAMP), Alexander Fleming, 105, 13083-881 Campinas, SP, Brazil
Full list of author information is available at the end of the article

Introduction

Since 1996, Brazil has had a public health system program that provides free antiretroviral therapy, laboratory tests, and procedures to HIV-infected patients. This program has been internationally recognized as a major initiative against HIV [1]. However, this program alone does not guarantee safety and effectiveness of treatment because HIV treatment requires long-term therapy. Treatment of HIV includes a large number of drugs and drug interactions, and requires careful monitoring of therapy, with the goal of decreasing viral resistance and drug-related problems [1-3].

Studies have investigated the effects of pharmaceutical care on the rational use of drugs in HIV-infected patients [4-6]. March et al. demonstrated that HIV-infected patients followed by a clinical pharmacist show significant improvements in CD4+ levels and viral load and a decrease in toxic effects related to treatment [7]. This reduction in toxicity improves the quality of life and treatment adherence of the patients [8]. In addition, a systematic analysis (including data from January 1980 to June 2011) revealed that providing pharmaceutical care to HIV-infected patients was associated with statistically significant improvements in treatment adherence and had a positive impact on viral suppression [9].

Despite the variety of pharmaceutical care studies conducted with HIV-infected patients, remarkably few include an economic analysis. There is a need to go beyond the investigation of clinical outcomes generated by pharmaceutical care. Studies that include the economic impact of pharmaceutical care are necessary to justify the implementation or expansion of pharmaceutical care services [10].

In addition to the lack of economic studies on pharmaceutical care conducted with HIV-infected patients, another limitation is that, even though the studies available demonstrate that pharmaceutical care practice can contribute to the reductions of costs, they focus only on the costs associated with drugs, physician appointments, and hospitalizations. The available literature does not present studies regarding the impact of pharmaceutical care on the costs associated with laboratory tests and procedures [9,11-13]. Moreover, the majority of pharmacoeconomic studies present many methodological limitations, such as the lack of a control group and non-inclusion of costs associated with pharmacist appointments [14]. Thus, it has become imperative to conduct well-designed studies in the area of pharmaceutical care in order to obtain a clearer comprehension of its economic impact [14]. Well-designed studies investigating economic impact should be encouraged because they enable the rationalization of resources in health care, where the available resources are limited [15].

This study was designed to perform a pharmacoeconomic analysis of the impact of pharmaceutical care on HIV-infected patients over a one-year period by measuring both clinical and health care system economic outcomes.

Methods

This was a one-year, ambispective, controlled study, with a systematic sample by quota controls, paired according to random characteristics. A retrospective chart review and a prospective pharmaceutical care follow-up were conducted. The study was conducted at a hospital in the state of São Paulo, Brazil. The Hospital Ethics Committee approved the research, and informed consent was obtained from all patients.

The inclusion criteria for the study were as follows: outpatients diagnosed with HIV/AIDS (Human Immunodeficiency Virus/Acquired Immunodeficiency Syndrome), aged between 18 and 60 years, having body mass index (BMI) lower than 30 kg/m^2, and receiving antiretroviral therapy (ART). Obese patients were not included because they present higher incidences of hyperlipidemia, hypertension, and insulin resistance, and because some HIV/AIDS medications such as protease inhibitors can cause weight gain and fat accumulation, it would not be possible to determine whether the weight gain was related to the medication or to the background disease in such patients [16-19]. Patients who were unable to return for later appointments/exams, who refused to participate, who have psychiatric disease (that unable them to follow the medical appointments schedule and the pharmacist interventions), and those who were pregnant were excluded. Patients were enrolled in the study from January 2009 to June 2011 and were assigned in a 1:1 ratio to either intervention or control group by the clinical pharmacy team. Control group patients were matched to intervention group patients according to gender and baseline CD4+ count.

For one year, the intervention group was followed by the clinical pharmacy staff, composed of two pharmacists trained by the hospital clinical pharmacy team regarding HIV/AIDS and pharmaceutical care, after routine medical appointments at the hospital, using a method developed and adapted to the reality of the hospital, based on the Pharmacist's Workup of Drug Therapy (PWDT) method [20]. The control group was not followed by the clinical pharmacy team, and its data were collected through review of medical charts encompassing the same period.

Initial and final pharmacotherapy problems were accounted for and classified as necessity, effectiveness, safety, or therapy compliance pharmacotherapy problems only for the intervention group [21]. The clinical pharmacy team performed written and verbal pharmacist interventions with the intervention group, which were accounted for and classified as pharmacist-patient or pharmacist-physician interventions and as resolutive pharmacotherapy problems, preventive pharmacotherapy problems, quality of life, or referral to other medical specialties interventions. The classifications used for pharmacotherapy problems and pharmacist interventions are in accordance with those used in another publication by the authors [22].

The five effectiveness outcomes were as follows: CD4+ count higher than 200 cells/mm^3, 350 cells/mm^3, and 500 cells/mm^3; viral load lower than 50 copies/ml; and absence of co-infections. The co-infections considered by the study were as follows: bacterial co-infections (urinary infection, shigellosis, infected sebaceous cysts, cellulitis, pneumonia, and hordeolums), viral co-infections (cytomegalovirus, influenza, *Herpes zoster, Herpes simplex*, human papillomavirus, viral conjunctivitis, and warts), parasitic co-infection (microsporidiosis, isosporiasis, coccidiosis, and neurocryptococcosis), and fungal co-infections (oral moniliasis, onychomycosis, and tinea pedis). Effectiveness outcomes were measured at six months and one year of study and were obtained through medical chart review for both groups. Additionally, using a decision tree model, we established the number of patients from both groups that achieved, after one year of study, an optimal immune response as characterized by viral load <50 copies/ml, absence of co-infection, and CD4+>500 cells/mm^3.

For cost analysis, we identified the number of appointments (medical/nursing/nutrition/physical therapy/speech therapy/dental), laboratory tests, procedures, and hospitalizations per patient in the first six months, the last six months, and in one year, for both groups, through review of their medical charts. For the intervention group, we also included the cost of the pharmacist appointment. The DATASUS database [23] provided the monetary values for all these items. Values were quoted in US dollars ($).

Cost analysis was performed for the one-year period, considering both the effectiveness and the costs of appointments, laboratory tests, procedures, hospitalizations, total cost, and total cost without procedures.

Statistical analysis of the results was performed by SAS System for Windows (Statistical Analysis System, version 9.2). For baseline characteristics analysis, chi-square, Fisher's exact, and Mann–Whitney tests were performed. For co-infection, CD4+ and viral load analysis and generalized estimating tests were performed. For costs analysis, ANOVA for repeated measures, with a transformation by positions, was performed. The significance level was set at 5% (P ≤0.050).

Results

The study screened 140 HIV-infected patients being treated at the hospital on an outpatient basis. Thirty-eight patients were excluded: two were pregnant; nine interrupted the treatment at the hospital; eight were transferred from the hospital; and nineteen had not returned for the second pharmaceutical appointment in the first six months of the study (Figure 1). Finally, 51 patients each were allocated to intervention and control groups. A medical chart review provided the demographic data and initial information for both study groups (Table 1). The two study groups had similar baseline characteristics, indicating homogeneity.

There were a total of 230 pharmaceutical appointments (143 in the initial six months and 87 in the final six months). During these appointments, 219 pharmacist interventions were performed. Among them, 185 (84.5%) were pharmacist-patient interventions and 34 (15.5%) were pharmacist-physician interventions; 116 (53.0%) were preventive interventions, 55 (25.1%) were resolutive interventions, 42 (19.2%) were quality of life interventions, and six (2.7%) were referral to other medical specialties

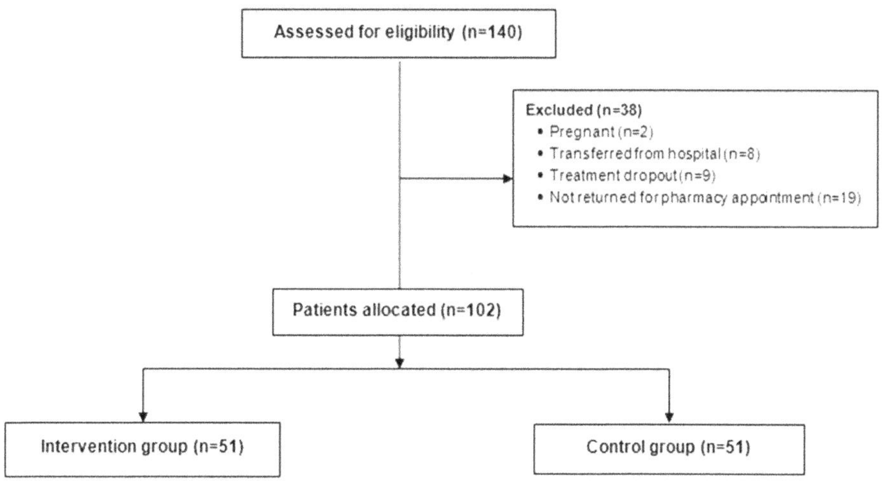

Figure 1 Flow diagram of the patients included in the study.

Table 1 Baseline characteristics of intervention group and control group

Characteristics	Control group N=51	Intervention group N=51	*P* value
Age (Mean [SD], years)	40.5 [9.2]	41.3 [8.8]	0.580[a]
Men - % (n)	66.7 (34)	66.7 (34)	1.000[b]
Ethnicity - % (n)			0.830[b]
Caucasian	70.6 (36)	68.6 (35)	
Black/ african descent	29.4 (15)	31.4 (16)	
HIV Diagnosis(Mean [SD], years)	7.5 [5.6]	8.3 [6.4]	0.690[a]
HIV Treatment Duration (Mean [SD], years)	5.7 [4.2]	6.5 [5.5]	0.780[a]
Number of tablets/day (Mean [SD])	9.3 [4.4]	10.1 [4.2]	0.250[a]
ART changes during the first 4 weeks of the study - % (n)	9.8 (5)	7.8 (4)	1.000[c]
CD4 + (Mean [SD], cells/mm^3)	304.0 [277.1]	310.4 [302.0]	0.980[a]
CD4 + >200 cells/mm^3 % (n)	56.9 (29)	54.9 (28)	0.840[b]
CD4 + >350 cells/mm^3 % (n)	31.4 (16)	33.3 (17)	0.830[b]
CD4 + >500 cells/mm^3 % (n)	15.7 (8)	17.7 (9)	0.800[b]
Viral load <50 copies/ml % (n)	60.8 (31)	64.8 (33)	0.190[b]
Number of Comorbidities (Mean [SD])	2.5 [1.6]	2.8 [2.1]	0.730[a]
Type of comorbidities % (n)			
Hepatitis C	23.5 (12)	21.6 (11)	0.630[b]
Tobaccoism	15.8 (8)	11.8 (6)	0.570[b]
Neurotoxoplasmosis	9.8 (5)	9.8 (5)	0.510[b]
Hypertriglyceridemia	3.9 (2)	9.8 (5)	0.440[c]
Pulmonary tuberculosis	13.7 (7)	3.9 (2)	0.160[c]
ART regimen % (n)			0.800[b]
TDF+3TC+EFV	17.6 (9)	21.6 (11)	
AZT+3TC+EFV	15.7 (8)	21.6 (11)	
AZT+3TC+LPV/r	9.8 (5)	7.8 (4)	
TDF+3TC+LPV/r	11.8 (6)	11.8 (6)	
Others	45.1 (23)	37.2 (19)	
Substance abuse % (n)			0.418[b]
Alcohol	19.6 (10)	29.4 (15)	
Tobacco	27.4 (14)	33.3 (17)	
Illicit drugs	13.73 (7)	7.8 (4)	

Note: [a]Mann-Whitney test; [b]Chi-square test;[c]Fisher's exact test.
Abbreviations: ART, antiretroviral therapy; AZT, zidovudine; CD4+, lymphocyte T CD4+; EFV, efavirenz; LPV/r, lopinavir/ritonavir; n, absolute number of patients; SD, standard deviation; TDF, tenofovir; 3TC, lamivudine.

interventions. We also observed significant decreases in total pharmacotherapy problems (from 248 to 145; 41.5%, P <0.001), necessity problems (from 55 to 26; 52.7%, P <0.001), and safety problems (from 161 to 96; 40.4%, P <0.001). A decrease in the other pharmacotherapy problems was also detected; however, it was not statistically significant: effectiveness problems (from 12 to 11; 8.4%, P =1.0000) and compliance problems (from 20 to 12; 40.0%, P =0.760).

Regarding clinical outcomes, in the initial six months, the intervention group contained higher percentages of patients without co-infections and of patients with CD4+ >500 cells/mm^3. At one year, the intervention group showed higher percentage of better clinical outcomes: absence of co-infection, viral load <50 copies/ml, CD4+ >200 cells/mm^3, CD4+ >350 cells/mm^3, and CD4+ >500 cells/mm^3 (Table 2). However, none of these differences was statistically significant. In addition, by using the decision tree model to establish the number of patients from each study group that achieved an optimal immune response (Figure 2), it was possible to infer that pharmaceutical care improves a patient's immune response.

At six months, the intervention group presented with two bacterial, five viral, and two fungal co-infections and, at one year, presented with two bacterial, one viral, two parasitic, and one fungal co-infections. At six months, the control group presented with five bacterial, three viral, two parasitic, and one fungal co-infections, and at one year, presented with one bacterial, five viral, and three parasitic co-infections.

At one year of study, the intervention group spent less per day on appointments, laboratory tests, and hospitalizations, but spent more on procedures and in total than the control group. Moreover, only the intervention group spent on pharmaceutical appointments. Compared with the control group, the intervention group annually generated savings per patient of $3.20 associated with appointments, $23.19 with laboratory tests, and $5.94 with hospitalizations. The intervention group also generated additional annual costs per patient of $50.60 associated with procedures, $12.88 with pharmaceutical appointments, and $31.13 with total costs (Table 3). However, the difference in costs between the groups was not statistically significant. The stark contrast in the costs associated with procedures was caused by two hip surgeries performed on patients from the intervention group, which together added $1,916.09 to the total expenses. This amount corresponds to 48.0% of the total spent on procedures in the first six months of the study ($3,991.04). Excluding the costs of these procedures from the total costs, the results demonstrate that compared with the control group, the intervention group would have spent $19.40 less per patient per year (Table 3).

Cost analysis identified the additional costs associated with procedures and total costs required to achieve each of the clinical outcomes outlined in the study (Table 4). Moreover, we found that, for each $1.00 spent on pharmaceutical care, there was a loss of $1.42 per day. However, when the costs associated with procedures were excluded

Table 2 Co-infection, viral load and CD4+ at baseline, 6 months, and at one year of study

	Control Group			Intervention Group			*P* value[a]
	N=51			N=51			
	Basal	6 months	1 year	Basal	6 months	1 year	
	% (n)	% (n)	% (n)	% (n)	% (n)	% (n)	
Absence of co-infection	/	72.6 (37)	56.9 (29)	/	76.5 (39)	64.7 (33)	0.092
Viral load <50 copies/ml	60.8 (31)	76.5 (39)	68.6 (35)	64.8 (33)	58.8 (30)	74.5 (38)	0.869
CD4+>200 cells/mm^3	56.9 (29)	68.6 (35)	74.5 (38)	54.9 (28)	70.8 (34)	78.4 (40)	0.793
CD4+>350 cells/mm^3	31.4 (16)	37.3 (19)	49.0 (25)	33.3 (17)	37.5 (18)	51.0 (26)	0.977
CD4+>500 cells/mm^3	15.7 (8)	17.7 (9)	19.6 (10)	17.7 (9)	20.8 (10)	27.5 (14)	0.599

Note: [a]Statistical significance value - Generalized estimating equations (GEE) test.
Abbreviation: CD4+, lymphocyte T CD4+.

from final costs, for each $1.00 spent on pharmaceutical care, there was a benefit of $2.51 per day. No relationship could be identified between the total daily costs generated by the patients and the reductions of pharmacotherapy problems (P =0.292; correlation R =0.15039; Spearman correlation coefficient test), or between the total costs and the number of pharmacist interventions (P =0.706; correlation R = −0.05412; Spearman correlation coefficient test).

Discussion

Pharmaceutical interventions were mostly of the pharmacist-patient type, which prevented therapy compliance errors (i.e., the patients needed clarifications regarding the use of medication, especially regarding dosage, drug interactions, and adherence). This type of intervention can help increase patient adherence to therapy. Hirsch et al. demonstrated in a cohort study with 2,234 patients that patients undergoing pharmaceutical care had greater adherence to antiretroviral therapy than patients not undergoing pharmaceutical care [6].

The decreases observed for all pharmacotherapy problem types are consistent with the literature. Studies have shown that pharmacist interventions can effectively identify, prevent, and solve pharmacotherapeutic problems [24,25]. Problems relating to safety were the most frequently encountered in our study. Other researchers have also identified a high frequency of issues related to inappropriate dosage and safety [5,26-29]. Carcelero et al. demonstrated that the most frequent issues with hospitalized HIV-infected patients are caused by combinations of contraindicated or not recommended drugs and by dosage errors, which happen in approximately one in five patients [5].

During one year of study, compared to the control group, the intervention group showed higher percentage of clinical outcomes, however there was no statistical difference. The better clinical response is associated with slower disease progression and a lower risk of complications, opportunistic infections, and co-infections [1,30-32]. We speculate that owing to these better clinical outcomes, the intervention group needed less hospitalization, laboratory tests, and medical appointments than the control group did.

Even though the difference in costs between the groups was not statistically significant, we can expect to see an overall, long-term cost analysis for the intervention group due its better clinical outcomes than the control group.

The lower costs associated with appointments and hospitalizations generated by the intervention group, compared with those of the control group, are consistent with the literature. Horberg et al. [13] and McPherson-Baker et al. [33] showed that the pharmacist's presence may decrease the number of appointments and, therefore, the costs for HIV-infected patients. A systematic review that included 32 articles pertaining to the impact of pharmaceutical care on HIV-infected patients showed that pharmaceutical care is associated with cost savings because it decreases the number of physician appointments, hospitalizations, and emergency visits [9]. A study in China found that total hospitalization costs in a group undergoing pharmaceutical care were significantly lower than those in a control group ($1,442.3 [684.9] vs. $1,729.6 [773.7], P <0.001) [34]. Furthermore, a Taiwanese study showed that the replacement of intravenous levofloxacin with its oral form, performed by a pharmacist, decreased hospital stays from 27.2 to 16.1 days (P =0.001), thereby lowering hospital costs [35]. Nevertheless, we found no studies in the literature that described the impact that pharmaceutical care has on the costs associated with laboratory tests and procedures.

In this study, an economic analysis that correlates the effectiveness and the costs of pharmacotherapy demonstrated that pharmaceutical care is dominant (less expensive and more effective), when we consider the effectiveness outcomes and the costs associated with appointments, laboratory tests, and hospitalizations. However, the intervention group generated higher costs associated with procedures and total costs than those of the control group. Furthermore, this study demonstrates

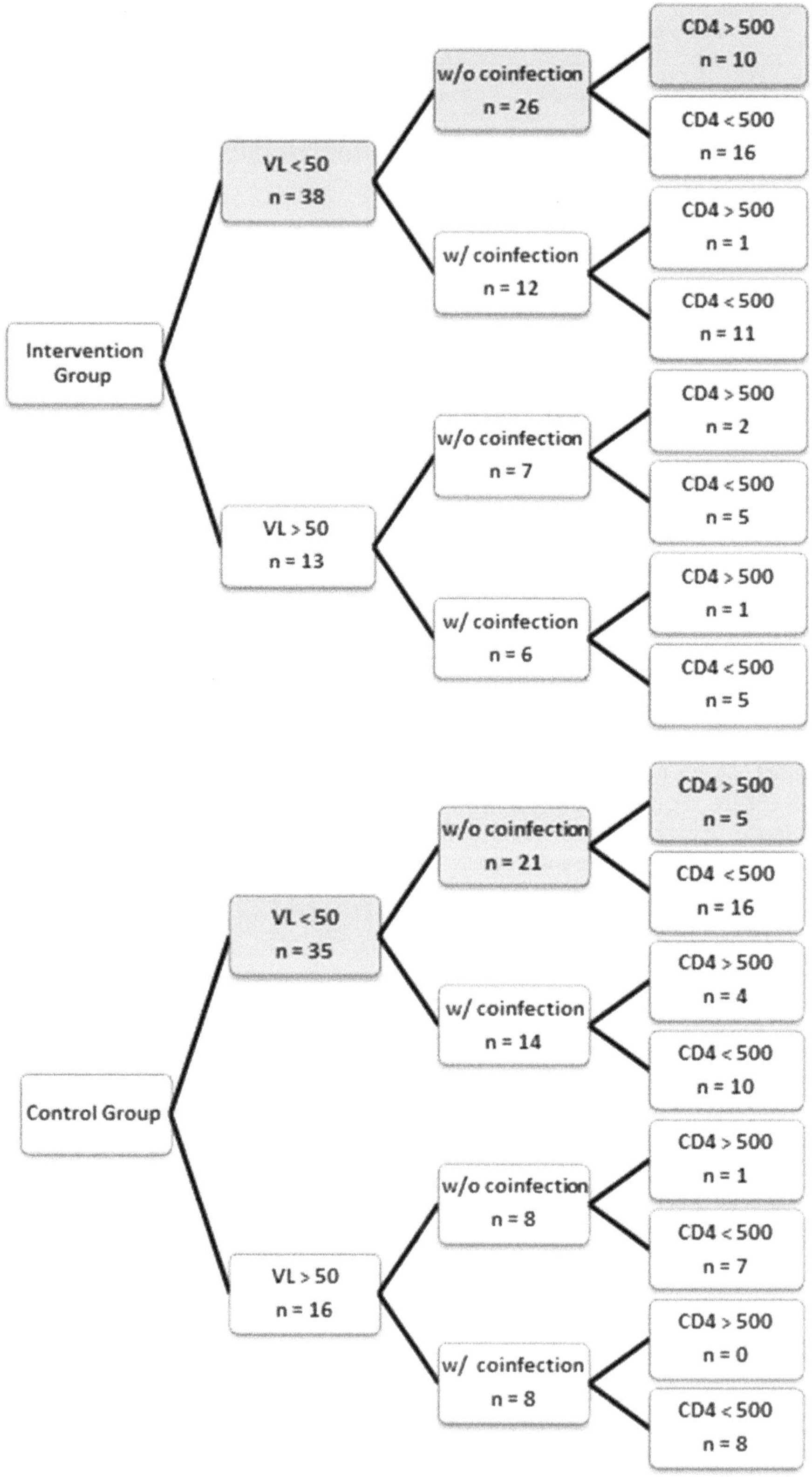

Figure 2 Optimal response immune for control and intervention groups. Abbreviation: CD4, CD4+ lymphocites; VL, viral load; w/o, without; w/, with.

Table 3 Study length of time and total daily costs (US$) for control and intervention groups

	Control Group			Intervention Group		
	N=51			N=51		
Study period	**6 m (i)**	**6 m (f)**	**Final**	**6 m (i)**	**6 m (f)**	**Final**
Length of time (mean [SD], days)	180.2[41.8]	190.5[6.4]	370.7[41.3]	196.8[29.3]	190.2[56.4]	387.0[39.8][a]
Appointments						
Total cost (US$) /day	8.65	6.49	**7.53**	8.01	6.12	**7.08**
Individual mean [SD] (US$)	0.17[0.08]	0.13[0.09]	**0.15[0.07]**	0.16[0.09]	0.12[0.08]	**0.14[0.07]**
Laboratory tests						
Total cost (US$) /day	38.07	25.35	**31.48**	33.33	22.96	**28.24**
Individual mean [SD] (US$)	0.75[0.74]	0.50[0.46]	**0.62[0.43]**	0.65[0.61]	0.45[0.43]	**0.55[0.44]**
Procedures						
Total cost (US$) /day	3.75	4.81	**4.29**	20.28	2.11	**11.36**
Individual mean [SD] (US$)	0.07[0.22]	0.09[0.21]	**0.08[0.17]**	0.40[1.11]	0.04[0.09]	**0.22[0.57]**
Hospitalization						
Total cost (US$) /day	2.62	2.53	**2.57**	2.30	1.17	**1.74**
Individual mean [SD] (US$)	0.05[0.30]	0.05[0.18]	**0.05[0.17]**	0.05[0.13]	0.02[0.10]	**0.03[0.09]**
Pharmacist						
Total cost (US$) /day	0.0	0.0	**0.0**	2.20	1.39	**1.80**
Individual mean [SD] (US$)	NA	NA	**NA**	0.05[0.02]	0.03[0.02]	**0.04[0.02]**
Total						
Final cost/day (US$)	53.09	39.18	**45.88**	66.13	33.74	**50.23**
Individual mean [SD] (US$)	1.04[0.99]	0.77[0.70]	**0.90[0.60]**	1.30[1.33]	0.66[0.55]	**1.00[0.81]**
Total excluding procedures						
Final cost/day (US$)	49.34	34.36	**41.58**	45.84	31.63	**38.87**
Individual mean [SD] (US$)	0.97[0.94]	0.67[0.63]	**0.82[0.56]**	0.90[0.71]	0.62[0.05]	**0.77[0.53]**

Note: [a] ANOVA results for repeated measures with a transformation by positions (P=0.057).
Abbreviations: 6m (i), initial 6 months; 6m (f), final 6 months; SD, Standard deviation.
Obs. The cost is the sum of the daily costs for all patients.

the importance of considering the costs associated with procedures. Here, if costs of procedures were disregarded when calculating the daily costs, the total costs of the intervention group would have been lower than those of the control group.

Table 4 Incremental Cost Effectiveness Ratio analysis per day for procedures and total costs (US$)

For each additional outcome of:	ICER (US $/day)	ICER (US$/day)
	Procedures	Total Cost (with procedures)
Viral load <50 copies/ml	2.36	1.45
Absence of co-infection	1.77	1.09
CD4+>200 cells/mm^3	3.53	2.18
CD4+>350 cells/mm^3	7.07	4.35
CD4+>500 cells/mm^3	1.77	1.09
Optimal immune response	1.41	0.87

Abbreviation: ICER, Incremental Cost Effectiveness Ratio.

Cost analysis identified a negative relationship when considering total cost, which contradicts the literature. According to Brennan et al., a $1.00 investment in pharmaceutical care showed a $3.00 return [36]. A meta-analysis demonstrated that 85% of the studies describe positive economic impacts of pharmaceutical care and concluded that the median benefit:cost ratio was 4.68:1 [10]. However, it should be noted that costs associated with laboratory tests and procedures were not included in these studies. In our study, by disregarding the procedures cost, the relationship becomes positive (2.51:1). Inclusion of costs associated with laboratory tests and procedures explains why this study showed different results than the results from the literature, and these differences clarify the need for well-designed studies that include the costs associated with procedures and laboratory tests, for a better understanding of the relationships among pharmaceutical care, HIV-infected patients, and the economy.

Limitations

This study has some limitations. There was no randomization of patients; the pharmacy staff was not blinded; pharmacotherapy problems were not verified for the control group (it was considered unethical to identify pharmacotherapy problems without providing any intervention); and the biggest limitation was our inability to retrieve the costs associated with the use of drugs, due to lack of information in the patient's medical charts. Several studies have analyzed the costs associated with the use of drugs [9,11-13,37] because they make a significant contribution to health care costs, especially in the context of hospital care, which represents 15%–25% of total health care costs. In a study conducted at the Maine Medical Center to guide the use of antibiotics, the pharmacist performed 74 interventions, which reduced the costs associated with antibiotics use, especially by replacing parenteral with oral formulations, generating savings of approximately $400.00 per patient and decreasing the length of hospital stay [38]. Therefore, with more comprehensive patient data, important additional savings regarding the use of drugs to treat co-infections could have been verified, since the intervention group had fewer co-infections than the control group did. For example, tuberculosis is common co-infection among HIV-infected patients and its treatment consists of a combination of rifampicin, isoniazid, and pyrazinamide [32], generating a cost of $316.56 per patient [39].

Conclusion

Our study presents important information about the impact that pharmaceutical care of HIV-infected patients can have on costs associated with procedure and laboratory tests. This information could not be found elsewhere in the literature, which indicates the need for well-designed and more complete studies.

This work demonstrated that pharmaceutical care of HIV-infected patients, for a one-year period, was able to decrease the number of pharmacotherapy problems. In addition, the intervention group presented higher percentage of better clinical outcomes and lower costs associated with appointments, laboratory tests, and hospitalizations than control group, however, there was no statistical difference; and, conversely, higher total costs and costs associated with procedures than those of the control group (no statistical significance). Additional pharmacoeconomic studies focused on pharmaceutical care are necessary to achieve a more comprehensive and reliable analysis.

Competing interests

The authors declare that they have no competing interests.

Authors' contributions

RCC, CGRCM, PGM and PM were responsible for concept and design. RCC and CGRCM collected data. RCC, CGRCM, PGM and PM interpreted data. RCC, MBV and PM were involved in the writing of manuscript. MBV and PM revised the manuscript. All authors read and approved the final manuscript.

Acknowledgments

The researchers would like to thank the hospital medical staff for their support and collaboration during the research, and Coordination for the Improvement of Higher Level Personnel (CAPES) and State of São Paulo Research Foundation (FAPESP) for financial support.

Author details

[1]Department of Clinical Pathology, Faculty of Medical Sciences (FCM), University of Campinas (UNICAMP), Alexander Fleming, 105, 13083-881 Campinas, SP, Brazil. [2]Faculty of Pharmaceutical Sciences (FCF), University of Campinas (UNICAMP), Sérgio Buarque de Holanda, 25, 13083-859 Campinas, SP, Brazil.

References

1. Brazil, Ministry of Health, Secretária de Vigilância em Saúde, Programa Nacional de DST e Aids: **Recomendações para Terapia Anti-retroviral em Adultos Infectados pelo HIV 2008** [http://www.ensp.fiocruz.br/portal-ensp/judicializacao/pdfs/491.pdf]
2. Dipiro J, Talbert R, Yees G, Matzke G, Wells B, Posey L: *Pharmacotherapy: A Pathophysiologic Approach*. 6th edition. Rio de Janeiro: Mcgraw Hill Companie; 2007.
3. Okie S: **Fighting HIV-Lessons from Brazil.** *N Engl J Med* 2006, **354:**1977–1981.
4. Ma A, Chen DM, Chau FM, Saberi P: **Improving adherence and clinical outcomes through an HIV pharmacist's interventions.** *AIDS Care* 2010, **22:**1189–1194.
5. Carcelero E, Tuset M, Martin M, De Lazzari E, Codina C, Miró J, Gatell J: **Evaluation of antiretroviral-related errors and interventions by the clinical pharmacist in hospitalized HIV-infected patients.** *HIV Med* 2011, **12:**494–499.
6. Hirsch J, Gonzales M, Rosenquist A, Miller T, Gilmer T, Best B: **Antiretroviral therapy adherence, medication use, and health care costs during 3 years of a community pharmacy medication therapy management program for Medi-Cal beneficiaries with HIV/AIDS.** *J Manag Care Pharm* 2011, **17:**213–223.
7. March K, Mak MM, Louie SG: **Effects of pharmacists' interventions on patient outcomes in an HIV primary care clinic.** *Am J Heal Syst Pharm* 2007, **64:**2574–2578.
8. Mocroft A, Youle M, Moore A, Sabin CA, Madge S, Lepri AC, Tyrer M, Chaloner C, Wilson D, Loveday C, Johnson MA, Phillips AN: **Reasons for modification and discontinuation of antiretrovirals: results from a single treatment centre.** *AIDS* 2001, **15:**185–194.
9. Saberi P, Dong BJ, Johnson MO, Greenblatt RM, Cocohoba JM: **The impact of HIV clinical pharmacists on HIV treatment outcomes: a systematic review.** *Patient Prefer Adherence* 2012, **6:**297–322.
10. Schumock GT, Butler MG, Meek PD, Vermeulen LC, Arondekar BV, Bauman JL: **Evidence of the economic benefit of clinical pharmacy services: 1996–2000.** *Pharmacotherapy* 2003, **23:**113–132.
11. Bozek PS, Perdue BE, Bar-Din M, Weidle PJ: **Effect of pharmacist interventions on medication use and cost in hospitalized patients with or without HIV infection.** *Am J Health Syst Pharm* 1998, **55:**1151–1155.
12. Engles-Horton LL, Skowronski C, Mostashari F, Altice FL: **Clinical guidelines and pharmacist intervention program for HIV-infected patients requiring granulocyte colony-stimulating factor therapy.** *Pharmacotherapy* 1999, **19:**356–362.
13. Horberg M, Hurley L, Silverberg M, Kinsman C, Quesenberry C: **Effect of clinical pharmacists on utilization of and clinical response to antiretroviral therapy.** *J Acquir Immune Defic Syndr* 2007, **44:**531–539.
14. De Rijdt T, Willems L, Simoens S: **Economic effects of clinical pharmacy interventions: a literature review.** *Am J Health Syst Pharm* 2008, **65:**1161–1172.
15. Areda CA, Bonizio RC, Freitas O: **Pharmacoeconomy : an indispensable tool for the rationalization of health costs.** *Braz J Pharm Sci* 2011, **47:**231–240.

16. Bavinger C, Bendavid E, Niehaus K, Olshen RA, Olkin I, Sundaram V, Wein N, Holodniy M, Hou N, Owens DK, Desai M: **Risk of cardiovascular disease from antiretroviral therapy for HIV : a systematic review.** *PLoS One* 2013, **8:**e59551.
17. Dube MP: **Disorders of glucose metabolism in patients infected with human immunodeficiency virus.** *Clin Infect Dis* 2000, **31:**1467–1475.
18. Friis-Møller N, Sabin CA, Data Collection on Adverse Events of Anti-HIV Drugs (DAD) Study Group, Weber R, D'Arminio Monforte A, El-Sadr WM, Reiss P, Thiébaut R, Morfeldt L, De Wit S, Pradier C, Calvo G, Law MG, Kirk O, Phillips AN, Lundgren JD: **Combination antiretroviral therapy and the risk of myocardial infarction.** *N Engl J Med* 2003, **349:**1993–2003.
19. Crum-Cianflone N, Roediger MP, Eberly L, Headd M, Marconi V, Ganesan A, Weintrob A, Barthel RV, Fraser S, Infectious Disease Clinical Research Program HIV Working Group, Agan BK: **Increasing rates of obesity among HIV-infected persons during the HIV epidemic.** *PLoS One* 2010, **5:**e10106.
20. Strand LM, Cipolle RJ, Morley PC: **Documenting the clinical pharmacists activities: back to basics.** *Drug Intell Clin Pharm* 1988, **22:**63–67.
21. **University of Minnesota College of Pharmacy. Pharmacy workup notes** [http://www.pharmacy.umn.edu/medmanagenotes/]
22. Molino CGRC, Carnevale RC, Rodrigues AT, Visacri MB, Moriel P, Mazzola PG: **Impact of pharmacist interventions on drug-related problems and laboratory markers in outpatients with human immunodeficiency virus infection.** *Ther Clin Risk Manag* 2014, **10:**631–639.
23. DATASUS: **SGTAP - Sistema de Gerenciamento da Tabela de Procedimentos, Medicamentos e OPM do SUS** [http://sigtap.datasus.gov.br/tabela-unificada/app/sec/inicio.jsp].
24. Ruiz I, Olry A, López MA, Prada JL, Causse M: **Prospective, randomized, two-arm controlled study to evaluate two interventions to improve adherence to antiretroviral therapy in Spain.** *Enferm Infecc Microbiol Clin* 2010, **28:**409–415.
25. Martin S, Wolters P, Calabrese S, Toledo-Tamula MA, Wood LV, Roby G, Elliott-DeSorbo DK: **The antiretroviral regimen complexity index. A novel method of quantifying regimen complexity.** *J Acquir Immune Defic Syndr* 2007, **45:**535–544.
26. Mok S, Minson Q: **Drug-related problems in hospitalized patients with HIV infection.** *Am J Health Syst Pharm* 2008, **65:**55–59.
27. Rastegar D, Knight A, Monolakis J: **Antiretroviral medication errors among hospitalized patients with HIV infection.** *Clin Infect Dis* 2006, **43:**933–938.
28. Pastakia S, Corbett A, Raasch R, Napravnik S, Correll T: **Frequency of HIV-related medication errors and associated risk factors in hospitalized patients.** *Ann Pharmacother* 2008, **42:**491–497.
29. Misson J, Clark W, Kendall M: **Therapeutic advances: protease inhibitors for the treatment of HIV-1 infection.** *J Clin Pharm Ther* 1997, **22:**109–117.
30. Osterberg L, Blaschke T: **Adherence to medication.** *N Engl J Med* 2005, **353:**487–497.
31. Langford SE, Ananworanich J, Cooper DA: **Predictors of disease progression in HIV infection : a review.** *Aids Res Ther* 2007, **4:**1–14.
32. Brazil, Ministry of Health, Secretaria de Vigilancia em Saúde, Departamento de DST Aids e Hepatites Virais: **Boletim Epidemiológico - AIDS e DST. 2012** [http://www.aids.gov.br/sites/default/files/anexos/publicacao/2011/50652/boletim_aids_2011_final_m_pdf_26659.pdf]
33. McPherson-Baker S, Malow RM, Penedo F, Jones DL, Schneiderman N, Klimas NG: **Enhancing adherence to combination antiretroviral therapy in non-adherent HIV-positive men.** *AIDS Care* 2000, **12:**399–404.
34. Shen J, Sun Q, Zhou X, Wei Y, Qi Y, Zhu J, Yan T: **Pharmacist interventions on antibiotic use in inpatients with respiratory tract infections in a Chinese hospital.** *Int J Clin Pharm* 2011, **33**(6):929–933.
35. Yen Y-H, Chen H-Y, Wuan-Jin L, Lin Y-M, Shen WC, Cheng K-J: **Clinical and economic impact of a pharmacist-managed i.v.-to-p.o. conversion service for levofloxacin in Taiwan.** *Int J Clin Pharmacol Ther* 2012, **50:**136–141.
36. Brennan TA, Dollear TJ, Hu M, Matlin OS, Shrank WH, Choudhry NK, Grambley W: **An integrated pharmacy-based program improved medication prescription and adherence rates in diabetes patients.** *Health Aff (Millwood)* 2012, **31:**120–129.
37. Lee AJ, Boro MS, Knapp KK, Meier JL, Korman NE: **Clinical and economic outcomes of pharmacist recommendations in a Veterans Affairs medical center.** *Am J Health Syst Pharm* 2002, **59:**2070–2077.
38. Janknegt R, Meer JWM van der: **Sequential therapy with intravenous and oral cephalosporins.** *J Antimicrob Chemother* 1994, **33:**169–177.
39. Brazilian Health Surveillance Agency (ANVISA): **Preços máximos de medicamentos por princípio ativo para compras públicas – monodrogas/ preços fábrica (PF) e preço máximo de venda ao governo (PMVG)** [http://portal.anvisa.gov.br/wps/wcm/connect/de29e2004baf729293c5dbbc0f9d5b29/LISTA_CONFORMIDADE_GOV_2012-06-19.pdf?MOD=AJPERES. Accessed July 12, 2014].

33

Effects of rutin on acrylamide-induced neurotoxicity

Vahideh Sadat Motamedshariaty[1], Sara Amel Farzad[1], Marjan Nassiri-Asl[2] and Hossein Hosseinzadeh[3*]

Abstract

Background: Rutin is an important flavonoid that is consumed in the daily diet. The cytoprotective effects of rutin, including antioxidative, and neuroprotective have been shown in several studies. Neurotoxic effects of acrylamide (ACR) have been established in humans and animals. In this study, the protective effects of rutin in prevention and treatment of neural toxicity of ACR were studied.

Results: Rutin significantly reduced cell death induced by ACR (5.46 mM) in time- and dose-dependent manners. Rutin treatment decreased the ACR-induced cytotoxicity significantly in comparison to control ($P < 0.01$, $P < 0.001$). Rutin (100 and 200 mg/kg) could prevent decrease of body weight in rats. In combination treatments with rutin (50, 100 and 200 mg/kg), vitamin E (200 mg/kg) and ACR, gait abnormalities significantly decreased in a dose-dependent manner ($P < 0.01$ and $P < 0.001$). The level of malondialdehyde significantly decreased in the brain tissue of rats in both preventive and therapeutic groups that received rutin (100 and 200 mg/kg).

Conclusion: It seems that rutin could be effective in reducing neurotoxicity and the neuroprotective effect of it might be mediated via antioxidant activity.

Keywords: Rutin, Acrylamide, MTT assay, Neural toxicity, Antioxidant

Introduction

Risk factors in food are either of chemical or microbiological origin, or a combination of both. Acrylamide (ACR), one such risk factor, is a possible human carcinogen [1]. It is an industrial chemical and has been known as an occupational hazard for decades [2,3]. However, in recent years, ACR has been found to form in fried and baked starchy foods during cooking [4,5]. This latter finding has greatly raised public concerns over ACR's potential health risk due to dietary exposure to people. ACR is a neurotoxic chemical and can cause peripheral and central neuropathy in humans and laboratory animals [6].

Early morphological studies suggested that both human and experimental neurotoxicities were mediated by cerebellar Purkinje cell injury and by degeneration of distal axons in the peripheral (PNS) and central nervous system (CNS) [7]. In addition to neurotoxicity, considerable experimental data from rodent studies has shown that ACR induces reproductive toxicity (e.g. reduced litter size) and genotoxic effects (e.g. DNA strand breaks, dominant lethal mutation) [3,8,9]. There are several reports that antioxidant agents could rescue neurotoxicity induced by ACR via increasing antioxidant activity [10-14].

Rutin (3, 3′, 4′, 5, 7 -pentahydroxyflavone-3-rhamnoglucoside) is a flavonoid of the flavonol type that is found in many typical plants, such as buckwheat, passion flower, apple and tea. It is also an important dietary constituent of foods and plant-based beverages [15]. Rutin has several pharmacological properties, including antioxidant, anticarcinogenic, cytoprotective, vasoprotective, cardioprotective and neuroprotective activities [16-23]. In humans, it attaches to the iron ion (Fe), preventing it from binding to hydrogen peroxide, which would otherwise create a highly reactive free radical that may damage cells [24].

The present study was therefore designed to investigate the protective effects of rutin in prevention and treatment of neural toxicity induced by ACR.

* Correspondence: hosseinzadehh@mums.ac.ir
[3]Pharmacodynamics and Toxicological Department, Pharmaceutical Research Center, School of Pharmacy, Mashhad University of Medical Sciences, Mashhad, Iran
Full list of author information is available at the end of the article

Materials and methods

Materials

RPMI 1640 and FBS were purchased from Gibco. (4,5-dimethylthiazol-2-yl)-2, 5-diphenyl tetrazolium (MTT), rutin hydrate ≥94% (HPLC), TBA (2-thiobarbituric acid), n-butanol, potassium chloride, phosphoric acid and ACR were obtained from Merck. Vitamin E was purchased in injectable form from Osveh Company, Iran.

Cell culture

PC12 cells were obtained from Pasteur Institute (Tehran, Iran). Cells were maintained at 37°C in a humidified atmosphere (90%) containing 5% CO_2. Cells were grown in RPMI 1640 medium supplemented with 10% (v/v) heat-inactivated foetal bovine serum, 100 U/ml penicillin and 100 µg /ml streptomycin.

Cell viability

The viability of cultured cells was determined by assaying the reduction of 3-(4,5-dimethyl thiazol-2-yl)-2,5- diphenyl tetrazolium bromide (MTT) to formazan [25]. Briefly, PC12 cells were cultured in a 96-well microliter plate at a density of 5000 cell/well. After pretreatment with rutin (0.5, 1, 1.5, 2.5, 5, 10, 20, 40, 80 and 160 µM/ml) for 24 h, ACR at concentration of 5.46 mM was added to each well. The cells were then incubated for 48 h and then treated with MTT solution (0.5 mg/ml PBS) for 1 h at 37°C. Upper mediate replaced with dimethyl sulfoxide (DMSO). The absorbance was measured at 570 nm (630 nm as reference) in a plate reader (TECAN infinit M200) [14].

Experimental animals

Male Wistar rats (200–270 g) were housed in colony rooms with 12/12 h light/dark cycle at 21 ± 2°C and had free access to food and water. All animal experiments were carried out in accordance with Mashhad University of Medical Sciences, Ethical committee Acts.

Experimental design

To induce neurotoxicity in rats, the animals were exposed to ACR at a daily dose of 50 mg/kg intraperitoneally (i.p.) [26]. All doses of rutin were selected as our previous work [18]. This daily dose and the corresponding route have been well characterized with respect to neuropathological expression and neurological deficits. For our study on the preventive effect, the rats were divided at random into 7 groups (n = 6 in each group) and treatment was given as follows:

1) Saline (negative control) for 14 days
2) ACR (50 mg/kg, i.p.) for 14 days
3) Rutin (50 mg/kg, i.p.) for 3 days alone and afterward rutin (50 mg/kg, i.p.) + ACR (50 mg/kg, i.p.) for 11 days
4) Rutin (100 mg/kg, i.p.) for 3 days alone and afterward rutin (100 mg/kg, i.p.) + ACR (50 mg/kg, i.p.) for 11 days
5) Rutin (200 mg/kg, i.p.) for 3 days alone and afterward rutin (200 mg/kg, i.p.) + ACR (50 mg/kg, i.p.) for 11 days
6) Rutin (200 mg/kg, i.p.) for 14 days
7) Vitamin E (200 mg/kg, i.p.) (positive control) for 3 days alone and afterward vitamin E (200 mg/kg, i.p.) + ACR (50 mg/kg, i.p.) for 11 days

Behavioural testing to assess preventive effects was performed on the 15th day [14].

After studying doses of rutin in preventing neurotoxicity, the most effective dose was used to assess its therapeutic effect. For our study, the rats were divided at random into 5 groups (n = 6 in each group) and treatment was given as follows:

1) Normal saline (negative control) for 14 days
2) ACR (50 mg/kg, i.p.) for 3 days alone and afterward ACR (50 mg/kg, i.p.) + rutin (200 mg/kg, i.p.) for 11 days
3) ACR (50 mg/kg, i.p.) for 3 days alone and afterward ACR (50 mg/kg, i.p.) + vitamin E (200 mg/kg, i.p.) for 11 days
4) ACR (50 mg/kg i.p.) for 7 days alone and afterward ACR (50 mg/kg, i.p.) + rutin (200 mg/kg i.p.) for 7 days
5) ACR (50 mg/kg i.p.) for 7 days alone and afterward ACR (50 mg/kg, i.p.) + vitamin E (200 mg/kg, i.p.) for 7 days

Behavioural testing was performed on the 15th day [14].

The behavioural index (gait scores) examination

After completion of treatment, the rats were placed in a clear plexiglass box and were observed for 3 min. Following observation, a gait score was assigned from 1 to 4, where 1 = a normal, unaffected gait; 2 = a slightly affected gait (foot splay, slight hind limb weakness and spread); 3 = a moderately affected gait (foot splay, moderate hind limb weakness, moderate limb spread during ambulation) and 4 = a severely affected gait (foot splay, severe hind limb weakness, dragging hind limbs, inability to rear) [27].

Biochemical assay

Furthermore, a test was conducted to determine lipid peroxidation by determining thiobarbituric acid reactive products (TBAR) of lipid peroxidation in brain tissue of rats [28,29]. Malondialdehyde (MDA) is the final product of lipid peroxidation and its complex with TBA is red and has maximum absorbance at 532 nm; MDA was assessed as the lipid peroxidation indicator. Briefly, the brain tissue was homogenized in cold KCl solution (1.5%) to obtain a homogenous suspension (10%). To a 10-ml tube, 0.5 ml of suspension was poured and 3 ml

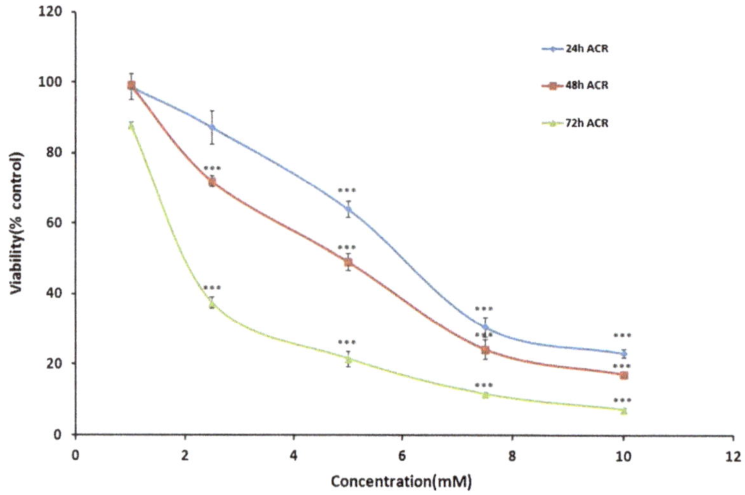

Figure 1 Cell viability of PC12 cells after exposure to different concentrations of acrylamide (ACR) for 24, 48 and 72 h. Cell viability was determined by MTT test. Data are expressed as mean ± SEM of 6 separate experiments. ACR was solubilised in PBS. For control cells PBS was used. ***P < 0.001 vs. control cells.

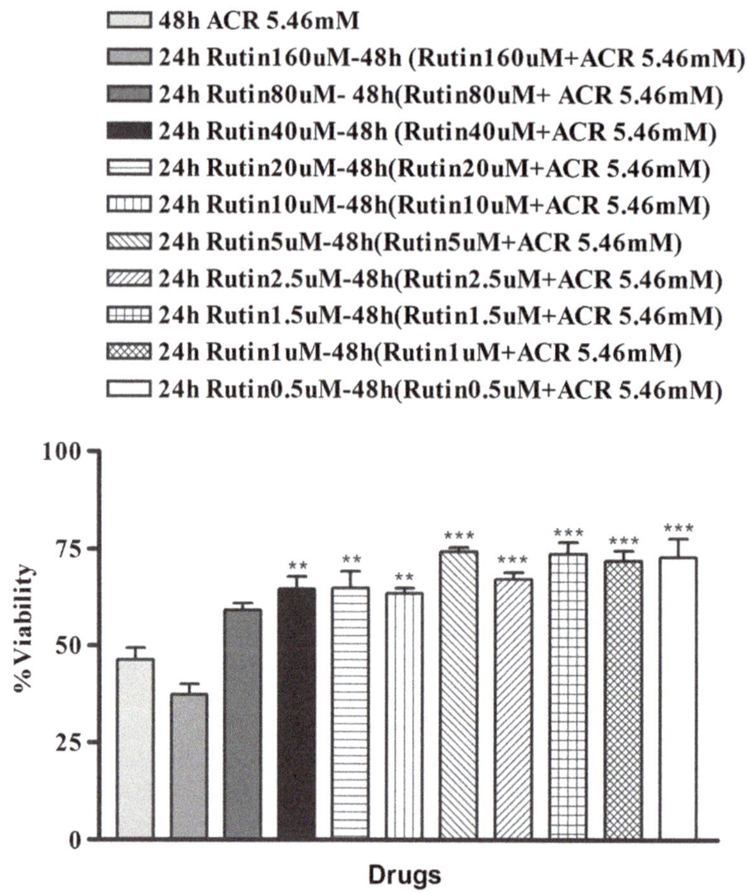

Figure 2 Effect of rutin on ACR-induced cytotoxicity in PC12 cells. Cells were pretreated with different concentration of rutin (0.5, 1, 1.5, 2.5, 5, 10, 20, 40, 80 and 160 μM/ml) for 24 h and ACR (5.46 mM) was added to each well later, followed by evaluation of cell viability using MTT assay. Data are expressed as the mean ± SEM of 6 separate experiments (n = 6). **P < 0.01, ***P < 0.001 vs. ACR-treated cells.

phosphoric acid (1%) and 1 ml TBA were added, following which the tube was placed in a boiling water bath for 45 min. Then, the suspension was cooled, 4 ml n-butanol added and the tube placed in vortex for complex mixing (1 min). Following this, the suspension was centrifuged (20000 rpm speed, 20 minutes) to separate the red-coloured upper phase and its absorbance was determined using the spectrophotometer. The standard curve for MDA (0–40 μM) was prepared [30].

Statistical analysis

Results are expressed as mean ± SEM. For in vitro assay, IC_{50} values were calculated using the method described by Litchfield and Wilcoxon method (PHARM/PCS software version 4). Statistical analyses were performed with ANOVA followed by the Tukey–Kramer test to compare the differences between means. Differences were considered statistically significant when $P < 0.05$.

Results

Effect of ACR in PC12 cells

The PC12 cells were treated with different concentration of ACR for 24, 48 and 72 h. Following this, the cell viability was measured using MTT test. Treatment of cells with ACR decreased viability in time- and dose-dependent manners, as shown in Figure 1. The IC_{50} (50% inhibitory concentration) value for treatment of PC12 cells with ACR for 48 h was 5.46 mM.

Effect of rutin on ACR-induced cytotoxicity in PC12 cells

PC12 cells were treated with different concentrations of rutin (0.5, 1, 1.5, 2.5, 5, 10, 20, 40, 80 and 160 μM/ml) for 24 h and then ACR (5.46 mM) was added to each well, followed by evaluation of cell viability using MTT assay. Rutin treatment decreased the ACR-induced cytotoxicity significantly in comparison to control (Figure 2).

Effect of ACR on rat body weight and the protective effect of rutin

The body weight of the ACR group decreased 33.6% after 14-day exposure to ACR (Figure 3). Treatment with rutin at a dose of 50 mg/kg failed to prevent weight loss caused by ACR. Therefore, body weight decreased after 14 days. However, rutin at doses of 100 and 200 mg/kg prevented decrease of body weight in rats. Vitamin E

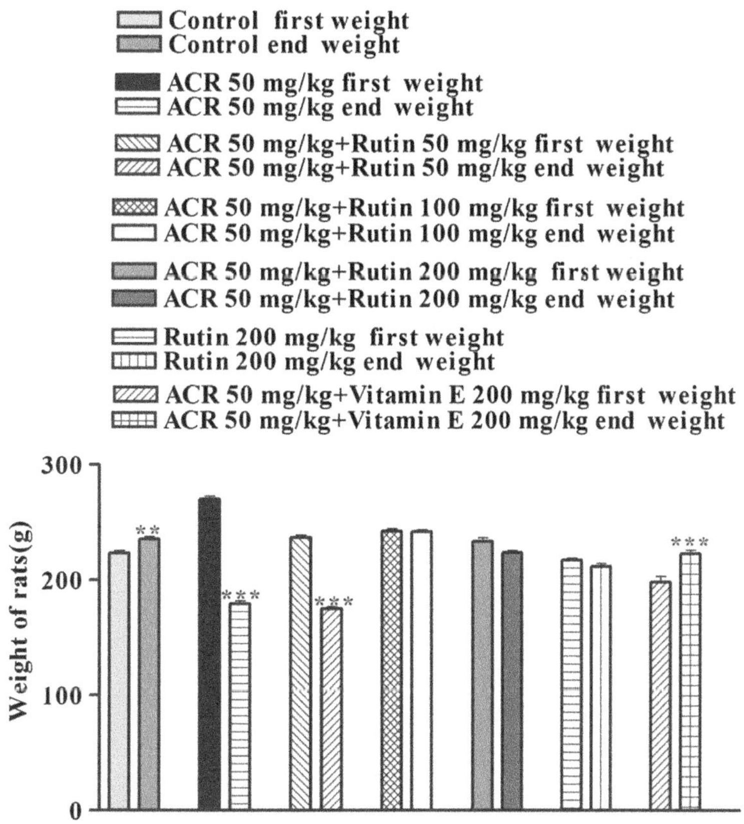

Figure 3 Protective effect of rutin (after 14 days of ACR exposure) by comparison between the initial and end weight of rats. Data are expressed as mean ± SEM, (n = 6), $^{**}P < 0.01$, $^{***}P < 0.001$ vs. first weight of each group treated with drugs.

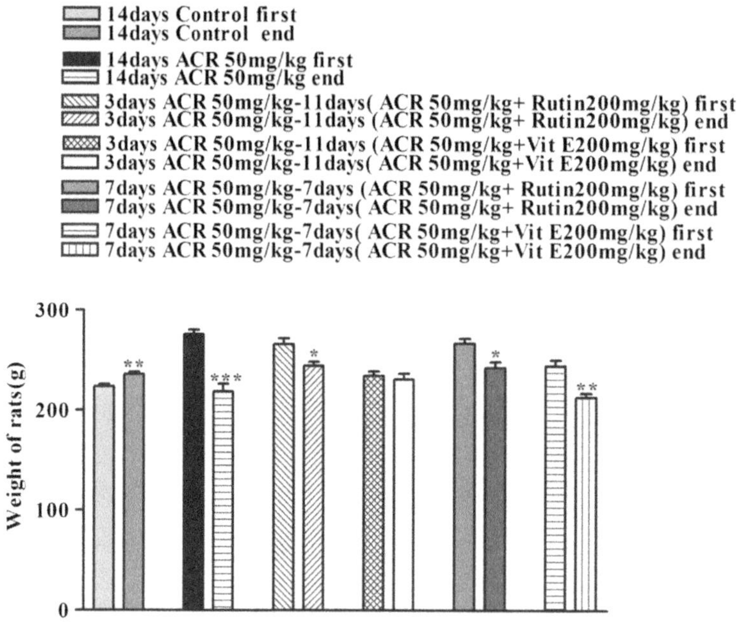

Figure 4 Therapeutic effect of rutin (after 14 days of ACR exposure) by comparison between the initial and end weight of rats. Data are expressed as mean ± SEM, (n = 6). *P < 0.05, **P < 0.01, ***P < 0.001 vs. first weight of each group treated with drugs.

(200 mg/kg) increased the body weight in rats (P < 0.001) (Figure 3).

Effect of ACR on rat body weight and the therapeutic effect of rutin

In the control group, only the body weight increased after 14 days compared with the first weight (P < 0.01). In other groups, the body weight significantly decreased compared with the first weight. However, in the group administered vitamin E, there was no significant change in body weight after 3 days (Figure 4).

Effect of ACR on the behavioural index (gait scores) in rats and the protective effect of rutin

Exposure to ACR (50 mg/kg, i.p.) for 14 days led to progressive gait abnormalities in rats, as shown in Figure 5. In groups of rats that were treated with combination of rutin (50, 100 and 200 mg/kg), vitamin E (200 mg/kg)

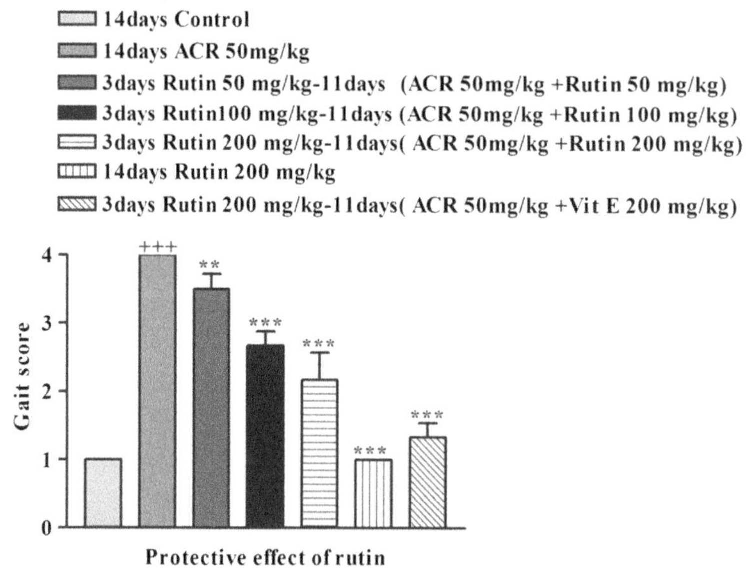

Figure 5 Protective effect of rutin on behavioural index (gait scores) in rats during treatment with ACR (50 mg/ kg, i.p.) for 14 days. Data are expressed as the mean ± SEM, (n = 6). +++P < 0.001 vs. control, *P < 0.05 **P < 0.01, ***P < 0.001 vs. ACR-treated animals.

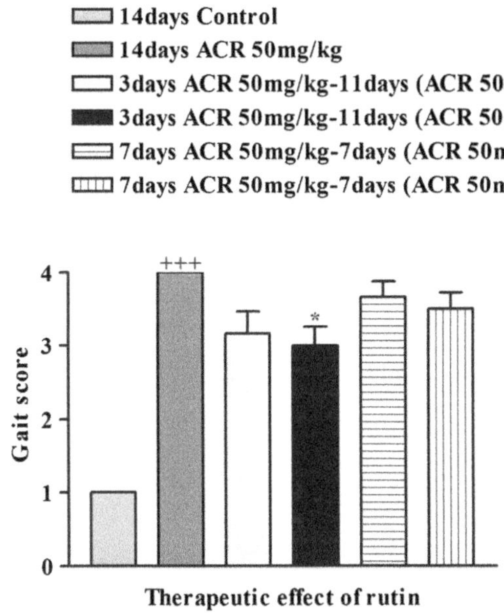

Figure 6 Therapeutic effect of rutin on behavioural index (gait scores) in rats during treatment with ACR (50 mg/ kg, i.p.) for 14 days. Data are expressed as the mean ± SEM, (n = 6). +++P < 0.001 vs. control, *P < 0.05 vs. ACR-treated animals.

and ACR, gait abnormalities significantly decreased in a dose-dependent manner (P < 0.01 and P < 0.001 vs. ACR-treated group) (Figure 5).

Effect of ACR on the behavioural index (gait scores) in rats and the therapeutic effect of rutin

The groups in which the therapeutic effect of rutin were evaluated, ACR was administered to the animals for 3 and 7 days and then treated 11 and 7 days with rutin and vitamin E with combination of ACR, respectively. In all groups, gait abnormalities decreased but the effect of vitamin E was only significant compared with ACR after 3 days treatment (P < 0.05) (Figure 6).

Effect of rutin in biochemical assay

There was an increase in the MDA levels following ACR administration compared with the control group (P < 0.001). The MDA levels significantly reduced dose dependently in all groups that were administrated rutin for preventive and therapeutic purposes (except on administration of 50 mg/kg rutin) (Tables 1 and 2).

Discussion

In this study, the neuroprotective effect of rutin on ACR-induced cytotoxicity in PC12 cells and ACR-induced neurotoxicity in rats was evaluated. Results showed that ACR could decrease cell viability in PC12 cells, which was

Table 1 Protective effect of rutin on lipid peroxidation following ACR administration

Groups	MDA concentration (nmol/g) tissue
14 days Control	45.75 ± 3.92
14 days ACR 50 mg/kg	92.58 ± 3.69^{+++}
14 days Rutin 200 mg/kg	75.52 ± 2.55***
3 days Rutin 50 mg/kg-11 days (ACR 50 mg/kg + Rutin 50 mg/kg)	69.39 ± 4.26
3 days Rutin 100 mg/kg-11 days (ACR 50 mg/kg + Rutin 100 mg/kg)	49.7 ± 7.77*
3 days Rutin 200 mg/kg-11 days (ACR 50 mg/kg + Rutin 200 mg/kg)	47.76 ± 3.05***
3 days Vit E 200 mg/kg-11 days (ACR 50 mg/kg + Vit E 200 mg/kg)	52.67 ± 4.38***

Values are mean ± SEM (n = 6). $^{+++}$P < 0.001 vs. control, *P < 0.05, ***P < 0.001 vs. ACR-treated animals.

Table 2 Therapeutic effect of rutin on lipid peroxidation following ACR administration

Groups	MDA concentration (nmol/g) tissue
14 days Control	45.75 ± 3.92
14 days ACR 50 mg/kg	92.58 ± 3.69^{+++}
3 days ACR 50 mg/kg-11 days (ACR 50 mg/kg + Rutin 200 mg/kg)	65.10 ± 5.03**
3 days ACR 50 mg/kg 11 days (ACR 50 mg/kg + Vit E 200 mg/kg)	60.75 ± 3.46***
7 days ACR 50 mg/kg-7 days (ACR 50 mg/kg + Rurin 200 mg/kg)	69.67 ± 5.630*
7 days ACR 50 mg/kg-7 days (ACR 50 mg/kg + Vit E 200 mg/kg)	68.87 ± 5.14*

Values are mean ± SEM (n = 6). $^{+++}$P < 0.001 vs. control, *P < 0.05, **P < 0.01, ***P < 0.001 vs. ACR-treated animals.

suppressed by administration of rutin. Also, rutin significantly inhibited behavioural index changes and body weight loss caused by ACR administration in rats. Also, the MDA levels significantly reduced in all groups of rutin.

ACR is known to induce apoptosis in time- and dose-dependent manners in neurons and astrocytes and significantly reduce the proliferation of neural progenitor cells and, in high concentrations [31]. In our study, ACR (5.46 mM) decreased cell viability in PC12 cells and pretreatment with rutin (0.5, 1, 1.5, 2.5, 5, 10, 20 and 40 μM/ml) increased the cell viability. According to previous studies, reactive oxygen species (ROS) have important role in the toxicity of ACR [31,32].

Antioxidant effects of rutin have been established in several studies [23,33]. Rutin and catechol-compounds are electron donors, and antioxidant activities of rutin and catechol and its derivatives indicate that they are potential antioxidants [34,35]. It seems that the protective effect of rutin in this model may be at least, in part, due to suppression of ROS generation because rutin has exhibited antioxidant effect in different studies [36].

ACR monomer is a potent neurotoxin and capable of inducing CNS and PNS damages in humans and animals. ACR induces ataxia, skeletal muscle weakness and weight loss in both occupationally exposed humans and experimental animal models [26,37]. Our results showed that treatment of animals with ACR (50 mg/kg, i.p.) for 11 days decreased body weight and caused gait abnormalities, and at the end of 14 days, ACR-exposed animals displayed severe abnormal gait (scores 4), but treatment of animals with rutin prevented the decrease in body weight and reduced abnormal gait.

In recent decades, there are several studies that have shown the neuroprotective effects of rutin [38-40]. Rutin has neuroprotective effect in brain ischemia and its administration attenuates ischemic neural apoptosis by inhibition of neurological deficit, lipid peroxidation, p53 expression and increase in endogenous antioxidant defence enzymes [41]. It was shown that the 4-oxo group and the 2,3 double bond in the C ring are common in rutin and that it may be related by its neuroprotective action [42]. Rutin has beneficial effects on hypoxic, glutamate and oxidative stress at concentrations as low as 1 nM on retinal ganglion cell. It appears that the sugar side chain of flavonoids may be important for neuroprotective activities [43].

The neuroprotective effect of vitamin E is related to its antioxidant activity [44,45]. For this reason, vitamin E was used was as a positive control in protection against ACR- induced neurotoxicity. As our results, vitamin E (200 mg/kg) increased the body weight compared to rutin as a preventive agent in rats.

It seems that the effect of vitamin E in the presence of ACR after 3 days treatment in inhibition of gait abnormalities is more than rutin (200 mg/kg). However, the protective and therapeutic effects of rutin (200 mg/kg) on lipid peroxidation following ACR administration are same as vitamin E (200 mg/kg).

It is possible that rutin by inhibiting neurological deficit could improve behavioral index of animals. Moreover, it was shown that rutin might be effective in treatment of tardive dyskinesia, an extrapyramidal movement disorder, through communicating the imbalance of dopaminergic transmission [46]. Pretreatment of rutin (100 and 200 mg/kg/day) for long-term caused behavioural and neurochemical changes in aged WAG male rats. It is possible that rutin may exert this effect by affecting brain dopaminergic and adrenergic systems [47]. Thus, there is another possibility that rutin could improve behavioral index of animals via modulating dopaminergic and adrenergic transmissions.

The results of the current study suggested that protective effect of rutin against ACR cytotoxicity in PC12 cells and rats was due to inhibition of ROS production in PC12 cells exposed to ACR or in the rat nervous system under ACR treatment.

Competing interests
The authors declare that they have no competing interests.

Authors' contribution
HH, designed the study, conducted, supervised experiment and prepared manuscript. SAF and VMS, conducted experiment and prepared manuscript. MNA, prepared manuscript. All authors read and approve the final manuscript.

Acknowledgments
The authors are thankful to the Vice Chancellor of Research, Mashhad University of Medical Sciences for financial support.

Author details
[1]Pharmaceutical Research Center, School of Pharmacy, Mashhad University of Medical Sciences, Mashhad, Iran. [2]Cellular and Molecular Research Centre, Department of Pharmacology, School of Medicine, Qazvin University of Medical Sciences, Qazvin, Iran. [3]Pharmacodynamics and Toxicological Department, Pharmaceutical Research Center, School of Pharmacy, Mashhad University of Medical Sciences, Mashhad, Iran.

References

1. Wenzl T, De La Calle MB, Anklam E: **Analytical methods for the determination of acrylamide in food products: a review.** *Food Addit Contam* 2003, **20**:885–902.
2. Bull RA, Hansman GS, Clancy LE, Tanaka MM, Rawlinson WD, White PA: **Norovirus recombination in ORF1/ORF2 overlap.** *Emerg Infect Dis* 2005, **11**:1079–1085.
3. Tyl RW, Friedman MA: **Effects of acrylamide on rodent reproductive performance.** *Reprod Toxicol* 2003, **17**:1–13.
4. Rosén J, Hellenäs KE: **Analysis of acrylamide in cooked foods by liquid chromatography tandem mass spectrometry.** *Analyst* 2002, **127**:880–882.
5. Tareke E, Rydberg P, Karlsson P, Eriksson S, Törnqvist M: **Analysis of acrylamide, a carcinogen formed in heated foodstuffs.** *J Agric Food Chem* 2002, **50**:4998–5006.
6. Barber DS, LoPachin RM: **Proteomic analysis of acrylamide-protein adduct formation in rat brain synaptosomes.** *Toxicol Appl Pharmacol* 2004, **201**:120–136.

7. Cavanagh J, Nolan CC: **Selective loss of Purkinje cells from the rat cerebellum caused by acrylamide and the responses of β-glucuronidase and β-galactosidase.** *Acta Neuropathol* 1982, **58:**210–214.
8. Sega GA, Alcota RP, Tancongco CP, Brimer PA: **Acrylamide binding to the DNA and protamine of spermiogenic stages in the mouse and its relationship to genetic damage.** *Mutat Res* 1989, **216:**221–230.
9. Working PK, Bentley KS, Hurtt ME, Mohr KL: **Comparison of the dominant lethal effects of acrylonitrile and acrylamide in male Fischer 344 rats.** *Mutagenesis* 1987, **2:**215–220.
10. Xichun Z, Min'ai Z: **Protective role of dark soy sauce against acrylamide-induced neurotoxicity in rats by antioxidative activity.** *Toxicol Mech Methods* 2009, **19:**369–374.
11. Alturfan AA, Tozan-Beceren A, Sehirli AO, Demiralp E, Sener G, Omurtag GZ: **Resveratrol ameliorates oxidative DNA damage and protects against acrylamide-induced oxidative stress in rats.** *Mol Biol Rep* 2012, **39:**4589–4596.
12. Shinomol GK, Raghunath N, Bharath MM, Muralidhara M: **Prophylaxis with Bacopa monnieri attenuates acrylamide induced neurotoxicity and oxidative damage via elevated antioxidant function.** *Cent Nerv Syst Agents Med Chem* 2013, **13**(1):3–12.
13. Mehri S, Abnous K, Mousavi SH, Shariaty VM, Hosseinzadeh H: **Neuroprotective Effect of Crocin on Acrylamide-induced Cytotoxicity in PC12 cells.** *Cell Mol Neurobiol* 2012, **32:**227–235.
14. Hosseinzadeh H, Tabeshpur J, Mehri S: **Effect of Saffron extract on Acrylamide- induced toxicity: In vitro and in vivo assessment.** *Chin J Integr Med* 2014. In Press.
15. Kuntić V, Pejić N, Ivković B, Vujić Z, Ilić K, Mićić S, Vukojević V: **Isocratic RP-HPLC method for rutin determination in solid oral dosage forms.** *J Pharm Biomed Anal* 2007, **43:**718–721.
16. Javed H, Khan MM, Ahmad A, Vaibhav K, Ahmad ME, Khan A, Ashafaq M, Islam F, Siddiqui MS, Safhi MM, Islam F: **Rutin prevents cognitive impairments by ameliorating oxidative stress and neuroinflammation in rat model of sporadic dementia of Alzheimer type.** *Neuroscience* 2012, **17:**340–352.
17. Richetti SK, Blank M, Capiotti KM, Piato AL, Bogo MR, Vianna MR, Bonan CD: **Quercetin and rutin prevent scopolamine-induced memory impairment in zebrafish.** *Behav Brain Res* 2011, **217:**10–15.
18. Nassiri-Asl M, Mortazavi SR, Samiee-Rad F, Zangivand AA, Safdari F, Saroukhani S, Abbasi E: **The effects of rutin on the development of pentylenetetrazole kindling and memory retrieval in rats.** *Epilepsy Behav* 2010, **18:**50–53.
19. Mellou F, Loutrari H, Stamatis H, Roussos C, Kolisis FN: **Enzymatic esterification of flavonoids with unsaturated fatty acids: effect of the novel esters on vascular endothelial growth factor release from K562 cells.** *Process Biochem* 2006, **41:**2029–3204.
20. Trumbeckaite S, Bernatoniene J, Majiene D, Jakstas V, Savickas A, Toleikis A: **The effect of flavonoids on rat heart mitochondrial function.** *Biomed Pharmacother* 2006, **60:**245–248.
21. Schwedhelm E, Maas R, Troost R, Böger RH: **Clinical pharmacokinetics of antioxidants and their impact on systemic oxidative stress.** *Clin Pharmacokinet* 2003, **42:**437–459.
22. Janbaz KH, Saeed SA, Gilani AH: **Protective effect of rutin on paracetamol and CCl4-induced hepatotoxicity in rodents.** *Fitoterapia* 2002, **73:**557–563.
23. La Casa C, Villegas I, Alarcon de la Lastra C, Motilva V, Martin Calero MJ: **Evidence for protective and antioxidant properties of rutin, a natural flavone, against ethanol induced gastric lesions.** *J Ethnopharmacol* 2000, **71:**45–53.
24. Afanas'ev IB, Dorozhko AI, Brodskii AV, Kostyuk VA, Potapovitch AI: **Chelating and free radical scavenging mechanisms of inhibitory action of rutin and quercetin in lipid peroxidation.** *Biochem Pharmacol* 1989, **38:**1763–1769.
25. Mousavi SH, Tavakkol-Afshari J, Brook A, Jafari-Anarkooli I: **Role of caspases and Bax protein in saffron-induced apoptosis in MCF-7 cells.** *Food Chem Toxicol* 2009, **47:**1909–1913.
26. LoPachin RM: **Acrylamide neurotoxicity: Neurological, morphological and molecular endpoints in animal models, in advances in experimental medicine and biology.** *Adv Exp Med Biol* 2005, **561:**21–37.
27. LoPachin RM, Ross JF, Reid ML, Das S, Mansukhani S, Lehning EJ: **Neurological evaluation of toxic axonopathies in rats: Acrylamide and 2,5-hexanedione.** *Neurotoxicology* 2002, **23:**95–110.
28. Hosseinzadeh H, Hosseini A, Nassiri-Asl M, Sadeghnia HR: **Effect of *Salvia leriifolia* Benth. root extracts on ischemia-reperfusion in rat skeletal muscle.** *BMC Complement Altern Med* 2007, **7:**23.
29. Unal D, Yeni E, Erel O, Bitiren M, Vural H: **Antioxidative effects of exogenous nitric oxide versus antioxidant vitamins on renal ischemia reperfusion injury.** *Urol Res* 2002, **30:**190–194.
30. Hosseinzadeh H, Sadeghnia HR, Ziaee T, Danaee A: **Protective effect of aqueous saffron extract (*Crocus sativus* L.) and crocin, its active constituent, on renal ischemia-reperfusion-induced oxidative damage in rats.** *J Pharm Pharm Sci* 2005, **8:**387–393.
31. Park HR, Kim MS, Kim SJ, Park M, Kong KH, Kim HS, Kwack SJ, Kang TS, Kim SH, Kim HS, Lee J: **Acrylamide induces cell death in neural progenitor cells and impairs hippocampal neurogenesis.** *Toxicol Lett* 2009, **193:**86–93.
32. Yousef MI, El-Demerdash FM: **Acrylamide-induced oxidative stress and biochemical perturbations in rats.** *Toxicology* 2006, **219:**133–141.
33. Kamalakkannan N, Stanely Mainzen Prince P: **Rutin improves the antioxidant status in streptozotocin-induced diabetic rat tissues.** *Mol Cell Biochem* 2006, **293:**211–219.
34. Anbazhagan V, Kalaiselvan A, Jaccob M, Venuvanalingam P, Renganathan R: **Investigations on the fluorescence quenching of 2,3-diazabicyclo [2.2.2]oct-2-ene by certain flavonoids.** *J Photochem Photobiol B* 2008, **91:**143–150.
35. Manivannan C, Sundaram KM, Renganathan R, Sundararaman M: **Investigations on photoinduced interaction of 9-aminoacridine with certain catechols and rutin.** *J Fluoresc* 2012, **22:**1113–1125.
36. Becker EM, Ntouma G, Skibsted LH: **Synergism between and antagonism between quercetin and other chain-breaking antioxidants in lipid systems of increasing structural organization.** *Food Chem* 2007, **103:**1288–1296.
37. Shipp A, Lawrence G, Gentry R, McDonald T, Bartow H, Bounds J, Macdonald N, Clewell H, Allen B, Van Landingham C: **Acrylamide: review of toxicity data and dose–response analyses for cancer and noncancer effects.** *Crit Rev Toxicol* 2006, **36:**481–608.
38. Javed H, Khan MM, Ahmad A, Vaibhav K, Ahmad ME, Khan A, Ashafaq M, Islam F, Siddiqui MS, Safhi MM, Islam F: **Rutin prevents cognitive impairments by ameliorating oxidative stress and neuroinflammation in rat model of sporadic dementia of Alzheimer type.** *Neuroscience* 2012, **210:**340–352.
39. Tongjaroenbuangam W, Ruksee N, Chantiratikul P, Pakdeenarong N, Kongbuntad W, Govitrapong P: **Neuroprotective effects of quercetin, rutin and okra (Abelmoschus esculentus Linn.) in dexamethasone-treated mice.** *Neurochem Int* 2011, **59:**677–685.
40. Yang YC, Lin HY, Su KY, Chen CH, Yu YL, Lin CC, Yu SL, Yan HY, Su KJ, Chen YL: **Rutin, a flavonoid that is a main component of Saussurea involucrata, attenuates the senescence effect in D-Galactose aging mouse model.** *Evid Based Complement Alternat Med* 2012, **2012:**980276.
41. Khan MM, Ahmad A, Ishrat T, Khuwaja G, Srivastawa P, Khan MB, Raza SS, Javed H, Vaibhav K, Khan A, Islam F: **Rutin protects the neural damage induced by transient focal ischemia in rats.** *Brain Res* 2009, **1292:**123–135.
42. Pu F, Mishima K, Irie K, Motohashi K, Tanaka Y, Orito K, Egawa T, Kitamura Y, Egashira N, Iwasaki K, Fujiwara M: **Neuroprotective effects of quercetin and rutin on spatial memory impairment in an 8-arm radial maze task and neuronal death induced by repeated cerebral ischemia in rats.** *J Pharmacol Sci* 2007, **104:**329–334.
43. Nakayama T, Yamada M, Osawa T, Kawakishi S: **Suppression of active oxygen-induced cytotoxicity by flavonoids.** *Biochem Pharmacol* 1993, **45:**265–267.
44. Yun JS, Na HK, Park KS, Lee YH, Kim EY, Lee SY, Kim JI, Kang JH, Kim DS, Choi KH: **Protective effects of vitamin E on endocrine disruptors, PCB-induced dopaminergic neurotoxicity.** *Toxicology* 2005, **216:**140–146.
45. Gümüştaş K, Meta Güzeyli FM, Atükeren P, Sanus GZ, Kemerdere R, Tanriverdi T, Kaynar MY: **The effect of vitamin E on lipid peroxidation, nitric oxide production and superoxide dismutase expression in hyperglycemic rats with ceberal ischemia- reperfusion injury.** *Turk Neurosurg* 2007, **17:**78–82.
46. Bishnoi M, Chopra K, Kulkarni SK: **Protective effect of rutin, a polyphenolic flavonoid against haloperidol-induced orofacial dyskinesia and associated**

behavioural, biochemical and neurochemical changes. *Fundam Clin Pharmacol* 2007, **21**:521–529.

47. Pyrzanowska J, Piechal A, Blecharz-Klin K, Joniec-Maciejak I, Zobel A, Widy-Tyszkiewicz E: **Influence of long-term administration of rutin on spatial memory as well as the concentration of brain neurotransmitters in aged rats.** *Pharmacol Rep* 2012, **64**:808–816.

Permissions

All chapters in this book were first published in DARU-JPS, by BioMed Central; hereby published with permission under the Creative Commons Attribution License or equivalent. Every chapter published in this book has been scrutinized by our experts. Their significance has been extensively debated. The topics covered herein carry significant findings which will fuel the growth of the discipline. They may even be implemented as practical applications or may be referred to as a beginning point for another development.

The contributors of this book come from diverse backgrounds, making this book a truly international effort. This book will bring forth new frontiers with its revolutionizing research information and detailed analysis of the nascent developments around the world.

We would like to thank all the contributing authors for lending their expertise to make the book truly unique. They have played a crucial role in the development of this book. Without their invaluable contributions this book wouldn't have been possible. They have made vital efforts to compile up to date information on the varied aspects of this subject to make this book a valuable addition to the collection of many professionals and students.

This book was conceptualized with the vision of imparting up-to-date information and advanced data in this field. To ensure the same, a matchless editorial board was set up. Every individual on the board went through rigorous rounds of assessment to prove their worth. After which they invested a large part of their time researching and compiling the most relevant data for our readers.

The editorial board has been involved in producing this book since its inception. They have spent rigorous hours researching and exploring the diverse topics which have resulted in the successful publishing of this book. They have passed on their knowledge of decades through this book. To expedite this challenging task, the publisher supported the team at every step. A small team of assistant editors was also appointed to further simplify the editing procedure and attain best results for the readers.

Apart from the editorial board, the designing team has also invested a significant amount of their time in understanding the subject and creating the most relevant covers. They scrutinized every image to scout for the most suitable representation of the subject and create an appropriate cover for the book.

The publishing team has been an ardent support to the editorial, designing and production team. Their endless efforts to recruit the best for this project, has resulted in the accomplishment of this book. They are a veteran in the field of academics and their pool of knowledge is as vast as their experience in printing. Their expertise and guidance has proved useful at every step. Their uncompromising quality standards have made this book an exceptional effort. Their encouragement from time to time has been an inspiration for everyone.

The publisher and the editorial board hope that this book will prove to be a valuable piece of knowledge for researchers, students, practitioners and scholars across the globe.

List of Contributors

Aida Kulo
Center for Clinical Pharmacology, University Hospitals Leuven, Leuven, Belgium
Institute of Pharmacology, Clinical Pharmacology and Toxicology, Faculty of Medicine, University of Sarajevo, Sarajevo, Bosnia Herzegovina

Anne Smits
Neonatal Intensive Care Unit, University Hospitals Leuven, Leuven, Belgium

Gunnar Naulaers
Neonatal Intensive Care Unit, University Hospitals Leuven, Leuven, Belgium

Jan de Hoon
Center for Clinical Pharmacology, University Hospitals Leuven, Leuven, Belgium

Karel Allegaert
Neonatal Intensive Care Unit, University Hospitals Leuven, Leuven, Belgium
Neonatal Intensive Care Unit, University Hospitals Leuven, Herestraat 49, Leuven, 3000 Belgium

Samaneh Bairami
Central Hospital Pharmacy of Imam Khomeini Hospital, Tehran, Iran

Sepideh Elyasi
Department of Clinical Pharmacy, Faculty of Pharmacy, Tehran University of Medical Sciences, Tehran, Iran

Hossein Khalili
Department of Clinical Pharmacy, Faculty of Pharmacy, Tehran University of Medical Sciences, Tehran, Iran

Saeed Reza Jamali-Moghadam
Department of Infectious Diseases, Imam Khomeini Hospital, Tehran, Iran

Shirin Farahyar
Department of Medical Mycology and Parasitology, School of Public Health, Tehran University of Medical Sciences, Tehran, Iran

Farideh Zaini
Department of Medical Mycology and Parasitology, School of Public Health, Tehran University of Medical Sciences, Tehran, Iran

Parivash Kordbacheh
Department of Medical Mycology and Parasitology, School of Public Health, Tehran University of Medical Sciences, Tehran, Iran

Sassan Rezaie
Department of Medical Mycology and Parasitology, School of Public Health, Tehran University of Medical Sciences, Tehran, Iran

Mahin Safara
Department of Medical Mycology and Parasitology, School of Public Health, Tehran University of Medical Sciences, Tehran, Iran

Reza Raoofian
Department of Medical Genetics, School of Medicine, Mashhad University of Medical Sciences, Mashhad, Iran

Mansour Heidari
Department of Medical Genetics, School of Medicine, Tehran University of Medical Sciences, Tehran, Iran

Lisha Jenny John
Lecturer, Department of Pharmacology, Gulf Medical University, Ajman, United Arab Emirates

Mohamed Arifulla
Professor and Head, Department of Pharmacology, Gulf Medical University, Ajman, United Arab Emirates

Jenny John Cheriathu
Lecturer and Specialist, Department of Pediatrics, Gulf Medical College Hospital and Research Center, Ajman, United Arab Emirates

Jayadevan Sreedharan
Professor and Assistant Director, Research Division, Gulf Medical University, Ajman, United Arab Emirates

Roya Mashayekhi
Faculty of Biomedical Engineering Department, Islamic Azad University, Science and Research Branch, Tehran, Iran
Iran Polymer and Petrochemical Institute, P.O. Box:14185/458, Tehran, Iran

Hamid Mobedi
Iran Polymer and Petrochemical Institute, P.O. Box:14185/458, Tehran, Iran

Jamal Najafi
Center of Veterinary, Tehran, Iran

Marjan Enayati
Pharmaziezentrum, Althanstrasse 14, Universität Wien, Raum 2D177, Wien, Austria

Hamid Reza Monsef-Esfahani
Department of Pharmacognosy, Faculty of Pharmacy, Tehran University of Medical Sciences, Tehran, Iran

Mohsen Amini
Department of Medicinal Chemistry, Faculty of Pharmacy, Tehran University of Medical Sciences, Tehran, Iran

Navid Goodarzi
Department of Pharmaceutics, Faculty of Pharmacy, Tehran University of Medical Sciences, Tehran, Iran
Nanotechnology Research Centre, Faculty of Pharmacy, Tehran University of Medical Sciences, Tehran, Iran

Fatemeh Saiedmohammadi
Department of Pharmacognosy, Faculty of Pharmacy, Tehran University of Medical Sciences, Tehran, Iran
Department of Pharmacology and Toxicology, Faculty of Pharmacy, Tehran University of Medical Sciences, Tehran, Iran

Reza Hajiaghaee
Pharmacognosy & Pharmaceutics Department of Medicinal Plants Research Center, Institute of Medicinal Plants, ACECR, Karaj, Iran

Mohammad Ali Faramarzi
Department of Pharmaceutical Biotechnology, Faculty of Pharmacy & Biotechnology Research Center, Tehran University of Medical Sciences, Tehran, Iran

Zahra Tofighi
Department of Pharmacognosy, Faculty of Pharmacy, Tehran University of Medical Sciences, Tehran, Iran

Mohammad Hossein Ghahremani
Nanotechnology Research Centre, Faculty of Pharmacy, Tehran University of Medical Sciences, Tehran, Iran
Department of Pharmacology and Toxicology, Faculty of Pharmacy, Tehran University of Medical Sciences, Tehran, Iran

Esmaeil Shahsavand Ananloo
Department of Genomic Psychiatry (DGP), Roozbeh Hospital, Tehran University of Medical Sciences (TUMS), Tehran, IRAN

Padideh Ghaeli
Roozbeh Hospital, Tehran University of Medical Sciences (TUMS), Tehran, IRAN

Mohammad-Zaman Kamkar
Fifth of Azar Hospital, Golestan University of Medical Sciences, Gorgan, IRAN

Majid Sadeghi
Psychiatry and Psychology Research Center, Roozbeh Hospital, Tehran University of Medical Sciences (TUMS), Tehran, IRAN

Sanaz Golbabaei
Department of Medicinal Chemistry, Faculty of Pharmacy and Medicinal Plants Research Center, Tehran University of Medical Sciences, Tehran, Iran

Roya Bazl
Department of Medicinal Chemistry, Faculty of Pharmacy and Medicinal Plants Research Center, Tehran University of Medical Sciences, Tehran, Iran

Sahand Golestanian
Department of Medicinal Chemistry, Faculty of Pharmacy and Medicinal Plants Research Center, Tehran University of Medical Sciences, Tehran, Iran

Farzaneh Nabati
Department of Medicinal Chemistry, Faculty of Pharmacy and Medicinal Plants Research Center, Tehran University of Medical Sciences, Tehran, Iran

Zinat Bahrampour Omrany
Department of Medicinal Chemistry, Faculty of Pharmacy and Medicinal Plants Research Center, Tehran University of Medical Sciences, Tehran, Iran

Behnam Yousefi
School of Advanced Medical Technologies, Tehran University of Medical Sciences, Tehran, Iran

Reza Hajiaghaee
Pharmacognosy & Pharmaceutics Department of Medicinal Plants Research Center, Institute of Medicinal Plants, ACECR, Karaj, Iran

Shamsali Rezazadeh
Pharmacognosy & Pharmaceutics Department of Medicinal Plants Research Center, Institute of Medicinal Plants, ACECR, Karaj, Iran

Massoud Amanlou
Department of Medicinal Chemistry, Faculty of Pharmacy and Medicinal Plants Research Center, Tehran University of Medical Sciences, Tehran, Iran

Subhabrata Paul
Department of Botany, University of Calcutta, 35, Ballygunge Circular Road, Kolkata 700019, India

Rita Kundu
Department of Botany, University of Calcutta, 35, Ballygunge Circular Road, Kolkata 700019, India

Abbas Kebriaeezadeh
Department of Pharmacoeconomics and Pharmaceutical Administration, Faculty of Pharmacy, Tehran University of Medical Sciences, P.O. Box 14155- 6451, Tehran 14174, Iran
Department of Toxicology and Pharmacology, Faculty of Pharmacy, Tehran University of Medical Sciences, P.O. Box 14155-6451, Tehran 14174, Iran

Nasser Nassiri Koopaei
Department of Pharmacoeconomics and Pharmaceutical Administration, Faculty of Pharmacy, Tehran University of Medical Sciences, P.O. Box 14155- 6451, Tehran 14174, Iran

Akbar Abdollahiasl
Department of Pharmacoeconomics and Pharmaceutical Administration, Faculty of Pharmacy, Tehran University of Medical Sciences, P.O. Box 14155- 6451, Tehran 14174, Iran

Shekoufeh Nikfar
Department of Pharmacoeconomics and Pharmaceutical Administration, Faculty of Pharmacy, Tehran University of Medical Sciences, P.O. Box 14155- 6451, Tehran 14174, Iran

Nafiseh Mohamadi
Management Information System Division, Osvah Pharmaceutical Company, Tehran, Iran

Parisa Fathi Rezaei
Molecular Research Lab, Department of Pharmacology and Toxicology, Faculty of Pharmacy, Tehran University of Medical Sciences, Tehran, Iran
Department of Microbiology and Molecular cell biology, Faculty of Science, University of Maragheh, Maragheh, Iran

Shamileh Fouladdel
Molecular Research Lab, Department of Pharmacology and Toxicology, Faculty of Pharmacy, Tehran University of Medical Sciences, Tehran, Iran
Research Institute for Islamic and Complementary Medicine, Tehran University of Medical Sciences, Tehran, Iran

Seyed Mahmood Ghaffari
Department of Biochemistry, IBB, University of Tehran, Tehran, Iran

Gholamreza Amin
Department of Pharmacognosy, Faculty of Pharmacy, Tehran University of Medical Sciences, Tehran, Iran

Ebrahim Azizi
Molecular Research Lab, Department of Pharmacology and Toxicology, Faculty of Pharmacy, Tehran University of Medical Sciences, Tehran, Iran

Fereshteh Haghighi
Department of Biology, Faculty of Science, Ferdowsi University of Mashhad, Mashhad, Iran

Maryam M Matin
Department of Biology, Faculty of Science, Ferdowsi University of Mashhad, Mashhad, Iran
Cell and Molecular Biotechnology Research Group, Institute of Biotechnology, Ferdowsi University of Mashhad, Mashhad, Iran

Ahmad Reza Bahrami
Department of Biology, Faculty of Science, Ferdowsi University of Mashhad, Mashhad, Iran
Cell and Molecular Biotechnology Research Group, Institute of Biotechnology, Ferdowsi University of Mashhad, Mashhad, Iran

Mehrdad Iranshahi
Biotechnology Research Center and School of Pharmacy, Mashhad University of Medical Sciences, Mashhad, Iran

Fatemeh B Rassouli
Department of Biology, Faculty of Science, Ferdowsi University of Mashhad, Mashhad, Iran

Azadeh Haghighitalab
Department of Biology, Faculty of Science, Ferdowsi University of Mashhad, Mashhad, Iran

Mohammad K Mohammadi
Faculty of sciences, Ahvaz Branch, Islamic Azad University, Ahvaz, Iran

Omidreza Firuzi
Medicinal and Natural Products Chemistry Research Center, Shiraz, University of Medical Sciences, PO Box 3288-71345, Shiraz, Iran

Mehdi Khoshneviszadeh
Medicinal and Natural Products Chemistry Research Center, Shiraz, University of Medical Sciences, PO Box 3288-71345, Shiraz, Iran

Nima Razzaghi-Asl
Departments of Medicinal Chemistry, School of Pharmacy, Shiraz University of Medical Sciences, Shiraz, Iran

Saghi Sepehri
Departments of Medicinal Chemistry, Faculty of Pharmacy, Isfahan University of Medical Sciences, Isfahan, Iran

Ramin Miri
Medicinal and Natural Products Chemistry Research Center, Shiraz, University of Medical Sciences, PO Box 3288-71345, Shiraz, Iran
Departments of Medicinal Chemistry, School of Pharmacy, Shiraz University of Medical Sciences, Shiraz, Iran

Roshanak Salari
Department of Drug and Food Control, School of Pharmacy, Mashhad University of Medical Sciences, Mashhad, Iran

BiBi Sedigheh Fazly Bazzaz
Department of Drug and Food Control, School of Pharmacy, Mashhad University of Medical Sciences, Mashhad, Iran Biotechnology Research Centre, School of Pharmacy, Mashhad University of Medical Sciences, Mashhad, Iran

Omid Rajabi
Department of Drug and Food Control, School of Pharmacy, Mashhad University of Medical Sciences, Mashhad, Iran
Targetted Drug Delivery Research Centre, School of Pharmacy, Mashhad University of Medical Sciences, Mashhad, Iran

Zahra Khashyarmanesh
Department of Drug and Food Control, School of Pharmacy, Mashhad University of Medical Sciences, Mashhad, Iran

Shekoufeh Nikfar
Department of Pharmacoeconomics and Pharmaceutical Administration, Faculty of Pharmacy, Tehran University of Medical Sciences, Tehran, Iran
Food & Drug Organization, Ministry of Health & Medical Education, Tehran, Iran

Abbas Kebriaeezadeh
Department of Pharmacoeconomics and Pharmaceutical Administration, Faculty of Pharmacy, Tehran University of Medical Sciences, Tehran, Iran

Rassoul Dinarvand
Department of Pharmacoeconomics and Pharmaceutical Administration, Faculty of Pharmacy, Tehran University of Medical Sciences, Tehran, Iran

Mohammad Abdollahi
Department of Pharmacoeconomics and Pharmaceutical Administration, Faculty of Pharmacy, Tehran University of Medical Sciences, Tehran, Iran
Faculty of Pharmacy, and Pharmaceutical Sciences Research Center, Tehran University of Medical Sciences, Tehran, Iran

Mohammad-Ali Sahraian
Department of Neurology, Sina Hospital, Tehran University of Medical Sciences, Tehran, Iran

David Henry
Institute for Clinical Evaluative Sciences, Toronto, Canada

Ali Akbari Sari
Department of Pharmacoeconomics and Pharmaceutical Administration, Faculty of Pharmacy, Tehran University of Medical Sciences, Tehran, Iran
Department of Health Management and Economics, School of Public Health, Tehran University of Medical Sciences, Tehran, Iran

Amir Hashemi Meshkini
Department of Pharmacoeconomics and Pharmaceutical administration, Faculty of pharmacy, Tehran University of Medical Sciences, 16th Azar st, Keshavarz Blvd, Tehran, Iran

Abbas Kebriaeezadeh
Department of Pharmacoeconomics and Pharmaceutical administration, Faculty of pharmacy, Tehran University of Medical Sciences, 16th Azar st, Keshavarz Blvd, Tehran, Iran

Rasoul Dinarvand
Department of Pharmacoeconomics and Pharmaceutical administration, Faculty of pharmacy, Tehran University of Medical Sciences, 16th Azar st, Keshavarz Blvd, Tehran, Iran
Department of Pharmaceutics, Faculty of Pharmacy, Tehran University of Medical Sciences, 16th Azar st, Keshavarz Blvd, Tehran, Iran

Shekoufeh Nikfar
Department of Pharmacoeconomics and Pharmaceutical administration, Faculty of pharmacy, Tehran University of Medical Sciences, 16th Azar st, Keshavarz Blvd, Tehran, Iran
Food & Drug Laboratory Research Center, Food & Drug Organization, Ministry of Health & Medical Education, Tehran 1314715311, Iran

MohammadGafar Habibzadeh
The Department of Law, human science faculty of Tarbiat Modarres University, Kargar Street, Tehran, Iran

Iman Vazirian
Department of Pharmaceutics, Faculty of Pharmacy, Tehran University of Medical Sciences, 16th Azar st, Keshavarz Blvd, Tehran, Iran

Khosro Keshavarz
Department of Pharmacoeconomics and Pharmaceutical administration, Faculty of pharmacy, Tehran University of Medical Sciences, Tehran, Iran

Abbas Kebriaeezadeh
Department of Pharmacoeconomics and Pharmaceutical administration, Faculty of pharmacy, Tehran University of Medical Sciences, Tehran, Iran

Amir Hashemi Meshkini
Department of Pharmacoeconomics and Pharmaceutical administration, Faculty of pharmacy, Tehran University of Medical Sciences, Tehran, Iran

Shekoufeh Nikfar
Department of Pharmacoeconomics and Pharmaceutical administration, Faculty of pharmacy, Tehran University of Medical Sciences, Tehran, Iran
Food & Drug Laboratory Research Center, Food & Drug Organization, Ministry of Health & Medical Education, Tehran, Iran

Iman Mirian
Department of Public Health, Faculty of Public Health, Hormozqan University of Medical Sciences, Bandar abbas, Iran

Hasan Khoonsari
Department of Clinical Pharmacy, Faculty of Pharmacy, Tehran University of Medical Sciences, Tehran, Iran

Fatemeh Soleymani
Department of Pharmacoeconomics and Pharmaceutical Management, Faculty of Pharmacy, Tehran University of Medical Sciences (TUMS), Tehran, Iran
National Committee on Rational Drug Use, Food and Drug Organization, Ministry of Health and Medical Education, Tehran, Iran

Arash Rashidian
Department of Pharmacoeconomics and Pharmaceutical Management, Faculty of Pharmacy, Tehran University of Medical Sciences (TUMS), Tehran, Iran
Department of Health Management and Economic, School of Public Health, TUMS, Tehran, Iran
Knowledge Utilization Research Center, TUMS, Tehran, Iran
National Institute of Health Research, Tehran University of Medical Sciences, No 78, Italia Ave, Tehran, Iran

Rassoul Dinarvand
Department of Pharmacoeconomics and Pharmaceutical Management, Faculty of Pharmacy, Tehran University of Medical Sciences (TUMS), Tehran, Iran
Department of Pharmaceutics, Faculty of Pharmacy and Nanotechnology Research Center, TUMS, Tehran, Iran

Abbas Kebriaeezade
Department of Pharmacoeconomics and Pharmaceutical Management, Faculty of Pharmacy, Tehran University of Medical Sciences (TUMS), Tehran, Iran
Department of Toxicology and Pharmacology, Faculty of Pharmacy and Pharmaceutical Sciences Research Center, TUMS, Tehran, Iran

Mostafa Hosseini
Department of Epidemiology and Biostatistics, School of Public Health, TUMS, Tehran, Iran

Mohammad Abdollahi
Department of Pharmacoeconomics and Pharmaceutical Management, Faculty of Pharmacy, Tehran University of Medical Sciences (TUMS), Tehran, Iran
Department of Toxicology and Pharmacology, Faculty of Pharmacy and Pharmaceutical Sciences Research Center, TUMS, Tehran, Iran

Hamid Nadri1,
1Department of Medicinal Chemistry, Faculty of Pharmacy and Neurobiomedical Research Center, Shahid Sadoughi University of Medical Sciences, Yazd 8915173143, Iran

Morteza Pirali-Hamedani
Faculty of Pharmacy and Pharmaceutical Sciences Research Center, Tehran University of Medical Sciences, Tehran, Iran

Alireza Moradi
Department of Medicinal Chemistry, Faculty of Pharmacy and Neurobiomedical Research Center, Shahid Sadoughi University of Medical Sciences, Yazd 8915173143, Iran

Amirhossein Sakhteman
Department of Medicinal Chemistry, Faculty of Pharmacy and Neurobiomedical Research Center, Shahid Sadoughi University of Medical Sciences, Yazd 8915173143, Iran

Alireza Vahidi
Herbal Medicine Center, Shahid Sadoughi University of Medical Sciences, Yazd 8915173143, Iran

Vahid Sheibani
Neuroscience Research Center, Kerman University of Medical Sciences, Kerman, Iran

Ali Asadipour
Neuroscience Research Center, Kerman University of Medical Sciences, Kerman, Iran

Nouraddin Hosseinzadeh
Drug design & Development Research Center, Tehran University of Medical Sciences, Tehran, Iran

Mohammad Abdollahi
Faculty of Pharmacy and Pharmaceutical Sciences Research Center, Tehran University of Medical Sciences, Tehran, Iran

Abbas Shafiee
Faculty of Pharmacy and Pharmaceutical Sciences Research Center, Tehran University of Medical Sciences, Tehran, Iran

Alireza Foroumadi
Neuroscience Research Center, Kerman University of Medical Sciences, Kerman, Iran
Drug design & Development Research Center, Tehran University of Medical Sciences, Tehran, Iran

Chioma A Anosike
Department of Biochemistry, University of Nigeria, Nsukka, Enugu State, Nigeria

Onyechi Obidoa
Department of Biochemistry, Kogi State University, Aiymgba, Kogi State, Nigeria

Lawrence US Ezeanyika
Department of Biochemistry, University of Nigeria, Nsukka, Enugu State, Nigeria

Hoda Lavasani
Biopharmaceutics and Pharmacokinetics Division, Department of Pharmaceutics, Faculty of Pharmacy, Tehran University of Medical Sciences, 14155-6451, Tehran, Iran

Behjat Sheikholeslami
Biopharmaceutics and Pharmacokinetics Division, Department of Pharmaceutics, Faculty of Pharmacy, Tehran University of Medical Sciences, 14155-6451, Tehran, Iran

Yalda H Ardakani
Biopharmaceutics and Pharmacokinetics Division, Department of Pharmaceutics, Faculty of Pharmacy, Tehran University of Medical Sciences, 14155-6451, Tehran, Iran

Mohammad Abdollahi
Department of Pharmacology and Toxicology, Faculty of Pharmacy, Tehran University of Medical Sciences, 14155-6451, Tehran, Iran
Pharmaceutical Sciences Research Centre, Faculty of Pharmacy, Tehran University of Medical Sciences, 14155-6451, Tehran, Iran

Lida Hakemi
Biopharmaceutics and Pharmacokinetics Division, Department of Pharmaceutics, Faculty of Pharmacy, Tehran University of Medical Sciences, 14155-6451, Tehran, Iran

Mohammad-Reza Rouini
Biopharmaceutics and Pharmacokinetics Division, Department of Pharmaceutics, Faculty of Pharmacy, Tehran University of Medical Sciences, 14155-6451, Tehran, Iran
Pharmaceutical Sciences Research Centre, Faculty of Pharmacy, Tehran University of Medical Sciences, 14155-6451, Tehran, Iran

Bardia Jamali
Department of Pharmaceutics, Biopharmaceutics and Pharmacokinetics Division, Faculty of Pharmacy, Tehran University of Medical Sciences, Tehran, Iran

Yalda Hosseinzadeh Ardakani
Department of Pharmaceutics, Biopharmaceutics and Pharmacokinetics Division, Faculty of Pharmacy, Tehran University of Medical Sciences, Tehran, Iran

Mohammad-Reza Rouini
Department of Pharmaceutics, Biopharmaceutics and Pharmacokinetics Division, Faculty of Pharmacy, Tehran University of Medical Sciences, Tehran, Iran

Alireza Foroumadi
Drug design and Development Research Center, Tehran University of Medical Sciences, Tehran, Iran

Salimeh Amidi
Department of Medicinal Chemistry, School of Pharmacy, Shahid Beheshti University of Medical Sciences, Tehran, Iran

Vahid Hossein Zadeh Aghdam
Central Research Laboratories, Shahid Beheshti University of Medical Sciences, Tehran, Iran

Farzad Kobarfard
Department of Medicinal Chemistry, School of Pharmacy, Shahid Beheshti University of Medical Sciences, Tehran, Iran

Bahador Mirrahimi
Department of Clinical Pharmacy, Faculty of Pharmacy, Tehran University of Medical Sciences, Tehran 1417614411, Iran

Hadi Hamishehkar
Department of Clinical Pharmacy, Faculty of Pharmacy, Tabriz University of Medical Science, Tabriz 1476651664, Iran

Arezo Ahmadi
Department of anesthesia and intensive care, Sina hospital, Tehran University of Medical Science, Tehran 1136746911, Iran

Mohamad Reza Mirjalili
Department of anesthesia and intensive care, Faculty of Medicine, Shahid Sadoghi University of Medical Science, Yazd 8915173143, Iran

Mostafa Aghamohamadi
Sina hospital, Tehran University of Medical Science, Tehran 1136746911, Iran

Atabak Najafi
Department of Toxicology and Pharmacology, Faculty of Pharmacy, and Pharmaceutical Sciences Research Center, Tehran University of Medical Sciences, Tehran 1417614411, Iran

Mohammad Abdollahi
Department of Toxicology and Pharmacology, Faculty of Pharmacy, and Pharmaceutical Sciences Research Center, Tehran University of Medical Sciences, Tehran 1417614411, Iran

Mojtaba Mojtahedzahed
Department of Clinical Pharmacy, Faculty of Pharmacy, Tehran University of Medical Sciences, Tehran 1417614411, Iran

Hossein Khalili, Simin Dashti-Khavidaki, Mohammad-Reza Shahidi, Zahra Jahangard-Rafsanjani and Azita-Hajhosssein Talasaz
Department of Clinical Pharmacy, Faculty of Pharmacy, Tehran University of Medical Sciences, Tehran, Iran

Alireza Abdollahi
Department of Pathology, Faculty of Medicine, Tehran University of Medical Sciences, Tehran, Iran

Sirous Jafari
Department of Infectious Diseases, Faculty of Medicine, Tehran University of Medical Sciences, Tehran, Iran

Elham Akhtari, Mansoor Keshavarz and Soodabeh Bioos
Department of Traditional Medicine, School of Medicine, Tehran University of Medical Sciences, Tehran, Iran

Mohammad Kamalinejad
Department of Pharmacognosy, School of Pharmacy, Shaheed Beheshti University of Medical Sciences, Tehran, Iran

Ali Ghobadi
Department of Traditional Medicine, School of Traditional Pharmacology, Tehran University of Medical Sciences, Tehran, Iran

Firoozeh Raisi
Psychiatry, Fellow of the European Committee of Sexual Medicine (FECSM), Roozbeh Psychiatric Hospital, Psychiatric and Clinical Psychology, Research Center, Tehran University of Medical Sciences, South Kargar Street, Tehran 13337, Iran

Hamed Hosseini
School of Public Health, Tehran University of Medical Sciences, Tehran, Iran
Clinical Trial Center, Tehran University of Medical Sciences, Tehran, Iran

Farnaz Sohrabvand
Department of Gynecology and Infertility, Imam Khomeini Hospital, Tehran University of Medical Sciences, Tehran, Iran

Maryam Abbasi
Department of Medicinal Chemistry, Faculty of Pharmacy, Pharmaceutical Science Research Center, Tehran University of Medical Science, Tehran, Iran
Department of Medicinal Chemistry, Faculty of Pharmacy, Isfahan University of Medical Sciences, 81746-73461 Isfahan, Iran

Fatemeh Ramezani and Massoud Amanlou
Department of Medicinal Chemistry, Faculty of Pharmacy, Pharmaceutical Science Research Center, Tehran University of Medical Science, Tehran, Iran

Maryam Elyasi
Medicinal & Natural Product Chemistry Research Center, Shiraz University of Medical Sciences, Shiraz, Iran

Hojjat Sadeghi-Aliabadi
Department of Medicinal Chemistry, Faculty of Pharmacy, Isfahan University of Medical Sciences, 81746-73461 Isfahan, Iran

Saeed Abbasi
Anesthesiology and Critical Care Research Center, Isfahan University of Medical Sciences, Isfahan, Iran

Shadi Farsaei
Department of Clinical Pharmacy and Pharmacy Practice, Isfahan University of Medical Sciences, Isfahan, Iran

Kamran Fazel
Department of Anesthesia and Critical Care Medicine, Bagiatalla University of Medical Sciences, Tehran, Iran

Samad EJ Golzari
Medical Education Research Center, Tabriz University of Medical Sciences, Tabriz, Iran

Ata Mahmoodpoor
Cardiovascular Research Center, Tabriz University of Medical Sciences, Tabriz, Iran

Marzieh Qaraaty and Mohsen Naseri
Traditional Medicine Clinical Trial Research Center, Shahed University, Tehran, Iran

Seyed Hamid Kamali
Department of Traditional Medicine, Faculty of Traditional Medicine, Shahid Beheshti University of Medical Sciences, Tehran, Iran

Fataneh Hashem Dabaghian
Research Institute for Islamic and Complementary Medicine, Iran University of Medical Sciences, Tehran, Iran

Nafiseh Zafarghandi
Department of Gynecology and Obstetrics, Faculty of Medical Sciences, Shahed University, Tehran, Iran

Roshanak Mokaberinejad
Department of Traditional Medicine, School of Traditional Medicine, Shahid Beheshti University of Medical Sciences, Tehran, Iran

Masumeh Mobli and Gholamreza Amin
Department of Traditional Pharmacy, Faculty of Traditional Medicine, Tehran University of Medical Sciences, Tehran, Iran

Mohammad Kamalinejad
Department of Pharmacognosy, School of Pharmacy Shahid Beheshti University of Medical Sciences, Tehran, Iran

Mohsen Amin
Department of Drug and Food control, Faculty of Pharmacy, Tehran University of Medical Sciences, Tehran, Iran

Azizeh Ghaseminejad
Department of Gynecology and Obstetrics, Tehran University of Medical Sciences, Tehran, Iran

Seyedeh jihan HosseiniKhabiri
Khatam Hospital, Tehran, Iran

Daryush Talei
Medicinal Plant Research Centre, Shahed University, Tehran, Iran

Talha Bin Emran
Department of Pharmacy, BGC Trust University Bangladesh, Chittagong 4000, Bangladesh
Department of Biochemistry and Molecular Biology, University of Chittagong, Chittagong 4331, Bangladesh

Md Atiar Rahman
Department of Biochemistry and Molecular Biology, University of Chittagong, Chittagong 4331, Bangladesh

Mir Muhammad Nasir Uddin
Department of Pharmacy, University of Chittagong, Chittagong 4331, Bangladesh
Raju Dash, Md Firoz Hossen, Mohammad Mohiuddin and Md Rashadul Alam
Department of Pharmacy, BGC Trust University Bangladesh, Chittagong 4000, Bangladesh

Hwan Hee Lee, Seulki Lee and Hyosun Cho
College of Pharmacy, Duksung Women's University, Seoul 132-714, Republic of Korea
Innovative Drug Center, Duksung Women's University, Seoul 132-714, Republic of Korea

Kanghyo Lee
Mushroom Research Division, National Institute of Horticultural and Herbal Science, Rural Development Administration,Eumseong 369-873, Republic of Korea

Yu Su Shin
Department of Medicinal Crop Research, National Institute of Horticultural and Herbal Science, Rural Development Administration, Eumseong 369-873, Republic of Korea

Hyojeung Kang
College of Pharmacy, Research Institute of Pharmaceutical Sciences and Institute for Microorganisms, Kyungpook National University, Daegu 702-701, Republic of Korea

Maryam Payan and Mohammad Reza Rouini
Biopharmaceutics and Pharmacokinetics Division, Department of Pharmaceutics, School of Pharmacy, Tehran University of Medical sciences, Tehran, Iran

Nader Tajik
Cellular and Molecular Research Center (CMRC), Iran University of Medical Sciences, Tehran, Iran

Mohammad Hossein Ghahremani
Department of Pharmacology and Toxicology, School of Pharmacy, Tehran University of Medical sciences, Tehran, Iran

Reza Tahvilian
Department of pharmaceutics, School of Pharmacy, Kermanshah University of Medical Sciences, Kermanshah, Iran

Renata Cavalcanti Carnevale, Caroline de Godoi Rezende Costa Molino, Marília Berlofa Visacri and Priscila Gava Mazzola
Department of Clinical Pathology, Faculty of Medical Sciences (FCM), University of Campinas (UNICAMP), Alexander Fleming, 105, 13083-881 Campinas, SP, Brazil

Patricia Moriel
Department of Clinical Pathology, Faculty of Medical Sciences (FCM), University of Campinas (UNICAMP), Alexander Fleming, 105, 13083-881 Campinas, SP, Brazil
Faculty of Pharmaceutical Sciences (FCF), University of Campinas (UNICAMP), Sérgio Buarque de Holanda, 25, 13083-859 Campinas, SP, Brazil

Vahideh Sadat Motamedshariaty and Sara Amel Farzad
Pharmaceutical Research Center, School of Pharmacy, Mashhad University of Medical Sciences, Mashhad, Iran

Marjan Nassiri-Asl
Cellular and Molecular Research Centre, Department of Pharmacology, School of Medicine, Qazvin University of Medical Sciences, Qazvin, Iran

Hossein Hosseinzadeh
Pharmacodynamics and Toxicological Department, Pharmaceutical Research Center, School of Pharmacy, Mashhad University of Medical Sciences, Mashhad, Iran